MW00612054

Best Practices for
Transradial Approach
in Diagnostic Angiography and Intervention

Best Practices for **Transradial Approach** in Diagnostic Angiography and Intervention

Olivier F. Bertrand, MD, PhD, FSCAI
Interventional Cardiologist
Quebec Heart–Lung Institute;
Associate Professor, Faculty of Medicine (Tenured)
Laval University;
Adjunct Professor, Department of Mechanical Engineering
McGill University;
Director
CAIC Transradial Interventions Working Group
International Chair on Interventional Cardiology and Transradial Approach
Quebec City, Quebec, Canada

Sunil V. Rao, MD
Associate Professor with Tenure
Duke University Medical Center;
Section Chief, Cardiovascular Medicine
Durham VA Medical Center
Durham, North Carolina

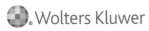. Wolters Kluwer

Philadelphia • Baltimore • New York • London
Buenos Aires • Hong Kong • Sydney • Tokyo

Acquisitions Editor: Julie Goolsby
Product Development Editor: Andrea Vosburgh
Production Project Manager: Bridgett Dougherty
Design Coordinator: Joan Wendt
Manufacturing Coordinator: Beth Welsh
Marketing Manager: Stephanie Manzo
Prepress Vendor: S4Carlisle Publishing Services

9 8 7 6 5 4 3 2 1

Printed in China (or the United States of America)

Library of Congress Cataloging-in-Publication Data

Best practices for transradial approach in diagnostic angiography and intervention / [edited by] Olivier F. Bertrand, Sunil V. Rao. — First Edition.
  p. ; cm.
  Includes bibliographical references.
  ISBN 978-1-4511-7725-1
  I. Bertrand, Olivier F., editor.   II. Rao, Sunil V., editor.
  [DNLM: 1. Coronary Angiography—methods.   2. Cardiac Catheterization—methods.   3. Cardiovascular Diseases—diagnosis.   4. Percutaneous Coronary Intervention—methods. WG 141.5.A3]
  RC683.5.C25
  616.1'207572—dc23

                                                                                    2014027076

CONTRIBUTORS

Eltigani Abdelaal, MD, MRCP (UK), CCT Cardiology (UK)
Interventional Cardiologist
Cardiac Catheterization Laboratories
Quebec Heart–Lung Institute
Quebec City, Quebec, Canada

Stephan Achenbach, MD
Professor
Department of Internal Medicine 2 (Cardiology)
University of Erlangen–Nuremberg
Erlangen, Germany

Pierfrancesco Agostoni, MD, PhD
Department of Cardiology
University Medical Center Utrecht
Utrecht, the Netherlands

Giovanni Amoroso, MD, PhD
Heart Center
Onze Lieve Vrouwe Gasthuis
Amsterdam, the Netherlands

Gérald Barbeau, MD, CSPQ, FRCPC, FACC
Interventional Cardiology and Advanced
   Cardiovascular Imaging
Institut Universitaire de Cardiologie et de
   Pneumologie de Quebec
Quebec City, Quebec, Canada

Ashok Gangasandra Basavaraj, MBBS, FRACP
Clinical Fellow, Interventional Cardiology
Department of Medicine
McMaster University, Hamilton Health Sciences
Hamilton, Ontario, Canada

Hakim Benamer, MD, ICPS
Institut Cardiovasculaire Paris Sud
Hopital privé Jacques Cartier
Massy, France;
Hopital Claude Galien
Quincy Sous Senart, France;
ICV-GVM, Hopital Européen de Paris
La Roseraie
Aubervilliers, France

Ivo Bernat, MD, PhD
Cardiology Department
University Hospital and Faculty of Medicine
Pilsen, Czech Republic

Olivier F. Bertrand, MD, PhD, FSCAI
Interventional Cardiologist
Quebec Heart–Lung Institute;
Associate Professor, Faculty of Medicine
   (Tenured)
Laval University;
Adjunct Professor, Department of Mechanical
   Engineering
McGill University;
Director
CAIC Transradial Interventions Working Group
International Chair on Interventional Cardiology
   and Transradial Approach
Quebec City, Quebec, Canada

Gurbir Bhatia, MD, MRCP
Birmingham Heartlands Hospital
Birmingham, West Midlands, United Kingdom

Giuseppe Biondi-Zoccai, MD, FSICI-GISE
Department of Medico-Surgial Sciences and
   Biotechnologies
Spaienza University of Rome
Rome, Italy

Marta Francesca Brancati, MD
Institute of Cardiology
Catholic University of the Sacred Heart
Rome, Italy

Francesco Burzotta, MD, PhD
Institute of Cardiology
Catholic University of the Sacred Heart
Rome, Italy

Warren J. Cantor, MD, FRCPC, FSCAI
Interventional Cardiologist
Southlake Regional Health Centre;
Associate Professor of Medicine
University of Toronto
Newmarket, Ontario, Canada

Asim N. Cheema, MD, PhD, FRCPC, FACC
Director, Interventional Cardiology Fellowship
    Program
St. Michael's Hospital;
Associate Professor of Medicine
University of Toronto
Toronto, Ontario, Canada

Mauricio G. Cohen, MD, FACC, FSCAI
Associate Professor of Medicine
Cardiovascular Division, Department of Medicine
University of Miami Miller School of Medicine;
Director, Cardiac Catheterization Laboratory
University of Miami Hospital
Miami, Florida

Nicholas Collins, BMed, FRACP
Cardiovascular Unit
John Hunter Hospital
Newcastle, New South Wales, Australia

John T. Coppola, MD, FACC, FSCA
Clinical Assistant Professor
Division of Cardiology
NYU Langone Medical Center
New York, New York

Johannes B. Dahm, MD
Department of Cardiology
Angiology Heart and Vascular Center
Neu Bethlehem
Gattingen, Germany

Vladimír Džavík, MD, FRCPC, FACC, FAHA
Peter Munk Cardiac Centre
University Health Network
Mount Sinai Hospital;
University of Toronto
Toronto, Ontario, Canada

Basem Elbarouni, MBBCh, FRCPC
Clinical Fellow, Interventional Cardiology
University of Toronto
Toronto, Ontario, Canada

Douglas G. Fraser, MB, Bchir, BA, DM, FRCP
Manchester Heart Centre
Central Manchester Foundation Trust
Manchester, United Kingdom

Run-Lin Gao, MD
Professor of Medicine
Department of Cardiology
Cardiovascular Institute and Fuwai Hospital
Chinese Academy of Medical Sciences
Beijing, China

Philippe Garot, MD, FESC
Institut Cardiovasculaire Paris Sud
Hopital privé Jacques Cartier
Massy, France;
Hopital Claude Galien
Quincy Sous Senart, France;
ICV-GVM, Hopital Européen de Paris
La Roseraie
Aubervilliers, France

Ian C. Gilchrist, MD, FACC, FSCAI, FCCM
Heart and Vascular Institute
MS Hershey Medical Center
Pennsylvania State University
Hershey, Pennsylvania

Rajiv Gulati, MD, PhD
Consultant
Division of Cardiovascular Diseases
Associate Professor of Medicine
College of Medicine
Mayo Clinic
Rochester, Minnesota

Thomas Hovasse, MD
Institut Cardiovasculaire Paris Sud
Hopital privé Jacques Cartier
Massy, France;
Hopital Claude Galien
Quincy Sous Senart, France;
ICV-GVM, Hopital Européen de Paris
La Roseraie
Aubervilliers, France

Yuji Ikari, MD, PhD
Professor
Department of Cardiovascular Medicine
Tokai University School of Medicine
Isehara, Japan

Sanjit S. Jolly, MD, MSc
Department of Medicine
Population Health Research Institute
McMaster University, Hamilton Health Sciences
Hamilton, Ontario, Canada

David E. Kandzari, MD, FACC, FSCAI
Chief Scientific Officer and Director
Interventional Cardiology
Piedmont Heart Institute
Atlanta, Georgia

Saibal Kar, MD, FACC, FSCAI
Director of Interventional Cardiac Research
Associate Professor of Medicine
Heart Institute, Cedars Sinai Medical Center
Los Angeles, California

Sasko Kedev, MD, PhD, FESC, FACC
Professor of Cardiology, Medical Faculty
University of St. Cyril and Methodius;
Director
University Clinic of Cardiology
Skopje, Macedonia

Ferdinand Kiemeneij, MD, PhD
Tergooi Hospital
Blaricum, the Netherlands

Ravikiran Korabathina, MD, FSCAI
Interventional and Clinical Cardiologist
Department of Cardiovascular Medicine
Bayfront Health System
St. Petersburg, Florida

Mikhailia W. Lake, MD
Cardiovascular Fellow
Cardiovascular Division, Department of Medicine
University of Miami Miller School of Medicine
Miami, Florida

Thierry Lefèvre, MD, FESC, FSCAI
Institut Cardiovasculaire Paris Sud
Hopital privé Jacques Cartier
Massy, France;
Hopital Claude Galien
Quincy Sous Senart, France;
ICV-GVM, Hopital Européen de Paris
La Roseraie
Aubervilliers, France

Yves Louvard, MD, FSCAI
Institut Cardiovasculaire Paris Sud
Hopital privé Jacques Cartier
Massy, France;
Hopital Claude Galien
Quincy Sous Senart, France;
ICV-GVM, Hopital Européen de Paris
La Roseraie
Aubervilliers, France

Josef Ludwig, MD, PhD
Director of Cathlabs
Department of Cardiology
University of Erlangen–Nuremberg
Erlangen, Germany

Jimmy MacHaalany, MD, FRCPC
Division of Cardiology
Humber River Regional Hospital
Sunnybrook Health Sciences Centre
Ontario, Canada

J. Tift Mann III, MD, FACC
Interventional Cardiologist
Wake Heart Associates
Raleigh, North Carolina

David Meerkin, MBBS
Director, Structural and Congenital Heart
    Disease Unit
Shaare Zedek Medical Center
Jerusalem, Israel

James Nolan, MBChB, MD, FRCP
University Hospital of North Staffordshire
Stoke-on-Trent, Staffordshire, United Kingdom

Samir B. Pancholy, MD
Program Director, The Wright Center for
    Graduate Medical Education
Associate Professor of Medicine
The Commonwealth Medical College
Scranton, Pennsylvania

Tejas Patel, MD, DM, FACC, FESC, FSCAI
Chairman, Chief Interventional Cardiologist
Apex Heart Institute
Ahmedabad, Gujarat, India

Amir H. Sadrzadeh Rafie, MD
Cardiology Fellow
Cedars Sinai Medical Center
Cedars Sinai Heart Institute
Los Angeles, California

Sunil V. Rao, MD
Associate Professor with Tenure
Duke University Medical Center;
Section Chief, Cardiovascular Medicine
Durham VA Medical Center
Durham, North Carolina

Sudhir Rathore, MD, MRCP, FACC, FESC
Consultant Interventional Cardiologist
Frimley Park Hospital NHS Foundation Trust
St. George's Hospital
London, United Kingdom

Karim Ratib, MB, ChB
University Hospital of North Staffordshire
Stoke-on-Trent, Staffordshire, United Kingdom

Harald Rittger, MD
Associate Professor
Medizinische Klinike 2
University Hospital Erlangen
Erlangen, Germany

Enrico Romagnoli, MD, PhD, FSICI-GISE, EAPCI
Interventional Cardiology Unit
Policlinico Casilino
Rome, Italy

Helen C. Routledge, FRCP, MD
Consultant Cardiologist
Worcester Royal Hospital
Worcester, United Kingdom

Neal Sawlani, MD
Department of Cardiovascular Medicine
University of Illinois, Chicago
Chicago, Illinois

Alessandro Sciahbasi, MD
Department of Interventional Cardiology
Sandro Pertini Hospital
Rome, Italy

Gioel Gabrio Secco, MD
Department of Clinical and Experimental
   Medicine
University of Eastern Piedmont;
Interventional Cardiology
Maggiore della Carita Hospital
Novara, Italy

Sanjay Shah, MD, DM
Assistant Professor, Department of Cardiology
Smt NHL Municipal Medical College
Sheth VS General Hospital;
Director, Department of Cardiology
Apex Heart Institute
Ahmedabad, Gujarat, India

Adhir Shroff, MD, MPH
Associate Professor
Department of Medicine
University of Illinois, Chicago
Jesse Brown VA Medical Center
Chicago, Illinois

Bernadette S. Speiser, BNS, MSN, CCRN
Nurse Manager, Cardiology Department
Jesse Brown Veteran's Administration Hospital
Chicago, Illinois;
National Cardiology Nurse Consultant
Patient Care Service
VA Central Office
Washington, DC

Carlo Trani, MD
Head, Interventional Cardiology Unit
Catholic University of the Sacred Heart
Rome, Italy

Thierry Unterseeh, MD
Institut Cardiovasculaire Paris Sud
Hopital privé Jacques Cartier
Massy, France;
Hopital Claude Galien
Quincy Sous Senart, France;
ICV-GVM, Hopital Européen de Paris
La Roseraie
Aubervilliers, France

Bo Xu, MBBS
National Center for Cardiovascular Diseases
Fu Wai Hospital
Beijing, China

Yue-Jin Yang, MD
Department of Cardiology
Cardiovascular Institute and Fuwai Hospital
Chinese Academy of Medical Sciences
Peking Union Medical College
Beijing, China

FOREWORD

The development of transradial coronary interventions (TRIs) can be divided into several phases or, speaking in more contemporary terms, several versions.

TRI beta-version

Just at the time when Dr. Lucien Campeau's paper on the results of 5F percutaneous transradial coronary angiography in 100 patients was published in 1989, we were trying to find a solid solution for the severe bleeding complications associated with transfemoral coronary stenting. Inspired by Dr. Campeau's work, transradial stenting appeared to me as *the* solution for these problems. However, we had to await the availability of 6F guiding catheters, in order to perform the first transradial coronary angioplasty in 1992. This is what I call the *TRI's beta-version*. It was a single-center try-out phase, not recommended for general use. At first this novel approach deserved thorough exploration, testing, and evaluation. This phase was characterized by absence of dedicated materials, unknown technical limitations, complications, pitfalls, and clinical potential. Colleagues and catheterization laboratory staff were trained internally, and data acquisition had to result in analysis of the potential benefits of TRI. The first lectures, abstracts, posters, and papers were prepared. There were no others to share information and experience, and a lot of convincing had to be done for the coming years.

TRI v.1.0

In 1993, a poster presentation on the results of the first 100 TRI patients at the 66th American Heart Association meeting for the first time attracted international attention. This resulted in the visit of internationally well-known cardiologists to the OLVG hospital (Amsterdam, the Netherlands), who actually could see with their own eyes that patients who had just underwent transradial coronary stenting had a simple pressure bandage immediately following the procedures and walked alone out of the catheterization laboratory. In 1994, Dr. Jean Fajadet, from Clinique Pasteur (Toulouse, France), performed a live demonstration of transradial coronary stenting at the TCT in Washington that went smoothly. This attracted serious international attention. From this moment on an international family of "radialists" started to develop. This phase initiated *TRI v.1.0*. This was characterized by multicenter exploration of indications and contraindications, development of dedicated materials, data collection, early publications of TRI results, finding solutions for problems and shortcomings, and teaching and preaching TRI's benefits. Radialists found each other as faculty members and as teachers at several platforms and initiated their own dedicated meetings and launched radial courses. Thanks to the contributions of these many early pioneers of TRI in all continents of the world, the technique slowly matured to what we have today.

TRI v.2.0

Today, TRI is a globally acknowledged technique. Over 1,400 positive papers have been published on TRI-related issues (Fig. 1). Most important, data are emerging pointing toward lower mortality rates in TRI patients, compared with those seen in TFI patients. This is the most important and conclusive end point, urging all centers to accept TRI as the default technique. Materials have been refined, technical borders have been explored, contraindications have been minimized, and TRI-related complications and problems have all been encountered, described, and analyzed. Excellent training centers are active worldwide. Pioneers have trained numerous radialists, and these doctors are currently training a "third generation." But this is still not the final version; a lot more has to be done.

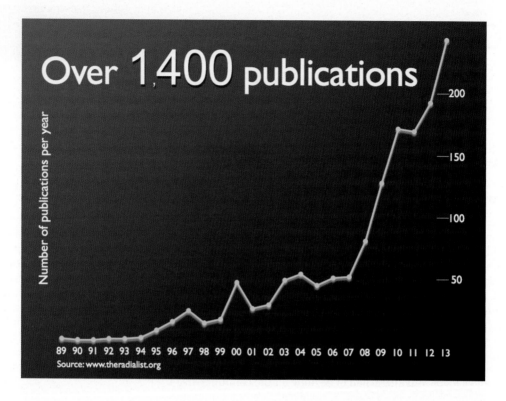

TRI v.3.0

When are we ready for the next version? Currently TRI is gaining in popularity throughout the United States and other countries. Once TRI becomes the default technique in countries that accepted TRI as the best way to access the coronary arteries relatively late, a new phase will be entered. Large-scale international multicenter studies can be designed to prove survival benefits and to further increase the safety and applicability of TRI. It will trigger the medical device industry even more to help us develop the best TRI-related products. It will motivate medical insurance companies to reward hospitals performing TRIs and to reimburse outpatient percutaneous coronary interventions. And finally, this version will be characterized by coordinated and structured international training activities and perhaps even accreditation.

How does this all relate to this book, *Best Practices for Transradial Approach in Diagnostic Angiography and Intervention*?

First of all, all pioneers and experts in this field have given their best contribution in order to cover all relevant aspects associated with transradial coronary access. Basic facts and latest insights are presented to beginning and advanced radialists, covering procedural aspects from A to Z, learning curve, and complications and specific clinical subsets. In addition, noncoronary interventions are covered as well. It is my strong conviction that this textbook will be an essential key to open the gate toward TRI v.3.0.

Last but not least, this joint effort shows that all radialists worldwide form an enthusiastic and motivated group of interventional cardiologists who jointly strive to optimize patient care in an elegant, efficient, and cost-effective manner. This book will serve as a solid basis to optimize patient care and patient benefit.

Ferdinand Kiemeneij

PREFACE

Interventional cardiology has now reached a phase of optimization—optimization for devices and techniques as well as for patient care. Percutaneous coronary intervention (PCI) has now moved from the crude technique of balloon angioplasty performed by femoral approach, 9F catheters, and heavy anticoagulation mimicked from the surgical operating room to a much more refined and miniaturized environment where each component has been modified through the years. Balloon angioplasty as the sole therapy has now been almost completely replaced by insertion of drug-eluting stents, and those endoprostheses are now becoming biodegradable. Six-French guiding catheter size is now the standard size for almost any type of simple or complex intervention, and a sizeable number of PCIs are nowadays performed with 5F guiding catheters. We are even witnessing efforts to continue to downsize catheters and equipment, with Japan leading the way with the so-called "slender techniques." Heavy anticoagulation has been replaced with weight adjustment, and new short-lived or reversible anticoagulants have been developed. Yet femoral access has remained the standard access throughout the world.

Everyday practice is now driven by "evidence-based medicine" instead of "personal experience-based" or "anecdotal" medicine. International guidelines are regularly published and continuously updated to provide to the busy practitioners guidance on how their practice should evolve over time. With the advance of the Internet and multimedia resources, patients and all health-care providers have better and faster access to the latest clinical data. With the lack of industry resources and general ignorance of many interventional cardiologists, it has taken almost 20 years for dedicated radial operators to perform and complete clinical trials and observational studies to demonstrate the clinical advantages and benefits of transradial approach compared with the standard femoral approach. According to PubMed, there have been more than 1,000 papers published since the initial description of radial approach and there are now more than 150 scientific articles dedicated to radial approach published every year.

The goal of this textbook is to provide an in-depth review and critical analysis of available data in the literature. In addition, the online version will provide unique illustrations and videos gathered over the years by the enthusiastic radialists always keen to share their experiences.

As editors, Sunil and I have been very fortunate to benefit from the collaboration of international radial experts who themselves have published many papers on the different topics. Finally, we are most grateful to Olivier Costerousse, PhD, who patiently helped us to collect and edit manuscripts, and to Julie Goolsby and Andrea Vosburgh from Wolters Kluwer Health Publishing, who supported us during this collaborative effort.

CONTENTS

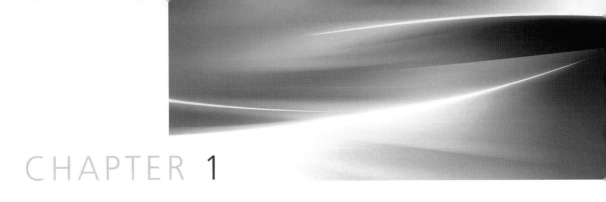

CHAPTER 1

Historical and Epidemiological Note

Josef Ludwig, Harald Rittger, and Stephan Achenbach

History

The history of radial artery access for angiography dates back to March 1947, when Radner[1] performed radial arteriotomy for thoracal aortography in Lund, Sweden (Fig. 1-1). The author reported a new technique for the visualization of the thoracic aorta. A catheter was introduced into the radial artery (cut-down) and guided under radioscopic control. Of note, a footnote in this paper states that "[t]he author is working on the angiography of the coronary blood vessels (...) the results of these investigations will be published later." It is also worth noting that like Werner Forssman, the Nobel Prize winner for the first catheterization in humans, Radner had performed the catheterization on himself (G. Olivecrona, personal communication) (Fig. 1-2).

In 1950, at the Cleveland Clinic, Zimmerman et al.[2] reported on retrograde left heart catheterization using the left ulnar artery. Of note, these early experiences were based on cut-down techniques with recommendation of suturing the vessels at the end of the procedure. Again in Sweden, Sven Seldinger from the Karolinska Institute reported a technique to access vessels percutaneously.[3] However, probably owing to catheter size and stiffness, distal artery access did not become popular.

In 1959, Sones et al.[4] performed selective coronary angiography via the much larger brachial artery, using a surgical cut-down. The Sones technique became the standard practice of care for more than two decades. The percutaneous transfemoral artery technique for coronary angiography was first introduced by Ricketts and Abrams[5] in 1961 and encouraged Judkins[6] in 1965 to create preshaped coronary right and left catheters designed especially for a femoral approach. At the same time, Bourassa et al.[7] and Amplatz et al.[8] also developed their preferred catheter curves to be used by femoral approach. Gruntzig's[9] first successful coronary angioplasty treatment on an awake human was performed in 1977. The growing interest in percutaneous coronary intervention around the world with the need of 8F to 9F guiding catheters made the femoral access the gold standard to reach the arteries of the heart.

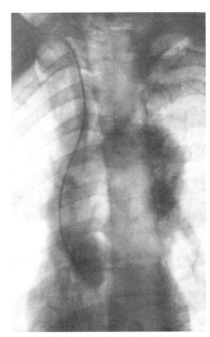

FIGURE 1-1 From the original publication by Radner[1] in *Acta Radiologica* (1948). (From Radner S. Thoracal aortography by catheterization from the radial artery: preliminary report of a new technique. *Acta Radiol.* 1948;29:178–180.)

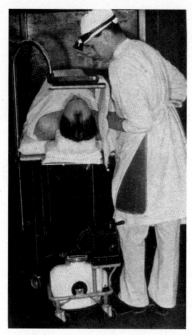

FIGURE 1-2 Dr. Stig Radner.

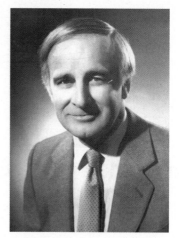

FIGURE 1-3 The man credited with pioneering transradial coronary angiography, Dr. Lucien Campeau (Montreal Heart Institute, Quebec, Canada), passed away on March 15, 2012, at the age of 82.

In Canada, Lucien Campeau had witnessed the efforts of his colleague, Martial Bourassa, struggling to design his own catheters to be used by the femoral approach. Starting in 1964, Campeau and Bourassa had begun to use the proximal radial artery instead of the brachial artery and they were completing the procedure by patiently suturing the radial artery, although they frequently noticed the absence of distal radial artery pulse after the procedure, which was performed with 7F catheters (M. Bourassa, personal communication). In 1974, Bertrand et al.,[10] in France, reported selective coronary angiography also using the proximal radial artery. At the end of the procedure, the radial artery was ligated and no symptom of distal ischemia was ever reported (M. Bertrand, personal communication).

Finally, in 1989, Campeau[11] reported a series of 100 diagnostic coronary angiographies using a percutaneous approach with the distal radial artery and 5F catheters (Fig. 1-3). Interestingly, in this pilot series, he could perform selective angiography in both coronary vessels in 88 patients, while he was unsuccessful in 12 cases because of puncture failure and in 2 cases for lack of selective cannulation. In 1992, Masaki Otaki in Osaka (Japan) applied the same percutaneous radial artery approach using 5F Judkins and Amplatz catheters in Japanese patients. Despite anticoagulation, both Campeau and Otaki reported cases of radial artery occlusion. However, these occlusion cases remained asymptomatic.

Thanks to the miniaturization of catheter materials, Kiemeneij and Laarman[12] from Amsterdam (Figs. 1-4 and 1-5), the Netherlands, set a milestone in coronary interventional cardiology in the early 1990s by performing balloon angioplasty as well as stent implantation through the radial artery. Furthermore, in the ACCESS study, Kiemeneij et al.[13] compared the radial approach with the brachial and femoral approaches in patients undergoing elective percutaneous transluminal coronary angioplasty, demonstrating that there were no significant differences between the three approaches in terms of success of coronary angiography or angioplasty or duration of the procedures. Interestingly, major access site complications were more frequently encountered after transbrachial and transfemoral percutaneous transluminal coronary angioplasty.

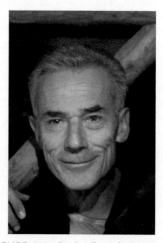

FIGURE 1-4 Dr. Ferdinand Kiemeneij.

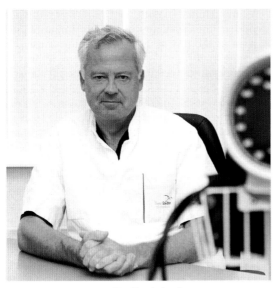

FIGURE 1-5 Dr. Gerrit Jan Laarman.

Although, since then, many countries produced at least one radial pioneer, as of today, the rate of use of radial access varies substantially between continents and even countries (see below). Following the pioneering work of a few dedicated "radialists" in Europe, then in the United States and Asia, radial access has been extended to acute coronary syndromes, including ST-segment elevation myocardial infarction, and also to noncoronary vascular territories (Fig. 1-6). Mann et al.[14] published the first randomized trial, radial versus femoral, in acute coronary syndrome patients in 1998 and concluded that coronary stenting from the radial approach is efficacious in these patients, access site bleeding complications are less,

and early ambulation results in a shorter hospital length of stay. Indeed, a 15% reduction in total hospital charge was reported in favor of the radial group. During the same period, Steg and Aubry[15] in Paris (France) reported two cases on radial approach for primary angioplasty in acute myocardial infarction in patients with contraindication to or impossible femoral access. In Germany, Josef Ludwig performed an observational study using radial access in patients referred for acute myocardial infarction. This experience was probably too premature for the period, as the paper was rejected by a high-impact factor journal, with a note stating that "the study raised significant ethical concerns." Years later, the preliminary experience from Josef Ludwig's center and Yves Louvard's center in France showed a significant reduction in access site bleeding and complications, with similar efficacy, compared with those in patients treated by femoral generation.[16]

In 2001, Scheinert et al.[17] published their experience in transradial renal artery stenting and stated that "transradial renal artery angioplasty and stenting is technically feasible and safe. Particularly in patients with unfavorable vessel anatomy, this new cranio-caudal approach is an attractive alternative technique." In 2002, Levy et al.[18] in the United States described the use of radial artery approach for cerebral angiography. The same year, Yoo et al.[19] reported on a case of transradial carotid stenting in a patient with Leriche syndrome. In 2004, Raghu and Louvard[20] from France reported on successful transradial approach for percutaneous transluminal angioplasty and stenting in the treatment of chronic mesenteric ischemia. In 2005, Flachskampf et al.[21] published one case of iliac artery stenting via the radial access route.

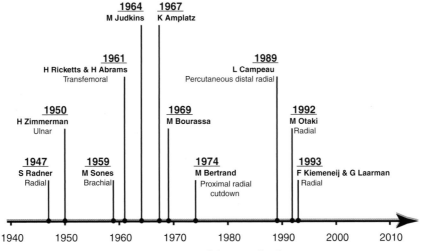

FIGURE 1-6 Radial access timeline.

Today, there have been reports of using the radial or ulnar approach as an access site for virtually all selective angiography or intervention in any artery throughout the body. More recently, radial approach has been described for tumor embolization or treatment, and renal denervation.[22,23]

The Adoption of Transradial Access in Invasive Cardiology

The use of radial artery approach still varies largely around the world. After initial description of clinical experience by the pioneers, radial approach grew mainly advocated by dedicated aficionados and early pioneers. In the 1990s, dedicated centers existed in the Netherlands, France, Canada, and the United States. In the early years of the new century, radial approach gained substantial popularity mostly in Europe and some Asian countries,

including India. Of note, the United States did not embrace the radial approach with similar enthusiasm as the rest of the world. Things started to change in 2010, when the detrimental impact of periprocedural bleeding began to be recognized and the surge of clinical trials brought important evidence-based medical information. Following the recent publication of large trials such as the RadIal Vs femorAL access for coronary intervention (RIVAL) trial and the possible mortality benefit associated with radial approach, this access site is now en route to becoming the default access for diagnostic angiography and coronary interventions.

Nowadays, it remains quite difficult to estimate the real practice of radial approach across the world. Overall, one has to rely on data provided by interventional cardiology societies, surveys, and industry. In the first report from the Society of Cardiovascular Angiography and Intervention published in 2011, a large variation was reported (Table 1-1).[24]

TABLE 1-1 Worldwide Transradial PCI Utilization by Country and Region

Source	National Database				Estimates 2009 (industry/personal/society)		Totals	
	PCI/year	% Radial	Year	Type	PCI/year	% Radial	PCI/year	% Radial
Germany					340,000	25		
France	115,000	55	2008	National				
UK	80,331	35	2008	National				
Spain					61,500	43		
Italy					132,000	25		
Poland	90,238	21.8	2008	National				
Countries (<50 K PCI/year)	16,527	15.7	2006	EAPCI/ SCAAR	66,000	37		
Europe's total	719,094	47.5	2009				1,069,202	29
USA		1.7	2008/9	NCDR	998,500			
Central/ South America					234,350	15		
Canada					60,000	50		
America's total							1,194,350	7
Japan					220,900	60		
India					143,000	32		
China					75,000	25		
Other (<50 K PCI/year)					143,000	32		
Asia's total							581,900	42
Africa/Middle East					245,000	1–3	245,000	1–3
Total worldwide							2,945,452	22

Data from Caputo RP, Tremmel JA, Rao S, et al. Transradial arterial access for coronary and peripheral procedures: executive summary by the transradial committee of the SCAI. *Catheter Cardiovasc Interv.* 2011;78:823–839.

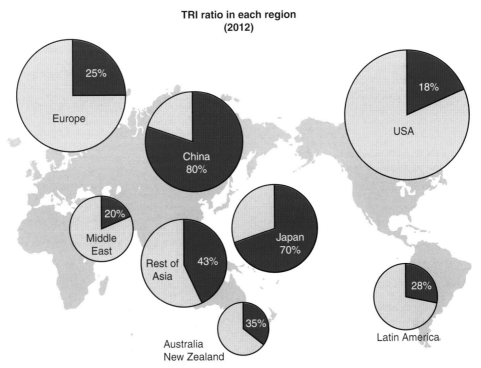

FIGURE 1-7   Transradial intervention rate in each region. (Courtesy Dr. S Saito and Terumo.)

From the industry (Terumo), here is a recent figure showing percentages of radial in the world (Fig. 1-7). Importantly, although the United States has lagged behind the rest of the world for a long time, there is now an exponential growth in radial use across the country, albeit radial being popular on the East Coast, compared with that on the West Coast (Fig. 1-8).

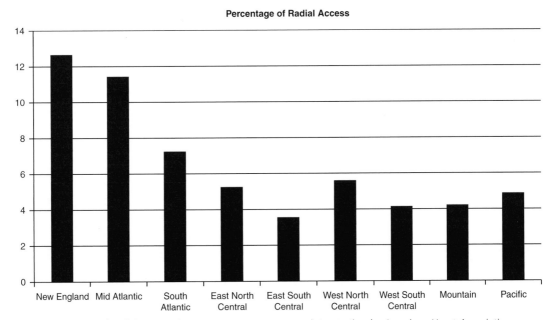

FIGURE 1-8   Use of radial approach to percutaneous coronary intervention by American Heart Association regions. (Data from Feldman DN, Swaminathan RV, Kaltenbach LA, et al. Adoption of radial access and comparison of outcomes to femoral access in percutaneous coronary intervention: an updated report from the national cardiovascular data registry (2007–2012). *Circulation*. 2013;127:2295–2306.)

Conclusion

Following the first reports of transradial coronary angiography by Lucien Campeau in 1989 and transradial percutaneous coronary stenting by Ferdinand Kiemeneij and Gert Laarman in 1992, there was initially limited use of transradial access around the world. With better recognition of the benefits of radial access, compared with that of femoral access, in all clinical scenarios, radial access is now positioning itself to become the preferred access site.

REFERENCES

1. Radner S. Thoracal aortography by catheterization from the radial artery; preliminary report of a new technique. *Acta Radiol.* 1948;29:178–180.
2. Zimmerman HA, Scott RW, Becker NO. Catheterization of the left side of the heart in man. *Circulation.* 1950; 1(3):357–359.
3. Seldinger SI. Catheter replacement of the needle in percutaneous arteriography; a new technique. *Acta radiol.* 1953; 39(5):368–376.
4. Sones FM Jr, Shirey EK. Cine coronary arteriography. *Mod Concepts Cardiovasc Dis.* 1962;31:735–738.
5. Ricketts HJ, Abrams HL. Percutaneous selective coronary cine arteriography. *JAMA.* 1962;181:620–624.
6. Judkins MP. Selective coronary arteriography, I: a percutaneous transfemoral technic. *Radiology.* 1967;89:815–824.
7. Bourassa MG, Lesperance J, Campeau L. Selective coronary arteriography by the percutaneous femoral artery approach. *Am J Roentgenol Radium Ther Nucl Med.* 1969;107:377–383.
8. Wilson WJ, Lee GB, Amplatz K. Biplane selective coronary arteriography via percutaneous transfemoral approach. *Am J Roentgenol Radium Ther Nucl Med.* 1967;100:332–340.
9. Gruntzig A. Transluminal dilatation of coronary-artery stenosis. *Lancet.* 1978;1:263.
10. Bertrand ME, Ketelers JY, Carre A, et al. A new approach in the hemodynamic exploration of the left cardiac cavities via the radial artery below the elbow. *Coeur Med Interne.* 1974;13:345–346.
11. Campeau L. Percutaneous radial artery approach for coronary angiography. *Cathet Cardiovasc Diagn.* 1989;16:3–7.
12. Kiemeneij F, Laarman GJ. Percutaneous transradial artery approach for coronary stent implantation. *Cathet Cardiovasc Diagn.* 1993;30:173–178.
13. Kiemeneij F, Laarman GJ, Odekerken D, et al. A randomized comparison of percutaneous transluminal coronary angioplasty by the radial, brachial and femoral approaches: the access study. *J Am Coll Cardiol.* 1997;29: 1269–1275.
14. Mann T, Cubeddu G, Bowen J, et al. Stenting in acute coronary syndromes: a comparison of radial versus femoral access sites. *J Am Coll Cardiol.* 1998;32:572–576.
15. Steg G, Aubry P. Radial access for primary PTCA in patients with acute myocardial infarction and contraindication or impossible femoral access. *Cathet Cardiovasc Diagn.* 1996;39:424–426.
16. Louvard Y, Ludwig J, Lefevre T, et al. Transradial approach for coronary angioplasty in the setting of acute myocardial infarction: a dual-center registry. *Catheter Cardiovasc Interv.* 2002;55:206–211.
17. Scheinert D, Braunlich S, Nonnast-Daniel B, et al. Transradial approach for renal artery stenting. *Catheter Cardiovasc Interv.* 2001;54:442–447.
18. Levy EI, Boulos AS, Fessler RD, et al. Transradial cerebral angiography: an alternative route. *Neurosurgery.* 2002;51:335–340; discussion 340–342.
19. Yoo BS, Lee SH, Kim JY, et al. A case of transradial carotid stenting in a patient with total occlusion of distal abdominal aorta. *Catheter Cardiovasc Interv.* 2002;56: 243–245.
20. Raghu C, Louvard Y. Transradial approach for percutaneous transluminal angioplasty and stenting in the treatment of chronic mesenteric ischemia. *Catheter Cardiovasc Interv.* 2004;61:450–454.
21. Flachskampf FA, Wolf T, Daniel WG, et al. Transradial stenting of the iliac artery: a case report. *Catheter Cardiovasc Interv.* 2005;65:193–195.
22. Fischman AM, Patel RS, Fung JW, et al. Introduction of the transradial technique into a busy metropolitan interventional radiology practice: the first 300 cases. *J Invasive Cardiol.* 2013;25:21.
23. Honton B, Pathak A, Sauguet A, et al. First report of transradial renal denervation with the dedicated radiofrequency iberis™ catheter. *EuroIntervention.* 2014;9(12):1385–1388.
24. Caputo RP, Tremmel JA, Rao S, et al. Transradial arterial access for coronary and peripheral procedures: executive summary by the transradial committee of the SCAI. *Catheter Cardiovasc Interv.* 2011;78:823–839.

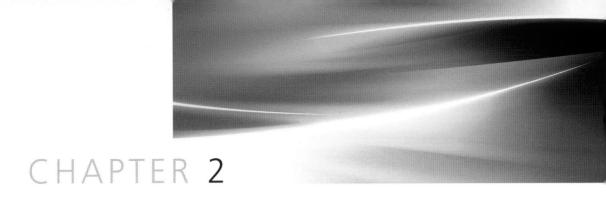

CHAPTER 2

Access Site Bleeding and Nonaccess Site Bleeding

Sunil V. Rao

Introduction

Clinical outcomes of interest related to percutaneous coronary intervention (PCI) include ischemia, bleeding, and vascular events. Ischemic outcomes include procedural events such as abrupt closure, slow or no reflow, or side branch occlusion; periprocedural events such as myocardial infarction (MI) or acute stent thrombosis; and long-term events such as restenosis, target vessel or lesion revascularization, or subacute, late, and very late stent thrombosis. Combination pharmacotherapy (antithrombin and antiplatelet therapies) is used to either prevent or treat these complications, and the evolution of antithrombotic therapy, along with the evolution in PCI equipment, has reduced the risk of ischemic complications and increased procedure success.[1]

Although large prospective randomized trials have compared the efficacy and safety of various antithrombotic drug permutations, it is clear that their use in the presence of an arteriotomy increases the risk of bleeding and vascular complications. These complications are associated with short- and long-term adverse events such as MI, stroke, stent thrombosis, and death, thus creating a "vicious cycle" of bleeding and ischemic events that are interrelated. Importantly, bleeding after PCI can occur at the vascular access site, remote from the access site, or at both sites. This chapter reviews the incidence of bleeding, the relative incidences of access site and nonaccess site bleeding, and the association between bleeding and outcomes as it relates to both access site and nonaccess site bleeding.

Incidence of Bleeding After PCI

The reported incidence of bleeding after PCI depends on three factors: the definition of bleeding used in the data source (clinical trials or registries),[2] the overall risk profile of the patients undergoing PCI,[3] and the pharmacological and vascular access approaches used.[4] Historically, clinical trials of antithrombotic therapies considered ischemic events—death, MI, and stroke—as the primary end point, with bleeding as a safety consideration. As such, the definitions of the individual components of major adverse cardiac events (MACE) were codified to be relatively consistent across clinical trials.[5] In contrast, the definitions of bleeding complications varied widely across studies[2]; however, as the number of therapeutic agents available to reduce MACE increased, safety concerns took on increasing significance. Choosing agents that provided enough antithrombotic effect to reduce MACE and yet did not increase bleeding risk has become a clinical priority. In this context, standardizing bleeding definitions may permit safety comparisons across different therapeutic strategies.[6] Another factor influencing the measured bleeding rate is the underlying risk of the population being studied. For patients undergoing PCI, those presenting with stable angina for elective PCI represent a low risk for ischemic and bleeding outcomes. The risk increases as the presenting syndrome becomes unstable (i.e., unstable angina [UA], non-ST-segment elevation MI [NSTEMI], ST-segment elevation MI [STEMI]) and the urgency of the procedure increases (urgent, emergent, salvage). The third variable that influences bleeding rates is the therapeutic approach used in terms of antithrombotic therapy (anticoagulation and antiplatelet therapy), vascular access strategy, and the use of other invasive procedures such as coronary artery bypass grafting (CABG). Taking these issues into account, the rate of bleeding measured in registries and clinical trials generally ranges from 1% to 10%,[2,7] but has been reported to be as high as 86% for CABG-related bleeding in some trials.[8] Among patients undergoing PCI in the modern era, there has been a temporal decrease in postprocedural bleeding complications, attributable to the adoption of targeted antithrombotic therapies rather than vascular access site strategies.[9]

Defining Bleeding

As mentioned earlier, the definition of bleeding significantly influences its reported incidence. Historically, there has been variation in the definition of hemorrhagic complications in studies of antithrombotic therapies for both acute coronary syndrome (ACS) and PCI. This presented significant challenges in determining the "comparative effectiveness" of different treatment strategies as they relate to safety. In order to create a more "apple to apples" comparison, two efforts were undertaken in an attempt to standardize the reporting of bleeding events across studies. The first, titled the Academic Bleeding Consensus (ABC) Working Group, outlined a set of recommendations related to the collection of bleeding data elements in registries and clinical trials.[10] The second, titled the Bleeding Academic Research Consortium (BARC), went further and created definitions that included both CABG-related and fatal bleeding (Table 2-1).[6] This set of definitions dispenses with qualitative terms such as "major" or "severe," and instead uses an ordinal numerical system. Several ongoing clinical trials are using the BARC definition of bleeding as the primary safety endpoint, and a post hoc analysis of clinical trial data has shown a relationship between BARC-defined bleeding and adverse outcomes.[11]

An important aspect of the BARC bleeding definition is that it does specify the location of the bleeding event, for example, gastrointestinal or vascular access site; however, some registries and clinical trials have included the location of bleeding as a data element in the bleeding definition. For example, the ACUITY trial included access

site hematoma >5 cm as part of the definition of major bleeding.[12] Similarly, the National Cardiovascular Data Registry (NCDR) CathPCI Registry, the largest ongoing PCI registry in the world, also specifies access site–related bleeding events, including retroperitoneal hematoma.[13] Among patients with ACS and those undergoing PCI, the most common site of nonaccess site bleeding is gastrointestinal.[14] Data from the NCDR CathPCI Registry show that the temporal decrease in bleeding is driven primarily by a decrease in access site bleeding; nonaccess site bleeding has remained relatively stable over time (Fig. 2-1).[9]

Relative Incidence of Access Site and Nonaccess Site Bleeding

For patients undergoing PCI, not only does the reported incidence of overall bleeding vary with the acuity of the presentation, but the proportion of bleeding events attributable to the vascular access site also varies (Fig. 2-2).[3] This is likely due to differences in the rate of PCI and aggressive antithrombotic therapy across the different syndromes. For example, approximately 55% to 60% patients with non-ST-segment elevation acute coronary syndrome (NSTE-ACS) will undergo PCI, while the proportion is much higher for patients with STEMI given the widespread use of primary PCI.[15] Therefore, the rate of access site bleeding is lower for patients with NSTE-ACS than for those with STEMI. These differences influence the relative impact of bleeding avoidance strategies (BAS) across patient subgroups—BAS that are access-site specific, such as radial access, should have greater impact among patients with STEMI. As described elsewhere in this text, this has been borne out in randomized trials where radial access has not been associated with a significant reduction in bleeding among patients with NSTE-ACS,[16] but does reduce bleeding and mortality in patients with STEMI.[17]

Bleeding Complications and Outcomes

Studies have consistently shown an association between bleeding complications and an increased risk for morbidity, mortality, and costs. Several observational and some prospective randomized trials have shown an association between BAS and reduced mortality among patients

TABLE 2-1 The Bleeding Academic Research Consortium (BARC) Definition of Bleeding Complications

Type 0 No bleeding

Type 1 Bleeding that is not actionable and does not cause the patient to seek unscheduled performance of studies, hospitalization, or treatment by a health-care professional

Type 2 Any overt, actionable sign of hemorrhage (e.g., more bleeding than would be expected for a clinical circumstance, including bleeding found by imaging alone) that *does not* fit the criteria for types 3, 4, or 5, but *does* meet at least one of the following criteria: (1) requiring nonsurgical, medical intervention by a health-care professional, (2) leading to hospitalization or increased level of care, and (3) prompting evaluation

Type 3

Type 3a

- Overt bleeding plus hemoglobin drop of 3 to <5[a] g/dL (provided hemoglobin drop is related to bleed)
- Any transfusion with overt bleeding

Type 3b

- Overt bleeding plus hemoglobin drop ≥5[a] g/dL (provided hemoglobin drop is related to bleed)
- Cardiac tamponade
- Bleeding requiring surgical intervention for control (excluding dental/nasal/skin/hemorrhoid)
- Bleeding requiring intravenous vasoactive drugs

Type 3c

- Intracranial hemorrhage (does not include microbleeds or hemorrhagic transformation; does include intraspinal)
- Subcategories; confirmed by autopsy or imaging or LP
- Intraocular bleed compromising vision

Type 4—CABG-Related Bleeding

- Perioperative intracranial bleeding within 48 hours
- Reoperation following closure of sternotomy for the purpose of controlling bleeding
- Transfusion of ≥5 units of whole blood or packed red blood cells within a 48-hour period[b]
- Chest tube output ≥2 L within a 24-hour period
- If a CABG-related bleed is not adjudicated as at least a type 3 severity event, it will be classified as "not a bleeding event."

Type 5—Fatal Bleeding

Type 5a

- Probable fatal bleeding: no autopsy or imaging confirmation, but clinically suspicious

Type 5b

- Definite fatal bleeding: overt bleeding or autopsy or imaging confirmation

LP, lumbar puncture; PRBC, packed red blood cells; Hgb, hemoglobin.
[a]Corrected for transfusion (1 unit PRBC or 1 unit whole blood = 1 g/dL Hgb).
[b]Only allogeneic transfusions are considered as transfusions for BARC type 4 bleeding. Cell saver products will not be counted.

with ACS[18] and with STEMI.[17,19] Table 2-2 lists selected studies that have examined the relationship between bleeding complications and short- and long-term outcomes among patients undergoing PCI. These outcomes have included clinical adverse events such as MACE, stent thrombosis, and mortality, as well as nonclinical events such as costs and hospital length of stay. In general, there is a strong, dose-dependent increase in the risk of adverse clinical and economic outcomes as bleeding severity increases.

Whether access site bleeding should take on the same significance as that of nonaccess site bleeding and thus be included in a "major" or "severe" bleeding definition is controversial.[6] At issue is that access site bleeding usually occurs within 24 hours of the PCI and is most commonly manifest as a hematoma. It is unlikely that such local bleeding is associated with an increased risk of mortality, and indeed some studies have shown that some types of access site bleeding, such as 5-cm groin hematomas, are not associated with

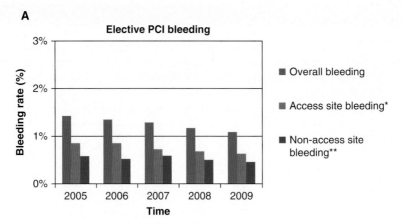

*P-value for temporal trend of access site bleeding: $P < 0.001$
**P-value for temporal trend of non-access site bleeding: $P = 0.104$

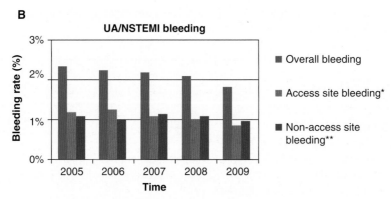

*P-value for temporal trend of access site bleeding: $P < 0.001$
**P-value for temporal trend of non-access site bleeding: $P = 0.827$

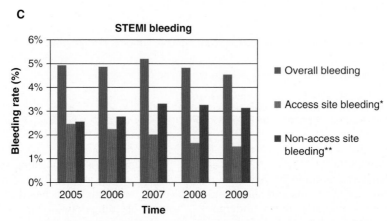

*P-value for temporal trend of access site bleeding: $P < 0.001$
**P-value for temporal trend of non-access site bleeding: $P < 0.001$

FIGURE 2-1 Temporal trends in postprocedural bleeding rates among patients with stable angina **(A)**, UA/NSTEMI **(B)**, and STEMI **(C)** undergoing PCI. *(Adapted from Subherwal S, Peterson ED, Dai D, et al. Temporal trends in and factors associated with bleeding complications among patients undergoing percutaneous coronary intervention: a report from the National Cardiovascular Data CathPCI Registry. J Am Coll Cardiol. 2012;59:1861–1869.)*

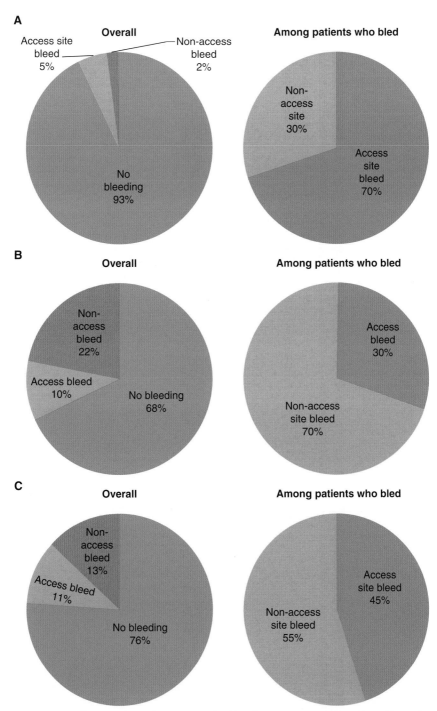

FIGURE 2-2   Proportion of access site and nonaccess site bleeding among patients with stable angina undergoing PCI **(A)**, NSTE-ACS undergoing invasive risk stratification **(B)**, and STEMI receiving fibrinolysis and cardiac catheterization **(C)**. *(Adapted from Rao SV, Cohen MG, Kandzari DE, et al. The transradial approach to percutaneous coronary intervention: historical perspective, current concepts, and future directions. J Am Coll Cardiol. 2010;55:2187–2195.)*

TABLE 2-2 **Selected Studies Showing an Association between Bleeding Complications and Adverse Outcomes**

| Study | Design | N | Outcomes in Patients with Bleeding vs No Bleeding | | | |
| | | | Early Deaths (in-hospital or at 30 days) | | Deaths up to 1 year | |
			Death Rates (%)	Adjusted Risk Ratio for Death (CI)	Death Rates (%)	Adjusted Risk Ratio for Death (CI)
Kinnaird et al. (2003)[20]	PCI, registry	10,974	7.5 vs 0.6	3.5 (1.9–6.7)	17.2 vs 5.5	Not significant
GRACE (2007)[21]	ACS, registry	40,087	20.9 vs 5.6	1.9 (1.6–2.2)	7.9 vs 5.2	0.8 (0.6–1.0)
REPLACE-2 (2007)[22]	PCI, RCT	6,001	5.1 vs 0.2	—	8.7 vs 1.9	2.7 (1.4–4.9)
Rao et al. (2005)[23]	Pooled data from NSTE-ACS trials	26,452	25.7 vs 2.9	10.6 (8.3–13.6)	35.1 vs 4.2	7.5 (6.1–9.3)
Eikelboom et al. (2006)[24]	NSTE-ACS, pooled data from trials/ registry	34,146	12.8 vs 2.5	9.8 (7.5–12.7)	4.6 vs 2.9	1.9 (1.3–2.8)
ACUITY (2007)[25]	NSTE-ACS, RCT	13,819	7.3 vs 1.2	7.6 (4.7–12.2)	—	3.5 (2.7–4.4)
Ndrepepa et al. (2008)[25]	PCI, meta-analysis of RCTs	5,384	—	—	12.2 vs 3.3	4.1 (2.1–8.3)
Amlani et al. (2010)[26]	STEMI, registry	1,389	19.7 vs 8.2	2.8 (1.8–14.3)	—	—

CI, confidence interval; RCT, randomized controlled trial.

adverse events.[27,28] On the other hand, more severe access site bleeding, such as retroperitoneal bleeding,[29] or access site hematomas[30] that require blood transfusion are associated with increased risk.[31]

Mechanisms

Studies examining the association between hemorrhagic complications and outcomes are largely observational. Indeed, although the concept of performing a trial comparing bleeding versus no bleeding may seem unethical and not feasible, such a trial has been completed. The iron (Fe) and Atherosclerosis Study Trial (FeAST) randomized 1,277 patients with symptomatic peripheral arterial disease to either "iron-reduction therapy" (i.e., phlebotomy) or usual care, on the basis of the hypothesis that reduction of excess iron accumulation will reduce all-cause mortality.[32] Patients in the iron reduction group underwent periodic scheduled phlebotomy with removal of a defined volume of blood at 6-month intervals. At 6 years of follow-up, there was no significant difference between the two groups with respect to all-cause mortality. Although this randomized trial may suggest that "bleeding" in itself is not associated with increased mortality, the data are not directly applicable to post-PCI bleeding in the clinical setting. Bleeding that occurs post-PCI is not similar to systematic planned removal of a volume of blood at defined intervals. However, this trial (FeAST) does underscore the possibility that many of the studies linking bleeding to other adverse outcomes are burdened by confounding. At the extremes, for example, exsanguination or intracranial hemorrhage, bleeding likely leads to death. These severe events are exceedingly rare after PCI, and the association between less severe bleeding events and outcomes requires further investigation into potential mechanisms.

Given that advanced age and renal dysfunction are significant predictors of bleeding after PCI,[13] it is possible that comorbidities that predispose patients to bleeding also predispose them to morbidity and mortality and that bleeding events are not causally related to adverse outcomes. In contrast, there may be other mechanisms at play. For example, bleeding events often lead to cessation of evidence-based antithrombotic therapy. From a clinical standpoint, the occurrence of a bleeding event among patients who are treated with parenteral antithrombotic agents leaves little choice but discontinuation of the therapy, leaving patients at risk for recurrent ischemic events. In the context of long-term antithrombotic therapy after PCI, bleeding events are associated with medication nonadherence. Roy et al.[33] examined the association between bleeding events and adherence to dual antiplatelet therapy among 2,360 unselected patients undergoing PCI with drug-eluting stents at a single center. The overall incidence of bleeding using the Serebruany classification[34] was 32.7%, with the majority (~85%) being classified as "nuisance" bleeding, defined as bruising, petechiae, or ecchymoses. The rate of discontinuation of thienopyridine therapy among patients with nuisance bleeding was 11%. These data may explain the association between bleeding complications and an increased risk for stent thrombosis.[35] In addition to the cessation of antithrombotic therapy, the use of blood transfusion among patients undergoing PCI may also increase the risk of recurrent MI, heart failure, and mortality.[4] Although transfusion may be necessary in extreme situations, its use as a routine therapy for anemic patients who are stable or as an "insurance policy" against bleeding is not recommended.[36] Although the exact mechanism by which transfusion is associated with adverse outcomes is not known, it may be related to the "storage lesion," whereby stored red blood cells undergo significant chemical changes such as depletion of nitric oxide that limit or eliminate their ability to increase oxygen delivery and may be associated with increased platelet aggregation and activation.[37]

Bleeding Avoidance Strategies and Outcomes

If bleeding complications are associated with an increased risk for mortality (regardless of the mechanisms involved), then reduced bleeding risk should be associated with reduced mortality. Reduction in bleeding risk can be achieved through the use of so-called BAS, which include both pharmacological approaches as well as access site approaches. Table 2-3 lists BAS that are supported by observational studies, randomized trials, or both.

Two pharmacological BAS are associated with reduced mortality—fondaparinux in NSTE-ACS and bivalirudin in primary PCI for STEMI. The OASIS 5 trial randomized 20,000 patients with high-risk NSTE-ACS to either enoxaparin or fondaparinux.[18] At 9 days, there was no significant difference in the incidence of death, MI, or refractory ischemia between the two arms. The rate of major bleeding at 9 days was 48% lower

TABLE 2-3 **Available Bleeding Avoidance Strategies**	
Strategy	**Example**
Appropriate dosing of antithrombotics	Adjustment of renally cleared agents for renal function
Avoiding potent antiplatelet agents in high-risk patients	Avoiding use of prasugrel in patients >75 years old, patients with prior stroke, body weight < 60 kg
Targeted anticoagulants	Bivalirudin for PCI; fondaparinux for NSTE-ACS
Access site strategies	Radial approach; femoral vascular closure devices

among patients assigned to fondaparinux. Moreover, there was a significant reduction in 30- and 180-day death in the fondaparinux arm. In the HORIZONS-MI trial, 3,602 patients with STEMI undergoing primary PCI were randomized to either bivalirudin with provisional glycoprotein IIb/IIIa (GPI) or unfractionated heparin with planned GPI.[19] At 30 days, the incidence of death, recurrent MI, or target vessel revascularization was similar between the two arms, but the rate of major bleeding was 40% lower in the bivalirudin arm. In addition, the rates of cardiac mortality and all-cause mortality were lower among patients assigned to the bivalirudin arm.

With respect to vascular access site strategies, the role of radial approach in clinical outcomes is detailed in the subsequent chapters in this textbook. Specifically, since the rate of bleeding is higher among patients with STEMI undergoing primary PCI, and because the proportion of access-site bleeding is relatively higher in this population compared with those who have NSTE-ACS, radial access should lead to significantly lower rates of bleeding, compared with femoral access among patients undergoing primary PCI. The RIFLE-STEACS trial, which randomized 1,001 patients with STEMI undergoing primary PCI to either radial or femoral access, showed that there was a 4% absolute decrease in BARC type 2 or greater bleeding in the radial arm.[17] This correlated with a 4% absolute decrease in 30-day mortality. These prospective randomized trials demonstrate that BAS, which maintain efficacy compared with control but significantly reduce bleeding risk, can improve survival in high-risk patients with ACS and those undergoing PCI.

Conclusion

Bleeding is the most common complication of PCI and occurs both at the vascular access site and remote from the access site. Multiple studies have consistently shown an association between bleeding complications and an increased risk for adverse clinical and economic outcomes. Strategies that reduce bleeding risk, whether they are directed at access site bleeding or nonaccess site bleeding, are associated with reduced mortality.

REFERENCES

1. Singh M, Rihal CS, Gersh BJ, et al. Twenty-five-year trends in in-hospital and long-term outcome after percutaneous coronary intervention: a single-institution experience. *Circulation*. 2007;115:2835–2841.
2. Steinhubl SR, Kastrati A, Berger PB. Variation in the definitions of bleeding in clinical trials of patients with acute coronary syndromes and undergoing percutaneous coronary interventions and its impact on the apparent safety of antithrombotic drugs. *Am Heart J*. 2007;154:3–11.
3. Rao SV, Cohen MG, Kandzari DE, et al. The transradial approach to percutaneous coronary intervention: historical perspective, current concepts, and future directions. *J Am Coll Cardiol*. 2010;55:2187–2195.
4. Doyle BJ, Rihal CS, Gastineau DA, et al. Bleeding, blood transfusion, and increased mortality after percutaneous coronary intervention: implications for contemporary practice. *J Am Coll Cardiol*. 2009;53:2019–2027.
5. Cannon CP, Battler A, Brindis RG, et al. American College of Cardiology key data elements and definitions for measuring the clinical management and outcomes of patients with acute coronary syndromes. A report of the American College of Cardiology Task Force on Clinical Data Standards (Acute Coronary Syndromes Writing Committee). *J Am Coll Cardiol*. 2001;38:2114–2130.
6. Mehran R, Rao SV, Bhatt DL, et al. Standardized bleeding definitions for cardiovascular clinical trials: a consensus report from the Bleeding Academic Research Consortium. *Circulation*. 2011;123:2736–2747.
7. Rao SV, Eikelboom JA, Granger CB, et al. Bleeding and blood transfusion issues in patients with non-ST-segment elevation acute coronary syndromes. *Eur Heart J*. 2007;28:1193–1204.
8. Wallentin L, Becker RC, Budaj A, et al. Ticagrelor versus clopidogrel in patients with acute coronary syndromes. *N Engl J Med*. 2009;361:1045–1057.
9. Subherwal S, Peterson ED, Dai D, et al. Temporal trends in and factors associated with bleeding complications among patients undergoing percutaneous coronary intervention: a report from the National Cardiovascular Data CathPCI Registry. *J Am Coll Cardiol*. 2012;59:1861–1869.
10. Rao SV, Eikelboom J, Steg PG, et al. Standardized reporting of bleeding complications for clinical investigations in acute coronary syndromes: a proposal from the academic bleeding consensus (ABC) multidisciplinary working group. *Am Heart J*. 2009;158:881–886.e1.

11. Ndrepepa G, Schuster T, Hadamitzky M, et al. Validation of the Bleeding Academic Research Consortium definition of bleeding in patients with coronary artery disease undergoing percutaneous coronary intervention. *Circulation.* 2012;125:1424–1431.

12. Stone GW, Bertrand M, Colombo A, et al. Acute Catheterization and Urgent Intervention Triage Strategy (ACUITY) trial: study design and rationale. *Am Heart J.* 2004;148:764–775.

13. Mehta SK, Frutkin AD, Lindsey JB, et al. Bleeding in patients undergoing percutaneous coronary intervention: the development of a clinical risk algorithm from the National Cardiovascular Data Registry. *Circ Cardiovasc Interv.* 2009;2:222–229.

14. Nikolsky E, Stone GW, Kirtane AJ, et al. Gastrointestinal bleeding in patients with acute coronary syndromes: incidence, predictors, and clinical implications: analysis from the ACUITY (Acute Catheterization and Urgent Intervention Triage Strategy) trial. *J Am Coll Cardiol.* 2009;54:1293–1302.

15. Roe MT, Messenger JC, Weintraub WS, et al. Treatments, trends, and outcomes of acute myocardial infarction and percutaneous coronary intervention. *J Am Coll Cardiol.* 2010;56:254–263.

16. Jolly SS, Yusuf S, Cairns J, et al. Radial versus femoral access for coronary angiography and intervention in patients with acute coronary syndromes (RIVAL): a randomised, parallel group, multicentre trial. *Lancet.* 2011;377:1409–1420.

17. Romagnoli E, Biondi-Zoccai G, Sciahbasi A, et al. Radial versus femoral randomized investigation in ST-segment elevation acute coronary syndrome: the RIFLE-STEACS (Radial Versus Femoral Randomized Investigation in ST-Elevation Acute Coronary Syndrome) study. *J Am Coll Cardiol.* 2012;60:2481–2489.

18. Fifth Organization to Assess Strategies in Acute Ischemic Syndromes Investigators; Yusuf S, Mehta SR, Chrolavicius S, et al. Comparison of fondaparinux and enoxaparin in acute coronary syndromes. *N Engl J Med.* 2006;354:1464–1476.

19. Stone GW, Witzenbichler B, Guagliumi G, et al. Bivalirudin during primary PCI in acute myocardial infarction. *N Engl J Med.* 2008;358:2218–2230.

20. Kinnaird TD, Stabile E, Mintz GS, et al. Incidence, predictors, and prognostic implications of bleeding and blood transfusion following percutaneous coronary interventions. *Am J Cardiol.* 2003;92:930–935.

21. Moscucci M, Fox KA, Cannon CP, et al. Predictors of major bleeding in acute coronary syndromes: the Global Registry of Acute Coronary Events (GRACE). *Eur Heart J.* 2003;24:1815–1823.

22. Feit F, Voeltz MD, Attubato MJ, et al. Predictors and impact of major hemorrhage on mortality following percutaneous coronary intervention from the REPLACE-2 Trial. *Am J Cardiol.* 2007;100:1364–1369.

23. Rao SV, O'Grady K, Pieper KS, et al. Impact of bleeding severity on clinical outcomes among patients with acute coronary syndromes. *Am J Cardiol.* 2005;96:1200–1206.

24. Eikelboom JW, Mehta SR, Anand SS, et al. Adverse impact of bleeding on prognosis in patients with acute coronary syndromes. *Circulation.* 2006;114:774–782.

25. Ndrepepa G, Berger PB, Mehilli J, et al. Periprocedural bleeding and 1-year outcome after percutaneous coronary interventions: appropriateness of including bleeding as a component of a quadruple end point. *J Am Coll Cardiol.* 2008;51:690–697.

26. Amlani S, Nadarajah T, Afzal R, et al. Mortality and morbidity following a major bleed in a registry population with acute ST elevation myocardial infarction. *J Thromb Thrombolysis.* 2010;30:434–440.

27. Mehran R. Impact of different bleeding types on mortality after PCI: results from a pooled analysis of the REPLACE-2, ACUITY, and HORIZONS-AMI trials. European Society of Cardiology, Barcelona, Spain, 2009.

28. White H, Aylward P, Gallo R, et al. Hematomas of at least 5 cm and outcomes in patients undergoing elective percutaneous coronary intervention: insights from the SafeTy and Efficacy of Enoxaparin in PCI patients, an internationaL randomized Evaluation (STEEPLE) trial. *Am Heart J.* 2010;159:110–116.

29. Ellis SG, Bhatt D, Kapadia S, et al. Correlates and outcomes of retroperitoneal hemorrhage complicating percutaneous coronary intervention. *Catheter Cardiovasc Interv.* 2006;67:541–545.

30. Yatskar L, Selzer F, Feit F, et al. Access site hematoma requiring blood transfusion predicts mortality in patients undergoing percutaneous coronary intervention: data from the National Heart, Lung, and Blood Institute Dynamic Registry. *Catheter Cardiovasc Interv.* 2007;69:961–966.

31. Verheugt FW, Steinhubl SR, Hamon M, et al. Incidence, prognostic impact, and influence of antithrombotic therapy on access and nonaccess site bleeding in percutaneous coronary intervention. *JACC Cardiovasc Interv.* 2011;4:191–197.

32. Zacharski LR, Chow BK, Howes PS, et al. Reduction of iron stores and cardiovascular outcomes in patients with peripheral arterial disease: a randomized controlled trial. *JAMA.* 2007;297:603–610.

33. Roy P, Bonello L, Torguson R, et al. Impact of "nuisance" bleeding on clopidogrel compliance in patients undergoing intracoronary drug-eluting stent implantation. *Am J Cardiol.* 2008;102:1614–1617.

34. Serebruany VL, Atar D. Assessment of bleeding events in clinical trials—proposal of a new classification. *Am J Cardiol.* 2007;99:288–290.

35. Manoukian SV, Feit F, Mehran R, et al. Impact of major bleeding on 30-day mortality and clinical outcomes in patients with acute coronary syndromes: an analysis from the ACUITY trial. *J Am Coll Cardiol.* 2007;49:1362–1368.

36. Bassand JP, Hamm CW, Ardissino D, et al. Guidelines for the diagnosis and treatment of non-ST-segment elevation acute coronary syndromes. *Eur Heart J.* 2007;28:1598–1660.

37. Rao SV, Califf RM. Is old blood bad blood? *Am Heart J.* 2010;159:710–712.

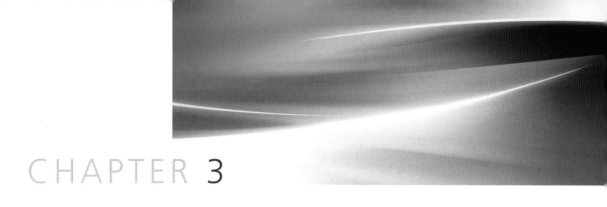

CHAPTER 3

General Overview, Patient Preparation, and Selection

Alessandro Sciahbasi, Giuseppe Biondi-Zoccai, and Enrico Romagnoli

General Overview

Coronary angiography and percutaneous coronary intervention (PCI) are a mainstay in the diagnostic workup, prognostication, and therapeutic management of patients with coronary artery disease.[1-4] Historically, coronary procedures were done via the brachial route (exploiting surgical cut-down) or the femoral route (using the Seldinger approach as refined by Judkins). The dominant role of these access sites for many years can easily be explained by several factors, including the availability at those specific times of devices with rather large diameters yet relatively poor torquability, a property that is difficult to define formally but is of utmost importance for practitioners.[5] Indeed, large and bulky devices call almost unanimously for large arteries and access sites that are more proximal (i.e., closer to the anatomic target), as is still typical for endografts and transcatheter aortic valve implantation (TAVI) devices.

Over such background, transradial coronary angiography was originally introduced by Campeau[6] in the late 1980s and transradial PCI was first proposed by Kiemeneij and Laarman[7] in the early 1990s. Such pioneering transradial efforts should be considered as even more paradigm shifting given the type and quality of diagnostic and interventional devices available, respectively in 1989 and 1993, which, for instance, included as coronary stents only the Wallstent and the Palmaz-Schatz devices.[6,7]

After more than two decades since these baby steps, transradial approach is the most common access site in several institutions worldwide, and is poised to gain further ground given its objective benefits on clinically relevant end points, its economic appeal, and patient preference.[8-12]

In this chapter, we strive to provide a comprehensive and updated perspective on transradial access for diagnostic and therapeutic cardiovascular procedures, emphasizing the key background data in support of this access site, as well as the crucial steps of patients selection and preparation for an effective and safe transradial approach.

Definition of Transradial Access

Defining transradial access might seem unnecessary in a book devoted wholeheartedly to this topic,[3] but for the purpose of this textbook, transradial access is considered any percutaneous transluminal access to the radial artery, almost invariably at a level higher than the anatomical snuffbox.[13] Identifying a proximal limit to the transradial access zone is conversely more difficult, as experienced operators can gain safe and effective access even close to the origin of the radial artery from the brachial artery at the elbow. Nonetheless, transradial access conventionally entails percutaneous transluminal access by means of standard (front- and back-wall puncture) or modified (front-wall-only puncture) Seldinger techniques at or above the wrist, but still in the distal third of the radial artery. Emphasis on transradial access rather than on radial access per se can be justified by the obvious percutaneous transluminal approach typically employed, at odds with the cut-down method, historically common for brachial access and still used for femoral procedures requiring very large devices. Finally, transradial access is often considered to comprise transradial access per se as well as transulnar access, which has some distinct features, but still shares many of the pros and cons typical of transradial access in comparison to transfemoral or transbrachial accesses.[14,15]

Pathophysiologic Rationale for Transradial Access

What are the theoretical advantages of gaining access to the arterial circulation through the radial artery? We propose several favorable theoretical features of this approach, which may (and actually do) directly translate into clinical benefits. First, the radial artery, similar to the common femoral artery and the brachial artery, runs in its distal tract above a bony landmark (i.e., the radius), and thus is easily found at the beginning of the procedure and compressed after the procedure or in case of complications. Moreover, given its superficial location, it can be easily managed by gentle compression to achieve hemostasis, without the need for very aggressive, diffuse, or prolonged compression efforts. Even in the case of local hematoma or bleeding, there is no nearby anatomic space or cavity that can be readily filled by a bleeding process (at odds with the peritoneal space), and this may self-limit the severity of access site bleeding. In addition, the small size of the radial artery and its tendency to spasm in case of trauma also concur to a much lower likelihood of bleeding. Nonetheless, the lack of an overt exit route for rapidly increasing hematomas may lead, on rare occasions, to compartment syndrome.[16]

The radial artery is not the only vessel feeding the distal upper limb, as the ulnar artery also provides blood flow to the hand. This means that in most patients even total radial occlusion is well tolerated and asymptomatic, a fact confirmed by ongoing experience of transradial operators who do not perform preliminary Allen test and by the well-established role of radial artery grafting during bypass surgery.[14,17]

Transradial access by definition does not limit ambulation, thus increasing comfort and autonomy of patients, enabling outpatient treatment, and thereby reducing workload for nurses and ancillary personnel.[18] Finally, its origin from the aortic arch and the typical path of this artery and other important potential therapeutic targets make transradial access an ideal choice for catheterization of selected vessels, such as the left internal mammary artery and the renal arteries, which are more easily reached from the radial artery rather than from the femoral artery.[19] This may translate into more favorable success rates and procedural times for such procedures.

Clinical Evidence in Support of Transradial Access

Since its introduction, a wealth of clinical evidence has accumulated on the risk–benefit and cost–benefit profiles of transradial access, actually, largely in its favor.[8,9,20,21] For the purpose of this work, we shall focus on the most important randomized trials (Tables 3-1 and 3-2) and systematic reviews (Table 3-3), largely disregarding case reports, series, and nonrandomized studies, which have nonetheless often important technical and clinical implications, given their real-world features and common focus on "off-label" approaches.[17,22,23] Specifically, Ghuran and colleagues[17] have provided robust evidence, through data on their 632-patient registry, including 662 PCI performed through the transradial route (right-sided in 97.6%) without checking preliminarily for a nonpathologic Allen test. Indeed, the presence of a palpable radial pulse was sufficient to attempt transradial artery cannulation. Notably, despite the large and real-world sample, there was no case of pseudoaneurysm, arterovenous fistula, bleeding requiring surgical repair, or upper limb ischemia.

The Prospective REgistry of Vascular Access in Interventions in Lazio region (PREVAIL) study has prospectively compared 509 patients undergoing transradial access with 543 receiving transfemoral access for coronary procedures (with 40% PCI rate) in the current era in nine high-volume Italian institutions.[23] In this study, Pristipino et al. showed that transradial access was associated with fewer major or minor in-hospital hemorrhages, strokes, or entry site complications (2.0% vs 4.2%, $P = 0.03$), as well as a lesser incidence of the composite end point of in-hospital death or myocardial infarction (0.6% vs 3.1%, $P = 0.005$). Notably, no specific threshold was identified in institutional volume, suggesting that once adequate experience in transradial access has accumulated, even relatively low procedural volumes are not associated with untoward events. Most recent data from the same study reporting on right versus left transradial access have also been provided.[24]

Finally, in the comprehensive report from the National Cardiovascular Data Registry, Feldman et al. have shown how much room for improvement

TABLE 3-1	**Patient Selection in Key Clinical Trials Focusing on Transradial Access**	
Study	**Inclusion Criteria**	**Exclusion Criteria**
ACCESS (1997)	Stable or unstable angina, palpable pulses in radial, femoral, and brachial arteries	Absence of pulse in femoral, brachial, or radial arteries, abnormal Allen test, failed prior transradial access, chronic total occlusion, acute myocardial infarction, expected need for intra-aortic balloon pump, right cardiac catheterization or temporary pacemaker, ad hoc PCI after prior transfemoral access, indwelling sheath from prior catheterization, planned primary stenting or atherectomy
OUTCLAS (2005)	Stable and unstable angina (Braunwald class 1 or 2), NHLBI type A and B lesions (type C lesions only if there was an intention and technical possibility to implant a stent), multivessel disease, multivessel PTCA (if not more than one treated vessel remained unstented)	Acute myocardial infarction, unstable angina Braunwald class 3, type C lesion, chronic total occlusion with anticipated difficult stenting, expected hemodynamic collapse in case of reocclusion, last remaining vessel or unprotected left main PTCA, intracoronary thrombus, any reason for using catheter equipment >6F (i.e., for nonballoon technique), non-PTCA-related reason for hospitalization, negative Allen test for adequate collateral blood supply of the hand, inability or refusal to give informed consent
RIFLE-STEACS (2012)	Suspected STEACS planned for early percutaneous revascularization strategy (within 24-h of symptom onset)	Contraindication to either radial or femoral vascular access (e.g., abnormal Allen test or known severe peripheral vascular disease), recent stroke (within 4 weeks), anticoagulant therapy assumption with an international normalized ratio >2, other severe bleeding diathesis
RIVAL (2011)	ACS with or without ST-elevation, invasive approach planned, the interventional cardiologist was willing to proceed with either radial or femoral access (and had expertise for both, including at least 50 radial procedures for coronary angiography or intervention within the previous year), dual circulation of the hand was intact as assessed by an Allen test	Cardiogenic shock, severe peripheral vascular disease precluding a femoral approach, or previous coronary bypass surgery using more than one internal mammary artery
TALENT (2011)	Palpable pulse in both radial arteries	Previous coronary artery bypass, hemodynamic instability, STEACS, need of >6F catheters, ischemic Allen test, simultaneous right ventricular catheterization, hemodialysis patients with an arteriovenous fistula, age <18 y
TEMPURA (2003)	Acute myocardial infarction within 12 h from onset, age >20 y, normal Allen test	Prior thrombolytic therapy, shock without valid radial pulse, prior coronary artery bypass grafting, lack of equipoise for feasibility of both transradial and transfemoral access, lack of evident culprit lesion, culprit lesion unsuitable for stenting

ACS, acute coronary syndrome; F, French; NHLBI, National Heart Lung and Blood Institute; PCI, percutaneous coronary intervention; PTCA, percutaneous transluminal coronary angioplasty; STEACS, ST-elevation acute coronary syndrome.

TABLE 3-2   Patient Preparation in Key Clinical Trials Focusing on Transradial Access

Study (Year)	Right-Sided Transradial Access	Preparation	Hemostasis
ACCESS (1997)	100%	34° abduction of the arm, with wrist hyperextension, and puncture with a 20–18G needle	Occlusive tourniquets
OUTCLAS (2005)	>95%	NA	Manual compression and a pressure bandage
RIFLE-STEACS (2012)	NA	Standard femoral preparation	Inflatable wrist band (TR Band) or pressure bandage with three elastic sticky straps
RIVAL (2011)	NA	NA	NA
TALENT (2011)	50%	Standard femoral preparation	Inflatable wrist band (TR Band) or pressure bandage with three elastic sticky straps
TEMPURA (2003)	NA	NA	NA

NA, not available or applicable.

TABLE 3-3   Systematic Reviews and Meta-analyses Focusing on Transradial Access

First Author (Year)	Studies	Patients	Selection Criteria	Main Findings
Agostoni (2004)	12	3,224	RCT comparing TRA vs TFA in patients undergoing coronary angiography or PCI	TRA reduced the risk of entry site complications (OR = 0.20 [0.09–0.42], $P < 0.001$), even if at the price of a higher rate of procedural failure (OR = 3.30 [1.63–6.71], $P < 0.001$)
Bertrand (2012)	76	761,919	RCT (15) and non-RCT (61) studies comparing TRA vs TFA in patients undergoing PCI	TRA reduced the risk of bleeding (OR = 0.22 [0.16–0.29]), transfusion (OR = 0.20 [0.11–0.32]), and short-term death (OR = 0.56 [0.45–0.67])
Biondi-Zoccai (2011)	5	3,210	RCT comparing right vs left TRA in patients undergoing coronary angiography or PCI	Right TRA increased the risk of failure leading to bail-out transfemoral access (RR = 1.65 [1.18–2.30], $P = 0.003$)
Jolly (2009)	23	7,020	RCT comparing TRA vs TFA in patients undergoing coronary angiography or PCI	TRA reduced major bleeding (OR = 0.27 [0.16, 0.45], $P < 0.001$) and hospital stay by 0.4 days (0.2–0.5, $P = 0.001$)
Joyal (2012)	10	3,347	RCT (10) comparing TRA vs TFA in patients with STEMI undergoing PCI	TRA increased survival (OR = 0.53 [0.33–0.84]) and reduced fewer vascular complications (OR = 0.35 [0.24–0.53]), but increased procedural times (WMD =1.76 min [0.59–2.92])

OR, odds ratio (95% confidence interval); PCI, percutaneous coronary intervention; RCT, randomized clinical trial; STEMI, ST-elevation myocardial infarction; TFA, transfemoral access; TRA, transradial access; WMD, weighted mean difference (95% confidence interval).

is still there in US practice, as far as transradial access is concerned, in comparison to that seen in other countries. Out of a total of 2,820,874 procedures, only 178,643 (6.3%) were done transradially.[22] Moreover, less than 1.6% of centers chose the transradial route in more than 40% of their cases. Nonetheless, such access site was still associated with fewer bleedings (odds ratio = 0.51 [95% confidence interval 0.49–0.54]) with increase in procedural success in comparison to transfemoral access (odds ratio = 1.13 [1.06–1.20]).

Randomized Trials

The first and most important randomized trial on transradial access is arguably the pioneering ACCESS trial, published by Kiemeneij et al.[25] in 1997. Notably, among the key exclusion criteria were the following: absence of pulse in femoral, brachial, or radial arteries, abnormal Allen test, failed prior transradial access, chronic total occlusion, acute myocardial infarction, expected need for intra-aortic balloon pump, right cardiac catheterization or temporary pacemaker, ad hoc PCI after prior transfemoral access, indwelling sheath from prior catheterization, planned primary stenting, or atherectomy. Patient setup was based on a right arm–supporting extension of the catheterization table enabling 45° abduction of the upper limb, with wrist hyperextension. Thereafter, local anesthesia with 2% Xylocaine was provided and the radial artery was punctured with a 20- or 18G needle at 1 cm proximal from the styloid process.

In this three-arm trial including 900 patients undergoing PCI and randomized to transradial (right-sided in all), transbrachial, or transfemoral access, procedural success (respectively 91.7%, 90.7%, and 90.7%, $P = 0.885$) and duration (40, 39, and 38 minutes, $P = 0.603$), fluoroscopy time (13, 12, and 11 minutes), catheter and balloon consumption, hospital stay, and one-month events (6.7%, 8.3%, and 5.3%, $P = 0.342$) were remarkably similar in the three groups. Conversely, transradial access appeared associated with significantly fewer major entry site complications (none vs 2.3% in the transbrachial group and 2.0% in the transfemoral group, $P = 0.035$). Nonetheless, asymptomatic radial occlusion occurred in 3.0% of cases.

Several trials have followed suit the ACCESS study, in large part confirming its findings, albeit increasing statistical precision as well as bolstering external validity. Such trials have been poignantly summarized by the available systematic reviews focusing on transradial access, but among the largest and most important are the OUTCLAS,[26] RIFLE-STEACS,[11] RIVAL,[10] TALENT,[27] and TEMPURA studies.[28]

The Transradial Approach (LEft vs right) aNd procedural Times during percutaneous coronary procedures (TALENT) trial randomized 1,540 patients undergoing diagnostic (1,467 subjects) or interventional (688 subjects) coronary procedures to right versus left transradial access.[27] Left transradial access was associated with a lower fluoroscopy time (149 seconds [1st–3rd quartile 95–270] vs 168 seconds [110–277], $P = 0.003$) and dose area product (10.7 Gy·cm^2 [6–20.5] vs 12.1 Gy·cm^2 [7–23.8], $P = 0.004$) in the diagnostic group, but not in the interventional cohort. Moreover, subgroups analyses showed that differences in fluoroscopy time and dose area product were significant only in older patients and with inexperienced operators.

The OUTpatient Coronary Low-Profile Angioplasty Study (OUTCLAS) trial compared transradial versus transfemoral access in 644 subjects eligible for outpatient management (i.e., discharged within 4 to 6 hours after PCI).[26] Indeed, 58.2% of those included in the trial were discharged as early as planned, yielding similar 1-month event rates in the transradial versus transfemoral group (2.2% vs 1.2%, $P = 0.361$). Outpatient management was not associated with an increased rate in adverse events (1.1% vs 2.6%, $P = 0.215$), and transradial access enabled outpatient management in a numerically higher proportion of patients (61.5% vs 55.0%, $P = 0.093$), mainly given its lower likelihood of causing (minor) bleedings.

The TEst for Myocardial infarction by Prospective Unicenter Randomization for Access sites (TEMPURA) study, conducted between 1999 and 2001, was the first to appraise the risk–benefit balance of transradial versus transfemoral access in 149 patients with ST-segment elevation myocardial infarction undergoing primary PCI.[28] Reperfusion success (thrombolysis in myocardial infarction 3 flow 96.1% vs 97.2%, $P = 0.624$) and in-hospital major adverse cardiac events (5.2% vs 8.3%, $P = 0.444$) were similar in the two groups, whereas one patient required cross-over access for failure at the first transfemoral attempt, and two patients had severe bleeding in the transfemoral group.

The RadIal Versus femorAL access for coronary intervention (RIVAL) trial is the largest study to date to compare transradial versus transfemoral access, eagerly awaiting the Italian Minimizing Adverse haemorragic events by TRansradia access site and systemic Implementation of angioX

(MATRIX) study.[10] This pivotal randomized trial included 7,021 patients with acute coronary syndromes, and specifically 1,958 subjects with ST-elevation myocardial infarction. The primary end point of the study was a composite of death, myocardial infarction, stroke, or noncoronary artery bypass grafting–related major bleeding at 1 month. Given its size, the RIVAL study could provide rather precise effect estimates also for important secondary end points and subgroups. The main results showed that transradial access was associated with a 3.7% risk of the primary end point, in comparison to a 4.0% risk for transfemoral access ($P = 0.50$). Notably, transradial access appeared more beneficial in high-volume radial centers (1.6% vs 3.2%, P for effect $= 0.015$, P for interaction $= 0.021$), emphasizing the importance of adequate transradial training, skills, and experience. In addition, transradial access appeared remarkably safer than transfemoral access in patients with suspected or confirmed ST-elevation myocardial infarction, with 3.1% risk of the primary end point (vs 5.2% in the transfemoral group, P for effect $= 0.026$, P for interaction $= 0.025$), and with an important and statistically significant survival benefit (1.3% vs 3.2%, P for effect $= 0.006$, P for interaction $= 0.001$).

The most recent Radial versus Femoral Randomized Investigation in ST-Elevation Acute Coronary Syndrome (RIFLE-STEACS) study, focusing only on patients with suspected ST-elevation myocardial infarction and involving only centers with an established expertise in transradial access, has confirmed the results of the RIVAL trial.[11] Specifically, the RIFLE-STEACS trial was a multicenter randomized trial including 1,001 patients with suspected ST-elevation myocardial infarction, and randomizing subjects to transradial versus transfemoral access. The primary end point was the 30-day rate of net adverse clinical events (NACE), defined as the composite of cardiac death, myocardial infarction, stroke, target lesion revascularization, and bleeding, which was met in 13.6% of subjects allocated to transradial access and 21.0% of those in whom transfemoral access was attempted ($P = 0.003$). Similar differences were found for 30-day cardiac mortality (5.2% vs 9.2%, $P = 0.020$), and bleeding (7.8% vs 12.2%, $P = 0.026$). Notably, transradial access did not come at the price of increased procedural times or lower likelihood of successful and timely myocardial reperfusion.

Meta-analyses

The first comprehensive and thorough review focusing on transradial access was reported by Agostoni and colleagues[8] in 2004. They focused only on randomized clinical trials comparing transradial versus transfemoral access for diagnostic or therapeutic coronary procedures. They included, after a detailed search involving The Cochrane Library, MEDLINE/PubMed, and mRCT, 12 trials (3,224 patients: 1,668 randomized to transradial access and 1,556 to transfemoral access). The main findings stemming from a random-effect analysis were that the risk of major adverse cardiac events was similar for transradial and transfemoral approach (odds ratio $= 0.92$ [0.57–1.48], $P = 0.7$). Instead, radial access was associated with a significantly fewer entry site complications (odds ratio $= 0.20$ [0.09–0.42], $P < 0.001$), even if at the price of a higher risk of procedural failure (odds ratio $= 3.30$ [1.63–6.71], $P < 0.001$).

The meta-analysis by Jolly et al.[9] is a comprehensive systematic review focusing on randomized trials of transradial versus transfemoral access in patients undergoing diagnostic or interventional coronary procedures. As many as 23 studies were included (7,020 patients), and provided insightful results in favor of transradial access, which significantly reduced major bleeding (odds ratio $= 0.27$ [0.16, 0.45], $P < 0.001$) and hospital stay by 0.4 days (0.2–0.5, $P = 0.001$). Moreover, favorable trends for transradial access were shown for death, myocardial infarction, or stroke (odd ratio $= 0.71$ [0.49–1.01], $P = 0.058$), as well as death (odds ratio $= 0.74$ [0.42–1.30], $P = 0.29$), despite a trend for higher rate of inability to the cross the lesion with wires, balloons, or stents (odds ratio $= 1.29$ [0.87, 1.94], $P = 0.21$).

Bertrand and colleagues[21] have pooled data from 15 randomized trials and 61 observational studies comparing transradial versus transfemoral access in 761,919 patients undergoing PCI. They found that transradial access significantly reduced bleedings (odds ratio $= 0.22$ [0.16–0.29]) and transfusions (odds ratio $= 0.20$ [0.11–0.32]). Moreover, transradial access was associated with significant reductions in early mortality (odds ratio $= 0.56$ [0.45–0.67]) and the composite of early death or myocardial infarction (odds ratio $= 0.69$ [0.55–0.84]).

Joyal et al.[29] have systematically reviewed 10 randomized trials comparing transradial versus transfemoral access in 3,347 patients undergoing PCI for ST-elevation myocardial infarction. They found that transradial access was associated with improved survival (odds ratio $= 0.53$ [0.33–0.84]) and fewer vascular complications (odds ratio $= 0.35$ [0.24–0.53]), as well as a trend toward reduced fewer bleedings (odds ratio $= 0.63$ [0.35–1.12]). However, transradial access led to longer procedural times (weighted mean difference = 1.76 minutes [0.59–2.92]).

Finally, Biondi-Zoccai et al.[20] have focused instead on the comparison between right versus left transradial access, pooling data from five randomized trials, including 3,210 patients. Right and left transradial accesses were associated with similar procedural times (weighted mean difference = 0.99 minutes [–0.53 to 2.51], $P = 0.20$), contrast use (weighted mean difference = 1.71 mL [–1.32 to 4.74], $P = 0.27$), fluoroscopy time (weighted mean difference = –35.79 minutes [–3.54 to 75.15], $P = 0.07$), or any major complication (relative risk = 2.00 [0.75–5.31], $P = 0.49$). Conversely, right transradial access was associated with a significantly higher risk of failure leading to bail-out transfemoral access (relative risk = 1.65 [1.18–2.30], $P = 0.003$)

Patient Selection

The use of transradial access is associated with some important advantages when compared to other access sites, such as a lower vascular complication rates and easier postprocedural management translating in early mobilization and shorter hospitalization.[8,9] These advantages should represent the primary reason to implement transradial approach in the catheterization laboratory and become more evident in selected patient categories summarized in Table 3-4. In particular, transradial use has been demonstrated successful and safe in patients with high bleeding risk and patients receiving anticoagulant therapies,[30-32] or glycoprotein IIb/IIIa inhibitors.[33] The reduction in vascular complications has also been confirmed in a large spectrum of high-risk patient classes such as women,[34] obese patients,[35] octogenarians,[36] and acute coronary syndrome.[9,10] In particular, two recent randomized studies have highlighted as radial approach in patient with acute ST-elevation myocardial infarction undergoing primary angioplasty is associated with an improved outcome in terms of morbidity and mortality.[10,11]

Radial use is also recommendable in patients with previous coronary artery bypass with single artery mammary graft. Indeed, retrograde ipsilateral

TABLE 3-4   **Practical Hints for Patient Selection for Transradial Access**

	Suitability	
	Inexperienced Operators	Experienced Operators
Ideal Situations for Transradial Access		
Acute coronary syndrome (especially ST-elevation myocardial infarction)	+/–	++
High bleeding risk (including anticoagulants)	++	++
Obese patients	++	++
Octogenarians	++	++
Previous bypass surgery (with single internal mammary graft)	+/–	++
Women	+/–	++
Situations in which transradial access may best be avoided		
End-stage renal failure or dialysis	+/–	++
Known innominate/subclavian axis anomalies	––	+
Patients candidate to bypass surgery in centers using radial grafts	+/–	+/–
Previous bypass surgery (with bilateral internal mammary graft)	––	+
Prior severely painful transradial access or radial spasm	––	+/–
Pulseless cardiogenic shock	––	+/–
Raynaud syndrome or small artery inflammatory disease	+/–	+
Very complex or high-risk PCI (e.g., on last remaining vessel)	––	+

++, highly recommended; +, recommended; +/–, possible; –, not recommended; ––, avoid; PCI, percutaneous coronary intervention.

approach for selective internal mammary artery has been demonstrated easier and rapid with significant reduction in procedural time.[37] Conversely, in patients with bilateral internal mammary grafts, the need for skilled catheter manipulation to engage contralateral mammary artery ostium should limit transradial approach to selected cases and to expert operators. Finally, radial approach should be carefully considered and implemented rather selectively in patients on dialysis treatment or candidate to bypass surgery in centers using radial grafts to not preclude the use of the artery (i.e. postprocedural occlusion risk).

Radial Artery Selection

One important criticism of transradial access is that it is technically more demanding and sometimes not feasible. In particular, radial cannulation represents the most challenging aspect, especially for beginners. Indeed, when compared to the femoral artery, the radial artery is smaller, more mobile, and prone to spasm. In the following paragraphs, we describe a useful methodological approach to the proper individuation of the ideal candidate for transradial approach.

Figure 3-1 shows a possible flowchart for the selection of radial over femoral access.

Identification of the Artery Pulse

Accurate evaluation of the radial artery focusing on strength, location, and course of vessel pulse is likely the more practical approach to identify which artery is suitable for catheterization with a good level of accuracy. Radial maximal pulse is generally located 1 to 2 cm below the styloid process and can be palpated over several centimeters in the distal part of forearm. The identification of the radial course in this tract could be very helpful to select the best point for the stick and to guide the operator after failure of the first cannulation attempt.

The contemporary evaluation of ulnar and radial pulses permits a more precise assessment of the hand circulation and allows to identify possible anatomic variants occurring in up to 15% of cases.[38] Indeed, both vessel tortuosity and anatomic anomaly are more commonly located in the proximal part of forearm and a radial pulse medially located or almost on the dorsal surface of the wrist are strongly suggestive of an

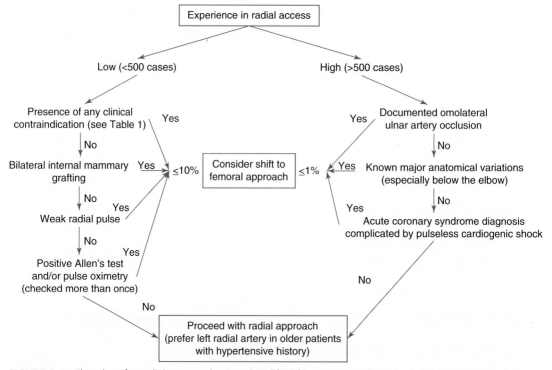

FIGURE 3-1 Flowchart for radial access selection. *(Modified from Romagnoli E, Mann T, Sciahbasi A, et al. Transradial approach in the catheterization laboratory: pros/cons and suggestions for successful implementation. Int J Cardiol. 2013;163(2):116–124.)*

unfavorable anatomic variant. At the same time, a radial pulse that appears significantly weaker than the ulnar pulse might suggest the presence of a remnant radial. Indeed, some operators use the wrist pulse "dominance" to select the radial or ulnar artery for initial cannulation.[39-42]

Preliminary duplex ultrasound evaluation of the radial artery could be important to identify viable radial arteries and to guide equipment sizing according to the artery diameter. Indeed, an artery to sheath size ratio >1.0 is associated with a reduced risk of peri-procedural vessel complications such as spasm and postprocedural artery occlusion.[43,44] This approach could be considered in the preliminary phase of a transradial training program to reduce frustration due to access failure and to accelerate operators' learning curve in the identification and management of the more challenging situations.

Left or Right Radial Artery?

It is good practice to assess both radial and ulnar arteries. Indeed, although several studies reported comparable vessel diameters between right and left radial vessels,[45-47] a difference in radial pulse strength and palpability can occasionally occur, depending on the patient's characteristics and clinical conditions. Moreover, the most challenging anatomical variants (e.g., tortuosity, loop) are not always bilateral and often differ for degree of complexity. The choice of radial side opposite to the patient handedness (i.e., left radial for right-handed patients) could represent a prudential approach to minimize the impact of postprocedural artery occlusion (up to 10% of cases), but it is not supported by any clinical evidence of advantage in patients with adequate collateral circulation via palmar arches. For these reasons, selection of the artery with the best radial pulse, as previously described, regardless of its side, is usually recommendable. Nonetheless, differences between right and left radial arteries in terms of the patient's preparation, operator's comfort, incidence of complex branching anomaly, catheter manipulation, and X-ray exposure[45] should be carefully considered by the operators, especially during their learning curve (see "Patient Preparation" section).

A Tiny Wrist Does not Necessarily Mean Small Radial Artery

Several angiographic and duplex ultrasound studies have demonstrated that in vivo the radial artery diameter ranges from 1.15 to 3.95 mm and its diameter is larger than a standard 5F vascular sheath in 83% of cases.[45] Variables typically associated with small radial diameters are female gender, diabetes mellitus, and older age, while hypertension does not seem to be associated with radial artery size, but with vessel tortuosity. According to these studies, there is not a tight correlation between wrist artery size and body weight parameters (i.e., body surface area or body mass index).[46-48] Consistently, postprocedural radial artery occlusion is correlated with the type and length of coronary procedure, but not with body surface area or radial artery diameter.[45]

Thus, a tiny wrist vessel should not discourage transradial approach differently from a weak radial pulse in a female diabetic patient. Also in these cases, accurate evaluation of the radial artery with adequate wrist hyperextension will facilitate the identification and correct evaluation of smaller and deeper arteries.

Can Anatomic Variants and Vessel Tortuosity Be Anticipated?

Anatomic variants of upper limb arteries together with artery spasm are the main causes of transradial access failure. In particular, radial artery anomalies, ranging from 7% up to 15% in different patient populations, are significantly associated with procedural failure even for skilled operators.[49,50]

The most frequent radial artery anomalies occur at level of the bifurcation with brachial artery and can be associated with vessel tortuosity and radial loop. Unfortunately, this type of anomaly cannot be anticipated. Indeed, there is no significant association of branching anomaly with the most common clinical risk factors (e.g., diabetes, hypertension), gender, body surface area, or age.[45] Nevertheless, procedural failure due to branching anomalies only is rare and insignificant if adequate radial expertise is provided.[45,49]

Conversely, older age and smaller body surface area are more frequently associated with vessel tortuosity. In particular, there is a significant correlation between age >70 years and subclavian- or innominate artery tortuosity, more evident when right transradial approach is attempted.

As previously described, accurate radial pulse evaluation in terms of location and strength is likely the best and practical way for the identification of the most challenging cases and can guide the access selection according to the operator's radial experience (Table 3-4).

Assessment of Collateral Circulation to the Hand

In patients with an adequate radial pulse, the next step is the evaluation of ulnar collateral circulation.[51] Indeed, the radial is not a terminal artery but contributes, together with the ulnar artery, to the palmar arch. In contrast to the brachial and axillary arteries, this collateral circulation minimizes the risk of ischemic hand injury in case of occlusion or damage of the radial artery. The assessment of collateral circulation between the ulnar and the radial arteries can be performed by mean of the Allen test or the more accurate pulse oxymetry and plethysmography. Most catheterization laboratories routinely use the Allen test; indeed, it is practical, legible, and can be performed by nursing staff. Nonetheless, it should be noted that some operators consider the assessment of hand collateral circulation not mandatory arguing that recruitment of collaterals from the median artery or the interosseous arterial system can provide an adequate hand circulation also in patients with ischemic Allen test.[51-54] Consistently, pulse oxymetry and plethysmography showed a valid collateral flow also in a significant percentage of patients with ischemic Allen test.[51] Nevertheless, congenital variations on the palmar arch arrangements are possible; specific studies showed that approximately 22% of the normal population has an incomplete superficial arch and 5% have their hand perfusion completely supplied by the radial artery due to ulnar absence.[52] Thus, routine testing of palmar collateral circulation is still recommended being an accurate predictor of symptomatic hand ischemia during transradial procedures and, if inadequate, should preclude the preventable radial artery cannulation.[53]

A practical guideline for the assessment of collateral hand circulation could be as follows:

- Check the Allen test bilaterally (rarely it is ischemic in both limbs).
- In case of ischemic or unclear response, repeat the Allen test several times (progressive collateral flow recruitment can be observed).
- In case of definite visual insufficiency of the hand collateral circulation, consider further evaluation with pulse oxymetry or plethysmography.

Patient Preparation

Patient preparation is an important step before performing a diagnostic or interventional coronary procedure. As in all cardiac catheterization procedures, advising the patient what to expect during and after the procedure is crucial: indeed, adequate patient education increases patient cooperation during and after the intervention. The patient should be asked for medication allergies, including prior reactions to contrast agents. Moreover, patients should receive explanation regarding the differences between transradial and transfemoral approaches, especially advantages and disadvantages of the procedure through transradial approach. In particular, the benefits of transradial approach should be highlighted: early ambulation, reduction in local pain, and reduction in major vascular complications, and that in a minority of cases, some forearm pain may develop as a consequence of radial spasm. Patients should be informed about the limitation of movement of their hand and wrist during the procedure and the immobilization should be explained as a safety measure. A previous study showed that the use of an audiovisual support before the procedure associated with the informed consent may increase patient information and makes patients more familiar with both the environment of the catheterization laboratory and the technical aspects of the procedures.[55]

Patient preparation for the diagnostic or interventional procedure through transradial approach can be divided into three steps: arm preparation, radial puncture, and "spasmolytic cocktail."

Arm Preparation

In the catheterization laboratory, it is important that both the patient and the operator feel comfortable and consequently the patient's arm should be adequately prepared.

First of all during patient preparation, the intravenous line should be placed in the upper extremity contralateral to where the transradial access is planned. If a line must be placed in the arm on the side of arterial access, it should be placed proximal to the wrist (preferably at the level of the elbow). This allows for free access to the wrist for the radial artery puncture. All jewelry and watches should be removed from the wrist area and rings should be removed from fingers. The wrist should be shaved (if necessary) and the femoral site should also be prepared in case it is needed, especially during the learning curve or in the presence of a weak radial pulse.

Either the right or the left radial access can be used, but, all around the world, the preferred access site for transradial approach is the right radial access.[56] In this case, with the patient lying supine, the arm should be maintained in neutral position with the palm up and the wrist adequately exposed. The patient's arm should be supported on the table and should remain as close to the body as possible. This will reduce radiation exposure to the operators and provide a more comfortable position for the patient. The patient's arm is generally placed along the patient's right side, and adducted with a hyper-extension of the wrist on the table next to the thigh. To maintain this position, the arm is immobilized with some tape across the palm to secure the hand. Hyperextension of the wrist to 30° to 60° using a rolled-up towel or a roll of gauze may allow easier cannulation of the radial artery by decreasing the tortuosity of the vessel (Fig. 3-2). Alternatively, some devices have been designed to optimally position and stabilize the hand, wrist, and forearm for arterial puncture and during radial artery catheterization as the "wrist splint" (Vascular Solutions, USA). In some cases, particularly with obese patients, most comfortable support for patient is achieved by placing an additional arm board or arm exten-sion under the patient's mattress along the table to provide a suitable flat working area.[57] Standard arm board extensions are included with most

catheterization laboratory X-ray systems: these additional arm boards may have different design but the most used are the "banjo" arm board and the rectangular one (Fig. 3-3). In some centers, using dedicated arm extensions (Fig. 3-3), the right arm is abducted and positioned at 60° or 90° angle, but this positioning exposes the operator to increased radiation exposure and makes inter-ventional procedures more cumbersome. In this case, the use of a transradial radiation protection board (TRPB) can significantly reduce radia-tion exposure for operators.[58] The TRPB consists of a 20-cm-high vertical shield (0.5-mm lead-equivalent rubber) slotted into a polycarbon-ate base that is placed under the supine patient. Another possibility to reduce the radiation dose for operators is the use of a disposable bismuth–barium radiation shield drape placed on the patient's arm around the area of sheath insertion and extended medially to the patient's body.[59] The use of this drape is significantly associated with a reduction in radiation dose absorbed by operators during right transradial approach par-ticularly at left wrist and thorax.

The right radial access technique, as depicted, allows to assume a very comfortable position for

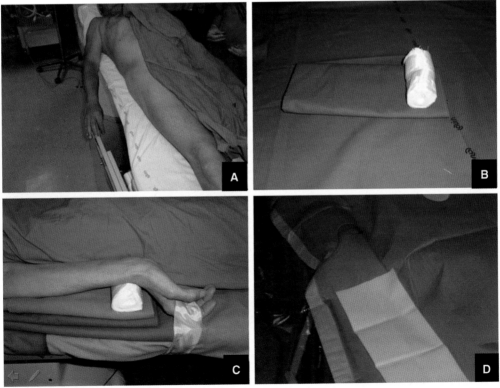

FIGURE 3-2 Patient preparation during right transradial approach. With the patient lying in supine position (**A**), the arm and wrist are placed over a roll of gauze (**B**). To maintain this position, the arm is immobilized with some tapes across the palm to secure the hand (**C**). Finally, a sterile drape is used to cover the patient (**D**).

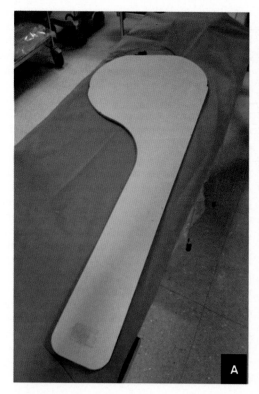
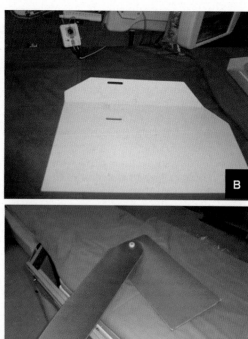
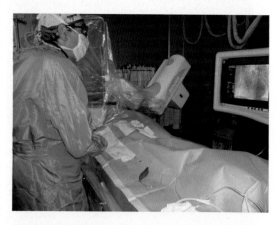

FIGURE 3-3 Different arm board used for transradial approach. The most used are the "banjo" arm board (**A**) and the rectangular one (**B**). In some centers, an articulated arm board is used in order to abduct the patient's arm to an angle of 60° or 90° (**C**).

operators (Fig. 3-4), and this position is very close to that assumed during transfemoral approach. Moreover, this technique does not need the catheterization laboratory room to be differently arranged, compared with that needed in transfemoral approach.

Transradial procedure can also be performed through the left radial approach. The use of left radial approach is associated with some important anatomical and technical advantages even if in some cases (short operators or in case of obese patients) might be more demanding for operators. The most important advantages of left radial approach are as follows:

- Catheter selection and manipulation similar to transfemoral approach.
- Better and easier cannulation of the left internal mammary artery in patients with previous coronary artery by pass.[37]
- Reduced frequency of severe tortuosity of subclavian artery.[27,60,61]
- Shorter learning curve.[62]
- Lower fluoroscopy times particularly in less experienced operators.[27]

FIGURE 3-4 Position taken by the operator during right transradial approach.

- Increased support during right coronary PCI.[63]
- Absence of transition through carotid vessels.
- Better patient comfort because most patients are right handed (patients are free to use his/her right hand immediately after the procedure).[64]

Many observational and randomized studies comparing left and right radial approach showed that either procedural time and fluoroscopy time were shorter using the left radial access.[27,43,44,61,65] In particular, the TALENT trial (the largest randomized trial comparing left and right radial access) showed a median of 19 seconds fluoroscopy times less during diagnostic procedures and 81 seconds less during PCIs with the left radial access.[27] Of note, these differences were mainly observed in operators at the beginning of their learning curve (not in expert operators) and in older patients (above 70 years).

Many physicians do not like the left radial access because it seems less comfortable for operators. The most important difference in performing the left radial access is that the operator must bend over the patient during the procedure increasing the workload to the back. To reduce operator discomfort, during left radial approach, it is very important to adequately place the patient's left arm. It is fundamental to uplift the left arm over (or at the same level) the patient's abdomen: we use some drapes or towels positioned under the patient's left arm that is placed over a dedicated arm board. Then the left arm should be fixed using some tape (Fig. 3-5). Another option to fix the left arm is to use a surgical cushion such as the VACUFORM Microspace System (BUW Schmidt GmbH, Garben, Germany) that adapts individually and ergonomically to the patient's arm, increasing the comfort for the patient and the operator (Fig. 3-6). This device is made of a flexible nonslip PVC plastic film, filled with air and polystyrene balls and equipped with one-piece valve. After positioning of the left arm, with the use of a dedicated pump, the air is extracted giving a lasting and effective support to the arm. The left arm position can be changed at any time by releasing the vacuum. Using one of these arrangements, radial puncture is easily performed from the right side of the patient even if some operators prefer cannulating the left radial artery on the left side of the patient. Catheter manipulation is comfortable for operators (Fig. 3-7), and during PCIs the guiding catheter can be placed over the patient's left leg to further increase the operator's comfort.

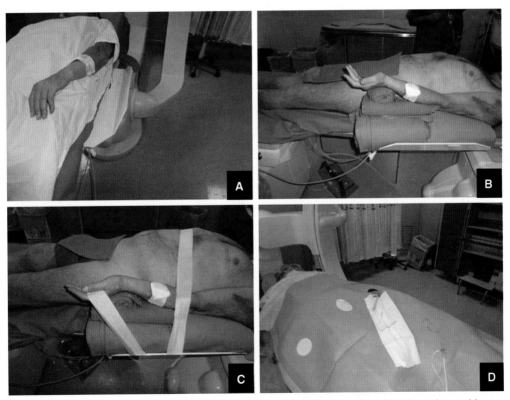

FIGURE 3-5   Patient preparation during left transradial approach. With the patient lying in supine position (**A**), the arm and wrist are placed over some drapes or towels to uplift the left arm over (or at the same level) the patient's abdomen (**B**). Then the left arm should be fixed using some tape (**C**) and finally a sterile drape is positioned over the patient (**D**).

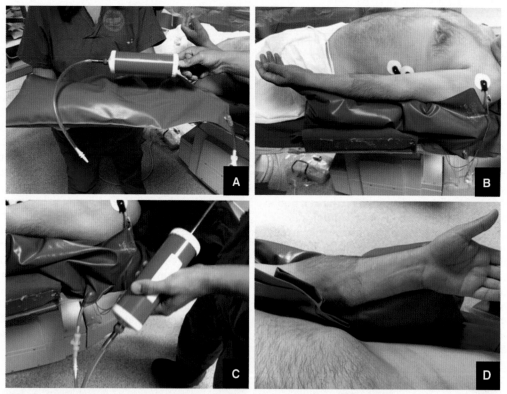

FIGURE 3-6 Patient preparation during left transradial approach using the VACUFORM Microspace System. This system is made of a plastic film filled with polystyrene balls and a vacuum pump (**A**). The patient is made to lie in supine position, and the arm and wrist are placed in a comfortable position for the patient (**B**). The air is removed from the system with the dedicated pump (**C**) and the left arm is ergonomically fixed (**D**). *(Courtesy Dr. F. Burzotta, Rome.)*

There are some concerns for a possible increased radiation dose for operators associated with the left radial approach. However, in the context of the TALENT trial, three expert operators were equipped with five pairs of dedicated dosimeters (at left wrist, at left shoulder, in

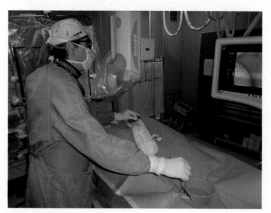

FIGURE 3-7 Position taken by the operator during left transradial approach.

the middle thorax outside the lead apron, in the middle thorax under the lead apron, and at thyroid level outside the lead collar) for the left or the right approach, and each month the radiation dose was evaluated.[66] There were no differences between the two radial accesses for radiation dose at thyroid, left shoulder, or thorax, with a possible advantage for the left approach at wrist level. Consequently, in our center, in particular conditions associated with increased rate of subclavian tortuosity (older patients, small patients), or in patients with coronary artery bypass, the left radial approach is our default approach for transradial procedures.[67]

Radial Puncture

The radial puncture is a very important step during transradial procedures and can be a major concern when performing a catheterization through the radial artery particularly at the beginning of the learning curve. Indeed when compared to femoral, the radial artery is sensibly smaller and mobile and an unsuccessful puncture, especially when the radial artery is incised, increases the risk of spasm.

Before radial puncture, the wrist area is prepared following sterile technique with a standard antiseptic scrub solution. A sterile drape is then used to cover the patient including the entire hand and the arm extension board. Standard femoral drapes can be used, positioning the hole over the wrist even if a dedicated multiaccess drape (Lulu Radial/Femoral Angiography Sheet, MCD, USA) with multiple precut holes consents access to either wrist or femoral site without a break in the sterile field (e.g., in case of simultaneous transradial access and intra-aortic balloon pump or temporary venous pacemaker).

To reduce patient discomfort during transradial puncture, generally a small amount of subcutaneous lidocaine 2% or an anesthetic cream composed of lidocaine 2.5% and prilocaine 2.5% is effectively used to reduce pain at puncture site. In particular, the anesthetic cream is able to halve cannulation pain and to reduce puncture failure, but the application time for the cream is between 1 and 3 hours before the procedures.[68] Because of the superficial location of the radial artery, small amount of anesthetics are required to obtain an acceptable anesthesia: it is important to avoid large amounts of lidocaine, as the wheal may obscure the pulse and make cannulation more difficult. Alternatively, some operators administer local anesthesia after radial puncture and prior the introduction of the sheath.[69] It might be useful in some cases to administer nitroglycerine subcutaneously or simply to mix nitroglycerin with xylocain (50/50) prior local anesthesia. In case of radial artery spasm, subcutaneous nitroglycerin might speed the return of radial artery pulse.

The course of radial artery is identified by palpation over several centimeters along the wrist. Some operators prefer cannulating the radial artery with the table placed at very low height and the operator comfortably positioned on a stool. Differently, most operators prefer performing radial puncture with the table elevated as high as possible, avoiding the need to bend over the puncture site. The point of puncture is approximately 2 to 3 cm cranial to the bony prominence of the distal radius (styloid process). Distal puncture sites (closer to the hand) are less convenient because the radial artery is smaller, more tortuous, and is partially located below the transverse carpal ligament. Differently proximal punctures (closer to the elbow) might be associated with more difficult hemostasis due to the

deeper position of the radial artery at this level. Radial puncture can be performed with a >45° needle inclination and with slow and gentle needle advancement using a little nonocclusive compression with the left hand in order to limit arterial movement (Fig. 3-8).

There are two methods for radial puncture: a beveled needle only and a needle-over-cannula puncture, with the first technique preferred by 60% of operators.[56] The bare needle method employs an open needle Seldinger-based technique with a front-wall puncture: the needle varies in length from approximately 2 to 5 cm and in caliber from 19G to 22G. Because the needles employed are generally small in caliber, the blood flow that accompanies the puncture is not necessarily pulsatile. Differently, the needle-over-cannula technique (Fig. 3-8) consists of a small-caliber metal needle that communicates with a transparent chamber and is inserted in a soft plastic cannula. With this device, the puncture is generally performed with the transfixion of the radial artery (through and through technique). When the metal needle pricks the artery, there is a flash of blood into the transparent hub chamber: at this point, the needle and cannula system is advanced in order to transfix the back wall of the artery. The metal needle is removed and the plastic cannula is gently and gradually withdrawn until the tip of the cannula reenters the lumen and a pulsatile arterial back flow is observed. In this position, the guidewire can be introduced through the cannula (Fig. 3-8). A wire that successfully enters the radial lumen will track smoothly with minimal force required to advance the wire up the vessel. If the wire does not exit easily from the tip of the needle, it is important to avoid forceful introduction maneuvers. Difficult advancement of the guidewire may be due to artery spasm or to access of the wire in a small branch vessel or to partial embedding of the needle in the vessel wall. In the first and second cases, the wire should be slightly withdrawn and advanced once more. Differently in the last situation (needle embedded in the vessel wall), the wire should be removed and the needle position modified to obtain a satisfactory bleed back before further attempts of wire introduction. If the problem still persists, the needle should be removed and the artery can be cannulated slightly more proximally.

Guidewires supplied with radial cannulation kits are optimized and specific for radial cannulation. These guidewires are usually small in caliber with soft atraumatic tips to facilitate tracking of the wire up the vessel. Guidewire may be

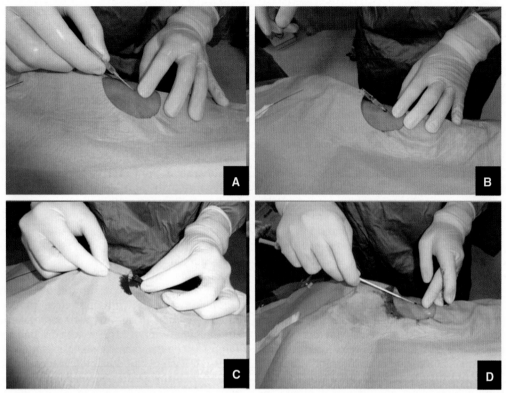

FIGURE 3-8 The needle-over-cannula technique for radial puncture. Radial puncture can be performed with a >45° needle inclination and with slow and gentle needle advancement using a little nonocclusive compression with the left hand in order to limit arterial movement (**A**). When the metal needle pricks the artery, there is a flash of blood into the transparent hub chamber: at this point, the needle and cannula system is advanced in order to transfix the back wall of the artery (**B**). The metal needle is removed and the plastic cannula is gently and gradually withdrawn until the tip of the cannula reenters the lumen and a pulsatile arterial back flow is observed. In this position, the guidewire can be introduced through the cannula (**C**). At this point, the cannula can be removed while leaving the guidewire in place. In this position, the sheath with the dilator can be introduced over the wire (**D**).

metallic wire (generally employed with the open needle techniques) or plastic and hydrophilic wires (generally employed with the needle-over-cannula technique) with different caliber (between 0.018″ and 0.025″). The wires are usually 30 to 50 cm and often have floppy tip and a more rigid shaft. Considering the small caliber of the artery, those wires with either a small angulation or even a straight tip seem to work better. J tips often get caught either in the sheath or in the proximal artery.

Once the guidewire has been smoothly advanced through the device, the cannula (or the needle) can be removed while leaving the guidewire in place. In this position, a small skin incision may facilitate sheath insertion, though, depending on the sheath used, it is not always necessary, particularly if a hydrophilic sheath is employed. At this point, the sheath with the dilator can be introduced over the wire: the use of a

gentle rotational motion while advancing may facilitate placement (Fig. 3-8). Then, the guidewire and the dilator assembly may be removed and the sidearm may be used for administration of medications.

There are a variety of sheaths available on the market that may be suitable for radial access, but there are some characteristics that may be desired in a radial sheath as a tapered edge that allows a smooth insertion of the sheath. Vascular sheaths may be hydrophilic or not and may have different lengths. The hydrophilic coating of vascular sheaths has been shown to be associated with less patient discomfort and local pain, and easy removal, particularly in the case of small-caliber radial artery.[70,71] However, there are some cases described of allergic reactions and noninfective granulomas associated with the use of these sheaths.[72-74] The ideal sheath length is not codified: some authors prefer short sheaths (7 to 12 cm) because they induce less trauma and endothelial injury in the radial artery, but they may be associated with an increased risk of radial spasm. Moreover, to avoid inadvertent removal of the sheath during catheter exchange or during catheter manipulation, in some centers an adhesive transparent tape is used to fix the sheath. Differently, long sheaths (23 to 25 mm) minimize the risk of radial spasm related to catheter manipulation and torquing manoeuvres, but they might increase vessel trauma. A possible compromise is to use an intermediate sheath length (16 cm) in order to reduce radial artery spasm without increasing the risk of vessel trauma.

Spasmolytic Cocktail

Sometimes the radial access is associated with radial spasm: the incidence varies about 10% and is caused by many factors. Independent predictors of radial spasm include the presence of radial artery anomalies, multiple catheter exchanges, pain during radial cannulation, diameter of the catheter employed, and radial diameter after administration of vasodilatory agents.[75] Radial spasm is documented by resistance during manipulation of intra-arterial equipment and by a patient complaining of pain in the forearm, generally, without clinical complications. Only rarely the spasm leads to serious complications such as radial eversion,[76] but it is commonly associated with procedural failure and patient discomfort. Consequently, many strategies have been developed to reduce spasm. First of all, it is essential that the patient is comfortable and relaxed: stress induces catecholamine release and increases the risk of spasm. To reduce the patient's anxiety, some centers use sedation medications (midazolam, fentanyl, etc.) even if in many hospitals premedication is not routinely used and it is reserved only in very selected cases.

In addition to premedication and local anesthesia, the use of intra-arterial administration of vasodilators (administered through the sidearm of the sheath immediately after obtaining radial access) might be of value particularly if a short sheath has been employed. Various spasmolytic cocktails have been tried,[77] but the most commonly used vasodilators are verapamil (2.5 to 5 mg, diluted up to 10 mL with saline) and nitrates (200 μg, diluted up to 10 mL with saline) used alone or in combination.[78,79] The patient should be warned of a transient burning sensation in the forearm during injection. Some of the discomfort encountered during injection is ameliorated by a slow injection and by withdrawing blood from the side arm into the cocktail, because blood buffers reduce the cocktail acidity (particularly due to verapamil), reducing the unpleasant sensation. Vasodilatation occurs immediately as documented using radial artery intravascular ultrasound, with only a moderate reduction in mean arterial pressure and no significant change in heart rate.[80] Other vasodilators such as diltiazem, papaverine, phentolamine, nicardipine, nicorandil, nitroprusside, or adenosine have also been tested, with variable results.[81–83] Magnesium sulfate has been evaluated as a spasmolytic agent with potential additional advantages of analgesia and absent hemodynamic changes.[84] Magnesium sulfate, administered as 150-mg intraarterial bolus over 1 minute, resulted in a 36% increase in radial artery diameter, with reduced hemodynamic effect compared to verapamil.

In a series of patients with radial spasm due to failed attempts at radial artery puncture,[85] three different options have been compared: the wait and see attitude, the administration of 400 μg of sublingual nitroglycerin or the injection of 200 μg of nitroglycerin solution on the medial and lateral aspects of the radial artery location. The mean time for the pulse to reappear was 18 ± 5, 8 ± 1, and 3 ± 1 minutes, respectively, and subsequently the rate of successful radial cannulation was 72%, 90%, and 100%. Bertrand et al.[86] refined the technique by routinely mixing 2% Xylocaine and nitroglycerin in the same syringe as the local anesthesia.

Despite all medications and techniques employed to prevent radial spasm, actually the best way for spasm prevention is a clear puncture and a gentle and smooth procedure. One important concept to bear in mind is that for transradial puncture the success on the first attempt always achieves the best results. If the radial artery is touched but missed during the first attempt, spasm, as well as hematoma formation, can occur. Finally, the incidence of spasm inversely relates to operator experience. Experienced operators use less catheters and manipulations, perform shorter and smoother procedures, increasing patient comfort and reducing the incidence of radial spasm.

REFERENCES

1. Wijns W, Kolh P, Danchin N, et al. Guidelines on myocardial revascularization. *Eur Heart J.* 2010;31:2501–2555.
2. Steg PG, James SK, Atar D, et al. ESC guidelines for the management of acute myocardial infarction in patients presenting with ST-segment elevation: the task force on the management of ST-segment elevation acute myocardial infarction of the European Society of Cardiology (ESC). *Eur Heart J.* 2012;33:2569–2619.

3. Romagnoli E, Mann T, Sciahbasi A, et al. Transradial approach in the catheterization laboratory: pros/cons and suggestions for successful implementation. *Int J Cardiol*. 2013;163:116–124.

4. Franchi E, Marino P, Biondi-Zoccai GG, et al. Transradial versus transfemoral approach for percutaneous coronary procedures. *Curr Cardiol Rep*. 2009;11:391–397.

5. Ceschinski H, Henkes H, Weinert HC, et al. Torquability of microcatheter guidewires: the resulting torsional moment. *Biomed Mater Eng*. 2000;10:31–42.

6. Campeau L. Percutaneous radial artery approach for coronary angiography. *Cathet Cardiovasc Diagn*. 1989;16:3–7.

7. Kiemeneij F, Laarman GJ. Percutaneous transradial artery approach for coronary stent implantation. *Cathet Cardiovasc Diagn*. 1993;30:173–178.

8. Agostoni P, Biondi-Zoccai GG, de Benedictis ML, et al. Radial versus femoral approach for percutaneous coronary diagnostic and interventional procedures: systematic overview and meta-analysis of randomized trials. *J Am Coll Cardiol*. 2004;44:349–356.

9. Jolly SS, Amlani S, Hamon M, et al. Radial versus femoral access for coronary angiography or intervention and the impact on major bleeding and ischemic events: a systematic review and meta-analysis of randomized trials. *Am Heart J*. 2009;157:132–140.

10. Jolly SS, Yusuf S, Cairns J, et al; RIVAL Trial Group. Radial versus femoral access for coronary angiography and intervention in patients with acute coronary syndromes (RIVAL): a randomised, parallel group, multicentre trial. *Lancet*. 2011;377:1409–1420.

11. Romagnoli E, Biondi-Zoccai G, Sciahbasi A, et al. Radial versus femoral randomized investigation in ST-segment elevation acute coronary syndrome: the RIFLE-STEACS (radial versus femoral randomized investigation in ST-elevation acute coronary syndrome) study. *J Am Coll Cardiol*. 2012;60:2481–2489.

12. Cooper CJ, El-Shiekh RA, Cohen DJ, et al. Effect of transradial access on quality of life and cost of cardiac catheterization: a randomized comparison. *Am Heart J*. 1999; 138:430–436.

13. Deepika K, Palaniappan D, Fuhrman T, et al. Anatomic snuffbox radial artery cannulation. *Anesth Analg*. 2010;111: 1078–1079.

14. Biondi-Zoccai G, Moretti C, Zuffi A, et al. Transradial access without preliminary Allen test—letter of comment on Rhyne et al. *Catheter Cardiovasc Interv*. 2011;78:662–663.

15. Agostoni P, Zuffi A, Biondi-Zoccai G. Pushing wrist access to the limit: homolateral right ulnar artery approach for primary percutaneous coronary intervention after right radial failure due to radial loop. *Catheter Cardiovasc Interv*. 2011;78:894–897.

16. Bertrand OF. Acute forearm muscle swelling post transradial catheterization and compartment syndrome: prevention is better than treatment! *Catheter Cardiovasc Interv*. 2010;75:366–368.

17. Ghuran AV, Dixon G, Holmberg S, et al. Transradial coronary intervention without pre-screening for a dual palmar blood supply. *Int J Cardiol*. 2007;121:320–322.

18. Kiemeneij F, Laarman GJ, Slagboom T, et al. Transradial Palmaz-Schatz coronary stenting on an outpatient basis: results of a prospective pilot study. *J Invasive Cardiol*. 1995;71:5A–11A.

19. Trani C, Tommasino A, Burzotta F. Transradial renal stenting: why and how. *Catheter Cardiovasc Interv*. 2009;74:951–956.

20. Biondi-Zoccai G, Sciahbasi A, Bodí V, et al. Right versus left radial artery access for coronary procedures: an international collaborative systematic review and meta-analysis

21. Bertrand OF, Bélisle P, Joyal D, et al. Comparison of transradial and femoral approaches for percutaneous coronary interventions: a systematic review and hierarchical Bayesian meta-analysis. *Am Heart J*. 2012;163:632–648.

22. Feldman DN, Swaminathan RV, Kaltenbach LA et al. Adoption of radial access and comparison of outcomes to femoral access in percutaneous coronary intervention: an updated report from the National Cardiovascular Data Registry (2007–2012). *Circulation* 2013;127:2295–2306.

23. Pristipino C, Trani C, Nazzaro MS, et al; Prospective REgistry of Vascular Access in Interventions in Lazio Region Study Group. Major improvement of percutaneous cardiovascular procedure outcomes with radial artery catheterisation: results from the PREVAIL study. *Heart*. 2009;95:476–482.

24. Pelliccia F, Trani C, Biondi-Zoccai GG, et al; Prospective Registry of Vascular Access in Interventions in Lazio Region (PREVAIL) Study Group. Comparison of the feasibility and effectiveness of transradial coronary angiography via right versus left radial artery approaches (from the PREVAIL study). *Am J Cardiol*. 2012;110:771–775.

25. Kiemeneij F, Laarman GJ, Odekerken D, et al. A randomized comparison of percutaneous transluminal coronary angioplasty by the radial, brachial and femoral approaches: the access study. *J Am Coll Cardiol*. 1997;29:1269–1275.

26. Slagboom T, Kiemeneij F, Laarman GJ, et al. Outpatient coronary angioplasty: feasible and safe. *Catheter Cardiovasc Interv*. 2005;64:421–427.

27. Sciahbasi A, Romagnoli E, Burzotta F, et al. Transradial approach (left vs right) and procedural times during percutaneous coronary procedures: TALENT study. *Am Heart J*. 2011;161:172–179.

28. Saito S, Tanaka S, Hiroe Y, et al. Comparative study on transradial approach vs. transfemoral approach in primary stent implantation for patients with acute myocardial infarction: results of the test for myocardial infarction by prospective unicenter randomization for access sites (TEMPURA) trial. *Catheter Cardiovasc Interv*. 2003;59:26–33.

29. Joyal D, Bertrand OF, Rinfret S, et al. Meta-analysis of ten trials on the effectiveness of the radial versus the femoral approach in primary percutaneous coronary intervention. *Am J Cardiol*. 2012;109:813–818.

30. Aguirre FV, Topol EJ, Ferguson JJ, et al. Bleeding complications with the chimeric antibody to platelet glycoprotein IIb/IIIa integrin in patients undergoing percutaneous coronary intervention. *Circulation*. 1995;91:2890–2892.

31. Hildick-Smith DJ, Walsh JT, Lowe MD, et al. Coronary angiography in the fully anticoagulated patient: the transradial route is successful and safe. *Catheter Cardiovasc Interv*. 2003;58:8–10.

32. Lo TS, Buch AN, Hall IR, et al. Percutaneous left and right heart catheterization in fully anticoagulated patients utilizing the radial artery and forearm vein: a two-center experience. *J Interv Cardiol*. 2006;19:258–263.

33. Choussat R, Black A, Bossi I, et al. Vascular complications and clinical outcome after coronary angioplasty with platelet 2b/3a receptor blockade: comparison of transradial vs. transfemoral arterial access. *Eur Heart J*. 2000;21:662–667.

34. Pristipino C, Pelliccia F, Granatelli A, et al. Comparison of access-related bleeding complications in women versus men undergoing percutaneous coronary catheterization using the radial versus femoral artery. *Am J Cardiol*. 2007;99:1216–1221.

35. Cox N, Resnic FS, Popma JJ, et al. Comparison of the risk of vascular complications associated with femoral and radial

access coronary catheterization procedures in obese versus nonobese patients. *Am J Cardiol.* 2004;94:1174–1177.

36. Louvard Y, Benamer H, Garot P, et al. Comparison of transradial and transfemoral approaches for coronary angiography and angioplasty in octogenarians (the OCTOPLUS study). *Am J Cardiol.* 2004;94:1177–1180.
37. Burzotta F, Trani C, Todaro D, et al. Comparison of the transradial and transfemoral approaches for coronary angiographic evaluation in patients with internal mammary grafts. *J Cardiovasc Med.* 2008;9:263–266.
38. Valsecchi O, Vassileva A, Musumeci G, et al. Failure of transradial approach during coronary interventions: anatomic considerations. *Catheter Cardiovasc Interv.* 2006;67:870–878.
39. Chiam PT, Lim VY. Transulnar artery approach for percutaneous coronary intervention: an alternative route in a patient with challenging transfemoral access and hypoplastic radial artery. *Singapore Med J.* 2010;51:e81–e84.
40. Roberts EB, Palmer N, Perry RA. Transulnar access for coronary angiography and intervention: an early review to guide research and clinical practice. *J Invasive Cardiol.* 2007;19:83–87.
41. Mangin L, Bertrand OF, De La Rochellière R, et al. The transulnar approach for coronary intervention: a safe alternative to transradial approach in selected patients. *J Invasive Cardiol.* 2005;17:77–79.
42. de Andrade PB, Tebet MA, de Andrade MV, et al. Transulnar approach: the rationale from the radialist's view. *Indian Heart J.* 2010;62:251–254.
43. Dominici M, Diletti R, Milici C, et al. Left radial versus right radial approach for coronary artery catheterization: a prospective comparison. *J Interv Cardiol.* 2012;25:203–209.
44. Fernández-Portales J, Valdesuso R, Carreras R, et al. Right versus left radial artery approach for coronary angiography: differences observed and the learning curve. *Rev Esp Cardiol.* 2006;59:1071–1074.
45. Yoo BS, Yoon J, Ko JY, et al. Anatomical consideration of the radial artery for transradial coronary procedures: arterial diameter, branching anomaly and vessel tourtuosity. *Int J Cardiol.* 2005;101:421–427.
46. Ashraf T, Panhwar Z, Habib S, et al. Size of radial and ulnar artery in local population. *J Pak Med Assoc.* 2010;60:817–819.
47. Loh YJ, Nakao M, Tan WD, et al. Factors influencing radial artery size. *Asian Cardiovasc Thorac Ann.* 2007;15:324–326.
48. Saito S, Ikei H, Hosokawa G, et al. Influence of the ratio between radial artery inner diameter and sheath outer diameter on radial artery flow after transradial coronary intervention. *Catheter Cardiovasc Interv.* 1999;46:173–178.
49. Lo TS, Nolan J, Fountzopoulos E, et al. Radial artery anomaly and its influence on transradial coronary procedural outcome. *Heart.* 2009;95:410–415.
50. Burzotta F, Brancati MF, Trani C, et al. Impact of radial-to-aorta vascular anatomical variants on risk of failure in trans-radial coronary procedures. *Catheter Cardiovasc Interv.* 2012;80:298–303.
51. Barbeau GR, Arsenault F, Dugas L, et al. Evaluation of the ulnar palmar arterial arches with pulse oximetry and plethysmography: comparison with the Allen's test in 1010 patients. *Am Heart J.* 2004;147:489–493.
52. Kieffer RW, Dean RH. Complications or intra-arterial monitoring. *Probl Gen Surg.* 1985;2:116–120.
53. Greenwood MJ, Della-Siega AJ, Fretz EB, et al. Vascular communications of the hand in patients being considered for transradial coronary angiography: is the Allen's test accurate? *J Am Coll Cardiol.* 2005;6:2013–2017.
54. Abu-Omar Y, Mussa S, Anastasiadis K, et al. Duplex ultrasonography predicts safety of radial artery harvest in the presence of an abnormal Allen test. *Ann Thorac Surg.* 2004;77:116–119.
55. Steffenino G, Viada E, Marengo B, et al. Effectiveness of video-based patient information before percutaneous cardiac interventions. *J Cardiovasc Med.* 2007;8:348–353.
56. Bertrand OF, Rao SV, Pancholy S, et al. Transradial approach for coronary angiography and interventions: results of the first international transradial practice survey. *J Am Coll Cardiol Interv.* 2010;3:1022–1031.
57. Freestone B, Nolan J. Transradial cardiac procedures: the state of the art. *Heart.* 2010;96:883–891.
58. Behan M, Haworth P, Colley P, et al. Decreasing operators' radiation exposure during coronary procedures: the transradial radiation protection board. *Catheter Cardiovasc Interv.* 2010;76:79–84.
59. Politi L, Biondi-Zoccai G, Nocetti L, et al. Reduction of scatter radiation during transradial percutaneous coronary angiography: a randomized trial using a lead-free radiation shield. *Catheter Cardiovasc Interv.* 2012;79:97–102.
60. Kawashima O, Endoh N, Terashima M, et al. Effectiveness of right or left radial approach for coronary angiography. *Catheter Cardiovasc Interv.* 2004;61:333–337.
61. Norgaz T, Gorgulu S, Dagdelen S. A randomized study comparing the effectiveness of right and left radial approach for coronary angiography. *Catheter Cardiovasc Interv.* 2012;80:260–264.
62. Sciahbasi A, Romagnoli E, Trani C, et al. Evaluation of the "learning curve" for left and right radial approach during percutaneous coronary procedures. *Am J Cardiol.* 2011;108:185–188.
63. Ikari Y, Masuda N, Matsukage T, et al. Backup force of guiding catheters for the right coronary artery in transfemoral and transradial interventions. *J Invasive Cardiol.* 2009;21:570–574.
64. Kiemeneij F. Left radial approach in cardiac catheterization: does it really matter. *Rev Esp Cardiol.* 2009;62:471–473.
65. Kim JY, Yoon J, Jung IH, et al. Transradial coronary intervention: comparison of the left and right radial artery approach. *Korean Circ J.* 2006;36:780–785.
66. Sciahbasi A, Romagnoli E, Trani C, et al. Operator radiation exposure during percutaneous coronary procedures through the left or right radial approach: the TALENT dosimetric substudy. *Circ Cardiovasc Interv.* 2011;4:226–231.
67. Cha KS, Kim MH, Kim HJ. Prevalence and clinical predictors of severe tortuosity of right subclavian artery in patients undergoing transradial coronary angiography. *Am J Cardiol.* 2003;92:1220–1222.
68. Kim SH, Kim EJ, Cheon WS, et al. Comparative study of nicorandil and a spasmolytic cocktail in preventing radial artery spasm during transradial coronary angiography. *Int J Cardiol.* 2007;120:325–330.
69. Ludwig J, Achenbach S, Flachskampft FA. Transradial approach: a modified puncture technique for arterial access. *EuroIntervention.* 2010;6:280–282.
70. Kiemeneij F, Fraser D, Slagboom T, et al. Hydrophilic coating aids radial sheath withdrawal and reduces patient discomfort following transradial coronary intervention: a randomized double-blind comparison of coated and uncoated sheaths. *Catheter Cardiovasc Interv.* 2003;59:161–164.
71. Rathore S, Stables RH, Pauriah M, et al. Impact of length and hydrophilic coating of the introducer sheath on radial artery spasm during transradial coronary intervention: a randomised study. *J Am Coll Cardiol Interv.* 2010;3:475–483.
72. Lim J, Suri A, Chua TP. Steroid-responsive sterile inflammation after transradial cardiac catheterisation using a sheath with hydrophilic coating. *Heart.* 2009;95:1202.

73. Kozak M, Adams DR, Ioffreda MD, et al. Sterile inflammation associated with transradial catheterisation and hydrophilic sheaths. *Catehter Cardiovasc Interv.* 2003;59:207–213.

74. Zellner C, Yeghiazarians Y, Ports TA, et al. Sterile radial artery granuloma after transradial cardiac catheterisation. *Cardiovasc Revasc Med.* 2011;12:187–189.

75. Ruiz-Salmerón RJ, Mora R, Vélez-Gimón M, et al. Radial artery spasm in transradial cardiac catheterisation: assessment of factors related to its occurrence, and of its consequences during follow-up. *Rev Esp Cardiol.* 2005;58:504–511.

76. Dieter RS, Akef A, Wolff M. Eversion endarterectomy complicating radial artery access for left heart catheterisation. *Catheter Cardiovasc Interv.* 2003;58:478–480.

77. Varenne O, Jégou A, Cohen R, et al. Prevention of arterial spasm during percutaneous coronary interventions through radial artery: the SPASM study. *Catheter Cardiovasc Interv.* 2006;68:231–235.

78. Kiemeneij F, Vajifdar BU, Eccleshall SC, et al. Evaluation of a spasmolytic cocktail to prevent radial artery spasm during coronary procedures. *Catheter Cardiovasc Interv.* 2003;58:281–284.

79. Rigattieri S, Di Russo C, Silvestri P, et al. Our technique for transradial coronary angiography and interventions. *Indian Heart J.* 2010;62:258–261.

80. Edmundson A, Mann T. Non occlusive radial artery injury resulting from transradial coronary interventions: radial artery IVUS. *J Invasive Cardiol.* 2005;17:528–531.

81. Ruiz-Salmerón RJ, Mora R, Masotti M, et al. Assessment of the efficacy of phentolamine to prevent radial artery spasm during cardiac catheterization procedures: a randomized study comparing phentolamine vs verapamil. *Catheter Cardiovasc Interv.* 2005;66:192–198.

82. Coppola J, Patel T, Kwan T, et al. Nitroglycerin, nitroprusside or both in preventing radial artery spasm during transradial artery catheterization. *J Invasive Cardiol.* 2006;18:155–158.

83. Kim JY, Yoon J, Yoo BS, et al. The effect of a eutectic mixture of local anesthetic cream on wrist pain during transradial coronary procedures. *J Invasive Cardiol.* 2007;19:6–9.

84. Byrne J, Spence M, Haegeli L, et al. Magnesium sulphate during transradial cardiac catheterisation: a new use for an old drug? *J Invasive Cardiol.* 2008;20:539–542.

85. Pancholy SB, Coppola J, Patel T. Subcutaneous administration of nitroglycerin to facilitate radial artery cannulation. *Catheter Cardiovasc Interv.* 2006;68:389–391.

86. Bertrand OF, Larose E, Rodes-Cabau J. Sub-cutaneous nitroglycerin: good example of the "KISS" rule! *Catheter Cardiovasc Interv.* 2006;70:161.

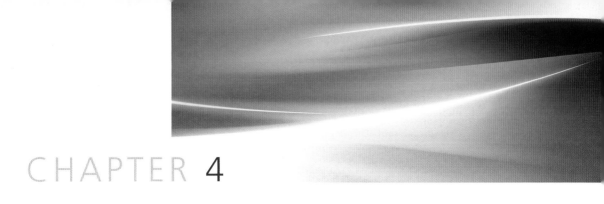

CHAPTER 4

Vascularization, Anatomy and Variants

Ian C. Gilchrist

Variability is the law of life.—Sir William Osler, 1903[1]

The vascular anatomy of the forearm is more diverse than that seen with femoral region. Developing an understanding of anatomical variations improves one's ability to obtain reliable success from the forearm, both arterial and venous accesses. The site of access in the forearm is in the distal region of the vasculature where collaterals are common and variability is the norm, with about 25% of patients showing some form of anomaly.[2-4] This diversity and redundancy of the vasculature is partially responsible for the safety of the transradial and similar forearm procedures, but can also be confusing to the operator and a potential source for complications.[5-7]

The goal of this chapter is to develop an understanding of the arm vasculature that will be relevant to the radial operator. Theories of embryologic development of the forearm will be reviewed, as presently understood, as this then provides an appreciation of why common variants are found in this regional circulation. Although the main part of this chapter deals with the arterial system, access to the venous system is attracting greater interest from cardiologists, and features of this part of the circulation will also be reviewed.

Arterial Anatomy

Embryology of Forearm Arteries

The embryologic development of the forearm vessels has been debated for years and continues to be a topic of some controversy. Initial models of growth envisioned vascular development similar to a root of a tree growing down the primordial limb; it has been referred to as the sprouting theory. Aberrant vasculature was considered just different routes followed by these nascent vessels. Unfortunately, this simple concept that had been described in many embryology textbooks is naive and the developmental sequence far more complicated. Instead, the forearm vasculature develops from a primordial capillary plexus in the arm that differentiates in a proximal-to-distal orientation through selective maintenance, regression, enlargement, and differentiation of certain capillary vessels.[8,9] This developmental sequence is highly conserved through man, primates, and even common ancestor tree shrews, as the variability in vascular anatomy in man is far less than that expected from random vascular development.[10]

Embryology of Central Upper Extremity Arteries

The upper arm vasculature in the subclavian region is derived embryologically from the aortic arches, with the right and left fourth arches contributing to the formation of the respective subclavian arteries. More distally, the subclavian arteries further develop with contributions from the seventh cervical segmental arteries that coalesce into the axillary, brachial, and then interosseous arteries.[8,9] Although aberrant subclavian vessels are rare, the *arteria luseria*, where the right or left subclavian artery passes retrograde to the esophagus to the contralateral side of the aorta, is the most common, occurring in 0.5% to 1.8% of the population. It has its origin in deviant development of the fourth aortic arch and has been traditionally associated with dysphagia and chronic cough.[11] With the advent of transradial procedures, it is apparent that most *arteria luseria* are asymptomatic except for posing a challenge to access the central aorta from the right radial when the right subclavian is involved.[12,13]

Embryology of Peripheral Upper Extremity Arteries

The arteries of the arm beyond the subclavian, such as the radial and ulnar, are derived from interactions between developing nervous, muscular, bone tissue and the capillary plexus that surrounds these embryologic structures. As the web of capillaries preferentially differentiates or regresses, the recognizable vascular structures consummate into their adult configuration. Abnormal vascular courses seen in adults are a result of persistent fetal patterns or anomalous development from the capillary plexus[8,9] and can be identified by Carnegie Stage 21[14] (52 days postovulation in humans) of embryonic growth.

The details of vascular embryology is beyond the scope of this chapter, but the net result is that the radial artery appears relatively late in the sequence of vascular development. It is derived not only from regions in the distal forearm, but also from contributions from branches that originally derived off the brachial or axillary artery. Many of the abnormalities experienced by radial operators can be defined simplistically by two characteristics: (1) the geographical location of the origin of the radial artery from the brachial/axillary artery and (2) the complexity of radial/brachial/ulnar connections in the antecubital fossa.

Normal morphology describes the ulnar and radial bifurcating from the brachial in the antecubital fossa, as shown in Figure 4-1. Persistence of upper forearm connections results in the common variants seen in the adult patients undergoing transradial catheterization that depend on anomalies in the geographic location of the radial/brachial bifurcation.[15] Variations in the development of the connection forming the bifurcation of the ulnar and radial arteries form the basis of many of the loops seen in this region that are often associated with variations in anterior or posterior course around forearm muscles and tendons.

The first factor to consider is the source of radial blood flow. Does the radial artery originate normally at the antecubital fossa, or is there a source of blood flow entering the radial distribution from higher up the brachial/axillary axis? Variations in the radial are 20 times more likely than analogous ulnar variations.[8,9] For the typical transradial operator, the ulnar variations have little material effect on the procedure using the radial artery, but it could be significant for the ulnar operator. The normal location for the radial takeoff is just slightly higher than the ulnar origin

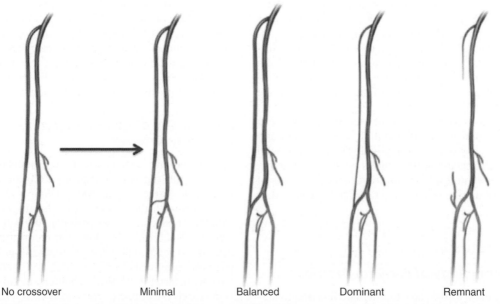

No crossover   Minimal   Balanced   Dominant   Remnant

FIGURE 4-1 Variations in arterial crossover between radial and ulnar arterial distributions in the forearm that can be encountered during arterial cannulation of the forearm. *(Adapted from Hamon M, McFadden E, eds. Transradial Approach for Cardiovascular Interventions. 2nd ed. Colombelles, France: ESM Eds; 2010.)*

in the bifurcation structure and is often noted as a simple inverted "Y" bifurcation in diagrams (Fig. 4-1), with the brachial artery being the sole source for blood flow.

Usually both the radial and the ulnar arteries then extend down to the wrist with contributions to interosseous systems and recurrent radial and ulnar vessels that can form collaterals between the upper and lower forearm. Another variant involves the median artery, which originates either as a continuation of the brachial in the forearm after the ulnar and radial have branched or as a branch of the interosseous artery. In the presence of the median artery, the radial or the ulnar or both may be diminished in size in view of the contribution provided by the median artery to distal perfusion.[16] Recent ultrasound measurements have suggested that the radial and ulnar arteries tend to be similar overall in size,[17] but there is variability both between arms and between people in the actual sizes of these vessels, ranging from a predominant radial system with remnant ulnar to a mirror image with dominant ulnar artery. Finally, both ulnar and radial arteries can be diminutive, with most of the blood flow to the hand arriving by a median artery or large interosseous system.

The other extreme to the normal inverse "Y" configuration is a radial artery that originates from a separate origin from either higher up on the brachial artery or even as far as the subclavian artery.

This forms a brachioradial artery or, in extreme cases, an axillioradial artery with no connection with the ulnar vessel in the antecubital region. Again, the sole source of blood for the radial is derived directly from the brachial artery. This variation typically has a course that appears unusual under fluoroscopy since the radial does not deviate medially to join the ulnar in the antecubital fossa, but rather continues up the arm to join the more proximal vessel. This variation, like the normal bifurcation, should not by itself result in a difficult passage unless the radial artery is otherwise diminutive or has developed tortuosity or disease.

Between the two extremes of radial origins are morphologies with dual blood sources for the radial. The upper origin is described as a duplication of the brachial artery known as the accessory brachial, with a region of merger to the true brachial at the antecubital fossa near the origin of the ulnar, and then continuation as the radial artery to the wrist. The precursor to these variants is the accessory brachial, which is basically a secondary branch of the brachial artery that rejoins the brachial above the antecubital fossa. This variant is problematic only when the accessory brachial is inadvertently entered (typically when using a hydrophilic wire) and there is a mismatch between the vessel and catheter size (Fig. 4-2).

If the accessory brachial continues to the antecubital fossa and becomes part of a dual source

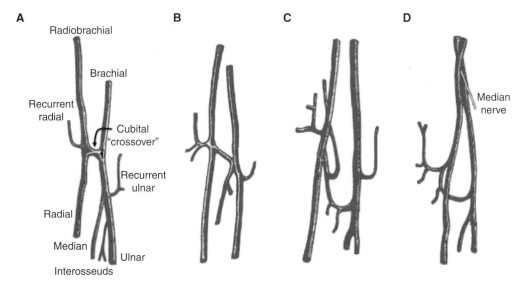

FIGURE 4-2 Anatomical variety found in crossover between radial and ulnar circulation in forearm before radial continues as a radiobrachial (accessory radial) to eventually rejoin the brachial artery at a more proximal location. **A**: Short cubital artery connecting radial and ulnar/brachial system. **B**: Elongated cubital artery between radial and ulnar/brachial system. **C**: A "U" course to cubital artery as it loops around muscle tendons between radial and ulnar/brachial system. **D**: An "Ω" (omega) course to cubital connection. Both this form and the "U" course in **C** may be especially problematic to passage of transradial catheters. *(Adapted from Cocchi A. Atti dell Accademia dei Fisocritici in Siena, Ser. 4, 3:247–261.)*

for radial artery flow along with collateral connections from the brachial artery itself, the situation becomes potentially more complex. There exists a continuum of vascular variations with interconnections both at the antecubital fossa and higher up on the brachial artery; most of these variations can be categorized as one of two variants. The first variant has a relatively balanced contribution with the radial providing similarly sized connection to both the anastomosis with the ulnar and then up the accessory radial to the upper brachial artery. This variant may allow access to the central system equally through either route or size differential may suggest one as a superior route in the case of larger-bore catheters.

The second variant exists as an asymmetric connection where most of the flow between the radial and brachial at the antecubital fossa originates from the distal brachial artery and only a remnant of the accessory brachial remains. The main connection itself is usually adequate for use, but the hazard is derived from the remnant accessory brachial allowing a small-diameter wire to enter but unable to accommodate a larger catheter. Likewise, the end of a long vascular sheath can inadvertently be placed into one of these remnant vessels and provide a nidus for vascular damage. This can result in disruption of the vessel and perforation. The inverse can also occur where the accessory brachial artery is dominant over the connection to the lower brachial artery, but once again the hazard exists if the smaller-diameter branch is inadvertently entered.

The other factor critical to passage up the arm is the geometry of the connection between the radial and ulnar/brachial region. If there is no remnant accessory radial, the radial/ulnar region usually provides the "Y" junction that is usually uneventful to cross. Occasionally, a loop may exist or a tortuosity may appear in the radial course that represents variability in the arterial pathway around tendons or nerves.[18] This is thought to have its origins in aberrant maturation of the primordial plexus around the muscles that ultimately coalesce into the varied adult arterial forms.

Once an accessory brachial exists and the radial has a dual source of blood flow, variation in the radial/brachial interconnection becomes more common. The simplest connection linking the accessory brachial with the radial and brachial arteries involves a straight linkage segment that results in the junction appearing in a "H" configuration. Typically this provides a relatively short and straight segment connecting the ulnar and radial vessels. Other than the sharp turn crossing the "H" from radial to ulnar side, this

variant is usually not too difficult to transverse as long as the segment being crossed is large enough to accommodate the wire and catheter.

As the connection between the radial/accessory radial and the ulnar/brachial system gets longer, complexities in its course arise. Tendons and muscles of the arm pass through this region, and a wide variety of looping vascular paths can develop as the artery system has formed during its development. Although gradual looping structures may be easily negotiable even with stable wires, others may take complex pathways or tight turns from a three-dimensional perspective that makes passage difficult. The simplest of these interconnections appear as "U"-shaped passages, while the more complex forms take on the form of an omega "Ω."[19] While solutions to these challenges can be obtained with persistence and thought, many opt to change access site to avoid the worst of these loops. The tendency to have complex antecubital connects is not associated with similar configuration in the contralateral arm; so given the propensity of the right arm to be more likely the location of a loop initially, the left radial often makes a good successful alternative.

A secondary hazard in the region of crossover between the accessory brachial–radial–brachial circulations is the potential for small branches originating in the region. Especially the recurrent radial or ulnar branches, small branches that span the region of the antecubital fossa, have a tendency to originate at the apex of turns made by these interconnections.[3] Complications such as perforation can then occur when a hydrophilic or other type of wire inadvertently enters one of these branches as the operator is attempting to negotiate the turns of the passage.

While the normal radial origin at the antecubital fossa appears like an inverse "Y," there are situations that result in complexities despite a single origin for the radial artery. Some of these perijunctional variants appear very similar to those seen with dual blood supplies to the radial and may actually represent remnant arterial structures after a legacy accessory brachial had atrophied. Often complex junctional anatomy is associated with recurrent radial branches and accessory vessels (Lo) that also suggest linkage to primordial accessory brachial vascular that had regressed.

Distal Forearm Artery Anatomy

The most commonly observed branches of the forearm for both the radial and ulnar arteries include a recurrent branch that circles back around the elbow region and may extend back up the humeral arm, and the muscular branches that penetrate the neighboring muscle groups. In addition, the proximal portion of the brachial–ulnar artery usually is the origin of the interosseous vessels, while the continuation of the brachial can result in a third artery extending to the hand, known as the median artery. Each of the two or three main branches terminates in the palmar arches of the hand. The interosseous, muscular, and recurrent branches can also add to the network of collateralizing vessels in this region.

The branches originating from the proximal end of both the radial and ulnar arteries would be only curiosities except for the potential they pose to trap angiographic wires being passed up the artery. This then results in the potential for perforation, spasm, or at worst disarticulation of the branch vessel is not recognized promptly. Distally, the radial artery divides into two or three subbranches as it enters the palmar arch. In 45% of subjects, this termination of the radial occurs normally after piercing into the region of the dorsal interossei at the base of the hand. In the majority of cases (52%), the first of the terminal branches of the radial artery has appeared before the artery reaches the dorsal interossi region and in 2% the radial has already trifurcated.[20] If this early branching occurs relatively high on the radial artery, it could become involved in the entry site of radial access and result in damage to one of this terminal branches. For this reason, entry into the radial artery is encouraged above the wrist crease to reduce the risk of branch vessel damage.[21]

While the usual circulation to the hand is relatively balanced between contributions from the radial and ulnar sources, there can be variations. Each of the three potential major branches to the wrist (radial, median, and ulnar) can be dominant and provide the majority of perfusion, leaving the other vessels small and unsuitable for catheter conduits. Perhaps the most extreme would be a palmar arch supplied primarily by the interossius arteries with minimal or no pulse in either the radial or ulnar arteries.[22]

Other causes for a diminished or atypical radial pulse would include a radial system that has bifurcated more proximally below the antecubital origin. The resulting reduced caliper of each subsequent branch may result in vessels that are too small to cannulate. Normally after leaving the bifurcation from the brachial artery, the radial passes distally under the belly of the brachioradialis muscle and surfaces to pass superficially a few centimeters from the wrist. If the radial courses on the anterior surface of the brachioradialis muscle, it is known as a superficial radial artery (or superficial brachioradial artery if the source is above the antecubital fossa) and its presence in the wrist may be more lateral than what would otherwise be expected.[18]

Loops and Tortuosity

Beyond anomalous courses to the radial artery and its origin that are relatively common, the arm arteries may also demonstrate a variety of tortuosity and looplike pathways. Most problematic involve variant origins to the radial artery and anastomosis at the antecubital fossa, but they can also occur more distally where the small diameter of the artery adds further to the risk of failure. Brachial and subclavian tortuosity and loops exist, but in general are a lesser source of procedural difficulty.[23]

The tortuosities in the vascular are usually the result of redundancy of the vessels to allow for extremity motion or the result of body mass loss in the elderly. Loops usually signify passage above or below a muscle group or tendon that is a variant of what one might consider a normal route. These abnormalities can occur anywhere along the subclavian–radial route; they most commonly pose problems when found in the radial artery. The forearm is also subject to degenerative changes from atherosclerosis and calcification that may also impede passage of catheters.[24] In addition, obstruction and collaterals may be present anytime acquired vascular disease such as atherosclerosis, arteritis, or trauma has affected the arm vasculature.

Axillary/Subclavian Region

In the upper arm and subclavian region, the greatest anatomical challenge involves tortuosities. These have been recognized since the early days of catheterization and are usually not appreciated by chest X-ray until engaged by the operator's wire or inability to advance a catheter along the atrial course.[25] While anomalous arterial courses isolated to the upper arm and subclavian region are less common than from the lower forearm, the one abnormality to recognize is the *arteria lusoria*. This is the result of a developmental flaw during embryology and has been reported in 0.2% to 1.7% patients.[26] The right subclavian fails to form a common trunk with the carotid artery on the right and originate from the aortic arch anterior to the esophagus. Instead, the right subclavian passes posterior to the esophagus and enters the aorta more distally, usually just beyond the arch and the insertion of the left subclavian. A similar aberration can occur with the left subclavian, but is rarer and of little consequence to transradial access. The diagnosis is often first noticed when the angiographic wire from the right radial artery appears to be persistently falling down the descending aorta from a potion slightly more distal along the arch of the aorta.[13] Such a sharp turn toward the ascending aorta and the retrograde course the catheter must travel to the ascending root to the location of the coronary ostia result in many operators switching to the left arm to continue the procedure. Like other abnormalities of the vasculature, this variant does not necessarily prevent continuation from the right arm, but skill and experience is needed. Fortunately, this is a rare abnormality, but will be seen eventually by most active operators.

Venous Anatomy

Introduction

The venous system is in many ways far more complex than the arterial system of the arm, but fortunately it is far more forgiving for the catheter passage. Veins are, by function, distensible, whereas arteries tend to spasm, and the pathways for redundancy and alternative routes are characteristic of the venous side. The veins are also thinner in structure, less forgiving to mechanical trauma, and therefore are more susceptible to puncture than the arterial tree.

Embryology of the Forearm Veins

The embryology of the upper extremity venous system is poorly understood. Simplistically, primitive veins are noted to exist initially along the borders of extremities. Venous capillary plexuses that exist around developing nerve and muscle structures further differentiate and integrate into these border veins. In the mature state, this results in venous drainage of the arm that is robust with collaterals and interconnections both superficially and around the deep structures.[27]

Veins Are Different from Arteries

Veins that have not been traumatized tend not to suffer from the tortuosity and loops of arteries, but do contain valves that at times can retard passage of the tip of a catheter. Veins are also more susceptible to trauma from events such

as broken bones or blunt trauma and collaterals may be readily found. In addition, veins can be the source of thrombus that may represent another challenge to passage. Finally, iatrogenic obstacles can exist. Pacemaker and defibrillator leads along with indwelling vascular ports can all impede passage of a catheter and alter the natural anatomy for the operator.

Anatomy of the Forearm Veins

Venous anatomy has not received the attention of arterial anatomy in the arm and relatively little literature describes its form. Essential all the venous drainage from the arm ends up in the subclavian vein, so potentially any vein entered will eventually bring the catheter to the central system, limited only by the catheter's length. Superficial veins commonly seen traversing the arm do not follow either the arterial tree or nerves, but rather have a wide range of individual variability. The deep veins of the arm do follow the courses of the major arteries and ultimately receive the drainage from the superficial veins.

Simplistically, the venous drainage can be defined as geographically serving either the radial or ulnar regions by several common venous conduits that inter connect at the antecubital fossa or bypass the region around medial or lateral regions of the elbow. Drainage that originates along the ulnar side of the arm, in general, will drain up the brachial vein. This blood then continues up the arm into the axillary and then subclavian veins. The veins draining the radial side of the forearm may drain into the brachial venous system, but they are just as likely to continue laterally up the cephalic system in the upper arm.[28] Interconnections are common even at the level of the humerus, but the main channel of the cephalic and brachial meet to form the axillary vein then pass under the clavicle to form the subclavian.

Basilic Vein

The basilic vein is functionally a direct extension of the subclavian and axillary vein and provides a straight route to the central system. It is a superficial vessel that runs along the medial aspect of the biceps muscle before joining with the deep brachial vein that accompanies the brachial artery and ultimately resulting in the axillary vein.

Cephalic Vein

The cephalic vein courses along the proximal forearm to the shoulder region. This course usually passes up the bicipital sulcus and along the deltoid pectoral triangle. At termination, the vein then passes into the deeper venous channel of the axillary vein. While interconnections are common between the superficial cephalic and basilic system, and interpersonal variability in courses exist along the upper arm, the terminal section of the cephalic is fairly uniform.[29] At the termination, the cephalic enters the axillary at a right angle described as a "T" junction. This junction may not preferentially lead the catheter to the central system, but rather may deflect it back down the arm via the brachial vein. As such, when passing a catheter up the arm, it is important to check its course at the shoulder to determine the route and redirect if necessary.

Alternatives to the classic "T" junction termination of the cephalic can be seen. Anatomically the cephalic, as defined as the vein entering the axillary to form the subclavian vein, has been reported absent in about 5% of cases.[30,31] In such cases, the cephalic drainage has entered the basilic vein prior to the shoulder and would not directly affect passage of arm catheters. Alternatively, interconnection with the external jugular vein is also possible instead of the traditional junction with the axillary.

While anatomical variation in arm veins is diverse, it rarely results in in clinical failure.[32] Similar to the lack of symmetry in the upper arterial system, the venous system also lacks symmetrical correlation. The sizes of venous structures vary greatly within individual patients and do not correlate to hand dominance or anthropomorphic indices.[33]

Natural Anomalies of the Venous System

Other than the wide variation in what one might consider normal venous anatomy along with variable populations of venous valves especially near junctions, the flow of blood up the veins favors passage up to the central system. One potential congenital venous anomaly, known as persistent left superior vena cava (PSVC), may be encountered if venous passage is practiced from the left arm.[34] This results in a variety of potential routes for venous drainage from the left arm to enter the heart, including the most common route to the right atrium via the coronary sinus and the less common route directly into the left atrium, resulting in the potential for systemic/venous shunting. While relatively rare (0.5%) in the normal population, the PSVC is reported in up to 11% of those with congenital heart syndromes.[35]

If entering the central venous system via the right arm, a PSVC may not be noticed, although there are variants of this anatomy that exist in 10% to 20% of cases where the right SVC may be absent.[36] From the left arm, catheters entering a PSVC will appear to pass inferiorly by the midline rather than the usual course to pass over to the upper right chest before descending into the right atrium. The PSVC commonly drains into the right heart via a variety of routes including the coronary sinus, or may be in some cases the source of shunting and hypoxemia when termination is in the left atrium or other left-sided structures. Observing a left venous catheter descending along a route more medially than expected should raise the suspicion of SVC. Likewise, in the case of an absent right SVC, the venous path from the right arm will appear to cross the midline to the left as it joins the remaining PSVC. Depending on the actually drainage pattern, completion of the right heart might require switching to the right arm in the case of a PSVC with preserved right SVC, or femoral vein when the right SVC is absent.

Iatrogenic Changes to the Venous System

The venous system is naturally more redundant than the arterial tree, but is also more susceptible to damage from trauma or thrombosis from indwelling devices. Prior arm, shoulder, or clavicle fractures, in addition to blunt trauma, may have altered or damaged the natural venous flow pattern even in patients who exhibit no external signs of venous obstruction. Likewise, pacing leads and indwelling intravenous catheters may also be thrombosed in place and offer little or no room for catheter passage. While prior trauma or device placement may not preclude normal passage of venous catheters, it can also portend the existence of collaterals that may or may not be friendly to venous catheter passage and the contralateral arm may be the better alternative.[37]

Breast Cancer Surgery and Lymphedema

Iatrogenic damage from either extensive dissection such as seen in breast cancer or extensive radiation therapy and subsequent lymphedema infers potentially significant damage to the normal vasculature. Consideration of this potential should be made in the setting of resistance to catheter passage. In the case of severe lymphedema, venous access may be problematic due to poor visualization and the use of the contralateral arm is probably the better option from the start.

The widely reported contraindication for vascular access in the ipsilateral arm as treated breast cancer is a topic of much emotional debate. The literature supporting many of the so-called prohibited actions such as no blood pressure cuffs, no intravenous lines, and no procedures is based on retrospective review and expert opinion with significant body of literature to refute such precautionary behavior.[38] Carpal tunnel surgery on the wrist ipsilateral to breast surgery with or without preexisting lymphedema has been reported successfully without any worsening of lymphedema in 15 women.[39] A second report[40] of hand surgery also ipsilateral to breast cancer surgery that used tourniquet-based local anesthesia, along with no preoperative antibiotics, showed no new lymphedema in 23 out of 25 women. In the remaining two, there was a patient perception of worsening of preexisting lymphedema. Finally, a survey of hand surgeons ($N = 606$) noted more than 95% have willingly performed hand surgery ipsilateral on patients with lymph node surgery or radiation, and 85% still operate with the presence of lymphedema.[41] There are no studies supporting the role of blood pressure measurement and the instigation of lymphedema. Beyond the potential for venous obstruction due to scarring from surgery that may physically alter the anatomy, there is no definitive data supporting the popularized prohibition from using the ipsilateral arm after breast cancer therapy.

Conclusion

Understanding the expected anatomy of the forearm and its rich variations is important to optimize catheter-based procedures from the forearm. Additionally, appreciating the embryologic basis, at least in general terms, adds a further basis to the understanding of why certain anatomical variations are present. Integrating this foundation understanding with considerations of the patient life experiences such as trauma or medical illness that might affect the forearm can reduce the chance of unexpected challenges for the operator and improve the overall efficiency and safety for forearm procedures.

REFERENCES

1. Osler W. On the educational value of the medical society [address to the New Haven Medical Association, January 6, 1903]. *Yale Med J.* 1903;9(10):327.

2. Fujii T, Masuda N, Tamiya S, et al. Angiographic evaluation of right upper-limb arterial anomalies: implications for transradial coronary interventions. *J Invasive Cardiol.* 2010;22(11):536–540.

3. Lo TS, Nolan J, Fountzopoulos E, et al. Radial artery anomaly and its influence on transradial coronary procedural outcome. *Heart.* 2009;95(5):410–415.

4. Uglietta JP, Kadir S. Arteriographic study of variant arterial anatomy of the upper extremities. *Cardiovasc Intervent Radiol.* 1989;12(3):145–148.

5. Burzotta F, Trani C, Mazzari MA, et al. Vascular complications and access crossover in 10,676 transradial percutaneous coronary procedures. *Am Heart J.* 2012;163(2):230–238.

6. Burzotta F, Brancati MF, Trani C, et al. Impact of radial-to-aorta vascular anatomical variants on risk of failure in trans-radial coronary procedures. *Catheter Cardiovasc Interv.* 2012;80(2):298–303.

7. Yokoyama N, Takeshita S, Ochiai M, et al. Anatomic variations of the radial artery in patients undergoing transradial coronary intervention. *Catheter Cardiovasc Interv.* 2000;49(4):357–362.

8. Rodríguez-Niedenführ M, Vázquez T, Nearn L, et al. Variations of the arterial pattern in the upper limb revisited: a morphological and statistical study, with a review of the literature. *J Anat.* 2001;199(pt 5):547–566.

9. Rodríguez-Niedenführ M, Burton GJ, Deu J, et al. Development of the arterial pattern in the upper limb of staged human embryos: normal development and anatomic variations. *J Anat.* 2001;199:407–417.

10. Matsumoto S, Kuhn HJ, Vogt H, et al. Embryological development of the arterial system of the forelimb in Tupaia. *Anat Rec.* 1994;240(3):416–422.

11. Kent PD, Poterucha TH, Poterucha TH. Aberrant right subclavian artery and dysphagia lusoria. *N Engl J Med.* 2002;346:1637.

12. Yiu K-H, Chan W-S, Jim M-H, et al. Arteria lusoria diagnosed by transradial coronary catheterization. *JACC Cardiovasc Interv.* 2010;3:880–881.

13. Abhaichand RK, Louvard Y, Gobeil JF, et al. The problem of arteria lusoria in right transradial coronary angiography and angioplasty. *Catheter Cardiovasc Interv.* 2001;54:196–201.

14. O'Rahilly R, Müller F. *Developmental Stages in Human Embryos.* Washington, DC: Carnegie Institution of Washington; 1987:637.

15. Rodríguez-Niedenführ M, Sañudo JR, Vázquez T, et al. Anastomosis at the level of the elbow joint connecting the deep, or normal, brachial artery with major arterial variations of the upper limb. *J Anat.* 2000;196(pt 1):115–119.

16. Rodríguez-Baeza A, Nebot J, Ferreira B, et al. An anatomical study and ontogenetic explanation of 23 cases with variations in the main pattern of the human brachio-antebrachial arteries. *J Anat.* 1995;187(pt 2):473–479.

17. Yan ZX, Zhou YJ, Zhao YX, et al. Anatomical study of forearm arteries with ultrasound for percutaneous coronary procedures. *Circ J.* 2010;74(4):686–692.

18. Jelev L, Surchev L. Radial artery course behind the biceps brachii tendon: significance for the transradial catheterization and a clinically oriented classification of the radial artery variations. *Cardiovasc Intervent Radiol.* 2008;31:1008–1012.

19. Yoo BS, Yoon J, Ko JY, et al. Anatomical consideration of the radial artery for transradial coronary procedures: arterial diameter, branching anomaly and vessel tortuosity. *Int J Cardiol.* 2005;101(3):421–427.

20. Gupta C, Ray B, Dsouza AS, et al. A morphological study of variations in the branching pattern and termination of the radial artery. *Singapore Med J.* 2012;53(3):208–211.

21. Caputo RP, Tremmel JA, Rao S, et al. Transradial arterial access for coronary and peripheral procedures: executive summary by the transradial committee of the SCAI. *Catheter Cardiovasc Interv.* 2011;78:823–839.

22. Poteat WL. Report of a rare human variation: absence of the radial artery. *Anat Rec.* 1986;214(1):89–95.

23. Louvard Y, Lefèvre T. Loops and transradial approach in coronary diagnosis and intervention. *Catheter Cardiovasc Interv.* 2000;51(2):250–252.

24. Moisiuc F, Kern MJ. Unusual radial artery calcification as contraindication to radial artery access? *Catheter Cardiovasc Interv.* 2013;81(4):742–743.

25. Bousvaros G, Sandler IA. Tortuosity of the innominate artery failure of retrograde catheterization of left side of heart by brachial arterial route. *JAMA.* 1968;205(6):214–215.

26. Valsecchi O, Vassileva A, Musumeci G, et al. Failure of transradial approach during coronary interventions: anatomic considerations. *Catheter Cardiovasc Interv.* 2006;67:870–878.

27. Zaleske DJ. Development of the upper limb. *Hand Clin.* 1985;1(3):383–390.

28. Chun HJ, Byun JY, Yoo S-S, et al. Tourniquet application to facilitate axillary venous access in percutaneous central venous catheterization. *Radiology.* 2003;226:918–920.

29. Bergman R, Thompson SA, Afifi AK. *Compendium of Human Anatomic Variation.* Baltimore, MD: Urban and Schwarzenberg; 1988:90–91, 431.

30. Reid CD, Taylor GI. The vascular territory of the acromiothoracic axis. *Br J Plast Surg.* 1984;37(2):194–212.

31. Le Saout J, Vallee B, Person H, et al. Anatomical basis for the surgical use of the cephalic vein (V. Cephalica). 74 anatomical dissections. 189 surgical dissections [in French]. *J Chir (Paris).* 1983;120(2):131–134.

32. Gilchrist IC, Moyer CD, Gascho JA. Trans-radial right and left heart catheterizations: a comparison to traditional femoral approach. *Catheter Cardiovasc Interv.* 2006;67:585–588.

33. Tan CO, Weinberg L, Peyton P, et al. Size variation between contralateral infraclavicular axillary veins within individual patients-implications for subclavian venous central line insertion. *Crit Care Med.* 2013;41(2):457–463.

34. Demos TC, Posniak HV, Pierce KL, et al. Venous anomalies of the thorax. *AJR Am J Roentgenol.* 2004;182(5):1139–1150.

35. Buirski G, Jordan SC, Joffe HS, et al. Superior vena caval abnormalities: their occurrence rate, associated cardiac abnormalities and angiographic classification in a paediatric population with congenital heart disease. *Clin Radiol.* 1986;37(2):131–138.

36. Bartram U, Van Praagh S, Levine JC, et al. Absent right superior vena cava in visceroatrial situs solitus. *Am J Cardiol.* 1997;80(2):175–183.

37. Gilchrist IC. Radial approach to right heart catheterization and intervention. *Indian Heart J.* 2010;62(3):245–250.

38. McLaughlin SA. Lymphedema: separating fact from fiction. *Oncology (Williston Park).* 2012;26(3):242–249.

39. Dawson WJ, Elenz DR, Winchester DP, et al. Elective hand surgery in the breast cancer patient with prior ipsilateral axillary dissection. *Ann Surg Oncol.* 1995;2:132–137.

40. Hershko DD, Stahl S. Safety of elective hand surgery following axillary lymph node dissection for breast cancer. *Breast J.* 2007;13:287–290.

41. Gharbaoui IS, Netscher DT, Thornby J, et al. Safety of upper extremity surgery after prior treatment for ipsilateral breast cancer: results of an American Society for Surgery of the Hand membership survey and literature review. *J Am Soc Surg Hand.* 2005;5:232–238.

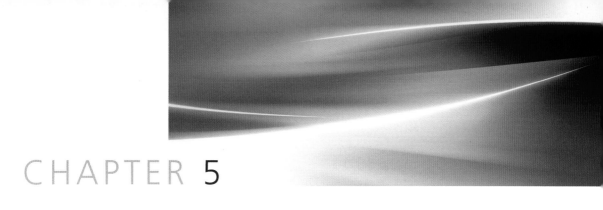

CHAPTER 5

Anatomy, Tortuosities, and Access Difficulties

Tejas Patel, Sanjay Shah, and Samir B. Pancholy

Background

Continuous refinement in the technique associated with revolution in technology, resulting from collaboration between cardiologists and engineers, has provided outstanding material for percutaneous treatment of cardiovascular diseases in daily practice. It has also resulted in a significant increase in the safety of diagnostic and interventional transradial procedures.

In this chapter, we have provided a stepwise guide to identify and deal with the issues related to transradial access. The issues related to transradial approach (TRA) can be divided into two categories:

1. those related to radial and brachial regions, and
2. those related to subclavian, innominate, and aortic arch regions.

Issues Related to Radial and Brachial Regions

Here is the normal anatomy of this region. The artery that supplies the upper limb continues as a single trunk from its origin down to the elbow. However, different parts of the artery have different names, depending on the regions through which they pass. The part of the artery that extends from its origin to the lateral border of the first rib is the subclavian artery. Beyond this point, to the lower border of axilla, is the axillary artery. From that point, to the bend of the elbow, is the brachial artery.

The radial artery (RA) commences at the bifurcation of the brachial artery, just below the bend of the elbow, and passes along the radial side of the forearm to the wrist. The RA extends from the neck of the radius to the front part of the styloid process. The upper part lies on the medial side of radius and the lower part lies on the bone. The upper part is deep and lies below the muscle (brachioradialis). The lower part is superficial, covered by skin and superficial and deep fascia. The RA is slightly smaller in caliber than the ulnar artery (Fig. 5-1).

Following are the important relevant issues:

- Radial artery spasm (RAS)
- Tortuosity
- Perforation
- Loops and curvatures

Radial Artery Spasm

Beginning radialists have apprehension to deal with RAS. True RAS is not as common as most interventionalists think. The overall incidence in experienced hands is about 5%, 0.5% of whom have severe spasm.[1-5]

Classification of Radial Artery Spasm

We have developed classifications of RAS (Box 5-1), which should be useful in clinical practice. This is a clinical and procedural outcome-related definition. Angiography should be performed in every instance of suspected spasm with exclusion of adverse anatomy as the underlying reason for above-mentioned circumstances. From length of spasm induced narrowed

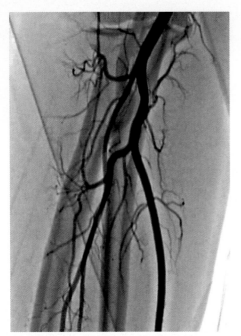

FIGURE 5-1   Normal anatomy of brachial, radial, and ulnar arteries.

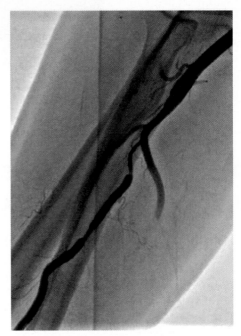

FIGURE 5-2   Focal spasm of RA.

segment it can be categorized as "focal" or "diffuse."

- Focal: narrowed segment <10 mm in length (Fig. 5-2)
- Diffuse: narrowed segment ≥10 mm in length (Fig. 5-3)

Identification and Management of Radial Artery Spasm

- If a patient complains of significant local pain in the region of RA during the passage of a guidewire and/or a catheter, RAS should be suspected.

- Perform a radial angiography through the side port of the introducer sheath or through the catheter itself to define the anatomy and detect spasm.
- If RAS is confirmed, an additional dose of spasmolytic cocktail should be given, and another radial angiography should be performed after a short period (30 seconds to 1 minute) to confirm that the spasm is relieved.
- If RAS contributes at this stage, the affected segment should be crossed carefully using a 0.025" J-shaped hydrophilic guidewire or a soft-tip 0.014" percutaneous transluminal coronary angioplasty (PTCA) guidewire.

BOX 5-1   Classification of Radial Artery Spasm

Grade I: Mild spasm
The patient experiences minimal pain and/or discomfort along the course of RA during and/or immediately after the procedure.

Grade II: Moderate spasm
The patient experiences significant pain and discomfort along the course of RA during and/or immediately after the procedure. However, catheter movement is possible to complete the procedure.

Grade III: Severe spasm
The patient experiences severe pain and discomfort along the course of RA during catheter movement despite the administration of at least two successive doses of spasmolytic cocktail, compelling the operator to terminate the procedure and cross over to other access site.

Grade IV: Very severe spasm
The patient experiences very severe pain and discomfort along the course of RA associated with catheter entrapment despite the administration of at least two successive doses of spasmolytic cocktail.

Once it is done successfully, a diagnostic or guide catheter should be negotiated over it. Instead of the usual pushing movement, use a slow, cork-screw movement to break the spasm. Once the tip of the catheter crosses the affected segment, the rest of the procedure can be completed in the regular manner.

- If spasm develops in RA with the initial catheter, downsizing the catheter (to a 4F instead of 5F diagnostic catheter, or a 5F instead of 6F guide catheter) helps to work past the spasm successfully.
- Beginners have relatively higher incidence of RAS. Multiple attempts for RA puncture are the most common cause. Sometimes the RA pulse becomes feeble or disappears because of severe spasm. Subcutaneous injection of nitroglycerine should be given; it helps return the RA pulse in most instances.
- Significant tortuosity, calcification, or atherosclerosis of RA segment may create difficulty in passing a guidewire and/or catheter. Repeated push of the assembly against this resistance is usually counterproductive and can lead to reactive focal or diffuse RAS. A repeat cocktail and the use of aforementioned steps to negotiate the assembly usually bring success.
- Anatomical variations of the RA, particularly the anomalous origin of the RA from high brachial or axillary artery and radio-brachial loops, are most commonly misinterpreted

as RAS. Whenever the RA has high brachial or axillary artery origin, its caliber is almost invariably small. This leads to significant resistance to passage of assembly through this segment. Downsizing the catheter resolves the problem to a great extent. The method of working through loops is discussed later in the chapter. Very rarely after completion of a diagnostic procedure or an intervention, the catheter is severely gripped in RAS segment. Even a gentle attempt to pull the catheter gives agonizing pain to the patient. In this rare situation, a short course of general anesthesia is helpful. Once the patient is anesthetized, the catheter can usually be easily removed without pain.

Tortuosity

Tortuosity is an important issue particularly while dealing with patients above 70 years, long-standing diabetics, hypertensives, and females[2,5-7] (Fig. 5-4).

- It is an important cause of resistance to the movement of a guidewire and/or a catheter.
- RA angiogram should define its severity and extent.
- Once it is diagnosed, it should be crossed using a 0.025″ or 0.032″ J-shaped hydrophilic guidewire or a 0.014″ soft-tip PTCA guidewire. The catheter should be negotiated slowly and

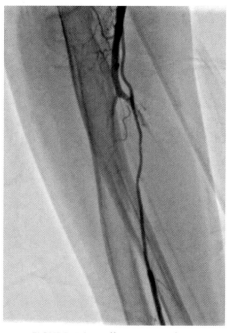

FIGURE 5-3   Diffuse spasm of RA.

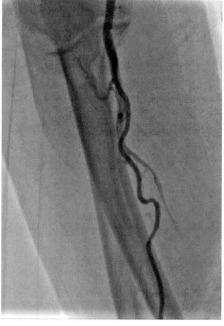

FIGURE 5-4   Severe tortuosity of RA.

carefully over the wire, using cork-screw movement under fluoroscopic guidance. Once the tortuous segment is crossed, the procedure can be completed in the usual manner.

- Sometimes, a repeat dose of cocktail helps working through a tortuous segment in small RA with or without spasm.[5,8]

Perforation

This complication should be identified and managed promptly, as it is the commonest cause of large forearm hematoma.[2,8-11] In our series, the incidence was 0.1%.[11]

Classification of Radial–Brachial Perforation

We have developed a classification for radial–brachial perforations (Box 5-2), which should be useful in clinical practice.

Identification and Management

- Resistance to the passage of a guidewire and/or a catheter felt by an operator associated with a complaint of significant local pain and discomfort in the radial and/or brachial region by a patient, with or without development of expanding forearm hematoma, makes this diagnosis.
- Immediate removal of the assembly and injection of diluted contrast through side port of an introducer sheath confirms the site and size of perforation.
- A radial operator might have an apprehension to work through it. In that case, we recommend abandoning the procedure, reversing the effect of heparin, and giving manual compression at the local site for a sufficiently

longer time to prevent a large hematoma. Sealing of perforation can be confirmed by injecting diluted contrast through the side port of the introducer sheath. The procedure may be completed after several hours or next day using a contralateral radial or a femoral route.

- We recommend the following technique to work past the perforation.[10] The steps are as follows (Fig. 5-5):
  - Identify the site and size of perforation by injecting diluted contrast through the side port of introducer sheath.
  - Use a floppy-tip 0.014″ PTCA wire and carefully cross the affected area. Park the wire higher in the brachial or axillary region.
  - Negotiate a diagnostic or guide catheter over the wire and stop when the tip of the catheter reaches the perforated segment.
  - Gently negotiate the catheter using a slow cork-screw movement (instead of the usual push) to reduce the friction in the perforated segment. Once the tip crosses the affected segment, the movement of the catheter becomes smooth and the procedure can be completed in the usual manner.
  - If there is resistance in the movement of the catheter tip at the perforation site, remove the catheter immediately and downsize it (i.e., a 4F diagnostic catheter instead of 5F, or a 5F guide catheter instead of 6F). This strategy facilitates the successful crossing of the affected segment with less friction.
  - Once the diagnostic or interventional procedure is over, the catheter is pulled back and an injection of diluted contrast is made through the catheter itself or the side port of introducer sheath, to confirm

BOX 5-2 **Classification of Radial–Brachial Perforation**

Grade I

Small perforation (<1 mm arterial rent, or side-branch diameter on radial angiography) confirmed by minimal extravasation of contrast, usually self-limiting and not associated with muscular infiltration and significant hematoma.

Grade II

Moderate perforation (1 to 2 mm arterial rent, or side-branch diameter on radial angiography) confirmed by significant extravasation of contrast and associated with muscular infiltration and expanding hematoma.

Grade III

Large perforation (>2 mm arterial rent or side-branch diameter on radial angiography) confirmed by rapid and significant extravasation of contrast and associated with large muscular infiltration and rapidly expanding hematoma.

Grade IV

Free RA rupture.

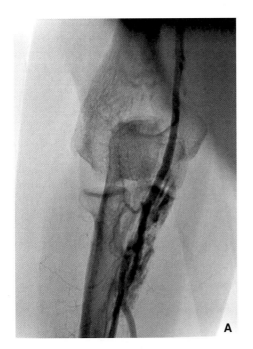

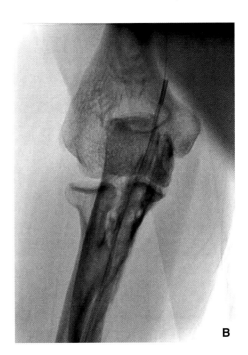

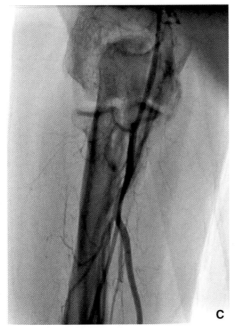

FIGURE 5-5   **A:** Grade II perforation with significant extravasation of contrast. **B:** It was crossed with a 0.014″ balance middleweight (BMW) PTCA guidewire and a 5F Judkins right no. 4 guide catheter. **C:** Postprocedure angiogram revealed completely sealed perforation.

appropriate sealing of the perforated segment. It is important to understand that the catheter functions as an internal hemostatic device to help seal the perforated segment.

Loops and Curvatures

These are important anatomical variations to understand and manage.[2,5–8,12] In our experience,

most of the times what we think is RAS is actually an anatomical variation in the form of tortuosity, loops, or curvatures. We strongly recommend keeping a low threshold for performing an RA angiography to define anatomy for working through vast majority of loops and curvatures.

Identification and Management

We have already developed a protocol to work through loops and curvatures.[5,8] It should reduce apprehension of a new radial operator and give additional confidence to an experienced operator. Following are the important steps to remember (Fig. 5-6).

- Define the task: When you encounter resistance in the movement of a wire and/or a catheter, inject diluted contrast to define the anatomy. If a simple loop is identified, you can work through it under fluoroscopic guidance. If it is a complex loop, take multiple views (i.e., right anterior oblique (RAO) and left anterior oblique (LAO), cranial, or caudal angulations). Identify the view that best defines the loop. The view that is chosen can then be used as a "road map" for working through it (Fig. 5-7).
- Downsize the guidewire: If you encounter resistance in the passage of a standard 0.032" or 0.035" guidewire while working through the loop, remove the wire, as repeated attempts

to negotiate it against the resistance can lead to perforation, spasm, and severe local pain. A flexible guidewire (i.e., 0.014" soft-tip PTCA guidewire or a 0.025" hydrophilic guidewire) should be used in place of a standard guidewire to cross the loop. The tip of a guidewire (especially of a 0.014" PTCA wire) can be shaped to the angle of the loop to facilitate crossing. When the guidewire crosses the loop, its tip is parked as high as possible (i.e., high brachial, axillary, or subclavian region). Then the catheter can be advanced over it. Sometimes, when these guidewires do not provide adequate support for the advancement of the catheters, the strategy should be changed (mentioned in the later part of this discussion) (Fig. 5-8).

- Use of buddy wire(s): When a single 0.014" PTCA guidewire provides inadequate support for a catheter to cross the loop, use of

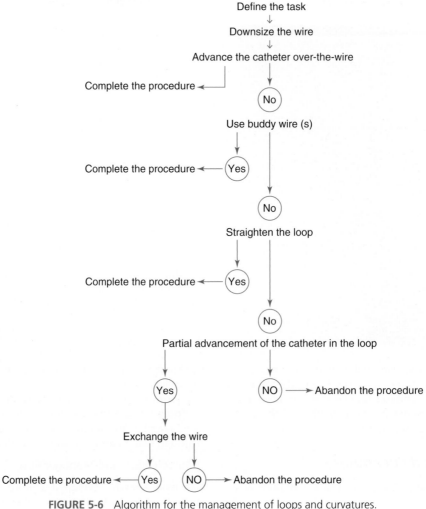

FIGURE 5-6 Algorithm for the management of loops and curvatures.

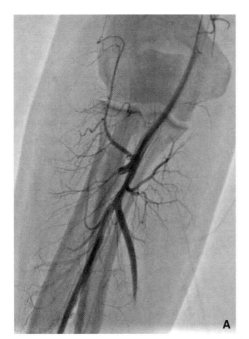 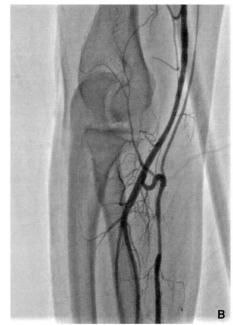

FIGURE 5-7 **A:** RA angiogram in anterio-posterior (AP) view revealed a complex loop with unclear anatomy. **B:** RA angiogram in LAO view revealed a double hair-pin loop.

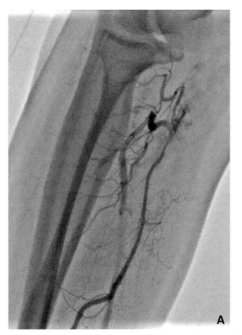 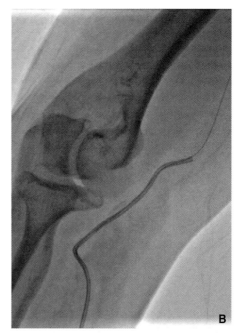

FIGURE 5-8 **A:** RA angiogram revealed RA with a small caliber with loop and Grade I perforation created by a standard 0.032″ guidewire. **B:** We downsized the 0.032″ guidewire to a 0.014″ soft-tip PTCA guidewire and crossed the affected segment with a 5F diagnostic catheter.

additional one or two such guidewires should facilitate the advancement of the catheter by adding additional support (Fig. 5-9).
- Straightening of the loop: Mostly the catheter can easily be negotiated over the wire

across a loop without disturbing the shape of the loop. When there is resistance in the passage of the catheter while working through the loop, this technique is useful. Push the catheter as far as possible into the

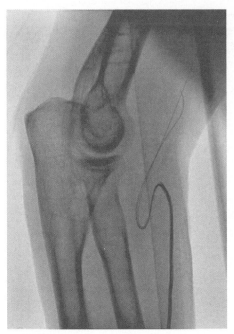

FIGURE 5-9 Use of a buddy wire to help the catheter crossing a complex double hair-pin loop.

loop, keeping the tip of the wire as high as possible (i.e., in high brachial, axillary, or subclavian region). Then, pull the entire assembly slightly back (i.e., the catheter along with the guidewire). This maneuver opens up the loop and straightens it. At this stage,

advancement of the catheter across the loop becomes easy (Fig. 5-10).

- Exchanging the guidewire: This technique is helpful in addressing the most difficult loops. It is used if the catheter is partly inside the loop, but has not crossed the entire loop and it is difficult to advance it any farther. Advance the catheter into the loop as far as possible. Exchange the thin guidewire with another guidewire to provide extra support. A 0.014″ PTCA guidewire can be exchanged with a 0.025″ hydrophilic guidewire and a 0.025″ hydrophilic guidewire can be exchanged with a standard 0.035″ guidewire, if necessary. Then, advance the catheter on the new wire. Avoid using a super-stiff guidewire unless you have crossed the loop and the tip of the catheter is well into the higher segment (i.e., high brachial, axillary, or subclavian region). This technique is useful in working through a difficult radio-cubital trunk and a 360° loop with very small diameter (Fig. 5-11).

Balloon-Assisted Tracking of a Catheter: A Must-Learn Technique

Sometimes, the operator encounters an RA with a smaller caliber, extreme tortuosity, or atherosclerotic lesions – each of which can lead to difficult tracking of a diagnostic or guide catheter. Repeated attempts to negotiate a catheter increase

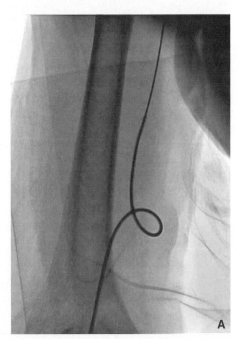

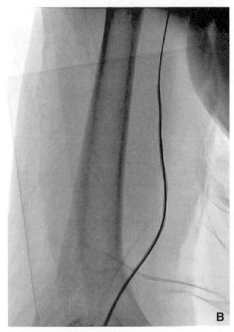

FIGURE 5-10 **A:** A 360° loop was crossed with a guidewire and a 5F diagnostic catheter. **B:** The loop was successfully straightened by gentle pull-back of the assembly.

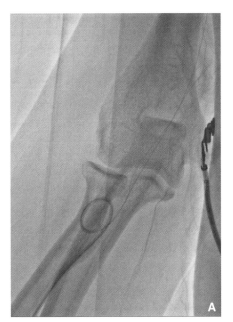
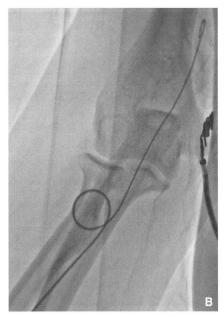

FIGURE 5-11   A: A 360° loop was crossed with a 0.014" soft-tip PTCA guidewire and a pigtail catheter was advanced over the wire. **B:** PTCA guidewire was exchanged with a 0.035" standard guidewire to advance the catheter over it.

the chances of spasm, pain, discomfort, and perforation, potentially leading to hematoma. An effective technique to work through this complexity is called "balloon-assisted tracking (BAT) of a catheter."[5,13] For BAT, define anatomy by contrast injection through the side port of the introducer sheath. Cross the segment with a 0.014" floppy-tip PTCA guidewire. A PTCA catheter of 1.5, 2.0, or 2.5 mm diameter should be selected, depending on the inner lumen of the diagnostic or guide catheter (5F, 6F, or 7F). The distal 4 to 5 mm segment of balloon should protrude outside the mouth of the catheter. The catheter is kept in the proximal segment. The balloon is inflated to 4 to 5 atm, and the assembly is tracked through the segment. Once the segment is crossed, the procedure is finished in the usual manner. This technique has the subtle advantage of avoiding friction and the "razor effect" while working through small and tortuous radial segments (Fig. 5-12).

Issues Related to Subclavian, Innominate, and Aortic Arch Regions

The anatomy differs on the right and left sides as far as the subclavian artery is concerned. On the right side, the subclavian artery arises from the innominate artery. On the left side, it arises from the arch of the aorta. Therefore, they differ in length, direction, and their relationship to neighboring structures in their proximal parts (Figs. 5-13 and 5-14).

The innominate–arch junction is unique to transradial procedures. Here the catheters and guidewires must take an obtuse-angle turn to enter into the ascending aorta.

In cases of normal anatomy, the turn is smooth and does not pose challenges in performing diagnostic or interventional procedures. In cases of abnormal anatomy due to dilation and/or distortion of the aorta, the procedure requires judicious use of guidewires (0.025" or 0.032" hydrophilic guidewires, standard 0.035" guidewires, and super-stiff guidewires) and catheters (unusual curves, if necessary) to complete the procedure.

Following are the important relevant issues:

- Tortuosity in subclavian region
- Severely dilated and distorted aortic route (pseudo-arteria lusoria)
- Arteria lusoria

Tortuosity in Subclavian Region

Tortuosity is divided into

- mild tortuosity (Fig. 5-15) and
- severe tortuosity (Fig. 5.16).

Old age, female gender, long-standing diabetes, and hypertension are the predictors for this issue.[2,14-18]

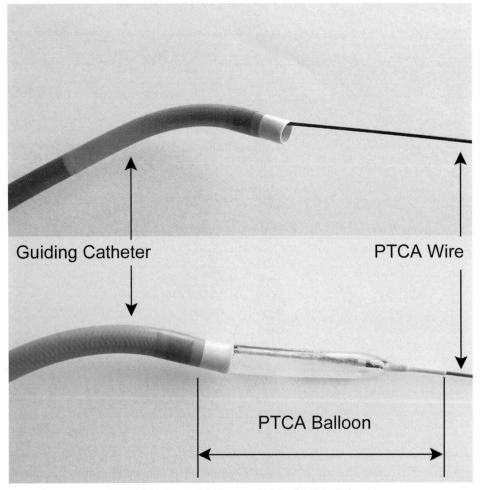

FIGURE 5-12 In vitro demonstration of BAT technique.

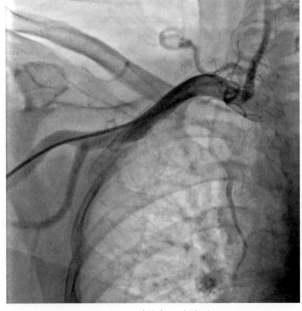

FIGURE 5-13 Normal right subclavian anatomy.

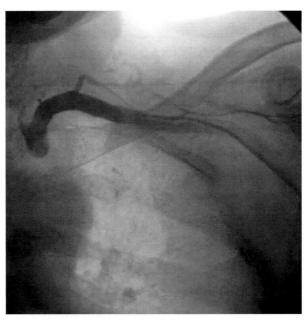

FIGURE 5-14   Normal left subclavian anatomy.

Identification and Management

- Resistance to a guidewire and/or a catheter movement in this region is an important clue.
- Gentle movement of assembly under fluoroscopic guidance leads to successful entry in ascending aorta particularly for mild tortuosity.

- The use of a super-stiff guidewire is avoided unless ascending or descending aorta is entered, as it can lead to injury and dissection in this region.
- At times, deep inspiration facilitates entry of a guidewire and catheter in ascending aorta.
- At times, in a case of severe tortuosity, despite optimal position of a guidewire in

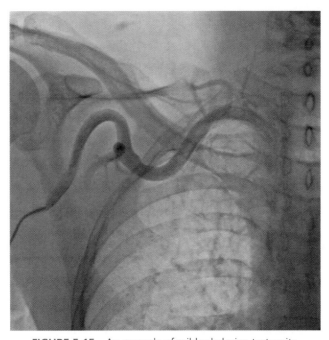

FIGURE 5-15   An example of mild subclavian tortuosity.

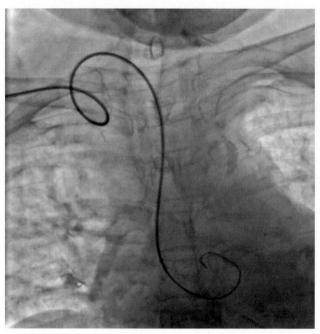

FIGURE 5-16   An example of severe subclavian tortuosity.

ascending aorta, there is severe resistance to the catheter movement at subclavian–innominate junction. At this stage, instead of pushing the catheter further over the wire, pulling the whole assembly slightly back straightens the tortuosity and allows its smooth entry in the ascending aorta.

- Always use fluoroscopic guidance while working through this region to prevent damage to origins of carotid, vertebral, or internal mammary artery.

Severely Dilated and Distorted Aortic Route (Pseudo-arteria Lusoria)

This is seen mainly in patients with advanced-stage, uncontrolled hypertension and long-standing severe aortic valve lesions. Dilatation and distortion of aorta leads to changes in the anatomy, particularly distances of origin of aortic arch branches and positions of coronary ostia[2,14–18] (Fig. 5-17).

Identification and Management

- Entry in ascending aorta is usually not so difficult; however, for coronary cannulation wider catheter curves are required.
- If the catheter has a tendency to enter the descending aorta, deep inspiration helps entry in ascending aorta.

- While working through the left radial approach, the catheter traverses through a wider angle and at times it has a tendency to slip in the descending aorta. Deep inspiration helps ascending aortic entry and wider catheter curves help coronary cannulation.

Working through Arteria Lusoria Using Right Transradial Approach

Arteria lusoria is a congenital anomaly of the right subclavian artery characterized topographically as follows: the artery originates below the left subclavian artery as the fourth main branch of the aortic arch and turns to the right behind the esophagus and in front of the vertebral column.[17–22] In over 35,000 transradial procedures, we have objectively documented arteria lusoria for 52 times (0.15%). It is a rare anomaly.

We have developed a protocol to work through this situation (Fig. 5-18).[21] It is divided into two parts: (1) entering the ascending aorta through arteria lusoria and (2) the cannulation of the coronary arteries.

1. **Entering the ascending aorta**
   - **Step 1:** The catheter and guidewire have a tendency to enter the descending aorta. If this happens, withdraw the catheter and the guidewire together as an assembly.

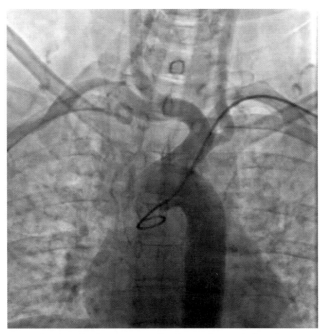

FIGURE 5-17   An example of pseudo-arteria lusoria.

After asking the patient to take a deep breath, gently push the 0.035″ standard guidewire. If the guidewire enters the ascending aorta effortlessly, you can then push the catheter over the guidewire.

- **Step 2:** If Step 1 is not successful, keep the guidewire in the descending aorta. Remove the Judkins right or left catheter, or the first catheter you tried. Take a 5F internal mammary artery (IMA) diagnostic catheter, put it into the descending aorta over the guidewire, and try the same maneuver. In many cases, you will be successful in entering the ascending aorta.
- **Step 3:** If the IMA catheter fails, then a 5F Simmon-1 catheter can be used to enter the ascending aorta.
- **Step 4:** If the 0.035″ standard guidewire has a tendency to slip into the descending aorta, the second choice is a 0.032″ or a 0.025″ hydrophilic guidewire. The slippery character of a hydrophilic guidewire facilitates relatively easy entry into the ascending aorta in challenging situations.
- **Note**
  - Prefer working in the 40° LAO view.
  - Do not use super-stiff guidewires unless you have entered the ascending aorta.
2. **Cannulation of the coronary arteries**
   Once the guidewire and the catheter are in the ascending aorta, cannulate the left or right

coronaries in the usual manner. It is relatively easy to cannulate the coronaries. If there is a challenge, follow these steps:

- **Step 1:** Remove the standard 0.035″ guidewire or the hydrophilic guidewire, keeping the catheter in the ascending aorta.
- **Step 2:** Using a 0.035″ super-stiff guidewire, make a loop of wire in the ascending aorta, and slowly slide the catheter over it so that you can make a loop of the assembly (catheter and guidewire).
- **Step 3:** Slowly pull the guidewire slightly inside the mouth of the catheter and pull the assembly back. This usually cannulates the left coronary artery.
  - For cannulation of the right coronary artery, slowly and gently rotate the assembly clockwise.
  - For diagnostic procedures, use a Judkins left, Optitorque TIG, or an Amplatz left catheter to cannulate the left coronary ostium. Sometimes, a 5F extra back-up guide catheter is useful to cannulate the left coronary ostium. Use a Judkins right or an Amplatz left catheter to cannulate the right coronary ostium.
  - For intervention in the left coronary arteries, choose any extra back-up guide catheter as your first choice. If this is not successful, use a Judkins left or an Amplatz left guide catheter.

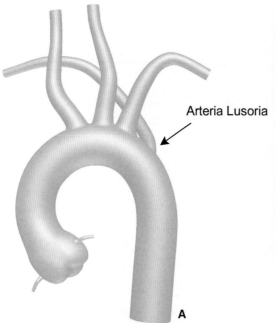

Arteria Lusoria

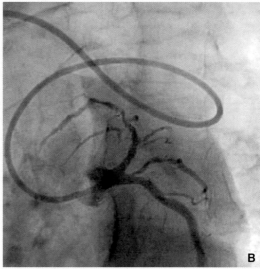

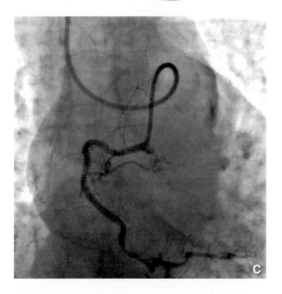

FIGURE 5-18 **A:** Schematic representation of arteria lusoria. **B:** Left coronary cannulation through arteria lusoria. **C:** Right coronary cannulation through arteria lusoria.

- For intervention in the right coronary arteries, Amplatz right is our first choice. If this does not succeed, a Judkins right or an Amplatz left catheter is used.
- **Note:** At any stage during cannulation of the coronary ostium, do not push too much or the assembly may flip into the descending aorta.

These steps may seem complicated, but arteria lusoria is very rare, and patience and perseverance can help you complete the procedure in the usual manner. If the first few attempts to enter the ascending aorta are unsuccessful, gracefully switch to the left radial or to the femoral route. Do not get discouraged. One day you will beat the learning curve and address this situation effortlessly.

Conclusion

During one's journey to become a radialist, one needs to go through a process of "a new learning curve." A new operator will take a longer time as compared to an experienced operator. One needs to understand normal vascular anatomy of the region, acquired variations, and congenital anomalies. If there are issues, they need to be resolved. In this chapter, we have done our best to resolve practically all important issues related to TRA. The tips and tricks discussed here shall help operators with different levels of experience.

Acknowledgment

The authors are thankful to Mr. Yash Soni and Mr. Chidambaram Iyer for their assistance during the preparation of this chapter.

REFERENCES

1. Coppola J, Patel T, Kwan T, et al. Nitroglycerin, nitroprusside, or both, in preventing radial artery spasm during transradial artery catheterization. *J Invasive Cardiol.* 2006; 18(4):155–158.
2. Gilchrist I. Transradial technical tips. *Catheter Cardiovasc Interv.* 2000;49(3):353–354.
3. Kiemeneij F. Prevention and management of radial artery spasm. *J Invasive Cardiol.* 2006;18(4):159–160.
4. Pancholy S, Coppola J, Patel T. Subcutaneous administration of nitroglycerin to facilitate radial artery cannulation. *Catheter Cardiovasc Interv.* 2006;68(3):389–391.
5. Patel T, Shah S, Pancholy S, et al. Radial and brachial regions: understanding and addressing the issues. In: *Patel's Atlas of Transradial Intervention: The Basics and Beyond.* Malvern, PA: HMP Communications; 2012:chap 5:37–60.
6. Barbeau G. Radial loop and extreme vessel tortuosity in the transradial approach: advantage of hydrophilic-coated guidewires and catheters. *Catheter Cardiovasc Interv.* 2003; 59(4):442–450.
7. Louvard Y, Lefèvre T. Loops and transradial approach in coronary diagnosis and intervention. *Catheter Cardiovasc Interv.* 2000;51(2):250–252.
8. Patel T, Shah S, Ranjan A. Radial region: addressing the issues. In: *Patel's Atlas of Transradial Intervention: The Basics.* Seattle, WA: Sea Script Company; 2007:chap 7:61–102.
9. Calviño-Santos R, Vázquez-Rodríguez J, Salgado-Fernández J, et al. Management of iatrogenic radial artery perforation. *Catheter Cardiovasc Interv.* 2004;61(1):74–78.
10. Patel T, Shah S, Sanghavi K, et al. Management of radial and brachial artery perforations during transradial procedures—a practical approach. *J Invasive Cardiol.* 2009;21(10):544–547.
11. Shah S, Patel T, Skelding K, et al. Complications and management. In: *Patel's Atlas of Transradial Intervention: The Basics and Beyond.* Malvern, PA: HMP Communications; 2012:chap 4:31–36.
12. Lo T, Nolan J, Fountzopoulos E, et al. Radial artery anomaly and its influence on transradial coronary procedural outcome. *Heart.* 2009;95(5):410–415.
13. Patel T, Shah S, Pancholy S. Balloon-assisted tracking of a guide catheter through difficult radial anatomy: a technical report. *Catheter Cardiovasc Interv.* 2013;81:E215–E218.
14. Caputo R, Simons A, Giambartolomei A, et al. Transradial cardiac catheterization in elderly patients. *Catheter Cardiovasc Interv.* 2000;51(3):287–290.
15. Cha K, Kim M, Kim H. Prevalence and clinical predictors of severe tortuosity of right subclavian artery in patients undergoing transradial coronary angiography. *Am J Cardiol.* 2003;92(10):1220–1222.
16. Dehghani P, Mohammad A, Bajaj R, et al. Mechanism and predictors of failed transradial approach for percutaneous coronary interventions. *JACC Cardiovasc Interv.* 2009;2(11):1057–1064.
17. Valsecchi O, Vassileva A, Musumeci G, et al. Failure of transradial approach during coronary interventions: anatomic considerations. *Catheter Cardiovasc Interv.* 2006;67(6):870–878.
18. Patel T, Shah S, Radadiya R. Subclavian, innominate and aortic arch regions: understanding and addressing the issues. In: *Patel's Atlas of Transradial Intervention: The Basics and Beyond.* Malvern, PA: HMP Communications; 2012:chap 6:61–82.
19. Abhaichand R, Louvard Y, Gobeil J, et al. The problem of arteria lusoria in right transradial coronary angiography and angioplasty. *Catheter Cardiovasc Interv.* 2001; 54(2):196–201.
20. Grollman J Jr. The many faces of the anomalous left aortic arch. *Catheter Cardiovasc Interv.* 2001;54(2):202–203.
21. Patel T. Right trans-radial approach-working through arteria lusoria. *Indian Heart J.* 2006;58(4):301.
22. Yiu K, Chan W, Jim M, et al. Arteria lusoria diagnosed by transradial coronary catheterization. *JACC Cardiovasc Interv.* 2010;3(8):880–881.

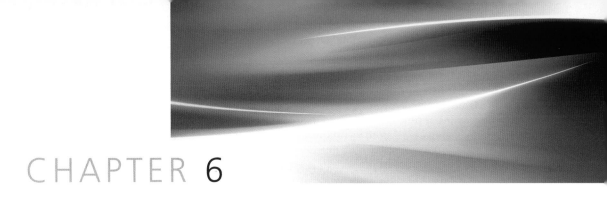

CHAPTER 6

Radial Artery versus Ulnar Artery Catheterization

Sasko Kedev

Background

Since its initial description as a safe and feasible access route for cardiac catheterization,[1,2] the radial artery access has increasingly been used for percutaneous cardiovascular procedures. The main advantage over the transfemoral approach (TFA) is a reduced risk of access site bleeding and major vascular complications, particularly in the presence of multiple antiplatelet and antithrombotic agents.[3,4]

While transradial angiography (TRA) is used in many catheterization laboratories worldwide, the ulnar artery approach has received very little attention as a potential access for cardiac catheterization.[5,6] The first efforts at retrograde arterial catheterization of the left ventricle involved the use of ulnar artery cut-down for arterial access. Zimmerman et al.[7] used this approach for the first successful retrograde catheterization of the left ventricle in 1949 in 11 patients with aortic insufficiency. The transulnar approach (TUA) for coronary angiography was first reported by Terashima et al.[8] in 2001, and a few preliminary reports on a small number of patients have suggested that the ulnar approach may be both feasible and safe for coronary angiography and percutaneous coronary intervention (PCI) in selected patients.[9-13]

Potential advantages of the ulnar approach are related to the reasons for failure of the radial approach. Specifically, anatomical variations of the radial artery such as loops and high bifurcations can complicate smooth passage of equipment through the arm,[14] and the TUA can be used in these cases as well as in cases of radial access failure due to small-caliber radial artery or severe radial artery spasm. In some of these difficult

transradial cases, ulnar artery cannulation may serve as a reasonable and useful alternative to the TRA because of its usual straight course. Transulnar cannulation has characteristics similar to those of the TRA, and a prospective, randomized trial by Aptecar et al. suggested that the procedures were equivalent. No difference was found regarding rates of access success, procedural success, procedure time, fluoroscopy time, and cardiac and access site complications with the two techniques. The TUA was also associated with low incidence of access site vascular complications, that is, minor bleeding, few asymptomatic artery occlusions, no hand ischemia, very rare arteriovenous fistula, and pseudoaneurysm.[14] In another randomized trial, Li et al. showed that the TUA is as safe and effective as the TRA for coronary angiography and intervention. In contrast, a randomized trial by Hahalis and colleagues compared radial with ulnar access in 902 patients at five centers and was stopped early because of inferiority of the ulnar approach with respect to access site crossover, major adverse cardiac events (MACE), and major arm vascular events.[15] This underscores that radial approach is the preferred approach for coronary angiography and intervention, and that ulnar approach can be considered a back-up technique. Furthermore, the relationship between ulnar approach and outcomes may be influenced by operator experience.[16]

Results of the First International Transradial Practice Survey showed that in cases of radial artery failure, the homolateral ulnar artery approach was preferred only by 3.3% of overall surveyed operators, and up to 9.1% by operators in China.[17] For institutions that use the radial approach routinely, with experienced high-volume operators, the TUA might be of particular benefit when the radial artery access site is not available or at high risk of failure or complications, mostly after repeated radial artery catheterizations.[16,18,19] Both techniques from the wrist share a high success rate, an extremely low incidence of entry site complications, reduced costs and length of hospital stay.

Anatomic Considerations

The radial artery and the ulnar artery are the two terminal branches of the brachial artery. The radial artery appears to be the continuation of the brachial artery. It commences at the bifurcation of the brachial, and passes along the radial side of the forearm to the wrist. Into the palm of the hand, it crosses the metacarpal bones and, at the ulnar side of the hand, unites with the deep palmar branch of the ulnar artery to form the deep palmar arch.

The *ulnar artery* is usually the larger (1.35/1 ratio to the radial artery)[20,21] and the less tortuous of the two terminal branches of the brachial artery, which makes it less prone to spasm. It begins below the bend of the elbow and, passing obliquely downward, reaches the ulnar side of the forearm at a point about midway between the elbow and the wrist. Then it runs along the ulnar border to the wrist, crosses the transverse carpal ligament on the radial side of the pisiform bone, and, immediately beyond this bone, divides into two branches, which enter into the formation of the superficial and deep palmar arches. At the wrist, the ulnar artery terminates in the superficial palmar arch, which is a major source of arterial inflow for fingers of the ulnar portion of the hand (Figs. 6-1 and 6-2).

About one inch below the origin of the ulnar artery, common *interosseous artery* arises and divides into anterior and posterior branches. In the instance of a high takeoff of the ulnar artery, the common interosseous artery in the majority of cases arises from the radial artery or from the brachial artery. In most patients with radial artery occlusion (RAO), anterior interosseous branches provide significant collateral flow distal to the RAO.

In the forearm, the ulnar artery is deeper and therefore less palpable than the radial artery; as it passes down the forearm, it lies just lateral (deep) to the ulnar nerve. Exactly above the middle of the forearm, the ulnar nerve joins the artery, lying to its ulnar side, and accompanies it down into the hand.

The superficial palmar arch (primarily ulnar) and *the deep palmar arch* (primarily radial) are functionally important arterial connections between the ulnar artery and the radial artery.[20,21] The superficial arch is much larger and more important

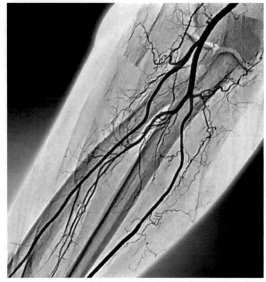

FIGURE 6-1   Normal anatomy of the forearm arteries.

than the deep palmar arch. The perfusion territory shows considerable overlap between the deep arch from the radial artery and the superficial palmar arch from the ulnar artery. However, the superficial arch is more often incomplete than the deep arch, as shown by anatomical studies[22,23] (Fig. 6-3).

Although the deep palmar arch is found to be angiographically complete in 95% of subjects, a complete superficial palmar arch is seen in only 40% to 80% of individuals, depending on the mode of study.[21] This probably explains the relatively

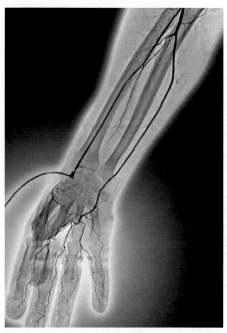

FIGURE 6-2   Superficial and deep palmar arch.

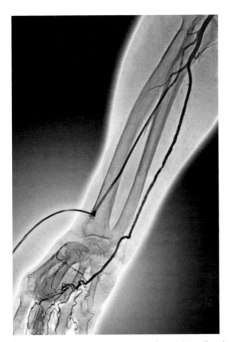

FIGURE 6-3   Superficial palmar arch—primarily ulnar.

high incidence of abnormal Allen test results,[24] an indication that ulnar collateral support to the hand is inadequate in a significant proportion of individuals. The high prevalence of a complete deep palmar arch suggests that radial collateral support is more frequently present, and that cannulation of the ulnar artery should be relatively safe (Fig. 6-4).[14]

Slogoff et al.,[25] reporting on the safety of radial and ulnar artery cannulation, described a subset of 22 patients who underwent ipsilateral ulnar artery cannulation after numerous failed attempts at radial artery cannulation. No patient experienced ulnar artery occlusion or signs and symptoms of hand ischemia. For the vast majority of patients, the smaller-caliber, more superficial radial artery is easier to palpate at the wrist than the ulnar artery; the radial artery is properly the target for access in these individuals.[26] However, in a small number of patients, the ulnar artery is palpably the larger vessel at the wrist and is the reasonable choice for cannulation (Figs. 6-5 and 6-6).

Similar to the radial artery, the ulnar artery can also have anatomical variation. The most common cases of *ulnar artery variations* (7.7%) are *ulnar artery with high takeoff* from the brachial or axillary artery. The brachial artery is the more frequent site of the ulnar artery takeoff, with the lower portion being more common than the upper portion.[27,28] The superficial ulnar artery is a rare variation of the upper limb arterial system that arises from the brachial or axillary artery and runs superficial to the muscles arising from the medial epicondyle. The variable incidence is about 0.7% to 7% (Figs. 6-7 and 6-8).[18]

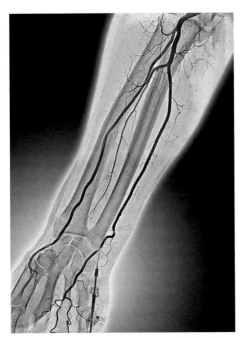

FIGURE 6-4   Incomplete superficial palmar arch: retrograde ulnar arteriography with cannula.

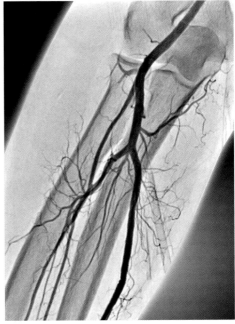

FIGURE 6-5   Hypoplastic radial artery and larger-size ulnar artery.

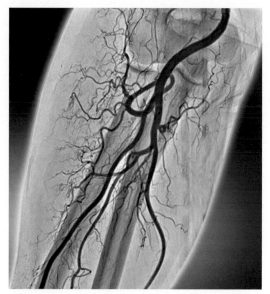

FIGURE 6-6 Very complex 360° loop of the radial artery distal to the bifurcation of the brachial artery.

Loops and curvatures of the ulnar artery are very rarely encountered in comparison to the radial artery equivalents.

Furthermore, the radial artery and the ulnar artery atherosclerosis and calcifications may be an important marker for extensive extracardiac

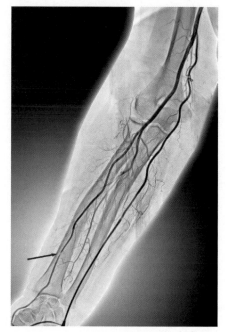

FIGURE 6-8 TUA with high takeoff of the ulnar artery from the midbrachial artery, after failed radial artery cannulation *(left arrow sign)*.

vascular disease. Many such patients were found to have severe brachiocephalic tortuosity that could not be navigated, leading to procedural failure, especially during the initial learning phase.[29]

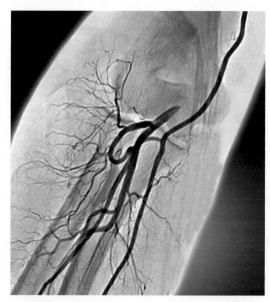

FIGURE 6-7 Radial artery loop and high takeoff of the ulnar artery.

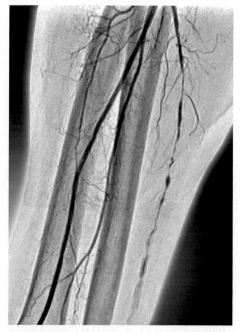

FIGURE 6-9 Severely atheromatous and calcified right ulnar artery.

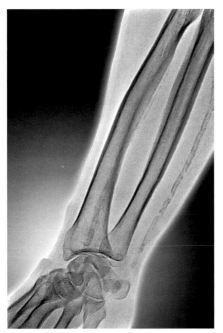

FIGURE 6-10 Calcifications of both right radial and ulnar arteries.

The early recognition of such anatomy at procedure outset is important for avoiding potential complications (Figs. 6-9 to 6-11).[30]

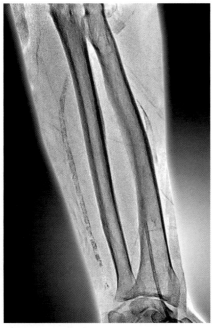

FIGURE 6-11 Left ulnar artery calcifications in the same patient.

Allen Tests, Pulse Oximetry, and Doppler Plethysmography

Allen test is done on the right or left wrist, and its purpose is to determine the ulnar artery patency and adequate radial–ulnar collaterals to the hand.

A reverse Allen test is performed by compressing both the radial and ulnar arteries and having the patient make fist clenches several times. In contrast to the Allen test, in which pressure on the ulnar artery is released, for the reverse Allen test, occlusion of the ulnar artery is maintained while pressure on the radial artery is released. If there is return of blush to the palm within 10 seconds, the test is considered positive and indicates adequate collateral supply to the hand.

The modified Allen test should be performed in order to assess the adequacy of the ulnar artery supply to the palmar arch. It can be conducted with the *pulse oximeter* sensor placed over the index finger. A normal waveform should be observed before arterial compression. The test is conducted in the same manner, but instead of observing hand color when releasing the ulnar artery, the pulse oximetry tracing is examined. The tracing is initially blunted or flat when both the radial and ulnar arteries are occluded. The tracing should return to the baseline within 10 seconds after releasing the ulnar artery for the test to be considered normal. The presence of an arterial waveform (even if delayed or with reduced amplitude) and a hemoglobin oxygen saturation >90% confirm the adequacy of the ulnar artery supply to the palmar arch.[31] The pulse oximetry method is preferred, because it is not as subjective as the traditional Allen test. For the *Doppler plethysmography test*, the radial and ulnar arteries are compressed sequentially while confirming normal audible signal intensity over the palmar arch. Doppler plethysmography and pulse oximetry are of particular importance for ensuring "patent hemostasis" after sheath removal.

Puncture Technique

Preprocedure evaluation of the wrist includes palpation of both the radial and the ulnar arteries, with access attempted of the more superficial vessel, provided there is demonstrated competent palmar collateral support to the hand by the ipsilateral complementary vessel.[9]

A large enough area should be prepared to cover both the radial and ulnar arteries, and to place the sterile drape so that it need not be moved in the event the ulnar artery is used.

The wrist is hyperextended and the skin is prepared with local anesthesia (1-mL lidocaine 2%) at the site where the pulse is strongest, usually 0.5 to 3 cm proximal to the pisiform bone for ulnar artery and 1 to 2 cm proximal from the styloid process for radial artery access. Compression of the ipsilateral radial artery could improve weak or hardly palpable ulnar artery pulsations and facilitate ulnar artery cannulation. The ideal ulnar artery puncture site is approximately 0.5 to 3 cm proximal to the flexor crease skinfold along the axis with the most powerful pulsation of the artery. The needle should be inserted at a 45° to 60° angle along the vessel axis and from lateral to medial, avoiding the ulnar nerve. The ulnar artery is preferentially punctured with a 20G plastic cannula using the Seldinger technique. When a good arterial "back bleed" is obtained, the 0.025" hydrophilic wire guidewire should be gently advanced and the hydrophilic sheath should be introduced over the guidewire (Fig. 6-12).

An intra-arterial vasodilator (most frequently 5-mg verapamil) is injected via the cannula or through the sidearm of the sheath to reduce ulnar artery spasm. In order to prevent the painful and burning sensations, blood is mixed with verapamil before injection. Immediately after sheath insertion, intravenous unfractionated heparin should be administered (50–70 U/kg, up to 5,000 units) to reduce the risk of radial artery thrombosis (Fig. 6-13).

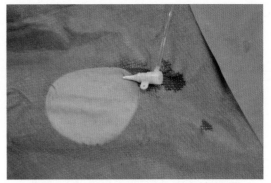

FIGURE 6-13 Short 5F sheath in the right ulnar artery.

Procedure failure for ulnar artery access is almost always related to the puncture, which can be more difficult than the radial artery puncture, because of the deeper ulnar artery course and lower intensity of pulsations.

Distal puncture of the ulnar artery: In cases when ulnar artery pulsations are weak but palpable at the distal wrist, it is safe to puncture the ulnar artery more distally, at the level of skinfolds (over the carpal bones). The risk of postprocedural hematoma is lower when puncturing the ulnar artery near the wrist's skinfolds (Fig. 6-14).

High puncture of the ulnar artery: Although the ideal site for puncture is 0.5 to 3 cm proximal to the pisiform bone, the ulnar artery can be punctured up to the midforearm as long as the pulsations can be felt. This approach may be useful for an experienced operator performing coronary or endovascular interventions requiring larger-bore devices. However, the ulnar nerve is very close to

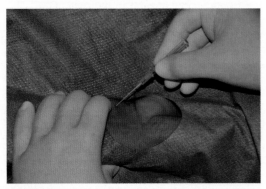

FIGURE 6-12 Puncture of the right ulnar artery with a 20G plastic cannula by the Seldinger technique.

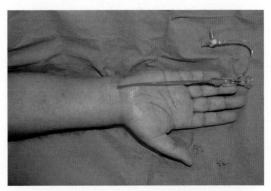

FIGURE 6-14 Distal cannulation of the right ulnar artery with 90-cm-long 6F (inner lumen) guiding sheath for carotid artery stenting.

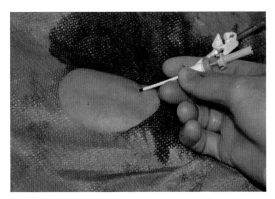

FIGURE 6-15   Initial ulnar artery cannulation with short 5F sheath, before exchanging with larger-bore dedicated sheathless guiding catheter.

the ulnar artery in that region, and so the puncture has to be very accurate and the operator has to be very cautious, avoiding accidental nerve damage.[18]

Once the sheath is in place, the transulnar procedure is performed in the same manner as the transradial catheterization.

Particular care should be undertaken while exchanging and upgrading sheaths of different sizes with dedicated sheathless guiding catheters, in order to avoid local bleeding complications related to the inappropriately sized devices. For example, this could be the case when the initial 6F introducer sheath is exchanged with 7.5F dedicated sheathless guiding catheter that has smaller outer lumen diameter. Therefore, a short 4F or 5F introducer sheath is recommended initially when complex procedures with larger-bore devices and sheathless guiding catheter exchanges are considered (Figs. 6-15 and 6-16).

Retrograde Arteriography of the Wrist

Radial and ulnar artery anomalies are relatively common and a cause of procedural failure even for experienced radial operators. Retrograde radial and ulnar arteriography helps to assess the diameter of the arteries and delineate underlying anomalies. By identifying patients with unfavorable anatomy, the operator could plan a strategy to overcome the anomaly or change access route with the potential to save time and avoid vascular complications.[29]

After administration of the arterial vasodilatator, a solution of 3 mL of contrast mixed with 7 mL of blood is injected briskly through the cannula or through the side arm of the sheath under fluoroscopy in anterior–posterior (AP) position to define the anatomy of arteries from the distal forearm to the brachial anastomosis (Fig. 6-17).

When high-bifurcating radial or ulnar artery origin is detected, a further arteriography is needed to identify higher up the point of anastomosis to the brachial or to the axillary artery.

If anomalous anatomy, tortuosity, or loops are identified, the operator can further plan the procedure on that basis. In most cases, crossing with hydrophilic coronary guidewire under

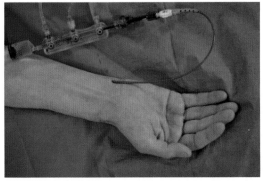

FIGURE 6-16   Right TUA for complex PCI with 7.5F (outer lumen) dedicated sheathless guiding catheter.

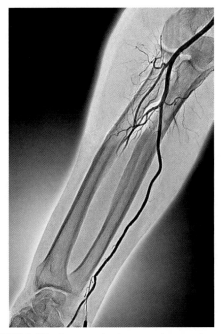

FIGURE 6-17   Retrograde ulnar arteriogram through a cannula.

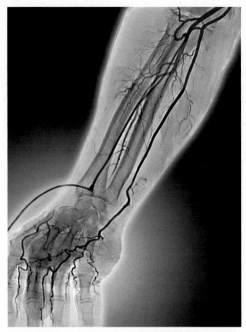

FIGURE 6-18 Road map from retrograde radial arteriogram in a patient with radial artery loop and high takeoff of the ulnar artery.

fluorography control is highly recommended (Fig. 6-18).

The acquisition of a radial and ulnar arteriogram requires only a minimal contrast load, a small

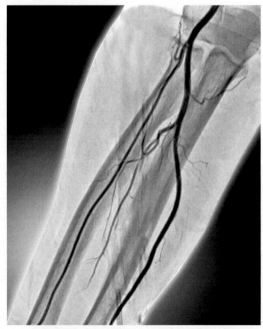

FIGURE 6-19 Right ulnar arteriogram showing larger-size ulnar artery eligible for large-bore 7F catheterization.

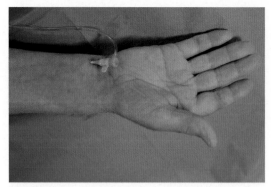

FIGURE 6-20 Right TUA with 7F sheath in place for complex PCI.

amount of additional radiation, and trivial extra procedural time. Retrograde angiogram of the wrist is of particular importance in patients with several previous transradial interventions. By providing important road map and estimating the artery dimension, it aids the operator to plan an optimal procedure with appropriately-sized catheters.

Moreover, an angiography of the wrist can be incorporated as a routine part of either transradial or transulnar catheterization, particularly in complex procedures requiring large-bore devices (Figs. 6-19 and 6-20).

Postprocedure Management

The sheath is removed immediately after the procedure, regardless of the level of anticoagulation, and a compressive dressing or compression device is applied. Several hemostatic devices have been proposed for selective compression of the target radial or ulnar artery. Care must be taken while compressing the target artery in order to prevent venous stasis and unnecessary contralateral artery occlusion.

Patent hemostasis has been proven as highly effective in reducing RAO after transradial catheterization.[32]

Capillary refill, index finger pulse oximetry, and Doppler plethysmography are used to monitor hand perfusion. Guided compression should be performed to maintain the target artery patency at the time of hemostasis and to prevent future radial or ulnar artery occlusion.

The technique of patent hemostasis after transulnar catheterization is the same as after the TRA. The sheath should be partially withdrawn and a plastic band placed around the forearm at the entry site. While a pulse oximeter sensor is placed over the index finger, the hemostasis

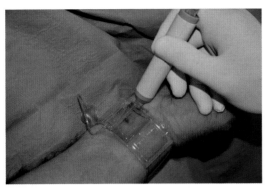

FIGURE 6-21 Doppler plethysmography after ensuring patent hemostasis at the right ulnar artery.

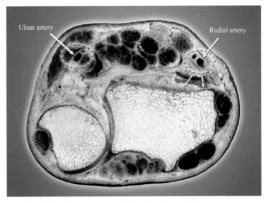

FIGURE 6-23 Cross section of the wrist: no underlying bone base for the ulnar artery.

device is tightened, and the sheath completely removed. The ipsilateral radial artery should be occluded and the device loosened until plethysmographic signal returned (confirming ulnar artery patency) or bleeding occurred. If bleeding occurs at the pressure required to maintain patency, the device should be tightened until bleeding stops.

Compression should be applied for approximately a 2- to 3-hour period (depending on the sheath size), with gradual relaxation of compression after the first hour (Figs. 6-21 and 6-22).

The absence of a good underlying bone base, as is the case with radial artery, makes the ulnar artery hemostasis slightly more difficult, particularly in cases with more proximal TUA.

More distal puncture, closer to the wrist's skin folds, is associated with more predictable hemostasis (over the carpal bones) and lower risk of hematomas (Fig. 6-23).

Compressive dressing is mandatory with a higher puncture site, because of the deeper artery location and greater risk of hematoma. The patient's arm should be closely monitored for signs and symptoms of local bleeding or hand ischemia.

Before discharge, patients should be instructed to keep the puncture site clean, dry, covered with an adhesive bandage until healed, and to limit use of the catheterized arm for 24 hours.

Potential Benefits of the Transulnar Approach

Repeat comparison with TFA showed a clear advantage of the TRA for minimizing or near eliminating vascular complications and suggested that the radial approach could also be associated with improved clinical outcomes.[33–37] The available clinical evidence summarized in a recent meta-analysis of 14 studies demonstrated that radial catheterization was favored over femoral catheterization in the cost–benefit analysis.[38]

However, the radial approach does not seem appropriate for 5% to 15% of patients undergoing cardiac catheterization for reasons including an abnormal Allen test[24]; significant anatomic variations such as loops, tortuous configurations, stenoses, hypoplasia, and aberrant origin[29,39,40]; and vasospasm, leading to radial artery access procedural failure (Figs. 6-24 and 6-25).[36,41,42]

Other reasons, such as local scarring, previous hand injury, granulomas, synovial cysts, local hematomas due to previous intravenous line placement, or artery punctures for blood gas

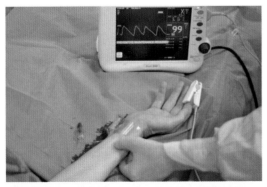

FIGURE 6-22 TUA patent hemostasis confirmed with ipsilateral RAO and plethysmographic signal with pulse oximetry (99%) from the sensor placed over the index finger.

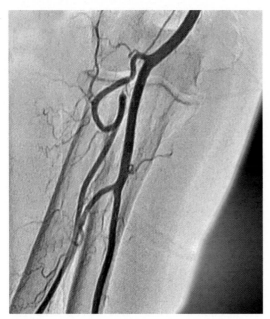

FIGURE 6-24 Radial artery loop, proximal to the brachial bifurcation.

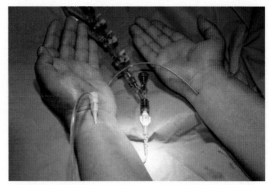

FIGURE 6-26 Bilateral wrist approach for CTO PCI: right TUA with 7.5F sheathless guiding catheter and left TRA with 5F sheath for contralateral injections.

measurement can preclude the use of the radial artery approach.

Thus, when the transradial access is not possible or fails, the TUA may be considered as a safe alternative before reverting to the TFA.[43,44] (See Fig. 6-8, TUA after failed radial artery puncture.)

Remarkably, even complex procedures requiring larger-bore devices, as is the case of the bifurcation PCI,[45] rotational atherectomy,[46] PCI for chronic total occlusions,[47] and carotid artery stenting,[18] can be safely performed through the ulnar access (Figs. 6-26 and 6-27).

The TUA might be particularly useful in patients with several previous transradial catheterizations associated with smaller-size radial artery lumen due to intimal hyperplasia (Figs. 6-28 and 6-29).

Furthermore, the ulnar artery approach may be valuable as a radial artery-sparing procedure in anticipation of its use as a coronary bypass conduit,[48] or dialysis fistula in patients with advanced renal failure.

There are several *potential benefits of using the ulnar artery approach* after an event of failed

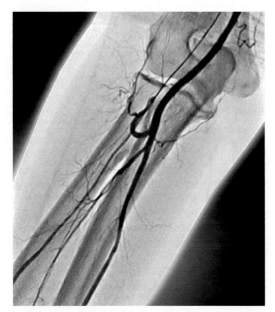

FIGURE 6-25 Small-size radial artery with loop and remnant artery arising from the loop.

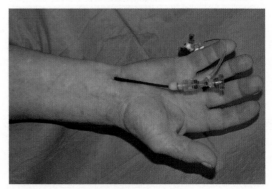

FIGURE 6-27 Right TUA with 6F/90-cm-long guiding sheath for carotid artery stenting.

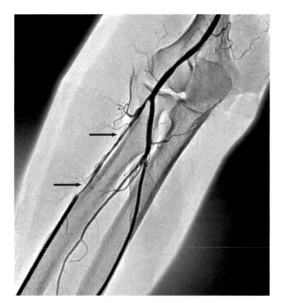

FIGURE 6-28 Smaller-size radial artery due to lumen loss related to several previous transradial catheterizations.

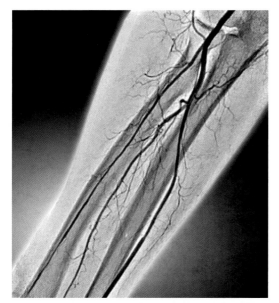

FIGURE 6-29 Right TUA after repetitive ipsilateral TRA procedures.

radial artery cannulation, but with confirmed radial artery patency:

- There is no time wasted in preparing the opposite arm or leg.
- The same sheath, wire, and needle can be used on the ulnar approach as for the radial access.

- Once the sheath is in place, manipulation of the coronary catheter with the ulnar approach is not different from the radial site.
- Even in the clinical setting of in which the avoidance of the TFA is likely to be of greatest benefit due to the aggressive concomitant antiplatelet/antithrombotic therapy and higher access site bleeding risk.[11,49,50]

Hence, homolateral ulnar access should be attempted only by very experienced high-volume radial operators with expertise in ulnar artery cannulation.[19]

The possible risks related to this kind of procedure, mainly specific bleeding complications and hand ischemia, should be considered. Currently, there is no large enough relevant scientific data available for recommending routine crossover to homolateral ulnar cannulation after failed radial access.

Limitations of the Transulnar Approach

The TUA can be more challenging when compared with TRA, with a *steeper learning curve.* However, for the extensively experienced transradial operator, the learning curve can be significantly shorter.[16] Although similar in size, the radial artery is more superficial and thus easier to palpate at the wrist than the ulnar artery. The limitation of the TUA could be due to the different anatomical orientation of the ulnar artery, which lies deeper around or just below the tendon of the muscle flexor carpi ulnaris.

In many cases, hyperextension of the wrist and transient compression of the radial artery markedly facilitate ulnar pulse perception and ulnar artery cannulation.

Since there is no underlying bone base, hemostasis of the ulnar artery is sometimes more challenging and requires more frequent control to prevent bleeding complications. Furthermore, the close proximity with the ulnar nerve can make the puncture very painful and rarely there is a chance of traumatic ulnar nerve injury.

Perioperative assessment of hand circulation by physical examination or by Doppler plethysmography is recommended, especially in patients with a history of previous TRA PCI. Multiple radial punctures may cause unilateral or bilateral RAO or atrophy. Therefore, before attempting the TUA, the operator should be aware of these

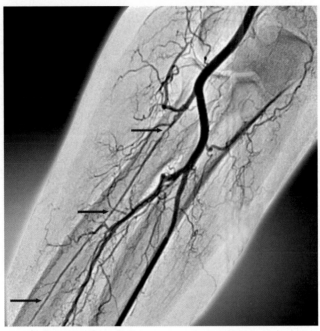

FIGURE 6-30 Right TUA in a patient with "shrinked" but patent ipsilateral radial artery from multiple TRA procedures.

considerations to avoid the extremely rare complication of hand ischemia after the transulnar intervention (Fig. 6-30).

Entry Site Complications

The radial and the ulnar artery approaches are associated with very low incidence (0.2%) of major vascular complications.[51]

Hematomas are usually minor, affecting only subcutaneous tissue.

RAO, although usually asymptomatic, is an important consequence of TRA, as it prohibits future ipsilateral radial access.[52] *Asymptomatic occlusion of the ulnar artery* is reported in less than 6% of patients.[14,16] Most frequently, it is related to the prolonged high-pressure compression, repeated ulnar artery interventions, and the use of larger sheath size compared to the ulnar artery diameter. It is almost never clinically significant because of the anatomy of the deep and superficial palmar arches that allow the radial and the interosseal arteries to deliver a collateral vascular supply to the hand. Every effort should be made to avoid occlusion of the ulnar artery, with the same strategy as for preserving the radial artery patency.

Ulnar artery spasm is less frequent than radial artery spasm and more common during the initial learning curve and is associated with multiple catheter exchanges and excessive manipulations.

Ulnar artery dissection/perforation and branch perforation resulting in forearm hematoma are rare minor complications linked to aggressive blind wire manipulation.

Although there is a theoretical basis for an increased risk of *ulnar nerve injury* with cannulation, clinical reports have failed to demonstrate any evidence of such trauma.[8,9,13,14,16]

However, patients may experience a "lightening-flash" sensation in the hand if the ulnar nerve is contacted with the micro puncture needle.

Granuloma formation at the access site has been associated with specific hydrophilic sheath use at the radial site. Cases of *arteriovenous fistula* and *pseudoaneurysm* are extremely rare.

Very uncommon potential complications are *compartment syndrome* and *hand ischemia,* where there is coexistent radial artery flow compromise or more commonly distal embolization of arterial thrombus.

It is important to remember that almost all potential complications are preventable by proper preprocedural evaluation, meticulous

TABLE 6-1 Advantages and Disadvantages of Transulnar Approach

Advantages
- All the associated benefits of transradial access: less complications, comfort, earlier ambulation, and patient's preference
- Larger diameter than the radial artery
- Straighter course than the radial artery
- Loops and curvatures are very rare
- Less prone to spasm than the radial artery
- The procedure after puncture is the same as transradial

Disadvantages
- Learning curve
- Puncture of the ulnar artery is more difficult than radial artery puncture
- Deeper position of the ulnar artery without underlying bone makes compression hemostasis more difficult
- Ulnar artery runs closely to the ulnar nerve
- High origin of the ulnar artery is more prone to spasm, thus making the procedure more challenging at times

TABLE 6-2 Potential Indications for Transulnar Access for Cardiovascular Interventions

- The stronger pulsation of the ulnar artery in patient with small-caliber radial artery or thin radial pulse
- Failed radial artery puncture (only puncture without sheath insertion)
- Confirmed complex most challenging loops and curvatures of the radial artery
- Previous multiple transradial interventions—but the patient must have positive reverse Allen test (<10 s)
- Previous large-bore (7F/8F sheath) transradial interventions with confirmed radial artery patency
- In patients requiring a large-bore device for complex PCI or CAS, after previous transradial interventions with confirmed radial artery patency
- If the radial artery has to be utilized for a bypass graft in patient with multivessel CAD or for dialysis fistula in patients with advanced renal failure

technique, and optimal postprocedural management (Tables 6-1 and 6-2).[53]

Conclusion

Considerable evidence supports conversion to radial access for most PCI procedures, with an emphasis on decreasing access site bleeding and vascular complications without compromising procedural outcome.

Besides the development of new more selective and safe antithrombotic agents, the use of radial access remains likely the best way to significantly minimize access site–related bleeding risk. The TUA for diagnostic catheterization and PCI can be considered a "second line" approach and can be a safe and effective alternative to the transradial access when used by experienced operators.

Therefore, the modern interventional cardiologist should go through a high-volume radial training program and after developing the optimal transradial and transulnar expertise to adopt "the wrist approach first" whenever possible. Femoral access will likely remain the viable alternative for patients not eligible for the wrist access.

Finally, it is important to remember that the choice of access site is only one aspect of improving the patient's outcome. All interventions should be performed according to the highest available standards, providing the best care for each individual patient, without sacrificing procedural success and long-term prognosis.

REFERENCES

1. Campeau L. Percutaneous radial artery approach for coronary angiography. *Cathet Cardiovasc Diagn.* 1989;16:3–7.
2. Kiemeneij F, Laarman GJ. Percutaneous transradial artery approach for coronary stent implantation. *Cathet Cardiovasc Diagn.* 1993;30:173–178.
3. Rao SV, Ou FS, Wang TY, et al. Trends in the prevalence and outcomes of radial and femoral approaches to percutaneous coronary intervention: a report from the National Cardiovascular Data Registry. *J Am Coll Cardiol Interv.* 2008;1:379–386.
4. Kiemeneij F, Laarman GJ, Odekerken D, et al. A randomized comparison of percutaneous transluminal coronary angioplasty by the radial, brachial and femoral approaches: the access study. *J Am Coll Cardiol.* 1997; 29:1269–1275.
5. Aptecar E, Dupouy P, Chabane-Chaouch M, et al. Percutaneous transulnar artery approach for coronary diagnostic and therapeutic interventions. *J Invasive Cardiol.* 2005;17:312–317.
6. Mangin L, Bertrand OF, De La Rochelliere R, et al. The transulnar approach for coronary intervention: a safe alternative to transradial approach in selected patients. *J Invasive Cardiol.* 2005;17:77–79.
7. Zimmerman HA, Scott RW, Becker NO. Catheterization of the left side of the heart in man. *Circulation.* 1950;1:357–359.
8. Terashima M, Meguro T, Takeda H, et al. Percutaneous ulnar artery approach for coronary angiography: a preliminary report in nine patients. *Catheter Cardiovasc Interv.* 2001;53:410–414.
9. Dashkoff N, Dashkoff PB, Zizzi JA Sr, et al. Ulnar artery cannulation for coronary angiography and percutaneous coronary intervention: case reports and anatomic considerations. *Catheter Cardiovasc Interv.* 2002;55:93–96.
10. Fu X. Feasibility of percutaneous coronary intervention via transulnar artery approach in selected patients with coronary heart disease. angiosoft.net
11. Limbruno U, Rossini R, De Carlo M, et al. Percutaneous ulnar artery approach for primary coronary angioplasty: safety and feasibility. *Catheter Cardiovasc Interv.* 2004;61(1):56–59.
12. Lanspa T, Reyes A, Oldemeyer J, et al. Ulnar artery catheterization with occlusion of corresponding radial artery. *Catheter Cardiovasc Interv.* 2004;61(2):211–213.
13. Lanspa TJ, Williams MA, Heirigs RL. Effectiveness of ulnar artery catheterization after failed attempt to cannulate a radial artery. *Am J Cardiol.* 2005;95:1529–1530.
14. Aptecar E, Pernes J, Chabane-Chaouch M, et al. Transulnar versus transradial artery approach for coronary angioplasty: the PCVI-CUBA study. *Catheter Cardiovasc Interv.* 2006;67(5):711–720.
15. Hahalis G, Tsigkas G, Xanthopoulou I, et al. Transulnar compared with transradial artery approach as a default strategy for coronary procedures: a randomized trial the transulnar or transradial instead of coronary transfemoral angiographies study (The AURA of ARTEMIS Study). *Circ Cardiovasc Interv.* 2013;6:252–261.
16. Li YZ, Zhou YX, Zhao YX, et al. Safety and efficacy of transulnar approach for coronary angiography and intervention. *Chin Med J.* 2010;123(13):1774–1779.
17. Bertrand OF, Rao SV, Pancholy S, et al. Transradial approach for coronary angiography and interventions: results of the first international transradial practice survey. *JACC Cardiovasc Interv.* 2010;3(10):1022–1031.
18. Kedev S. Transulnar approach: pros and cons. In: Patel T, ed. *Patel's Atlas of Transradial Intervention: The Basics and Beyond.* Malvern, PA: HMP Communications; 2012:221–232.
19. Kedev S, Zafirovska B, Dharma S, et al. Safety and feasibility of translunar catheterization when ipsilateral radial access is not available. *Catherization and Cardiovascular Interventions.* 2014;83: E51–E60.
20. Gray H. *Anatomy of the Human Body.* 38th ed. London, England: Churchill Livingstone; 1995:1542–1544.
21. Vogelzang RL. Arteriography of the hand and wrist. *Hand Clin.* 1991;7:63–86.
22. Jaschtchinski S. Morphologie und topography des Arcus volaris sublimes und profundus des Menschen. *Anat Hefte.* 1897;7:161–168.
23. Koman LA, Urbaniak JR. Ulnar artery thrombosis. In: Brunelli G, ed. *Textbook of Microsurgery.* Milan, Italy: Masson; 1988:75–83.
24. Benit E, Vranckx P, Jaspers L, et al. Frequency of a positive modified Allen's test in 1,000 consecutive patients undergoing cardiac catheterization. *Cathet Cardiovasc Diagn.* 1996;38:352–354.
25. Slogoff S, Keats AS, Arlund C. On the safety of radial artery cannulation. *Anesthesiology.* 1983;59:42–47.
26. Vassilev D, Smilkova D, Gil R. Ulnar artery as access site for cardiac catheterization: anatomical considerations. *J Interv Cardiol.* 2008;21(1):56–60.
27. Rodriguez-Baeza A, Nebot J, Ferreira B, et al. An anatomical study and ontogenetic explanation of 23 cases with variations in the main pattern of the human brachio-antebrachial arteries. *J Anat.* 1995;187(pt 2):473–479.
28. Rodriguez-Niedenfuhr M, Vazquez T, Nearn L, et al. Variations of the arterial pattern in the upper limb revisited: a morphological and statistical study, with a review of the literature. *J Anat.* 2001;199(pt 5):547–566.
29. Lo TS, Nolan J, Fountzopoulos E, et al. Radial artery anomaly and its influence on transradial coronary procedural outcome. *Heart.* 2009;95:410–415.
30. Louvard Y, Lefevre T. Loops and transradial approach in coronary diagnosis and intervention. *Catheter Cardiovasc Interv.* 2000;51:250–252.
31. Barbeau GR, Arsenault F, Dugas L, et al. Evaluation of the ulnopalmar arterial arches with pulse oximetry and plethysmography: comparison with the Allen's test in 1010 patients. *Am Heart J.* 2004;147:489–493.
32. Pancholy S, Coppola J, Patel T, et al. Prevention of radial artery occlusion-patent hemostasis evaluation trial (PROPHET study): a randomized comparison of traditional versus patency documented hemostasis after transradial catheterization. *Catheter Cardiovasc Interv.* 2008;72:335–340.
33. Jolly SS, Yusuf S, Cairns J, et al; RIVAL Trial Group. Radial versus femoral access for coronary angiography and intervention in patients with acute coronary syndromes (RIVAL): a randomised, parallel group, multicentre trial. *Lancet.* 2011;377:1409–1420.
34. Valgimigli M, Saia F, Guastaroba P, et al. Transradial versus transfemoral intervention for acute myocardial infarction: a propensity score-adjusted and -matched analysis from the REAL (REgistro regionale AngiopLastiche dell'Emilia-Romagna) multicenter registry. *J Am Coll Cardiol Interv.* 2012;5:23–35.
35. Romagnoli E, Biondi-Zoccai G, Sciahbasi A, et al. Radial versus femoral randomized investigation in ST-segment elevation acute coronary syndrome: the RIFLE-STEACS (Radial Versus Femoral Randomized Investigation in ST-Elevation Acute Coronary Syndrome) study. *J Am Coll Cardiol.* 2012;60: 2481–2489. http://dx.doi.org/10.1016/j.jacc.2012.06.017.
36. Agostoni P, Biondi-Zoccai GGL, De Benedictis ML, et al. Radial versus femoral approach for percutaneous

coronary diagnostic and interventional procedures. *J Am Coll Cardiol.* 2004;44:349–356.

37. Bertrand OF, Bélisle P, Joyal D, et al. Comparison of transradial and femoral approaches for percutaneous coronary interventions: a systematic review and hierarchical Bayesian meta-analysis. *Am Heart J.* 2012;163:632–648.

38. Mitchell MD, Hong JA, Lee BY, et al. Systematic review and cost-benefit analysis of radial artery access for coronary angiography and intervention. *Circ Cardiovasc Qual Outcomes.* 2012;5:454–462.

39. McCormack LJ, Cauldwell EW, Anson BJ. Brachial and ante-brachial arterial patterns: a study of 750 extremities. *Surg Gynecol Obstet.* 1953;96:43–54.

40. Chiam P, Lim V. Transulnar artery approach for percutaneous coronary intervention: an alternative route in a patient with challenging transfemoral access and hypoplastic radial artery. *Singapore Med J.* 2010;51(5):81–84.

41. Yoo BS, Yoon J, Ko JY, et al. Anatomical consideration of the radial artery for transradial coronary procedures: arterial diameter, branching anomaly and vessel tortuosity. *Int J Cardiol.* 2005;101:421–427.

42. Valsecchi O, Vassileva A, Musumeci G, et al. Failure of transradial approach during coronary interventions: anatomic considerations. *Catheter Cardiovasc Interv.* 2006;67:870–878.

43. Knebel AV, Cardoso CO, Correa Rodrigues LH, et al. Safety and feasibility of transulnar cardiac catheterization. *Tex Heart Inst J.* 2008;35:268–272.

44. Layton KF, Kallmes DF, Kaufmann TJ. Use of the ulnar artery as an alternative access site for cerebral angiography. *Am J Neuroradiol.* 2006;27(10):2073–2074.

45. Deftereos S, Giannopoulos G, Tousoulis D, et al. Sheathless transulnar versus standard femoral arterial access for percutaneous coronary intervention on bifurcation lesions. *Int J Cardiol.* 2011;149:398–400. doi:10.1016/j.ijcard.2011.03.028.

46. Deftereos S, Giannopoulos G, Tousoulis D, et al. Feasibility and safety of transulnar access for performing rotational atherectomy. *Int J Cardiol.* 2011;147:285–286. doi:10.1016/j.ijcard.2010.12.022.

47. Hussein H, Gan H, Fang H, et al. Bilateral percutaneous ulnar artery approach for retrograde chronic total occlusion intervention. *Int Heart J.* 2010;51(2):137–140.

48. Kamiya H, Ushijima T, Kanamori T, et al. Use of the radial artery graft after transradial catheterization: is it suitable as a bypass conduit? *Ann Thorac Surg.* 2003;76:1505–1509.

49. Andrade PB, Tebet MA, Andrade MV, et al. Primary percutaneous coronary intervention through transulnar approach: safety and effectiveness. *Arq Bras Cardiol.* 2008;91:e49–e52, e41–e44.

50. Agostoni P, Zuffi A, Biondi-Zoccai G. Pushing wrist access to the limit: homolateral right ulnar artery approach for primary percutaneous coronary intervention after right radial failure due to radial loop. *Catheter Cardiovasc Interv.* 2011;78:894–897.

51. Burzotta F, Trani C, Mazzari MA, et al. Vascular complications and access crossover in 10676 transradial percutaneous coronary procedures. *Am Heart J.* 2012;163(2):230–238.

52. Sakai H, Ikeda S, Harada T, et al. Limitations of successive transradial approach in the same arm: the Japanese experience. *Catheter Cardiovasc Interv.* 2001;54:204–208.

53. Bernat I, Bertrand OF, Rokyta R, et al. Efficacy and safety of transient ulnar artery compression to recanalize acute radial artery occlusion after transradial catheterization. *Am J Cardiol.* 2011;107:1698–1701.

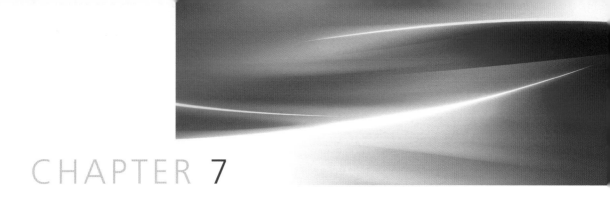

CHAPTER 7

Tips and Tricks for Diagnostic Angiography and Intervention

Mikhailia W. Lake and Mauricio G. Cohen

Introduction

During the transradial learning curve, the operator is expected to gain expertise in radial vascular access, become familiar with the upper extremity vasculature and its most frequent anomalies, and learn a different catheter manipulation technique. As opposed to the femoral approach, in which the tip of preformed catheters virtually "fall" into the coronary ostia without much manipulation, during transradial angiography (TRA), the operator needs to actively torque the catheters "seeking" the coronary ostia. In addition, owing to increased resistance at the level of the subclavian and innominate arteries (with right radial access), the catheters accumulate rotational tension and usually do not stay engaged in the coronary ostia. This may require the operator to apply continued torque force at the level of the catheter hub while performing the angiographic procedure.[1] In order to perform TRA efficiently, with the lowest number of catheter exchanges and reduced radiation exposure, expert operators apply a number of "tips and tricks" related to negotiation of the upper extremity vasculature and engagement of the native coronary arteries, saphenous vein grafts (SVGs), internal mammary grafts, and vessels in other vascular territories. Knowledge of these "tips and tricks" for overcoming potential procedural challenges is key for the operator who chooses to use the radial approach; these play an important role in ensuring procedural success. Importantly, since

the introduction of TRA by Campeau[2] in 1989, when he first published a study involving a series of 100 patients in whom cardiac catheterization via the left radial artery was attempted, newer tools that are specifically designed for TRA procedures have been developed.

Anatomical Considerations

It is obvious that the course of the catheters through the femoral and radial approach is different. The right and the left radial approaches also differ. From the femoral approach, the catheter usually courses up the descending aorta, then into the aortic arch along its superior wall, and finally into the ascending aorta along the right wall (Fig. 7-1C).[3] The curvature of the aortic arch is a potential area of resistance as the catheter is passed into the ascending portion of the aorta. This is usually inconsequential in the performance of the procedure. The left subclavian artery arises directly from the aorta; therefore, the catheter course with left TRA is somewhat similar to that in transfemoral angiography (TFA), with one area of resistance at the origin of the left subclavian artery, resulting in less complex catheter manipulation and greater control (Fig. 7-1B). The left radial approach should be considered in patients who have undergone coronary artery bypass grafting (CABG), as it provides direct access to the left internal mammary artery (LIMA). However, with the right radial

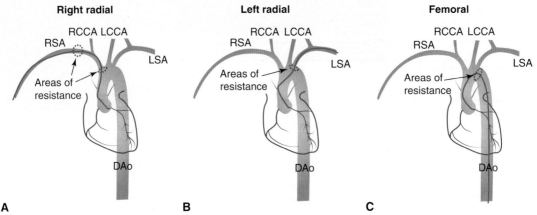

FIGURE 7-1 Areas of resistance. **A:** Two areas of resistance are met with right TFA. **B:** One area of resistance is/ met with left TRA. **C:** One area of resistance is met with TFA. DAo, descending aorta; RSA, right subclavian artery; RCCA, right common carotid artery; LCCA, left common carotid artery; LSA, left subclavian artery; TRA, transradial access; TFA: transfemoral access. (From Patel T, Shah S, Rihal CS, et al. Cannulation of the coronary ostia. In: *Patel's Atlas of Transradial Intervention: The Basics and Beyond.* 2nd ed. Malvern, PA: HMP Communications, 2012.)

approach, entry into the ascending aorta occurs via the subclavian artery and subsequently the innominate artery (brachiocephalic trunk) before entering the ascending aorta, leading to two areas of resistance. The course may be tortuous as the catheter passes through the subclavian artery, and the angle between the aorta and the innominate artery causes the body of catheter to assume a more central position in the ascending aorta (Fig. 7-1A).[4] For this reason, when using Judkins left (JL) catheters to engage the left main coronary artery, a shorter secondary curve, usually by 0.5 cm, may be needed for successful cannulation. A typical example is the need for a JL 3.5 instead of a JL 4.0 catheter for successful left coronary artery (LCA) cannulation, as depicted in Figure 7-2. In addition, the winding course of the subclavian artery often poses difficulty in keeping

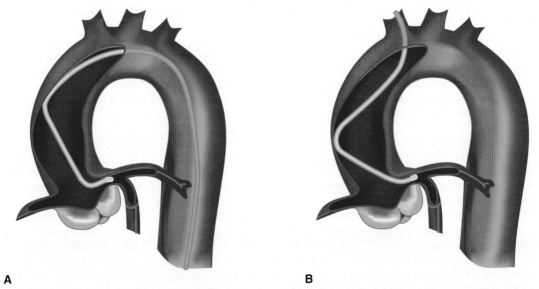

FIGURE 7-2 Differential catheter course through transfemoral **(A)** and transradial **(B)** vascular access. Because of the curvature between the brachiocephalic trunk and the ascending aorta, a shorter secondary curve, usually by 0.5 cm, is needed for successful cannulation of the LCA with a JL catheter. The operators should use a JL 3.5 **(B)** instead of a JL 4.0 **(A)**. (Courtesy of Medtronic.)

the catheter engaged in the coronary once angiography has begun. As a consequence of this, it requires the operator to employ small torquing movements from the fingers when cannulating the coronary, as opposed to larger torquing movements from the wrist when TFA is being performed. This may also require the operator to hold the catheter in place for longer periods of time. Furthermore, catheter stability during TRA procedures is affected by the movements of the diaphragm, as opposed to TFA procedures, in which the catheter position is stable throughout inspiration and expiration.

The anatomic differences between the left and right TRAs have practical implications, especially during the learning curve. Randomized data comparing right versus left radial access suggest that the initial adoption of left TRA is associated with a significantly shorter learning curve, with progressive reductions in cannulation and fluoroscopy times as the operator volume increases.[5,6] After the initial 50 to 100 cases, operators can transition to right TRA, which is ergonomically more convenient without the need to lean over the patient to reach the left upper extremity.

Given the occasional anatomical challenges, maintaining access to the ascending aorta is important. This can be done by using an exchange-length (260 cm) guidewire or by using a standard-length guidewire and constantly flushing the catheters with saline during catheter removal so that the tip of the guidewire stays in place.

Use of Respiration

Vessel tortuosity, particularly in older patients with long-standing hypertension, can pose a challenge in the delivery of the catheter to the ascending aorta, and this accounts for about half of all percutaneous coronary intervention (PCI) failures via the TRA.[7] At times, the wire may preferentially enter the descending aorta, and deep inspiration may facilitate motion of the wire into the ascending aorta by changing the angle of the innominate artery as it branches from the aorta (Fig. 7-3).[8] In the event that this is unsuccessful, the catheter can be advanced over the wire until it reaches the aortic arch; then it can be rotated until it points toward the ascending aorta. From there, the wire can be advanced into the aortic root. Alternatively, the use of a hydrophilic wire and repeating the inspiratory maneuver can help. Inspiration may also be useful in cases where deep engagement of the coronary is desired to facilitate PCI. In these situations, the patient is instructed to take a deep breath as the catheter is rotated into the ostium of the artery.[9]

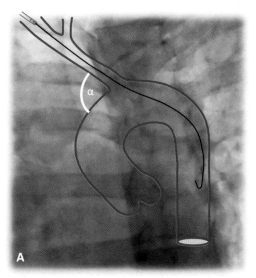 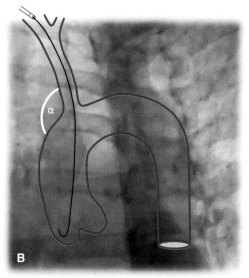

FIGURE 7-3   Effect of Inspiration. **A:** During expiration there is a more acute angle (α) between the brachiocephalic trunk and the ascending aorta; therefore, the wire takes a more horizontal direction toward the descending aorta. **B:** During deep inspiration, the diaphragm lowers the heart and straightens the angle (α) between the brachiocephalic trunk and the ascending aorta. The wire takes a more vertical direction toward the ascending aorta.

Catheter Selection for Diagnostic Coronary Angiography

Initially, the catheters used to perform TRA catheterization were those mainly developed for TFA (Judkins, Amplatz, and multipurpose). However, with better understanding of the anatomic challenges and the more central position within the ascending aorta that the catheters adopt when advanced from the upper limb, new catheters were developed that can be used to cannulate both coronary arteries. Newer catheters have a large loop at their distal end to move the catheters away from the central position within the aorta. Incorporation of a flat portion within the loop of the catheter provides sufficient support against the aorta; this is particularly important to maintain catheter stability especially during percutaneous interventions, and allows the operator to more easily keep the catheter in place. Figure 7-4 displays the most commonly used catheter shapes for TRA procedures.[10,11]

Catheters originally designed for TFA can be used to perform TRA catheterization; in fact, the Judkins catheters may be the easiest catheters to use in the early learning stages. The operator should be aware, however, of the potential of the JL catheter to cause injury to the left main artery when used via the TRA, because of the upward force stored by the tip of this catheter. If this catheter is used, downsizing the curve of the JL catheter from 4.0 to 3.5 may be required; very

careful manipulation is also necessary to avoid any trauma to the coronary arteries (Fig. 7-2). One drawback to the use of "femoral catheters" is the almost obligatory exchange of catheters, which may increase procedural and fluoroscopy times. This may be avoided by the use of a single universal catheter approach to selectively engage both coronaries. This approach may be technically more challenging at first. An example of a "radial" catheter is the Tiger catheter, made with stainless steel incorporated with polyurethane. The loop at the end of the catheter moves the body of the catheter from the central position that occurs naturally as a result of the angle between the innominate artery and the aorta. A flat segment in the third portion of the loop rests on the contralateral aortic wall to the coronary that is being engaged. This gives the catheter extra support and stabilizes it against the aorta. Engaging the coronaries can be done at 30° to 45° in either the left anterior oblique (LAO) or the anterior–posterior (AP) views. The catheter may be delivered under fluoroscopy to the ascending aorta and advanced to the level of the aortic valve with the use of a standard 0.035-inch J- or hydrophilic wire, which should be held in place below the LCA. With the catheter tip facing left, the catheter may spontaneously enter the LCA with slow pullback of the wire. It is important to retract the wire slowly, as a rapid retraction may cause the catheter to flip upward into the ascending aorta. If the catheter does not spontaneously enter the LCA upon pullback of the wire, slight

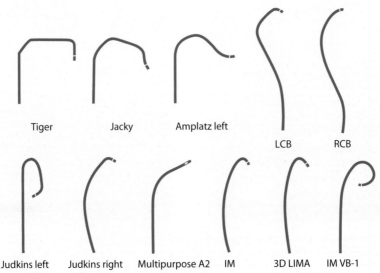

FIGURE 7-4 Most frequently used diagnostic coronary catheter shapes in transradial coronary angiography.

clockwise or counterclockwise torquing may be needed. Slight pullback of the catheter usually disengages it from the LCA. With clockwise motion, the catheter tip should enter the right sinus of Valsalva and engage the right coronary artery (RCA). In a minority of cases, the Tiger catheter may fail to engage the LCA and this catheter may be exchanged for a JL catheter. The RCA can also be successfully engaged with the Tiger catheter.[3,8] The operator should be aware that this catheter does have a tendency to easily disengage from the coronary ostium, particularly the left coronary, when a forceful injection of contrast is given; however, this nuisance is easily overcome with operator awareness, maintained finger torque at the hub of the catheter, and a smoother injection.

A few studies have compared the efficiency of the single- versus dual-catheter technique. A Canadian observational study assessed fluoroscopy time, radiation dose, and the number of crossovers with these techniques in 1,384 patients undergoing TRA native coronary angiography by 14 different operators. Most cases (85%) were performed with Judkins catheters (dual-catheter technique), while a number of different catheters, including Amplatz, Barbeau, and multipurpose, were used for the single-catheter technique. The average fluoroscopy time was 2.6 minutes. The dual-catheter technique was associated with fewer crossovers, lower radiation exposure (2,933 vs 3,352 cGy · cm^2, $P = 0.0001$), and shorter fluoroscopy time (2.6 vs 2.8 minutes, $P = 0.03$). It should be noted that the majority of cases were performed with two Judkins catheters and that the only "radial-specific catheter" in this study was the Barbeau catheter, which is currently not widely utilized in practice. A randomized study comparing Judkins (JL and JR) and the Tiger catheters demonstrated a significant reduction in procedural and fluoroscopy times by 40% and 33%, respectively, with the Tiger catheter. Technique crossover was rare, and RCA and LCA angiographies were completed in 100% and 98% of cases with the Tiger catheter, and in 91% and 95% with Judkins catheters.[3]

For patients with prior CABG, the left radial approach may be preferred because it allows easier cannulation of the LIMA. For SVGs, left TRA offers a similar experience as TFA; however, right TRA is usually associated with lengthier catheter manipulation and procedural time. In patients whose SVGs are not marked, it is advisable to perform ascending aortography in order to visualize the origin of the grafts in the aorta and select the catheters accordingly. Figure 7-5 provides guidance on the choice of catheters for selective cannulation of SVGs according to the location of the proximal anastomosis in the ascending aorta and whether the procedure should be more conveniently performed from left or right TRA. Multipurpose or JR 4 catheters can be used to cannulate right-sided SVGs usually to the RCA. Amplatz left (AL) catheters are well suited for grafts arising from the anterior or left walls of the aorta usually to the LCA. There is an area in the right wall of the aorta, adjacent to the origin of the innominate artery, that is difficult to reach, especially through right TRA, and catheters with more acute curves may be needed, such as extra backup or hockey stick.[12]

Adequate angiographic imaging of a patent internal mammary artery (IMA) graft is essential in the evaluation of patients with prior coronary bypass surgery. An important theoretical advantage of the TRA for IMA cannulation is the absence of catheter manipulation in the aortic arch, which potentially reduces the incidence of consequent cerebrovascular embolization and stroke. Homolateral TRA is associated with significant reductions in times to cannulation and visualization compared with TFA.[13] An important detail to keep in mind is that with the homolateral TRA approach, the take-off angle of the IMA is more frequently acute, as opposed to the obtuse angle that is encountered from the femoral approach. In most cases, the IMA can be successfully engaged with a regular IM catheter. However, when this angle is sharper, a more acute catheter curve such as the IM-VB1 may be needed (Fig. 7-6). Sharp angles are particularly frequent with the right IMA.[12]

The left IMA can be selectively cannulated and imaged from the contralateral right TRA. Although this technique is routinely used by some expert operators, the procedure involves more complex manipulation with multiple catheter exchanges because of the complex angles of both subclavian arteries in relation to the aortic arch.[14] To cannulate the contralateral IMA, a 0.035-inch wire is placed in the descending aorta and a catheter with a distal bend, such as JL 3.5, left coronary bypass (LCB), or Jacky/Tiger, is advanced over the wire. The wire is removed and the tip of the catheter rotated such that the tip points upward toward the left subclavian artery. Then a 0.035-inch or 0.032-inch exchange-length soft-angled-tip hydrophilic wire is advanced into the left subclavian artery and the tip positioned as far as possible beyond the brachial artery. The distal end of the wire can then be trapped by inflating

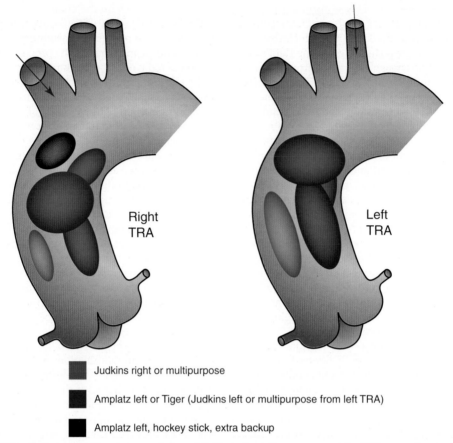

Right
TRA

Left
TRA

■ Judkins right or multipurpose

■ Amplatz left or Tiger (Judkins left or multipurpose from left TRA)

■ Amplatz left, hockey stick, extra backup

FIGURE 7-5   Catheter selection for cannulation of SVGs to the left coronary and the RCA according to right or left transradial approach. (Adapted from Burzotta F, Trani C, Hamon M, et al. Transradial approach for coronary angiography and interventions in patients with coronary bypass grafts: tips and tricks. *Catheter Cardiovasc Interv.* 2008;72(2):263–272.)

a blood pressure cuff in the left arm or by asking the patient to flex the forearm.[14] The initial catheter used to direct the wire is then exchanged for a 4F IMA or 3D LIMA catheter. The use of smaller 4F catheters is usually recommended because these catheters are malleable and can track over the wire without prolapsing into the descending aorta. The catheter is then advanced into the subclavian artery beyond the origin of the left IMA. The hydrophilic wire is removed. Then, maneuvering very gently, the catheter is rotated counterclockwise and carefully pulled back seeking the origin of the left IMA. Figure 7-7 illustrates each one of these procedural steps. The operator needs to keep in mind that catheter manipulations to engage the contralateral IMA are time-consuming, especially in the elderly with tortuous vessels, and if the catheter is pulled proximal to the IMA origin and/or falls into the aortic arch,

the whole process has to be reinitiated. Cha and colleagues published a study involving a series of 184 patients who underwent cardiac catheterization with left IMA angiography through right TRA.[15] They specifically designed a modified Simmons catheter with a 0.5-cm modified tip bent 80° laterally and 80° anteriorly. Left IMA was selectively cannulated in 164 (89%) patients, and subselectively in the remaining patients. There were no reported complications. The average time from catheter introduction to successful left IMA engagement was 3.7 minutes.

In practice, there is a wide variation in preference for diagnostic catheters as depicted in Figures. 7-8 and 7-9. A large survey including 874 interventional cardiologists from all over the world demonstrated that almost half of operators prefer using two Judkins catheters for engagement of native coronary arteries, JL 3.5 and JR 4.0 for

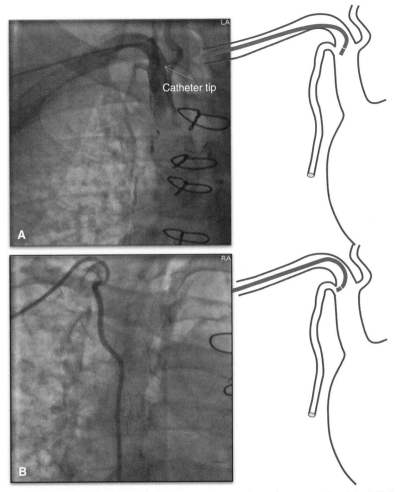

FIGURE 7-6 Right IMA angiography. **A:** The IM catheter cannot selectively engage the right IMA because of its sharp origin angle providing suboptimal images. **B:** A more angulated catheter, such as the IM-VB1, can selectively cannulate the right IMA without difficulty providing optimal angiographic opacification of the vessel.

the LCA and RCA, respectively. The most popular single-catheter technique choice seems to be the Tiger catheter, used in approximately 15% of cases. Other less frequent choices (<10%) include multipurpose and Amplatz catheters. A similar variation in choice is observed for saphenous bypass grafts. About half of operators prefer the JR 4.0 for left and right SVGs. Operators also appreciate the features of the AL catheters for SVGs to the LCA (23%) and the multipurpose for SVGs to the RCA (24%).[16]

TRA should not be limited to coronary angiography. Over the past few years, a larger number of patients are now referred to the catheterization laboratory for evaluation of aortic stenosis due to the inception of transcatheter valve therapies.

When indicated, crossing the aortic valve can be challenging regardless of the access approach. In TFA procedures, the AL 1.0 and the JR 4 catheters are the most widely used to direct the wire through a stenotic aortic valve. However, these catheters hardly assume a central aortic position when advanced from right TRA. We have found that the Amplatz right 1.0 catheter, with a shorter curve and a tip pointing inferiorly, usually takes a central position in the root of the aorta, ideal to direct a straight wire through a stenotic aortic valve. The MIV catheter (Merit Medical) is a specially designed pigtail catheter for use from the radial artery. It has an additional proximal bend, allowing it to avoid the noncoronary cusp and cross the aortic valve.

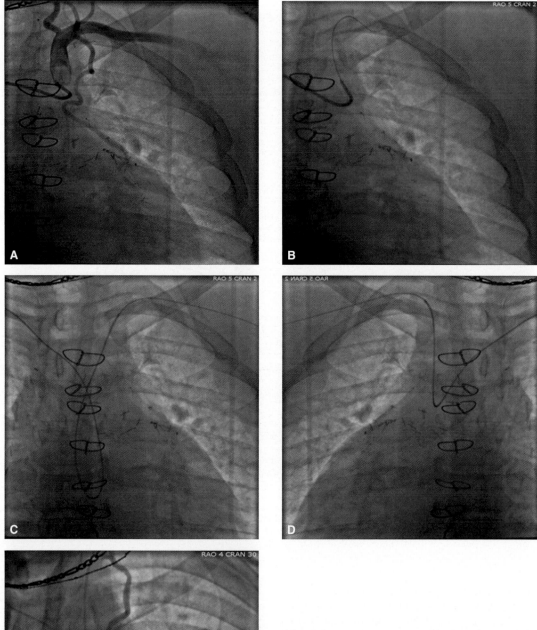

FIGURE 7-7 Contralateral LIMA cannulation. In **A,** a Jacky catheter points toward the left subclavian artery, then a floppy-angled-tip hydrophylic wire is advanced into the left subclavian and the tip positioned at beyond the brachial artery **(B)**. The wire can be stabilized by inflating a blood pressure cuff or asking the patient to flex the elbow. Then a 4F IM catheter is advanced very carefully to avoid prolapsing into the descending aorta. Sometimes the catheter will find support in the coronary sinuses **(C)**. Once the tip of the catheter is adjacent to the origin of the LIMA, the catheter is pulled gently and the wire removed **(D)**. Gentle torquing while carefully pulling the catheter will allow selective LIMA cannulation **(E)**.

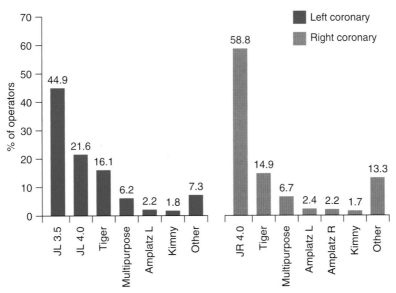

FIGURE 7-8 Catheter preference for engagement of native coronary arteries during TRA diagnostic procedures. TRA, transradial access; JL, Judkins left; JR, Judkins right; L, left; R, right.

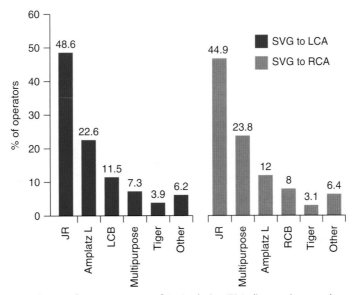

FIGURE 7-9 Catheter preference for engagement of SVGs during TRA diagnostic procedures. TRA, transradial access; JR, Judkins right; L, left; R, right; LCB, left coronary bypass; RCB, right coronary bypass.

Catheter Selection for Percutaneous Coronary Interventions

One impediment to the widespread use of transradial PCI has been the perception that the radial approach does not provide sufficient backup. In addition, the inability to upsize to larger diameter catheters for complex procedures involving bifurcation stenting or larger rotational atherectomy burrs may also contribute to operators' reluctance to use TRA for complex PCI. However, with modern equipment, most interventions can be performed through 6F guiding catheters, including bifurcations and calcified lesions requiring rotational atherectomy (maximum burr size ≤ 1.75 mm). Table 7-1 displays device compatibility according to catheter size.

TABLE 7-1	**Guiding Catheters and Device Compatibility**		
Catheter Size	**Device**	**Kissing Balloon**	**Kissing Stents**
5F	Balloon ≤ 5 mm	No	No
	Stent ≤ 4.5 mm		
	Intravascular ultrasound		
	Rotational atherectomy (1.25-mm burr)		
6F	All balloon sizes	Yes	No
	All stent sizes, including JoMed covered stents		
	Intravascular ultrasound		
	Optical coherence tomography		
	Rotational atherectomy (1.5- and 1.75-mm burr)		
	Aspiration thrombectomy catheters		
	Embolic protection devices for SVG interventions		
	Catheter extensions (mother–child/GuideLiner)		
7F	Rotational atherectomy (>1.75-mm burr)	Yes	Yes

SVG, saphenous vein graft.
Adapted from MacHaalany J, Abdelaal E, Bertrand OF. Guide catheter selection for transradial PCI. *Cardiac Interv Today*. 2013;7:45–48.

The lack of support can be overcome by the use of "active backup catheters" and guiding catheter extensions, such as telescoping a smaller 4F catheter through 6F guiding catheter for deep intubation (mother–child system) or the GuideLiner device.[17-19]

Guiding catheter selection is based on important characteristics including backup support, capacity for coaxial engagement, and stability after the target vessel is cannulated. As with diagnostic angiography, most catheters designed for TFA are suitable for TRA interventions. In fact, a large international survey demonstrated that the majority of operators choose to use extra backup curves for the left coronary and Judkins right catheters for the RCA. Similarly, for SVGs most operators usually choose either AL or Judkins right for left-sided bypasses and Judkins right or multipurpose for right-sided SVGs.[16] It is worth noting that universal catheters are not used as frequently in PCI as with diagnostic coronary angiography (Figs. 7-10 and 7-11).

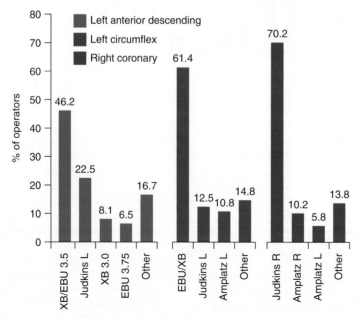

FIGURE 7-10   Catheter preference for engagement of native coronary arteries during TRA coronary interventions. TRA, transradial access; L, left; R, right.

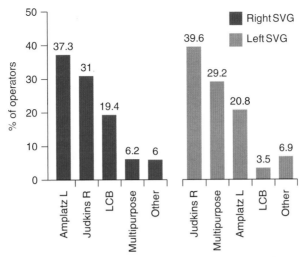

FIGURE 7-11   Catheter preference for engagement of SVGs during TRA coronary interventions. TRA, transradial access; L, left; R, right; LCB, left coronary bypass.

Passive Backup Support Catheters

For the LCA, extra backup catheters (EBU, Voda, or XB) usually provide excellent "passive" support, which means that the backup relies on the properties of the shaft and tip to maintain stable position. These catheters require minimal manipulation once seated in the coronary ostium (Fig. 7-12).

To engage the left main coronary artery, the catheter is advanced over the wire and rotated clockwise as it descends through the aorta pointing it toward the left coronary cusp. Then, the catheter can be advanced, forcing the tip to move up toward the ostium while the primary catheter curve is seated in the contralateral coronary sinus. If the catheter is pulled back gently, the contralateral wall of the aorta will push the tip forward into the left main, providing an even more stable position. Some operators may place the stiff backend of a regular 0.035-inch J-wire just proximal to the catheter tip to enhance catheter torquing and modify the catheter curve to facilitate selective engagement (Fig. 7-13).

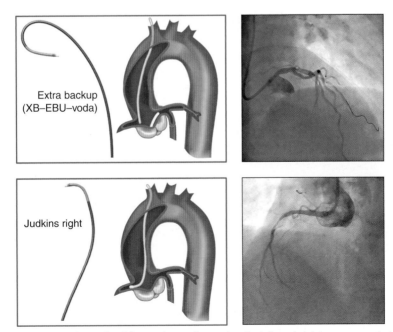

FIGURE 7-12   Most commonly used guiding catheter shapes for the left and right coronary arteries. (Courtesy of Medtronic.)

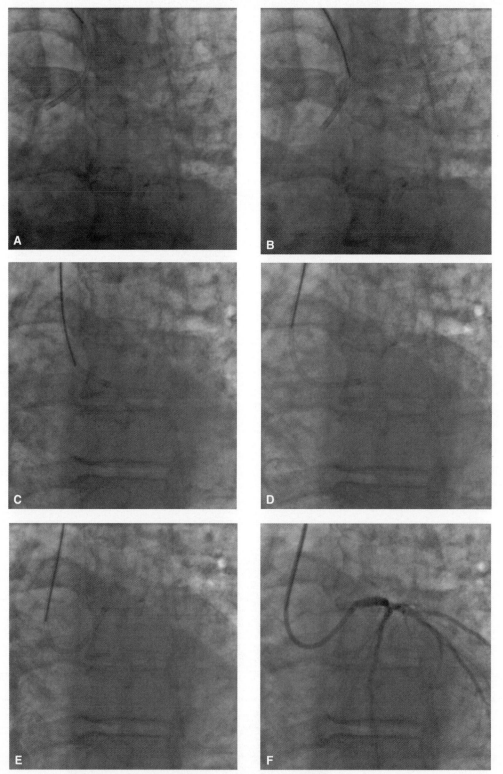

FIGURE 7-13 LCA selective cannulation with an extra backup catheter assisted with the backend of a regular 0.035-inch wire. Once the extra backup catheter reaches the ascending aorta, the J-wire is removed and reinserted backward **(A)**. The stiff backend of the wire straightens the catheter **(B)**. The catheter is easily rotated clockwise and advanced toward the left coronary sinus **(C and D)**. The wire is pulled a few centimeters, allowing the catheter to regain its original curvature **(E)**. The tip points up and engages the left coronary ostium from below. Note that the catheter curve is now seated on the contralateral coronary cusp, providing stability and backup support **(F)**.

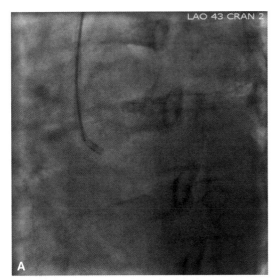 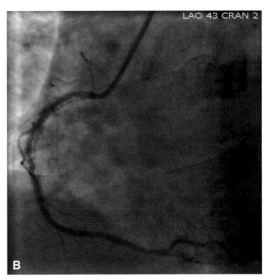

FIGURE 7-14   Right coronary engagement with a JL 3.5 guiding catheter. The JL 3.5 assumes a shape similar to that of a JR 4 catheter when the stiff backend of a 0.035″ J-wire is advanced proximal to the tip **(A)**. The catheter is pulled back gently while clockwise torque is applied to the hub to engage the right coronary ostium **(B)**. The wire is removed and the catheter assumes a stable position. The secondary curve of the JL 3.5 and the contralateral wall of the aorta provide excellent backup support.

For the RCA, Judkins right catheters are usually reliable for successful cannulation. To engage the right coronary ostium, a regular J-wire is looped in the root of the aorta. The catheter is advanced over the guidewire and once positioned in the right cusp, the wire is removed and the catheter pulled back slowly while applying clockwise torque to the hub. The catheter tip will turn and selectively engage the ostium. AL or hockey stick may be the preferred catheters in right coronaries with shepherd crook morphology. An alternative method for right coronary engagement is to use a JL 3.5 guiding catheter. To successfully perform this procedure, the stiff backend of a 0.035-inch J-wire is advanced into the JL 3.5 to a distance of approximately 2 cm proximal to the tip. The wire straightens the secondary curve and the catheter assumes a shape similar to that of a JR 4 catheter (Fig. 7-14). Then, with gentle pullback while applying clockwise torque, the right coronary ostium is engaged. Once the catheter is in place, the wire is removed and the secondary curve of the JL 3.5 catheter resting on the contralateral wall of the aorta will provide excellent backup support. During engagement, all manipulations need to be carefully performed as the forces stored in the catheter can easily dissect the right coronary ostium. In addition, contrast should be injected carefully because the JL 3.5 catheter has a tendency to deep-seat in the RCA or selectively engage the conus branch. A study of 100 patients performed in Spain showed that with this strategy, both coronary arteries can be optimally imaged in 94% of cases, without significant differences in procedural time compared to a control group of 20 cases performed with two Judkins catheters (16.9 ± 6.9 vs 15.8 ± 6.7 minutes; $P =$ NS).[20] The backend of the wire technique is also useful to straighten the curves of catheters, with a tendency to selectively cannulate the conus branch of the RCA, such as the Tiger catheter.[1]

Prevention of Catheter Kinking and Knotting

The operator should be aware that catheter kinking and knotting can occur with excessive clockwise torquing, especially while attempting to selectively engage the RCA. Because of its thinner wall and larger lumen, guiding catheters are more vulnerable to kinking than diagnostic catheters. Once a catheter is knotted, it is almost impossible to pass a wire through its lumen; in fact, if excessive force is applied to the wire, catheter and vessel perforation can occur. A knotted catheter can break, embolize, or cause vascular trauma.

Knots usually occur within the vasculature of the upper limb in patients with excessive subclavian tortuosity, needing laborious catheter manipulation. To successfully reduce a knot, it is important to fixate the distal portion of the catheter. If the knot is located in the arm or forearm, the catheter can be fixated by either applying manual pressure or a blood pressure cuff to the arm over the brachial artery; however, if the knot is located in the axillary artery or more centrally, the tip needs to be snared from the femoral approach. Once the distal portion is fixated, gentle counterclockwise rotation can be applied to the proximal portion of the catheter to untangle the knot.[21] To prevent kinking and knotting, the 0.035-inch wire should always be kept inside the guiding catheter during engagement manipulations.

Active Backup Support Catheters

These types of catheters use the aortic root to accomplish a desired shape and to provide support, which requires a fair amount of active manipulation by the operator to obtain a stable coaxial position. With the transradial approach, active guiding catheters play a more important role than with the standard femoral approach. Active support becomes even more relevant with 5 F catheters that can be deep-seated in the coronary arteries with less risk of vessel trauma or dissection.

The Ikari left catheter, exclusively designed for TRA interventions, can also be used for both the LCA and the RCA and is therefore considered a universal catheter. The Ikari left is similar in shape as that of the JL, but has three modifications consisting of a shorter secondary bend, followed by a straight portion of approximately 20 mm that lies in contact with the contralateral wall of the aorta providing strong backup support, a tertiary bend, and a proximal curve to better fit the angle between the innominate artery and the aorta (Fig. 7-15). Comparative assessments in plastic aorta models demonstrated that the Ikari left provides better backup force than the JL catheter. The Ikari left comes in three different curve sizes (3.5, 3.75, and 4), and the general recommendation is to use the same curve size as if using a JL catheter.[11] The physics of the Ikari left catheter have also been studied for RCA cannulation, showing that the backup force is comparable to that of the AL and higher than the Judkins right catheter. It should be noted that when a regular 0.035-inch wire is

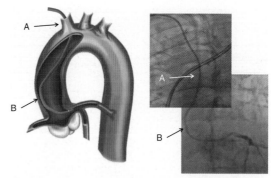

FIGURE 7-15   Ikari left catheter. Curve (A) to fit angle of innominate artery. Straight portion (20 mm) (B) to gain support from the contralateral aortic wall and generate backup.

placed in the Ikari left, the catheter assumes a shape similar to that of a Judkins right catheter.[22]

Left coronary engagement with the Ikari left is basically the same as with the JL catheter from TRA. In contrast with the Judkins catheter, when the Ikari left is pushed forward, backup force increases substantially and the catheter deep-seats in the coronary artery. Engagement maneuvers for RCA engagement with the Ikari left catheter are similar to the Judkins right catheter; however, when the guidewire is removed, the additional curves in the Ikari left generate stronger backup force and a more stable position.[22]

Universal Catheters versus Regular Catheters for Percutaneous Coronary Intervention

In contrast to diagnostic angiography, in which universal catheters can potentially save time and catheter exchanges, in PCI, universal catheters are not as needed because the operator already knows the anatomy and origin location of the target vessel and can choose the catheter that best suits the anatomy. However, there is one clinical scenario in which universal guiding catheters may provide added value: primary PCI for ST-elevation myocardial infarction. Being able to image both coronaries during primary PCI is important for clinical decision making and the use of a universal guide catheter may reduce unnecessary delays. An observational study from Canada including 1,900 patients compared diagnostic angiography of the noninfarct-related arteries (non-IRA), followed by PCI of the IRA (70% of cases), with PCI of the IRA, followed by diagnostic angiography of the non-IRA (30% of cases). The latter strategy was associated with a reduction of 8 minutes in door-to-balloon time (32 vs 40 minutes, $P < 0.001$). There were no differences in clinical outcomes between groups; however, the immediate PCI strategy was an independent predictor of door-to-balloon time $\leq$ 90 minutes, an important metric not only used to assess ST-elevation myocardial infarction (STEMI) care, but also a core performance measure that reflects overall institutional quality.[23,24]

A universal catheter that allows quick angiographic views of both coronary arteries and provides good backup support is a valuable option during primary PCI potentially saving time. An observational study from Korea compared TFA ($n = 102$) versus TRA with two catheters ($n = 109$) and TRA with a single catheter ($n = 31$) in STEMI patients undergoing primary PCI. The operators used a locally designed RM catheter, an active-support catheter with a shape similar to that of the Ikari left catheter. Door-to-balloon times were 89.5, 91, and 68.5 minutes, $P = 0.008$, respectively. Of note, with a single-catheter strategy, the proportion of patients achieving door-to-balloon time $\leq$ 90 minutes increased by approximately 50%.[25]

Saphenous Vein Grafts

Lesions located in SVGs are often complex and optimal backup support is needed. In general, the choice of guiding and diagnostic catheter recommendations for SVGs is similar. For left coronary grafts, AL curves provide a better support than the Judkins right and are the preferred option. For right coronary grafts, the recommended choices are Judkins right and multipurpose catheters.[12,16] For PCI of the IMA, the general recommendation is to access the ipsilateral radial artery for simplicity and better backup support. The catheter choices are either an IM or a modified IM catheter such as the IM VB1 (Fig. 7-6).

Guiding Catheter Extensions

In challenging PCI cases, including extreme proximal tortuosity, heavy calcification, chronic total occlusions, or SVG intervention, the use of the "mother–child" technique or a guiding catheter extension such as the GuideLiner can provide deep coronary intubation for extra support.[17-19]

The mother–child technique consists of telescoping a 5 or 4F long catheter of 120 cm, which is 20 cm longer than a regular 6F guiding catheter. The use of a "4-in-6" system is preferred to a "5-in-6" system because of better trackability and higher backup support. In a study including 51 patients undergoing complex TRA PCI with the mother–child technique, procedural success was achieved in 48 (94%) cases and stent delivery was successful in 40 of the 44 cases in which it was attempted.[19]

The GuideLiner catheter is a "rapid-exchange" version of the mother–child system. It consists of a 20-cm soft-tipped catheter connected with a metal collar to a 115-cm stainless steel shaft for advancement and positioning. The "5-in-6" version has an internal diameter of 0.056-inch. Compared to the mother–child technique with two catheters, the GuideLiner is simpler because it does not require the removal of the hemostatic valve for placement or the use of long coronary wires for catheter removal or exchange. The GuideLiner is useful in native coronary and SVG intervention.[17,18] Figure 7-16 displays the use of a GuideLiner device in a complex left anterior descending (LAD) intervention.

The use of a guide catheter extension allows the operator to stent in a proximal-to-distal manner in cases where this may be desired, as the device can be passed through stented areas.[26] As a caveat, this system is better suited for the delivery of stents less than 4 mm in size, as larger stents may be damaged as they pass through the metal collar of the system.[27] The operator should be extremely careful in retrieving an undeployed stent through a guiding catheter extension system because of significant risk of dislodgement upon withdrawal. A practical recommendation is not to attempt retrieval of an undeployed stent through a catheter extension. In fact, the catheter extension should be removed first or as a unit together with the stent. Moreover, in the case of slight resistance to passing a stent through a guiding catheter, the operator should also consider removing the guiding catheter first to prevent stent dislodgment and embolization.[19] One should also be mindful that deep-seating of the vessel with this system could result in pressure dampening and ischemia. In addition, careful withdrawal of the balloon after stent deployment is advised, as abrupt withdrawal could result in unanticipated catheter advancement causing vessel dissection.[28]

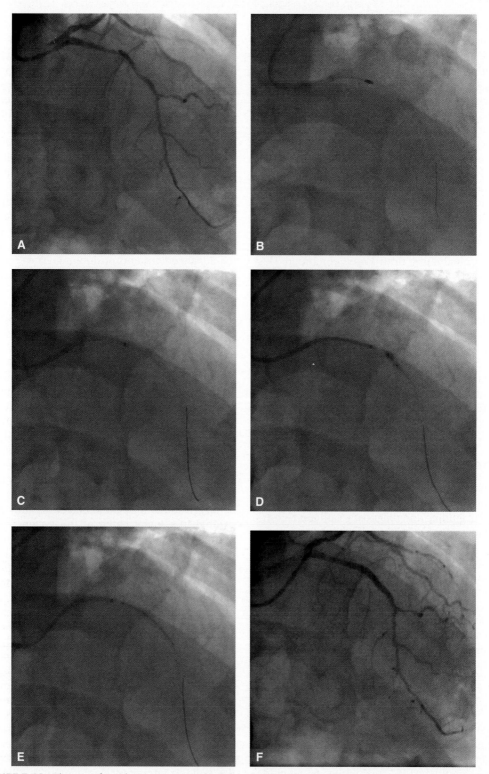

FIGURE 7-16 The use of GuideLiner in a complex left anterior coronary artery intervention. The left anterior descending, engaged with an extra backup catheter, has a complex long and calcified lesion **(A)**. To perform the intervention, the lesion is initially treated using rotational atherectomy with a 1.5-mm burr **(B)**. Subsequently a GuideLiner 5-in-6 is inserted to facilitate device deployment **(C)**. The most severe part of the lesion had to be dilated with a short 3.5- × 9-mm noncompliant balloon **(D)**. Once the lesion was dilated, a 3.5- × 28-mm stent was delivered and deployed **(E)** with optimal angiographic result **(F)**.

TABLE 7-2   **Tips and Tricks to Ensure Successful Transradial Catheterization**
1. Minimize radiation. After successful radial cannulation, avoid the use of fluoroscopy while advancing a 0.035-inch wire. Ideally, use a wire with a small J tip (1.5-mm tip curve radius) to avoid selection of vessel subbranches.
2. Minimize vessel trauma. Avoid forceful wire or catheter advancement. Observe the passage of the wire or the catheter under fluoroscopy and/or perform a limited angiogram to ensure tracking in the right direction.
3. Always introduce and remove catheters over a guidewire.
4. Use a hydrophilic-coated guidewire to negotiate significant tortuosity in the upper extremity or intrathoracic vessels. A stiff-shaft wire may help straighten tortuous brachiocephalic trunks.
5. All catheter exchanges should be performed over exchange-length guidewires (260 cm), especially in patients with tortuous radial, brachial, or subclavian anatomy.
6. Deep inspiration facilitates wire and catheter access to the ascending aorta.
7. Maintain the guidewire within the catheter to avoid kinking in case of difficult manipulation to engage the coronary arteries.
8. Use left transradial access for patients with left internal mammary grafts.
9. When using JL catheters from the right radial approach, downsize the secondary curve by 0.5 cm (use JL 3.5 instead of JL 4).
10. Consider a universal guiding catheter to decrease door-to-balloon time in TRA primary PCI.

Conclusion

TRA is different from TFA and left TRA is different from right TRA. A thorough understanding of catheter physics for cannulation and backup support is crucial. Knowledge of available equipment including wires and catheter shapes is important for successful completion of TRA procedures. Table 7-2 displays a number of tricks and tips to simplify and expedite TRA procedures. In this chapter, we provided a number of recommendations for successful coronary cannulation, though, in general, operators will decide on set of catheters that will provide the best results for their technique and practice.

REFERENCES

1. Patel T, Shah S, Rihal CS, et al. Cannulation of the coronary ostia. In: *Patel's Atlas of Transradial Intervention: The Basics and Beyond*. Malvern, PA: HMP Communications, 2012.
2. Campeau L. Percutaneous radial artery approach for coronary angiography. *Cathet Cardiovasc Diagn.* 1989;16:3–7.
3. Kim SM, Kim DK, Kim DI, et al. Novel diagnostic catheter specifically designed for both coronary arteries via the right transradial approach: a prospective, randomized trial of tiger ii vs. Judkins catheters. *Int J Cardiovasc Imaging.* 2006;22:295–303.
4. Ochiai M, Ikari Y, Yamaguchi T, et al. New long-tip guiding catheters designed for right transradial coronary intervention. *Catheter Cardiovasc Interv.* 2000;49:218–224.
5. Sciahbasi A, Romagnoli E, Burzotta F, et al. Transradial approach (left vs right) and procedural times during percutaneous coronary procedures: talent study. *Am Heart J.* 2011;161:172–179.
6. Sciahbasi A, Romagnoli E, Trani C, et al. Evaluation of the "learning curve" for left and right radial approach

during percutaneous coronary procedures. *Am J Cardiol.* 2011;108:185–188.
7. Dehghani P, Mohammad A, Bajaj R, et al. Mechanism and predictors of failed transradial approach for percutaneous coronary interventions. *JACC Cardiovasc Interv.* 2009;2:1057–1064.
8. Freestone B, Nolan J. Transradial cardiac procedures: the state of the art. *Heart.* 2010;96:883–891.
9. Burzotta F, Hamon M, Trani C, et al. Direct coronary stenting by transradial approach: rationale and technical issues. *Catheter Cardiovasc Interv.* 2004;63:215–219.
10. Ikari Y, Ochiai M, Hangaishi M, et al. Novel guide catheter for left coronary intervention via a right upper limb approach. *Cathet Cardiovasc Diagn.* 1998;44:244–247.
11. Ikari Y, Nagaoka M, Kim JY, et al. The physics of guiding catheters for the left coronary artery in transfemoral and transradial interventions. *J Invasive Cardiol.* 2005;17:636–641.
12. Burzotta F, Trani C, Hamon M, et al. Transradial approach for coronary angiography and interventions in patients with coronary bypass grafts: tips and tricks. *Catheter Cardiovasc Interv.* 2008;72(2):263–272.
13. Burzotta F, Trani C, Todaro D, et al. Comparison of the transradial and transfemoral approaches for coronary angiographic evaluation in patients with internal mammary artery grafts. *J Cardiovasc Med.* 2008;9:263–266.
14. Patel T, Shah S, Patel T. Cannulating LIMA graft using right transradial approach: two simple and innovative techniques. *Catheter Cardiovasc Interv.* 2012;80:316–320.
15. Cha KS, Kim MH. Feasibility and safety of concomitant left internal mammary arteriography at the setting of the right transradial coronary angiography. *Catheter Cardiovasc Interv* 2002;56:188–195.
16. Bertrand OF, Rao SV, Pancholy S, et al. Transradial approach for coronary angiography and interventions: results of the first international transradial practice survey. *JACC Cardiovasc Interv.* 2010;3:1022–1031.
17. Mamas MA, Fath-Ordoubadi F, Fraser DG. Distal stent delivery with guideliner catheter: first in man experience. *Catheter Cardiovasc Interv.* 2010;76:102–111.
18. Farooq V, Mamas MA, Fath-Ordoubadi F, et al. The use of a guide catheter extension system as an aid during

transradial percutaneous coronary intervention of coronary artery bypass grafts. *Catheter Cardiovasc Interv.* 2011;78:847–863.

19. Takeshita S, Shishido K, Sugitatsu K, et al. In vitro and human studies of a 4f double-coaxial technique ("mother-child" configuration) to facilitate stent implantation in resistant coronary vessels. *Circ Cardiovasc Interv.* 2011;4:155–161.

20. Rondan J, Lozano I, Moris C, et al. Cardiac catheterization via the right radial artery with a Judkins left catheter: a prospective study. *Rev Esp Cardiol.* 2005;58:868–871.

21. Patel T, Shah S, Pancholy S. A simple approach for the reduction of knotted coronary catheter in the radial artery during the transradial approach. *J Invasive Cardiol.* 2011;23:E126–E127.

22. Ikari Y, Masuda N, Matsukage T, et al. Backup force of guiding catheters for the right coronary artery in transfemoral and transradial interventions. *J Invasive Cardiol.* 2009;21:570–574.

23. Plourde G, Abdelaal E, Bataille Y, et al. Effect on door-to-balloon time of immediate transradial percutaneous coronary intervention on culprit lesion in ST-elevation myocardial infarction compared to diagnostic angiography followed by primary percutaneous coronary intervention. *Am J Cardiol.* 2013;111:836–840.

24. Bonow RO, Masoudi FA, Rumsfeld JS, et al. American College of Cardiology, American Heart Association Task Force on Performance Measures. ACC/AHA classification of care metrics: performance measures and quality metrics: a report of the American College of Cardiology/American Heart Association Task Force on Performance Measures. *J Am Coll Cardiol.* 2008;52:2113–2117.

25. Moon KW, Kim JH, Kim JY, et al. Reducing needle-to-balloon time by using a single guiding catheter during transradial primary coronary intervention. *J Interv Cardiol.* 2012;25:330–336.

26. Cola C, Miranda F, Vaquerizo B, et al. The guideliner catheter for stent delivery in difficult cases: tips and tricks. *J Interv Cardiol.* 2011;24:450–461.

27. Murphy JC, Spence MS. Guideliner catheter—friend or foe? *Catheter Cardiovasc Interv.* 2012;80:447–450.

28. Seto A, Kern M. The guideliner: keeping your procedure on track or derailing it? *Catheter Cardiovasc Interv.* 2012;80:451–452.

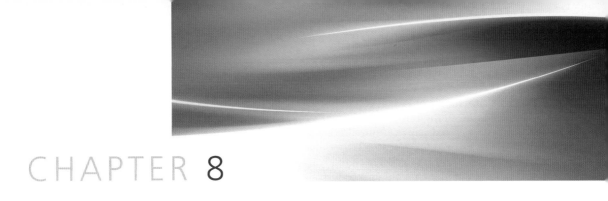

CHAPTER 8

Slender Catheters and Techniques

Yuji Ikari

Introduction

Bleeding complications following percutaneous coronary intervention (PCI) were once thought of as a minor complication. However, recent data have made it evident that resulting cases of death are on the rise. Less invasive strategy is favorable in coronary revascularization to reduce bleeding complications and to improve clinical outcomes. Dr. Gruntzig invented PCI as a less invasive strategy when compared with bypass surgery. A number of new devices and technologies have been invented, such as coronary stents and drug-eluting stents. Device companies have strived for miniaturization such that today almost all PCI can be performed using 6F catheters and a significant number using 5F catheters (see Chapter 14). Yet further reductions in size might be foreseeable. One of the future directions is transradial intervention (TRI) using smaller-size guiding catheter, sheathless techniques, 0.010-inch wires, and very small-sized coronary balloons, that is, 1.0 mm in diameter.

In 1999, Dr. Motomaru Masutani, Dr. Fuminobu Yoshimachi, and Dr. Takashi Matsukage launched the "Slender Club Japan" (Fig. 8-1). Their goal to collaborate with the industry to produce "slender devices and cool intervention" has rapidly become popular in Japan, with several live case sessions organized throughout the year. Overall, several people still have negative feelings about TRI because of its unsteadiness. Slender PCI such as TRI using a 5F or smaller guiding catheter may be even worse. At this stage, we must recognize that slender techniques are still technically more challenging, with some limitations.

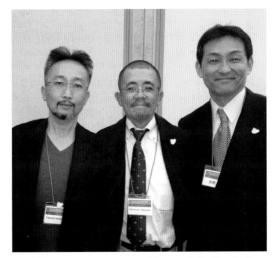

FIGURE 8-1 Dr. Motomaru Masutani, Dr. Fuminobu Yoshimachi, and Dr. Takashi Matsukage.

Yet we believe that emerging slender PCI is the future direction of PCI because of its less invasive nature. In this chapter, the new techniques, new devices, and current results of slender PCI are discussed.

What Is Slender Percutaneous Coronary Intervention?

PCI started as an alternative to coronary artery bypass surgery (CABG) in treating coronary artery disease. Despite the long-term superiority of bypass surgery as shown in many comparative studies, the use of PCI has increased over CABG for the last three decades. This is probably due to the less invasive nature of PCI. CABG required general anesthesia, sternotomy, and sometimes cardiac arrest assisted by cardiopulmonary pump. However, PCI required local anesthesia, a small skin incision, and no need for cardiac arrest. It is natural that patients prefer a less invasive strategy.

PCI also has several complications, such as bleeding or embolic complications. Bleeding at the puncture site, such as retroperitoneal bleeding, causes a critical event.[1] Even minor bleeding at the puncture site decreases the quality of life of the patient. Although the clinically positive cerebral infarction rate after PCI is reported to be less than 1%, minor cerebral infarction detected by diffusion weight imaging of magnetic resonance after regular PCI was between 10% and 15%.[2,3] Cholesterol embolism is a rare complication, but it is critical.[4] It may be more frequent in transfemoral intervention (TFI) than in TRI because thick and diffuse atherosclerotic plaques in the descending aorta are the origin of cholesterol embolism in many cases.[5] Although it is true that PCI is less invasive than CABG, we need to think of a further less invasive strategy to reduce the complications of PCI. To reduce bleeding complications and cholesterol embolism, the use of a slender guiding catheter in TRI can be an option.

In a narrow sense, "slender PCI" is defined as the use of a smaller device than the routinely used PCI devices. In a broader sense, slender PCI includes all the pursuits of a less invasive strategy of coronary revascularization. Recently launched in Europe by Dr. Ferdinand Kiemeneij and Dr. Shigeru Saito, Slender Club Europe intends to explore new technologies as well as change in practice in order to optimize PCI results. Beyond device miniaturization, this involves risks minimization of any complication, reduction of PCI costs, and same-day discharge.

Device Compatibility in Slender Guiding Catheters

In the early 1990s, balloon angioplasty required 8F guiding catheters. The first Palmaz–Schatz stent was 9F guiding catheter compatible; then its size was reduced to 8F compatible. The first directional coronary atherectomy required a 10F guiding catheter; then there was a gradual downsize to 8F compatible. In the late 1990s, coronary

stent size was reduced to 6F guiding compatible. Device compatibility changes all the time, and each size has its own limitations. Thus, we need to choose catheter size according to the required technique for each patient. If access site complication could be ignored, using a bigger catheter might have no technical limitations. However, recent studies have shown that access site bleeding complications relate with worse hard end points; we need to use a guiding catheter as slender as possible. Careful selection of appropriate-size guiding catheter on the basis of the PCI plan for the patient is a modern PCI approach. Specific to radial techniques, slender PCI brings the hope of risk minimization of radial artery occlusion postcatheterization and/or interventions.

New Devices in Slender Percutaneous Coronary Intervention

To achieve slender PCI, we introduce new slender PCI systems.

Downsizing in Regular 0.014 Inch Balloons

Regular 0.014-Inch compatible balloons are getting slender. Previously, the King Ghidorra technique (KGT), that is, simultaneous inflation of three balloons for complex trifurcations, required an 8F guiding catheter. Using new smaller-size balloons, we can do KGT with a 7F guiding catheter.

0.010-Inch Guidewire and Compatible Balloon System

A 0.010-inch wire and compatible balloon system could have a significantly big impact to downsize PCI materials. The 0.010-inch coronary wire system was available at the beginning of the 1990s, but its popularity fell and almost disappeared. Thus, the 0.010-inch system is not new but rather a revival. However, the current 0.010-inch system is smaller than that of the 1990s. The distal tip of some slender balloons is 0.012 inch compatible, that is, smaller than the regular 0.014-inch guidewire. Thus, the passing ability of the device is excellent. Furthermore, the small diameter of those slender balloons made the kissing balloon technique (KBT) possible within a 5F guiding catheter[6] and the KGT possible within a 6F guiding catheter.[7] With the standard 0.014-inch system, the KBT still requires 6F guiding catheter and the KGT requires 8F guiding catheter.

The IKAzuchi TEN (IKATEN) registry study showed the safety and feasibility of routine use of the 0.010-inch system in the real-world PCI, with a clinical success rate of 99%.[8] The passing ability of the balloon was also excellent. However, the 0.010-inch guidewire did not allow stents to pass a bended lesion due to less supporting ability. Despite this, the 0.010-inch guidewire had a high success rate in passing through chronic total occlusion (CTO), a fact supported by Masutani et al.,[9] who reported the efficacy of the 0.010-inch system for CTO lesions.

The Prospective multicenter registry of IKAzuchi-X for CHronic total occlUsion (PIKA-CHU) registry study[10] was then conducted to show the efficacy of the 0.010-inch system for CTO lesions. About 68% of lesions were successfully treated only with 0.010-inch system from the antegrade approach, whereas 86% of lesions were successfully treated using any devices including the 0.014-inch system. The 68% success rate was notable only from the antegrade approach. Recently, we have started the G-FORCE study, which is a multicenter prospective randomized trial, to show the superiority of the guidewire having a distal tip size of 0.010 inch or less for the CTO treatment. This study intends to show the superiority of using slender guidewires for CTO lesions.

Small-Size Intravascular Ultrasound Catheter

In a 5F guiding catheter, it is impossible to use the Atlantis pro-intravascular ultrasound (IVUS) catheter (Boston Scientific, Marlborough, MA) with a 0.014-inch guidewire. However, it is possible if the guidewire is 0.010 inch. Interestingly, two 0.010-inch guidewires can be passed through the Atlantis pro-IVUS catheter, even though a single 0.014-inch guidewire cannot. On the contrary, the Eagle eye IVUS catheter (Volcano, San Diego, CA) can be used with a 0.014-inch guidewire. Boston Scientific has recently launched a new version of its IVUS catheter which is now compatible with 5F guiding catheters.

The View-it IVUS catheter (Terumo) can also be used with a 0.014-inch guidewire in a 5F guiding catheter. Thus, some Japanese IVUS-oriented PCI operators turned to slender PCI because the View-it system has the same ability as the Atlantis IVUS catheter. The View-it IVUS system is available only in Japan. IVUS guide parallel wire technique for complex CTO PCI requires an 8F guiding catheter. However, it can be downsized to a 7F using the View-it IVUS catheter.

New Techniques in Slender Percutaneous Coronary Intervention

Bifurcation Treatment in Slender Percutaneous Coronary Intervention

Bifurcation lesions remain a challenge in today's PCI[11] (see Chapter 18). Crush stenting requires an 8F guiding catheter because two stents should be inserted in a guiding catheter (Table 8-1). The crush stent technique is simple and easy. However, it is not widely performed currently because of low long-term patency at the side branch.[12,13] If we do not perform the crush technique, we can reduce the guiding catheter size. Except for the backup problems, device compatibility is similar between 6F and 7F in bifurcation treatment. As it is impossible to perform KBT in a 5F guiding catheter without a 0.010-inch system,[6] it has been a limitation of 5F for bifurcation lesions. The clinical impact of KBT is more debatable now, but many operators still use it routinely. As far as KBT is concerned, the 0.010-inch system has great impact on the bifurcation treatment.[6] Then, left main bifurcation can be treated in TRI[14] even using 5F.[6] Furthermore, the KGT is now possible within a 6F guiding catheter using the 0.010-inch system.[7]

Chronic Total Occlusion

Many operators treat CTO lesions in TRI.[15] However, it requires strong backup force to pass a balloon or a microcatheter into the CTO lesion. Thus, many operators prefer larger guiding catheter to treat CTO. Some easy CTO lesions such as those with no calcification, short lesions, and straight lesions with low J-CTO score[16] can be treated using a 5F catheter. Some operators are interested in a 5F guiding catheter for retrograde approach because a microcatheter passage like corsair is enough for the retrograde catheter. At present, a 5F guiding catheter has many limitations in treating CTO (e.g., impossible parallel wire technique).

TABLE 8-1	**Bifurcation Treatment Technique**				
	Without 0.010" System		**With 0.010" System**		
Catheter Size	*Available Technique*	*Available Device*	*Available Technique*	*Available Device*	
8F	Crash stent	2 Stents	Crash stent	2 Stents	
	Culotte stent		Culotte stent		
	T stent		T stent		
	KGT	3 Balloons	KGT	3 Balloons	
	KBT	2 Balloons	KBT	2 Balloons	
7F	Crash stent	2 Stents	Crash stent	2 Stents	
	Culotte stent		Culotte stent		
	T stent		T stent		
	KGT	3 Balloons	KGT	3 Balloons	
	KBT	2 Balloons	KBT	2 Balloons	
6F	Crash stent	2 Stents	Crash stent	2 Stents	
	Culotte stent		Culotte stent		
	T stent		T stent		
	KGT	3 Balloons	KGT	3 Balloons	
	KBT	2 Balloons	KBT	2 Balloons	
5F	Crash stent	2 Stents	Crash stent	2 Stents	
	Culotte stent		Culotte stent		
	T stent		T stent		
	KGT	3 Balloons	KGT	3 Balloons	
	KBT	2 Balloons	KBT	2 Balloons	

KGT, King Ghidorra technique; KBT, kissing balloon technique.

Masutani et al.[9] suggested the 0.010-inch system for CTO lesions. The PIKACHU registry study was then conducted to show the efficacy of the 0.010-inch system for CTO lesions.[10] The success rate was as high as 68% for lesions treated only with 0.010-inch system from the antegrade approach because small-size distal tip could track the microchannels in CTO lesions. Thus, the major limitation of 5F catheter for CTO is the backup problem in a small guiding catheter. However, mother-and-child technique is now feasible with 4F catheters, which greatly enhance the support and can be very useful for cacified or CTO lesions.

Distal Protection in Slender Percutaneous Coronary Intervention

Distal protection occlusion balloon (PercuSurge, Medtronics, Fridley, MN) can be used in a 5F guiding catheter. However, it is suggested that this be used in a larger guiding catheter (because of the aspiration catheter) as the distal protection occlusion balloon (PercuSurge) requires aspiration after stenting. To this day, the smallest aspiration catheter still requires 6F or larger size. Interestingly, Yoshimachi et al.[17] used a 5F guiding catheter as an aspiration catheter. He deeply engaged the guiding into the vessel and aspirated using the 5F guiding catheter. Some cases have been performed using the Angiojet aspiration catheter with 5F guiding catheter, but contrast injection was not feasible with the Angiojet inside the guiding. The exact benefit of routine thrombectomy in acute ST-elevation myocardial infarction is still unclear, but if ongoing studies such as RIVAL confirm the potential, this will be a strong incentive for device companies to develop <6F compatible thrombectomy catheters.

Intravascular Ultrasound Catheter in 4F Guiding Catheter

IVUS during PCI is very popular among Japanese operators. In some cases, PCI can be performed through 4F guiding catheters. However, at this time, there is no possibility to perform IVUS through 4F guiding catheter, yet Yoshimachi reported the technique of IVUS in a 4F guiding catheter as guideless insertion of an IVUS catheter. The 4F guiding catheter was removed without removing a guidewire from the right coronary artery. Because an IVUS catheter can pass through a 4F sheath equal to 6F guiding catheter, the IVUS catheter was inserted through a 4F sheath without any guiding catheter. The bare IVUS catheter passed through the arteries into the coronary artery without a guiding catheter. This was called Emperor's New Clothes technique.

Sheathless System

Currently, the outer diameter of arterial sheath has 2F size up (see Chapter 20). For example, a 5F sheath has a 5F inner diameter, but the outer diameter is equal to 7F guiding catheter. Sheathless system can significantly reduce the size.[18-30] Recently, a 5F sheathless system has been developed by Medikit, but is still only available in Japan. This is equal to a 7F guiding catheter's inner diameter, but the outer diameter is 5F sheath. Table 8-2 lists actual inner and external diameters of current slender diagnostic and PCI catheters. It must be remembered that the French unit design outer diameters should be converted to millimeters by dividing the F value by 3; that is, 6F is equivalent to 6/3 = 2 mm outer diameter. Although often ignored, similar F values might in fact represent different values in millimeter. This is why the notion of « virtual » F has been proposed.

Virtual 3F/Virtual 2F

Today, the smallest commercially available guiding catheter size in Japan is 4F. However, we might still require smaller guiding catheters, such as 3F. The inner diameter of a 3F sheath is equal to the inner diameter of a 5F guiding catheter. Thus, a very long 3F sheath can be inserted up to the coronary artery.[19,31,32] The skin and arterial injury is of the same size as when the 3F sheath is used; however, the inner diameter is equal to a 5F guiding catheter. It is also possible to use a 5F guiding catheter instead of a 3F sheath. This is the same as the virtual 3F technique because the skin injury is equal to that when using the 3F sheath. Similarly, virtual 2F means 4F guiding catheter without

sheath.[33] The smallest diagnostic catheter is of 3F size. If we use the catheter without the sheath, it can be called virtual 1F. Measuring the size, the virtual 3F is equal to 19G needle size. It can reduce the size of the incision (very small) and the hemostasis time.

Minimum Contrast Technique

One of the benefits of 5F guiding catheter is the reduction of contrast dye volume, compared with that when using a larger guiding catheter, because of its smaller dead space. In case of severe chronic kidney disease, this may allow to reduce contrast dye to the minimum. This is why an exclusive IVUS-assisted PCI technique has been tested.[34] Every single step of PCI was validated solely by IVUS findings without any angiography except for the initial and final injections. Since angiography is performed only once at the beginning and once at the end of PCI, the contrast volume is generally less than 10 mL. Whether this IVUS-based PCI technique can significantly reduce the risks of contrast-induced kidney injury compared to other contrast sparing techniques remains to be proven.

Conclusion and Future Perspective

There are two main limitations with slender PCI techniques (Table 8-3). One is the limited device compatibility. The other limitation is weaker backup force of guiding catheters. The backup force of the guiding catheter is one of the keys for successful PCI. We have to say that it is the biggest limitation of slender PCI. Thus, operators of slender PCI must have deep consideration of backup force mechanics.

Recently, Dr. Saito and colleagues reported the results of the NAUSICA trial (Novel Angioplasty USIng Coronary Accessor) (clinicaltrials. gov identifier No. NCT00815997). In this multicenter randomized trial, all sorts of coronary lesions were treated using a 4F guiding catheter or standard 6F catheters. Overall, procedural success was similar in both groups (99%), but access site–related complications were significantly reduced in the 4F group, compared to 6F group (0% vs 6%, $P = 0.02$). Of note, hemostasis time was significantly reduced in the 4F group, and there was a trend for less radial artery

TABLE 8-2 Slender Conversion Table

Market Size	3Fr		4Fr		5Fr		6Fr		7Fr		8Fr	
	Diag.	PCI	Diag.	PCI	Diag.	PCI	Diag.	PCI	Diag.	PCI	Diag.	PCI
TERUMO OD			1.35 (0.053')	1.43 (0.056')	1.68 (0.066')	1.73 (0.068')	2.00	2.06 (0.081')		2.36 (0.093')		2.80 (0.110')
TERUMO ID			1.12 (0.044')	1.27 (0.050')		1.50 (0.059')		1.80 (0.071')		2.06 (0.081')		2.27 (0.089')
MEDIKIT OD	1.15 (0.043')		1.40 (0.55')	1.43 (0.056')		1.76 (0.070')						
MEDIKIT ID	0.85 (0.033')		1.05 (0.041')	1.26 (0.050')		1.50 (0.059')						
Virtual Fr	1Fr Sheathless		2Fr Sheahless		3Fr Sheathless							
ASAHI OD				1.50 (0.059')				2.16 (0.085')		2.49 (0.098')		2.80 (0.110')
ASAHI ID				1.28 (0.050')				1.78 (0.070')		2.06 (0.081')		2.27 (0.089')
Virtual Fr							6.5Fr		7.5Fr		8.5Fr	
Theoretical Fr size in mm (OD)*	1.0		1.33		1.666		2.0		2.333		2.66	

*OD = outer diameter. ID = internal diameter. By convention, French size represents the outer diameter and it is calculated as x Fr : 3 = OD in mm (for example, a 6Fr guiding is 6 : 3 = 2mm OD). In reality, sheaths and catheters have variable sizes according to manufacturers. The concept of virtual Fr sizes has been introduced by Japanese operators to describe the approximate OD of sheathless guiding catheters.

Name	Detail	Reference
5F de Percu	PercuSurge distal protection in a 5F guiding catheter	17
5F de Filter	Filter protection within a 5F guiding catheter	NA
5F de Kiss	KBT in a 5F guiding catheter	6
6F de KGT	KGT (simultaneous triple balloon inflation) in a 6F guiding catheter	7
5F de CTO	CTO treatment using a 5F guiding catheter	9, 10
Emperor's new clothes	IVUS is too big to pass within a 4F guiding catheter. Perform IVUS after removing the 4F guiding catheter	NA
Virtual 3F	Outer diameter of 5F guiding catheter is equal to 3F sheath. Insert 5F guiding without sheath	19, 31, 32
Virtual 2F	Outer diameter of 4F guiding catheter is equal to 2F sheath. Insert 4F guiding without sheath	33
MINICON PCI	IVUS guide PCI using minimum contrast volume to reduce contrast-induced nephropathy	34

TABLE 8-3 **New Techniques in Slender PCI**

NA, not available; CTO, chronic total occlusion; IVUS, intravascular ultrasound; MINICON PCI, minimum contrast PCI.

occlusion (assessed by pulse) in the 4F group (0% vs 4%, $P = 0.08$).

Interestingly, there are now two types of 4F guiding catheters (inner lumen = 0.050") which can be used as "mother-and-child" techniques and greatly enhance 5F or 6F guiding catheter support.[35,36]

REFERENCES

1. Eikelboom JW, Mehta SR, Anand SS, et al. Adverse impact of bleeding on prognosis in patients with acute coronary syndromes. *Circulation.* 2006;114(8):774–782.
2. Busing KA, Schulte-Sasse C, Flüchter S, et al. Cerebral infarction: incidence and risk factors after diagnostic and interventional cardiac catheterization—prospective evaluation at diffusion-weighted MR imaging. *Radiology.* 2005;235(1):177–183.
3. Lund C, Nes RB, Ugelstad TP, et al. Cerebral emboli during left heart catheterization may cause acute brain injury. *Eur Heart J.* 2005;26(13):1269–1275.
4. Karalis DG, Quinn V, Victor MF, et al. Risk of catheter-related emboli in patients with atherosclerotic debris in the thoracic aorta. *Am Heart J.* 1996;131(6):1149–1155.
5. Khoury Z, Gottlieb S, Stern S, et al. Frequency and distribution of atherosclerotic plaques in the thoracic aorta as determined by transesophageal echocardiography in patients with coronary artery disease. *Am J Cardiol.* 1997;79(1):23–27.
6. Yoshimachi F, Masutani M, Matsukage T, et al. Kissing balloon technique within a 5 Fr guiding catheter using 0.010 inch guidewires and 0.010 inch guidewire-compatible balloons. *J Invasive Cardiol.* 2007;19(12):519–524.
7. Matsukage T, Masuda N, Ikari Y. Simultaneous triple-balloon inflation technique within a 6 Fr guiding catheter for a trifurcation lesion. *J Invasive Cardiol.* 2008;20(7):E210–E214.
8. Matsukage T, Yoshimachi F, Masutani M, et al. A new 0.010-inch guidewire and compatible balloon catheter system: the IKATEN registry. *Catheter Cardiovasc Interv.* 2009;73(5):605–610.
9. Masutani M, Yoshimachi F, Matsukage T, et al. Use of slender catheters for transradial angiography and interventions. *Indian Heart J.* 2008;60(1)(suppl A):A22–A26.
10. Matsukage T, Masutani M, Yoshimachi F, et al. A prospective multicenter registry of 0.010-inch guidewire and compatible system for chronic total occlusion: the PIKACHU registry. *Catheter Cardiovasc Interv.* 2010;75(7):1006–1012.
11. Pinkerton CA, Slack JD. Complex coronary angioplasty: a technique for dilatation of bifurcation stenoses. *Angiology.* 1985;36(8):543–548.
12. Colombo A, Bramucci E, Saccà S, et al. Randomized study of the crush technique versus provisional side-branch stenting in true coronary bifurcations: the CACTUS (Coronary Bifurcations: Application of the Crushing Technique Using Sirolimus-Eluting Stents) study. *Circulation.* 2009;119(1):71–78.
13. Costa RA, Mintz GS, Carlier SG, et al. Bifurcation coronary lesions treated with the "crush" technique: an intravascular ultrasound analysis. *J Am Coll Cardiol.* 2005;46(4):599–605.
14. Cheng CI, Wu CJ, Fang CY, et al. Feasibility and safety of transradial stenting for unprotected left main coronary artery stenoses. *Circ J.* 2007;71(6):855–861.
15. Saito S, Tanaka S, Hiroe Y, et al. Angioplasty for chronic total occlusion by using tapered-tip guidewires. *Catheter Cardiovasc Interv.* 2003;59(3):305–311.
16. Morino Y, Abe M, Morimoto T, et al. Predicting successful guidewire crossing through chronic total occlusion of native coronary lesions within 30 minutes: the J-CTO (Multicenter CTO Registry in Japan) score as a difficulty grading and time assessment tool. *JACC Cardiovasc Interv.* 2011;4(2):213–221.
17. Yoshimachi F, Ikari Y, Matsukage T, et al. A novel method of PercuSurge distal protection in a five French guiding catheter without an export aspiration catheter. *J Invasive Cardiol.* 2008;20(4):168–172.
18. Mamas MA, Fath-Ordoubadi F, Fraser DG. Atraumatic complex transradial intervention using large bore sheathless guide catheter. *Catheter Cardiovasc Interv.* 2008;72(3):357–364.

19. Takeshita S, Saito S. Transradial coronary intervention using a novel 5-Fr sheathless guiding catheter. *Catheter Cardiovasc Interv.* 2009;74(6):862–865.

20. From AM, Gulati R, Prasad A, et al. Sheathless transradial intervention using standard guide catheters. *Catheter Cardiovasc Interv.* 2010;76(7):911–916.

21. Liang M, Puri A, Linder R, Transradial simultaneous kissing stenting (SKS) with sheathless access. *Catheter Cardiovasc Interv.* 2010;75(2):222–224.

22. Mamas M, D'Souza S, Hendry C, et al. Use of the sheathless guide catheter during routine transradial percutaneous coronary intervention: a feasibility study. *Catheter Cardiovasc Interv.* 2010;75(4):596–602.

23. Bayard YL, Jakob D, Meier B. All comers 5 French transfemoral percutaneous coronary intervention without sheath. *Catheter Cardiovasc Interv.* 2011;78(1):47–51.

24. Chiam PT, Liu B, Wong AS, et al. Comparison of novel 6.5 Fr sheathless guiding catheters versus 5 Fr guiding catheters for transradial coronary intervention. *EuroIntervention.* 2011;7(8):930–935.

25. Deftereos S, Giannopoulos G, Tousoulis D, et al. Sheathless transulnar versus standard femoral arterial access for percutaneous coronary intervention on bifurcation lesions. *Int J Cardiol.* 2011;149(3):398–400.

26. From AM, Bell MR, Rihal CS, et al. Minimally invasive transradial intervention using sheathless standard guiding catheters. *Catheter Cardiovasc Interv.* 2011;78(6): 866–871.

27. Sciahbasi A, Mancone M, Cortese B, et al. Transradial percutaneous coronary interventions using sheathless guiding catheters: a multicenter registry. *J Interv Cardiol.* 2011;24(5):407–412.

28. James D, Huang Y, Kwan TW. Percutaneous coronary intervention via transulnar sheathless approach. *J Invasive Cardiol.* 2012;24(7):E157–E158.

29. Kwan TW, Cherukuri S, Huang Y, et al. Feasibility and safety of 7F sheathless guiding catheter during transradial coronary intervention. *Catheter Cardiovasc Interv.* 2012;80(2):274–280.

30. Kwan TW, Ratcliffe JA, Huang Y, et al. Balloon-assisted sheathless transradial intervention (BASTI) using 5 Fr guiding catheters. *J Invasive Cardiol.* 2012;24(5):231–233.

31. Matsukage T, Yoshimachi F, Masutani M, et al. Virtual 3 Fr PCI system for complex percutaneous coronary intervention. *EuroIntervention.* 2009;5(4):515–517.

32. Mizuno S, Takeshita S, Taketani Y, et al. Percutaneous coronary intervention using a virtual 3-Fr guiding catheter. *Catheter Cardiovasc Interv.* 2010;75(7):983–988.

33. Tanaka A, Saito S. Percutaneous coronary intervention with a virtual 2-Fr system. *Catheter Cardiovasc Interv.* 2010;76(5):684–686.

34. Ogata N, Matsukage T, Toda E, et al. Intravascular ultrasound-guided percutaneous coronary interventions with minimum contrast volume for prevention of the radiocontrast-induced nephropathy: report of two cases. *Cardiovasc Interv Ther.* 2011;26:83–88.

35. Honda T, Fujimoto K, Miyao Y. Successful percutaneous coronary intervention using a 4-in-3 "slender mother and child" PCI technique. *Adv Interv Cardiol.* 2013;9(3):286–290.

36. Tobita K, Takeshita S, Saito S. The 4-in-5 mother-child technique: 5 Fr transradial coronary intervention for complex lesions using a 4 Fr child catheter. *J Invasive Cardiol.* 2013;25(8):406–408.

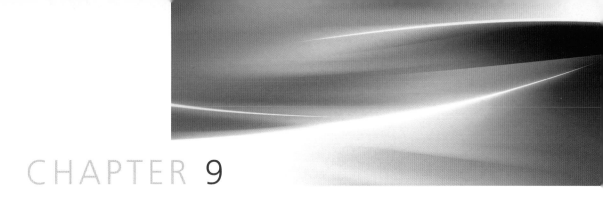

CHAPTER 9

Radial Artery Spasm and Abnormal Flow Reserve

Sudhir Rathore

The incidence of radial artery spasm (RAS) during transradial procedures has been reported to be around 10% to 20%, and in about 2% to 5% of the patients, this prevents the successful completion of the procedure by the transradial route.[1-4] RAS has been mainly defined in literature as the patient discomfort encountered during manipulation of arterial sheath or guide catheter in a radial artery and is also associated with considerable amount of friction. This friction is mainly due to mismatch between the outer diameter of the radial sheath or the guide and the inner diameter of the radial artery. This mismatch can be caused by smaller radial artery diameter as compared to the radial sheath size or due to the true RAS. There are several other factors that can also play a role in this mismatch (e.g., fixed atherosclerotic lesions, vessel tortuosity, and entry into the small aberrant arteries).

The occurrence of RAS during transradial coronary procedure could play a role in the patient's and/or physician's preference when choosing between the transradial and the transfemoral approaches.

The radial artery is a muscular artery with a prominent medial layer that is largely dominated by α1-adrenoreceptor function.[5] Much of the discomfort and difficulty of the transradial procedure is related to the vasospasm induced by the introduction of a sheath or catheter into the radial artery.[1-3] Circulating levels of catecholamine also play a role in RAS[6]; therefore, local anesthesia and adequate sedation to control anxiety, which would reduce circulating catecholamines during catheter insertion, may be important preventative measures.

Pathologic Basis of Radial Artery Spasm and Vascular Function

The radial artery is a thick-walled muscular artery. The intima has one layer of the endothelial cells beneath which multiple layers of subendothelial cells and a small number of myocytes are present. The internal elastic lamina has multiple fenestrations, and the media is composed of many leiomyocytes, elastic and collagen fibers, fibroblasts, and rare macrophages. The external elastic lamina is less individualized than the internal lamina. There is some evidence that the vaso vasorum, nerves, and lymphatic vessels are confined to the adventitia, and do not join the medial layer within the structure of the adventitia.[7]

The radial artery has a thicker wall as compared to other arteries and has higher density of muscle cells with the same amount of elastic tissue in its media[8] (Fig. 9-1). Moreover, in the radial artery, the myocytes are organized into multiple tight layers, and this, together with the wider thickness of the media, may at least in part explain the propensity of the radial artery to spasm.[7] Kaufer et al.[9] has investigated the pathology of the radial artery in 102 patients undergoing coronary artery bypass surgery. In their study, the intima-to-media ratio of more than 0.25 was noted in 54% of the patients as compared to 23% in the left internal mammary artery (LIMA) specimens. They analyzed the correlation between the degree of atherosclerosis and the various demographic factors. They found weak but statistically significant correlation between the degree

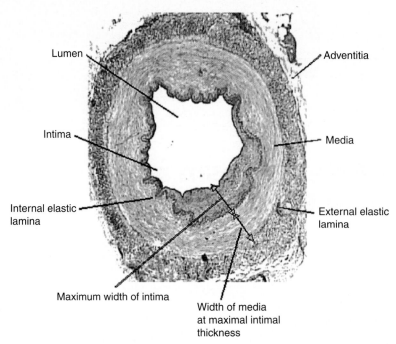

Lumen

Adventitia

Intima

Media

Internal elastic lamina

External elastic lamina

Maximum width of intima

Width of media at maximal intimal thickness

FIGURE 9-1   Different layers of the radial artery.

of atherosclerosis and diabetes ($r = 0.2061$; $P = 0.038$), male sex ($r = 0.3224$; $P = 0.001$), and advanced age ($r = 0.3262$; $P = 0.001$). The atherosclerotic involvement of the radial artery would reduce the lumen of the artery and could be one factor in predisposing the artery to spasm and endothelial dysfunction.

A similar study by Vanson et al.[7] has also shown that the radial artery is a muscular artery and the intima-media thickness is around 529 ± 52 μm, which may predispose the artery to spasm, causing occlusion and ischemia in patients undergoing bypass surgery. The radial artery is prone to accelerated intimal hyperplasia following endothelial injury or focal damage to the intima.

Physiologic Basis of Radial Artery Spasm and Vascular Function

According to the functional classification of the arterial grafts,[7] the radial artery belongs to type 3, a type of graft that is more spastic than type 1 arteries. To further investigate the spasmogenic nature of the radial arteries, He and Yang[10] investigated the subtype of adrenoreceptors found in the human radial artery in an ex vivo study. They, for the first time, were able to demonstrate that the radial artery is an α-1-adrenoceptor-dominant artery with little β-adrenoceptor function and that the post-α-1-adrenoceptor is dominant, although α-2 functions also exist. Therefore, circulating catecholamines will primarily contract the radial arteries through the α-1 mechanism, and the use of β-blockers will be unlikely to evoke radial artery contraction or spasm during or after coronary artery bypass surgery. RAS can result in the occlusion of radial artery in some cases. This understanding of radial artery physiology is important in the pathophysiology of RAS and occlusion and their avoidance and treatment.

Definition of Radial Artery Spasm

Radial artery vasospasm is induced by the introduction of a sheath or catheter into the radial artery and is usually manifest as difficulty in manipulating the catheter and/or the experience of discomfort in the forearm or upper arm by the patient. This is usually caused by the friction between the outer lining of the arterial sheath and the radial artery wall or pressure due to the overstretching of the arterial wall. Several operator- and patient-specific questionnaires have been developed and used to qualitatively assess RAS. These questionnaires rate the difficulty perceived by the operator and the discomfort experienced by the patient during the procedure. Some investigators have tried to quantify RAS using an automated pull-back device.[11] They have shown that all patients who experienced clinical RAS, as assessed subjectively by the difficulty perceived by the operator or pain perceived by the patient during the procedure, had a mean pull-back force of greater than 1 kg, while all other patients without a clinical spasm had a mean pull-back force of less than 1 kg. Similarly, Saito et al.[12] tested in vitro friction resistance as a surrogate for RAS. They concluded that a hydrophilic coating on the introducer sheath results in significantly less friction resistance. Objective methods of assessing RAS are cumbersome and impractical in a clinical setting.

Several studies have used a combination of definitions using operator- and patient-completed questionnaires used in previous studies[2-4,11] to quantify RAS both objectively and subjectively. Kiemeneij et al.,[11] using 6F 23-cm-long radial sheaths, have shown a direct correlation between the patient's assessment of pain during withdrawal of the radial artery sheath and the maximum pull-back force using an automated pull-back device. In a previous study,[11] these scores correlate with significant RAS measured objectively.

Measurement of Radial Artery Spasm

In clinical practice, RAS is mainly described as increased resistance during manipulation of the intra-arterial equipment and may or may not be associated with the patient complaining of pain in the forearm. Researchers have used a combination of operators and patients questionnaires to measure the extent of RAS. There have also been attempts to quantify the RAS objectively by the use of an automatic pull-back device (APD) for removal of the arterial sheath.[11] This device consists of a motorized trolley that railroad over a fixed platform. The trolley houses a digital force gauge (DFG) and a controller unit, which are connected to a personal computer for system control and data collection. The controller unit guides the movement of the trolley as per the commands set by the operator, and the DFG makes multiple instantaneous recordings during the pullback. With the use of this device, the researchers have shown, in 50 consecutive patients, the mean maximal pull-back force was 0.53 ± 0.52 kg (range, 0.1–3.0 kg). In 48 patients, the maximal pull-back

force was reached within the first 5 seconds of the pullback. All patients with clinical RAS, as assessed by the combination of operators and patients questionnaires, had a maximum pull-back force greater than 1.0 kg, while the remaining patients had a maximum pull-back force of less than 1.0 kg. In this study, clinical RAS was defined as the pain perceived by the patient and/or difficulty perceived by the operator during sheath insertion, removal, or catheter manipulation.

As mentioned above, there are quantitative and qualitative methods of assessing RAS during transradial procedures. However, the quantitative methods can only measure the spasm during sheath withdrawal, but this is not the clinical spasm that may prevent completion of the procedure. The clinical spasm during the procedure and the pull-back force needed to remove the sheath may be related. There is no way of quantifying the spasm that grips the catheter and makes torsion difficult during the procedure. Therefore, there is the need to use qualitative definition of spasm for our study. The qualitative definition of RAS has been used widely by several researchers to assess the efficacy of different drugs and equipment used during transradial procedures, and their impact on RAS.

Mechanism of and Factors Predisposing to Radial Artery Spasm

The radial artery has a prominent medial layer, composed of smooth muscle, which is largely dominated by α-1-adrenoreceptor function.[13] Thus, increased levels of circulating catecholamines predispose the artery to RAS.

It has also been well established that the vascular endothelium synthesizes and releases potent vasoactive factors that play active roles in vascular biology and pathophysiology. Among the various compounds formed in the endothelium are nitric oxide (NO) and endothelin-1 (ET-1), vasoactive factors that strongly influence the modulation of vascular tone.[14] In the intact blood vessel wall, there is a continuous basal release of both NO and ET-1. Mechanical forces such as shear stress and the activation of various receptors regulate the release of these vasoactive substances.[15] However, the balance between the two antagonistic substances, together with other released factors and the reactivity of smooth muscle cells, play an important role in the determination of vascular tone and various other physiologic processes.

In the vascular wall, endothelial cells and smooth muscle cells also generate superoxide, which is involved in the pathogenesis of RAS through its effects on NO scavenging, on peroxynitrite generation, and on redox-sensitive cell-signaling pathways.[16] An in vitro study by Aksungar et al.[17] has shown that basal and thrombin-stimulated release of NO from the internal mammary artery is higher than from the radial artery, while the release of ET-1 from the internal mammary artery is less than from the radial artery. This observation shows the functional difference between the two arterial beds and the higher tendency to spasm in the radial artery in reaction to various stimuli. Similarly, a better understanding of the contractile properties of radial artery smooth muscle will help address the critical question of RAS and its pathogenesis. Vascular smooth muscle tone is directly dependent on intracellular calcium concentration, which in turn is largely determined by the regulation of calcium influx through voltage-gated calcium channels. Potassium and calcium currents also play important roles in regulating the vascular tone. Several factors, including stretching and injury to the radial artery following radial artery manipulation, could affect ion channel function and subsequently interfere with the vasomotor response. It is known that potassium channel function is intricately regulated by endothelium-released autocoids, including prostaglandin I_2, NO, and endothelium-derived hyperpolarizing factors.[18]

Local anesthesia and adequate sedation to control anxiety during sheath insertion and catheter manipulation are potentially important preventative measures. Moreover, the friction or pressure caused by the mismatch between the outer diameter of the introducer sheath and the inner diameter of the radial artery could result in RAS by the various mechanisms discussed above. Therefore, increasing the mismatch between the size of the radial artery and the radial sheath could potentially cause more irritation, damage, and stimulation of the endothelium and smooth muscle cells. This would result in increased secretion of procoagulant and other vasoactive agents (ET-1 and superoxide radicals) causing RAS and injury. The length and coating of the introducer sheath could also have an impact on the occurrence of RAS. A long sheath, extending into the larger-diameter brachial artery, allows insertion, manipulation, and withdrawal of multiple catheters, without friction between the moving catheter and the surface of the radial artery. This results in less mechanical stimulation of the wall and also less irritation and damage to

the endothelium and smooth muscle cells, and therefore could be associated with less spasm. However, if spasm develops, it could be more difficult to retrieve a longer sheath. Sheaths with hydrophilic or lubricious coating may be easier to retrieve in the event of spasm.

Patient-related factors might play a role in the genesis of RAS (e.g., fixed atherosclerotic lesions,[19-21] vessel tortuousity, reduced radial artery diameter, or erroneous entrance into small side branches).

Impact of Vasodilator Agents on Radial Artery Spasm

It has been demonstrated in isolated radial artery ring segments that nitroglycerine and verapamil are effective agents in preventing arterial spasm.[22] A study using the APD has shown that an intra-arterial cocktail of verapamil and nitroglycerine reduces the incidence of pain from 14% to 34%. The mean pull-back force was also significantly lower (0.53 ± 0.52 kg vs 0.76 ± 0.45 kg) as compared to that in the patients not receiving any vasodilating drug.[12] In this study, clinically important RAS was seen in 8% of patients receiving a spasmolytic cocktail as compared to 22% in the control group ($P = 0.029$).

Salmeron et al. have shown, in a randomized controlled trial, that verapamil is more effective in preventing RAS than is phentolamine.[3] Both vasodilator agents induced a significant increase in radial artery diameter (2.22 ± 0.53 to 2.48 ± 0.57 mm for verapamil and 2.20 ± 0.53 to 2.45 ± 0.53 mm for phentolamine). However, verapamil was more effective in preventing RAS (13.2% vs 23.2% in phentolamine-treated patients) measured qualitatively.

SPASM study[23] group randomized patients to placebo, molsidomine, verapamil, or a combination of both verapamil and molsidomine, administered via the radial sheath. They concluded that the incidence of RAS was lowest in patients receiving verapamil and molsidomine (4.9%) than in patients receiving verapamil 2.5 or 5 mg (8.3% and 7.9%), molsidomine 1 mg (13.3%), or placebo (22.2%) ($P < 0.0001$). Filho et al.[24] have also shown in a randomized double-blind trial of 50 patients that the use of diltiazem, as an adjunctive drug to isosorbide mononitrate, administered through the transradial sheath, decreases the rate of vascular complications. Coppola et al.[25] have shown that the addition of nitroprusside to nitroglycerine did not further reduce the incidence of spasm. However, after multivariate analysis, the following variables were found to be independent predictors of RAS: radial artery diameter (RD)/height index ($P = 0.005$), RD/body surface area (BSA) index ($P = 0.012$), and sheath outer diameter (OD)/RD index ($P = 0.024$). The sex of the patient, presence of diabetes, BSA, and smoking history did not play any role in predicting the occurrence of RAS.

Similarly, Chen et al.[26] have shown the effectiveness of heparin and nitroglycerine combination in preventing RAS. In this study, there was no difference seen in the incidence of RAS between heparin + nitroglycerine+ verapamil and heparin + nitroglycerine groups. Recently, Kim et al.[27] have shown the effectiveness of nicorandil in preventing RAS. In a randomized study comparing 4 mg of nicorandil and 200 μg of nitroglycerine, the authors concluded that both agents induced a significant radial artery vasodilatation. Nicorandil caused a significant increase in the mean radial artery diameter compared to the cocktail at the midsegment of the radial artery (0.32 ± 0.23 mm for nicorandil and 0.24 ± 0.15 mm for nitroglycerine, $P < 0.05$). There was no significant difference between the rates of RAS, defined as discomfort during pullback of the sheath (50.7% vs 50.2%).

Fukuda et al.[28] have examined the incidence of RAS by radial arteriography immediately after and 5 months after the procedure in 48 patients. They quantified RAS by the degree of stenosis in the radial artery as compared to between the first (performed just after the transradial procedure) and the second arteriography (performed 5 months after the procedure using transbrachial approach). The radial artery diameter soon after the transradial procedure may be small because of RAS, and the investigators compared the radial artery diameter with baseline radial artery diameter on arteriography few months after the procedure. In this study, the authors defined more than 75% stenosis in the radial artery, 25% to 75% stenosis, and less than 25% stenosis as severe spasm, moderate spasm, and mild spasm, respectively. They concluded that some degree of radial spasm was seen in all patients, with severe spasm seen in 50% patients, moderate spasm in 23%, and mild spasm in 27%. They also found that the diameters of both the proximal and distal radial arteries in the severe spasm group were significantly smaller than those in the mild and moderate spasm groups (proximal site: severe group 2.39 ± 0.70 mm vs mild group 2.98 ± 0.46 mm, $P < 0.05$, and moderate group 2.96 ± 0.77 mm, $P < 0.05$; distal

site: severe group 2.26 ± 0.60 mm vs mild group 2.73 ± 0.47 mm, $P < 0.05$, and moderate group 2.86 ± 0.71 mm, $P < 0.05$). This study showed a correlation between severe spasm and the diameter of the artery.

Impact of the Introducer Sheath on Radial Artery Spasm

There are several different types of transradial introducer sheaths available from different manufacturers. The introducer sheaths from different manufacturers differ in sheath design and physical properties of the sheath. Broadly they can be divided into two groups: sheaths with different length and sheaths with or without hydrophilic coating.

The force required to remove an introducer sheath from the radial artery is the summative effect of various different forces: friction between the outer wall of the sheath and the inner radial artery wall, and friction between the outer wall of the sheath and the skin and the subcutaneous connective tissue. The former depends on the ratio of the inner luminal diameter of the vessel to the outer diameter of the sheath and the tone of the arterial wall musculature (anxiety and repeated punctures increase the tone and spasm) at the time of the procedure. The force required to insert or remove the sheath also depends on the surface properties of the two surfaces (hydrophilic coating might reduce friction) and also the surface area of contact between two surfaces (impact of length of sheath in contact with radial artery wall).

Therefore, the potential advantage of a long sheath may be the free movement of the guide and the guide wire in relation to the radial artery wall. This less mechanical stimulation of radial wall might be associated with less RAS and endothelial injury. However, if the spasm develops, it might be difficult to retrieve the long sheath. The opposite may be true for the short-length introducer sheath; they may be easier to retrieve in the event of spasm but could provide more substrate for the spasm because of the mechanical stimulation between the guide catheters and the guide wires. Similarly, the introducer sheaths coated with lubricious material could be easier to retrieve in the event of spasm because of less frictional force.

Saito et al.[12] have tested in vitro the static friction resistance between the introducer sheath with the hydrophilic coating and without the hydrophilic coating and also tested the durability of the lubricant. For the experiment, the sheath introducers were fixed to a strain gauge, and the glass tube filled with water and plugged by silicon rubber was slowly removed. The static friction resistance between the sheath introducer and the silicon rubber plug was defined as the maximum force between the glass tube moved away from the sheath introducer. They have also assessed the incidence of clinical RAS in both the groups. The researchers used a 6F (outer diameter 2.6 mm), 16-cm-long sheath from Terumo, Japan. Hydrophilic coating caused a 70% decrease in the friction force in the in vitro model (1,060 ± 105 to 312 ± 40 g force, $P < 0.0001$). Dynamic friction resistance, measured during 200 repeated forward and backward movements of the sheath introducers at a constant rate of 1,000 per minute, was highest in both groups at the beginning of the tests and was preserved during the tests. At all time points during the tests, dynamic friction resistance was significantly lower in sheaths with hydrophilic coating. The easiness of sheath insertion into the radial artery was not different in either group. The position stability of the sheath introducer was worse in hydrophilic group ($P = 0.0242$). The easiness of sheath removal was better in hydrophilic group ($P = 0.00003$). RAS occurred in one patient in the hydrophilic group (2.7%) and in four patients in the uncoated group (11%), $P = 0.15$. They concluded that the hydrophilic coating of the introducer sheath is useful during the transradial procedures.

Dery et al.[29] have assessed the impact of hydrophilic coating in a small randomized study of 90 patients. They used 6F, 19-cm-long hydrophilic-coated sheath or a 6F, 21-cm-long uncoated sheath, both from Cook, Inc, Bloomington, IN, USA. The researchers assessed the peak traction force by electronic traction gauge and quantification of pain at the time of removal of the introducer sheath. The mean ± SD peak traction force at sheath removal was 265 ± 167 g and 865 ± 318 g in the coated and uncoated groups, respectively (69% reduction; $P < 0.001$). Mean maximal pain score was 0.6 ± 1.2 and 4.8 ± 2.9 in the coated and uncoated groups, respectively (88% reduction; $P < 0.0001$). They concluded that the use of the hydrophilic-coated introducer sheath considerably reduces the traction force and the pain experienced by the patient during sheath removal.

Keimeneij et al.[30] also assessed the effects of hydrophilic-coated sheaths on the incidence of the RAS. All patients received 6F and 25-cm-long radial sheaths from Terumo and the vasodilator cocktail of heparin and nitroglycerine was used routinely. The APD as described before was used for sheath removal at the end of the procedure. Three patients (7%) in the coated group experienced discomfort during sheath removal, compared to 12 patients (27%) in the uncoated group ($P = 0.02$). The maximal pull-back force was significantly lower in the coated group than in the uncoated group (0.24 ± 0.31 vs 0.44 ± 0.33 kg; $P = 0.003$). Similarly, the mean pull-back force was significantly lower in the coated group (0.14 ± 0.23 vs 0.32 ± 0.24 kg; $P < 0.001$). They concluded that the removal of the coated Terumo transradial sheath requires less traction force than an identical uncoated sheath. The coated sheath was also associated with the less discomfort for the patient.

Koga et al.[31] assessed the impact of hydrophilic-coated catheters on the incidence of RAS during transradial procedures. They concluded that there was a reduced incidence of RAS, with the use of the hydrophilic-coated catheters (1% vs 11%, $P = 0.007$).

Therefore, there are a number of studies investigating the effect of hydrophilic coating on the introducer sheath in patients undergoing transradial coronary procedures. The available data suggest the usefulness of the hydrophilic-coated sheaths. However, these studies are small; some of them are nonrandomized and had routine use of vasodilator cocktail during the procedure. More recently, Rathore et al.[4] have studied the impact of length and hydrophilic coating of introducer sheath on RAS following transradial procedures in large randomized study involving 790 patients. The spasmolytic drugs were not used routinely in this study and were used in the event of RAS to assess the true impact of introducer sheath length and coating on RAS. The study shows that operator-defined RAS was observed in 230 (29.4%) of the patients and 172 (21.8%) patients reported discomfort of moderate or severe intensity. There was significantly less clinical RAS (relative reduction 50%) observed in patients randomized to a hydrophilic sheath. There was significantly less RAS (19.0% vs 39.9%, odds ratio [OR]: 2.87; 95% confidence interval [CI]: 2.07–3.97, $P < 0.001$) and patient-reported discomfort (15.1% vs 28.5%, OR: 2.27; 95% CI: 1.59–3.23, $P < 0.001$) observed in patients receiving a hydrophilic sheath. No significant difference was observed between the groups receiving long and short sheaths. An interaction test was applied to investigate the interaction between length and coating of the introducer sheath. There was no significant interaction observed between the length and coating for operator-defined RAS ($P < 0.108$) and patient-assessed RAS ($P < 0.631$).

The Potential Effects of Radial Artery Spasm on Other Complications

The above-mentioned studies have shown that RAS can cause discomfort to the patient and difficulty in retrieving the sheath at the end of the procedure. Spasm occurring during the procedure could cause increased friction between the sheath and the inner lining of the radial artery, resulting in damage to the endothelial lining of the radial artery. This interaction could result in the sustained endothelial damage and be a precursor for thrombus formation. Potentially, this can increase the incidence of nonocclusive and occlusive radial artery injury. This is a hypothesis, and although there is no proof of this, there is some evidence to support a link between vasospasm and subsequent neointimal hyperplasia. In the coronary vasculature, there is limited data supporting a relationship between vasospasm and neointimal hyperplasia.[31,32] Suzuki et al.[32] have found a high incidence (in 68% patients) of neointimal hyperplasia, thrombus formation, and intimal hemorrhage at the site of spasm from coronary atherectomy samples. They concluded that coronary vasospasm may provoke vascular injury that leads to the formation of neointima in these patients similar to that seen with restenosis. A study by Rathore et al.[4] has shown a high incidence of RAO in patients with documented spasm during their procedure (14.5% vs 7.4%, $P < 0.003$).

Predictors of Radial Artery Spasm

A recent study by Rathore et al.[4] has identified younger age, female sex, diabetes mellitus, smaller wrist circumference, low body mass index, and the use of uncoated introducer sheaths as predictors of RAS in univariate analysis. Younger age, female sex, diabetes mellitus, smaller wrist circumference, and low body mass index remained significant independent predictors of clinical RAS in multivariate analysis.

Previous studies have also identified younger age[23,25] and female sex[23,26] as independent predictors of RAS. Coppola et al.[25] also identified radial artery size, radial artery size to height ratio, radial artery size to sheath diameter ratio, and radial artery size to body mass index ratio as predictors of RAS. Our results are similar to those of these studies, and we identified additional predictors of RAS such as wrist size, diabetes mellitus, and body mass index. However, for simplicity, we did not measure the size of radial artery; so we cannot comment on morphometric indices involving measured artery size.

Morphometric indices might reflect mismatch between the radial artery size and the outer diameter of the introducer sheath, resulting in more friction resistance and overstretching, thereby causing more RAS and patient discomfort. Younger patients could be more anxious with higher resting sympathetic tone, and this could play a role in inducing RAS. Female patients generally have smaller wrist circumference and a smaller radial artery diameter, and this could predispose them to RAS. Whether differences in hormone status, pain tolerance, or anxiety between men and women will lead to different levels of catecholamine release, resulting in different rates of RAS, is unknown. Similarly, in diabetic patients, there could be a smaller internal diameter of the radial artery due to generalized atherosclerosis or increased intima-media thickness, which could predispose to RAS.

Physiologic Changes in the Radial Artery Following Transradial Procedures

The radial artery is a muscular artery and therefore more prone to spasm. The size of the radial artery is smaller and similar to the dimensions of the catheter and sheath used for transradial procedures, predisposing the vessel wall to injury during transradial procedures. These procedures can result in disruption and damage to endothelium and potentially cause injury to internal elastic laminae and tunica media, resulting in neointimal proliferation and arterial remodeling.

A small study has examined by ultrasound both endothelium- and nonendothelium-mediated vasodilatation of the radial artery before and after transradial catheterization.[33] The study group consisted of 18 patients, and a short sheath (7–12 cm) with no hydrophilic coating was used. They found that, at the baseline, mean radial artery diameter was 2.56 ± 0.45 mm. The mean diameter significantly increased to 2.86 ± 0.48 mm at 24 hours ($P = 0.001$). At 1 week, it was 2.75 ± 0.44 mm ($P = 0.03$), compared to baseline. At 1 month, the radial artery diameter was similar to baseline (2.60 ± 0.27 mm; $P = 0.95$). The maximum diameter, achieved after 0.4 mg sublingual nitroglycerine, was similar throughout the study period. Overall, there was a small vasodilatory response to postischaemic hyperemia (flow-mediated dilatation [FMD] 92.7% $\pm$ 4.7% at baseline), suggesting a high prevalence of endothelial dysfunction in this population. The response did not change significantly throughout the study period (3.4% $\pm$ 3.7%, 3.5% $\pm$ 3.9%, and 4.8% $\pm$ 4.7% at 1 day, 7 days, and 30 days, respectively). Nitroglycerine-induced vasodilatation decreased significantly at 24 hours, with a return to baseline at 7 days (14.1% $\pm$ 7.9% at baseline and 6.6% $\pm$ 8.4% at 1 day, 9.8% $\pm$ 8.5% at 7 days, and 13.0% $\pm$ 8.9% at 30 days). This study showed that hyperemia-induced vasodilatation did not change significantly, whereas nitroglycerine-induced vasodilatation was significantly attenuated at 24 hours, and had improved at 1 week and 1 month. This is probably related to local trauma provoked by the sheath and catheters. The study was performed on a mixed group of patients using different diameter sheaths (ranging from 4F to 6F) and majority of patients were males. The radial artery diameter was measured with ECG-gated ultrasound measurements, and there is a potential for error and intraobserver variability. The exact extent of endothelial damage and its impact on radial artery physiology in the long term are not known.

More recently, Burstein et al.[34] assessed the impact of radial artery cannulation for coronary angiography and angioplasty on radial artery function. They studied 22 patients using 6F short-length sheath with routine use of a vasodilator cocktail. Baseline radial artery diameters were 2.36 $\pm$ 0.9 mm in the cannulated arm and 2.38 $\pm$ 1.1 mm in the noncannulated arm. There were no significant changes in the noncannulated arm immediately after the procedure and at 9 week follow-up, whereas the radial artery diameter in the cannulated arm increased after the procedure (2.89 ± 0.9 mm, $P < 0.01$) and nearly returned close to its original size 9 weeks after the procedure (2.46 ± 0.9 mm, $P = 0.51$). The average FMD of the cannulated arm before the procedure was 13.2%. The average FMD of the cannulated arm immediately after the procedure was significantly decreased at 3.6% ($P < 0.01$). The average FMD of the cannulated arm at follow-up remained blunted at 0.2% and was significantly decreased compared with that before the procedure ($P < 0.01$). In comparison, there was no difference in the noncannulated arm across the study periods. Nitrate responsiveness in the cannulated arm before the procedure was 18.9%. This was significantly decreased immediately after the procedure ($3.7\%, P < 0.01$) and at follow-up ($8.6\%, P < 0.05$). No changes were seen in nitrate responsiveness in the noncannulated arm. They concluded that there was impaired vascular function of the radial artery up to 9 weeks following the transradial procedures.

Rathore and colleagues[35] have investigated the effect of transradial catheterization on vascular function and have shown that there was no significant difference in FMD or glyceryl trinitrate (GTN) between arms precatheterization (Fig. 9-2). There was a significant reduction in FMD at both the sheath ($P < 0.01$) and catheter sites ($P < 0.01$) in the catheterized arm (Fig. 9-2), but FMD was not completely abolished at either site. Similarly, there was a significant decrease to GTN postprocedure in

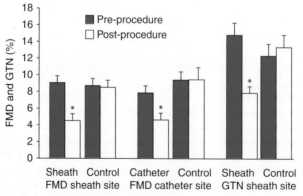

FIGURE 9-2   Changes in FMD (%) within the area of the sheath (sheath site, $n = 17$) and above the area of the sheath (catheter site, $n = 13$) and changes in GTN (%) within the area of the sheath ($n = 15$) in the catheterized and noncatheterized (control) arms pre- and postprocedure. Results are presented as means $\pm$ SEM. *Significantly different from pre-procedure ($P < 0.05$).

the sheath segment of the catheterized arm. These decreases had returned toward preprocedure values by 3 to 4 months after the catheterization (Fig. 9-2). In contrast, there was no change in FMD or GTN across any of the time points in the control arm (Fig. 9-2).

These studies show significant effect on FMD and similar effect on nitrate responsiveness of radial artery in cannulated arm following transradial procedures. The impaired FMD is probably a result of an endothelial damage and disruption during introducer sheath and catheter exchanges. However, the endothelial function should improve over time with endothelial repair. The impaired nitrate responsiveness could be explained due to impairment of smooth muscle function of the radial artery.

This impairment of vascular function as a result of injury sustained to the radial artery could theoretically be different with introducer sheaths of different sizes and lengths. These sheaths will cause different extents of injury to the radial artery and therefore could have different effect on the vascular function of the radial artery. Long sheaths will be in contact with a larger area of radial artery endothelium and therefore there is potential for more endothelial injury. Catheters are smaller in size than radial artery and may induce less damage because they are not in contact with the arterial wall. Similarly, shorter sheaths will be in contact with smaller area of radial artery endothelium and will cause less injury. However, in smaller-size radial arteries, where the catheter is in contact, there will be more radial artery irritation at the time of catheter exchanges with the use of shorter-length introducer sheath. There is also more endothelial irritation and disruption in the event of RAS as it is difficult to retrieve the introducer sheath and needs more manual traction.

These physiologic changes in the radial artery can have important implications for the patients. The radial artery is an important bypass conduit and also needed for arteriovenous fistula in patients requiring hemodialysis. Further research in reducing the extent of vascular impairment of the radial artery following transradial procedures will help this group of patients.

The Use of Radial Artery as Graft Conduit and Vascular Function

The use of radial artery as a conduit for coronary artery bypass surgery was first introduced over three decades ago. However, the use of this conduit was almost completely abandoned after 1976 because of high failure rates. These high failure rates were mainly due to intimal hyperplasia and hyperspasticity seen in radial artery grafts. In the early 1990s, interest in the use of radial artery was revived because of improved harvesting procedures and the use of aspirin and vasodilators. As there has been increasing interest in total arterial revascularization in coronary surgery, there has been resurgence in the use of the radial artery as an alternative arterial conduit.[36] With increasing use of the radial artery as the access site for percutaneous coronary intervention, there have been concerns raised and reluctance to use the radial artery after transradial procedures as a bypass conduit by cardiac surgeons. There is not much scientific data to support or examine this issue.

Kamiya et al. reported in a retrospective cohort study that there was significant intimal hyperplasia (68% vs 39%, $P = 0.046$) and reduced early graft patency (77% vs 98%) in patients in whom the radial artery had previously been used as an access route.[33] This was a retrospective cohort of 67 consecutive patients who underwent isolated coronary artery bypass grafting using the radial arteries. They further performed a subanalysis on 18 patients to investigate the relationships between the occurrence of graft stenosis or occlusion and preoperative transradial catheterization. Among the introducer size, number, and interval since previous catheterization, the number of previous transradial catheterizations was the most likely factor affecting the graft patency ($P = 0.07$). This study also demonstrated that the distal sites of the radial artery suffered from greater intimal hyperplasia after preoperative transradial catheterization compared with those without transradial catheterization. They concluded that preoperative transradial catheterization deteriorated early graft patency and caused intimal hyperplasia in the radial artery. However, this did not affect early clinical outcomes. The authors concluded that the use of the radial artery as a bypass conduit after transradial catheterization should be undertaken cautiously, particularly when multiple previous procedures have been performed. The impact of endothelial damage and long-term outcome following the use of radial artery as a bypass conduit is not yet known in prospective studies.

There are some data from surgical literature that examines the anatomy, pathology, and physiologic changes in radial artery in context with its use as a bypass conduit. It is well known that the radial artery is a thick-walled muscular artery and is more prone to suffer from intimal hyperplasia and arteriosclerotic change than is the internal mammary artery, which is an elastic artery.[37] Oshima et al.[38] examined the intravascular ultrasound images of the radial artery in the patients going for coronary artery bypass surgery. In a study of 58 patients, the mean luminal diameter was 3.28 ± 0.69 mm and 3.00 ± 0.70 mm at the proximal and distal segments, respectively, with a minimal diameter of 2.58 ± 0.73 mm. A plaque area greater than 50% was seen in five radial arteries (8.6%), whose average plaque length was 26.4 ± 30.8 mm. Five of these radial arteries showed calcification and were considered unsuitable for grafting. This study shows that the radial arteries in patients with coronary artery disease are not normal and could influence the results of transradial procedures.

The Physiologic Basis of Radial Artery Vascular Function and Endothelial Function

The endothelium is a single layer of cell lining covering the internal surface of blood vessels, cardiac valves, and numerous body cavities (Fig. 9-3). The location of the endothelium allows it to sense changes in the hemodynamic forces and blood-borne signals and respond by releasing vasoactive substances. A critical balance between endothelium-derived relaxation and contracting factors maintains vascular hemostasis. When this balance is disrupted, it predisposes the vasculature to vasoconstriction, leucocyte adherence, platelet activation, mitogenesis, pro-oxidation, thrombosis, impaired coagulation, vascular inflammation, and atherosclerosis.

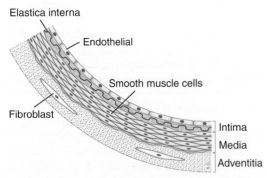

FIGURE 9-3   Layers of the radial artery. (In Voltz D. Artery. *New World Encyclopedia*. 2008. Available at http://www.newworldencyclopedia.org/p/index.php?title=Artery&oldid=786799.)

A transradial procedure has the potential to cause endothelial injury to the radial artery and results in the endothelial dysfunction. Radial sheaths can cause a mechanical insult to the lining and the muscular wall of the radial artery, cascading the above-mentioned effects as seen by other stimuli. Moreover, different length and coating of the sheath might cause different degrees of endothelial injury, and there are several patient-related factors that play a significant role in causing radial artery injury.

Optimization of Vascular Function after Transradial Procedures

Previous studies have shown that transradial procedures cause endothelial injury and various degrees of vascular function impairment. All efforts should be made during or before the procedure to optimize vascular function and minimize the vascular injury. Heiss et al.[39] have assessed the impact of smoking and catheter changes on vascular function of brachial artery during transradial catheterization. They have shown that transradial catheterization significantly decreased FMD in the radial artery (overall mean 8.5% ± 1.7% to 4.3% ± 1.6%) and the upstream brachial artery (overall mean 4.4% ± 1.6% to 2.9% ± 1.6%) at 6 hours. Subgroup analysis showed that FMD of both arteries at 6 hours was significantly lower in active smokers and that it only remained impaired at 24 hours in this group, whereas nonsmoker FMD fully recovered. The degree of brachial artery FMD but not radial artery FMD dysfunction was related to the number of catheters used, with no change after two catheters, 1.9% ± 1.2% decrease (6 hours) and recovery (24 hours) after three catheters, and 3.9% ± 1.2% decrease (6 hours) without recovery (24 hours) after 4 to 5 catheters. Park group[40] has evaluated the effect of trimetazidine (TMZ) on the functional recovery after transradial catheterization by measuring FMD. They have shown that in the TMZ group of the cannulated arm, the difference in FMD between baseline and post-TRCAG was also significant (11.3% ± 3.5% vs 6.3% ± 4.0%, $P < 0.01$). However, at 10-week follow-up, FMD was improved to 10.4% ± 3.4%, and there was no difference in FMD between baseline and 10-week follow-up (11.3% ± 3.5% vs 10.4% ± 3.4%, $P = 0.26$). Similarly, the size of the introducer sheath can have an impact on endothelial injury and vascular function as shown by Lei et al.[41] They have shown significant reduction in the radial artery diameter with the use of 6F sheath as compared to 4F group (2.51–3.3 mm, $P < 0.001$, and 2.49–2.45 mm, $P > 0.05$). More recently, Rathore and colleagues[42] have evaluated the impact of introducer sheath coating on endothelial function following transradial procedures in a randomized study. FMD in the catheterized arm decreased from 10.3% ± 3.8% to 5.3% ± 3.3% and 8.1% ± 2.4% to 5.2% ± 3.7% in the coated and uncoated groups, respectively ($P < 0.01$). These values returned to baseline levels 3 months later (coated: 6.4% ± 1.4%; uncoated: 9.4% ± 4.1%; $P < 0.05$) versus postprocedure. Glyceryl trinitrate decreased from 14.8% ± 7.2% to 9.5% ± 4.1% ($P < 0.05$) in the coated group and from 12.2% ± 4.6% to 7.5% ± 4.2% ($P < 0.01$) in the uncoated group. Values returned to baseline at 3 months (coated: 16.6% ± 5.6%; uncoated: 12.1% ± 3.9%; $P < 0.05$). This study failed to show any difference in the magnitude of decrease in FMD or GTN function between coated and uncoated groups.

It is also possible that optimizing the function and size of the artery before its cannulation may improve the outcome and recovery of the artery and reduce the chance of graft failure if the artery is removed for coronary artery bypass.[43] To this end, exercise training has been shown to improve arterial function and induce outward remodeling,[44–48] both of which might improve the health and recovery of the artery after the procedure. This hypothesis was tested by Dawson et al.[49] in a small study group, and the effect of exercise training on radial artery dilator and constrictor function was evaluated. They assessed the effect of local handgrip exercise training on radial artery vascular function in 18 subjects and randomized 9 subjects to a 6-week handgrip exercise training program. It was found that FMD and low-flow-mediated constriction (L-FMC) were preserved in the exercise group (FMD-pre: 6.84% ± 0.79%, FMD-post: 6.85% ± 1.16%; L-FMC-pre: −2.14% ± 1.42%, L-FMC-post: −3.58% ± 1.04%), but lower in the control group (FMD-pre: 8.27% ± 1.52%, FMD-post 4.66% ± 0.70%, $P = 0.06$; L-FMC-pre: −3.26% ± 1.19%, L-FMC-post: −1.34% ± 1.27%, $P < 0.05$). They have demonstrated for the first time that exercise training has beneficial impacts on radial artery vasodilator and constrictor function.

Future Directions

All efforts should be made during transradial catheterization to prevent RAS and radial artery injury and thereby reducing patient discomfort and vascular complications. Patients should be profiled preprocedure to identify their risk of RAS and tailor the need for optimal size radial artery sheath and catheters. Further studies are required to assess and compare the effects of novel vasodilators such as nicorandil, NO agonists, sodium nitroprusside, or oral vasodilators loading preprocedure to further reduce the occurrence of RAS. Research into novel coatings and reduction in the diameter of the introducer sheaths without compromising on the lumen are needed to assess their impact on RAS and injury. The use of sheathless guide catheters and hydrophilic guide catheters is shown to reduce RAS, and further research is needed to study their impact on vascular dysfunction. Reversible endothelial injury to the radial artery is commonly seen following transradial procedures and potentially triggers vascular complications like RAS, stenosis, and thrombosis. Preliminary studies have shown beneficial effects of systemic vasodilators and exercise training in optimizing endothelial dysfunction following transradial catheterization. This could further be translated into reducing RAS and other vascular complications following these measures. Large-scale clinical studies are needed to further test this hypothesis and improve the vascular health of radial artery. The ramifications of RAS and injury are not only in patients undergoing repeat coronary procedures, but also in the patients in whom the radial artery may be used as a conduit for coronary artery bypass surgery or in patients needing an arteriovenous fistula for hemodialysis. Future research and technological development should seek to minimize the effects of the catheter and the sheath on the vasculature.

Conclusion

The transradial approach for coronary procedures has become more popular over the years and has been used in all clinical situations. RAS is the most commonly encountered complication and can result in discomfort to the patient and procedural failure in some patients. Adequate sedation, analgesia, and the use of vasodilator agents and hydrophilic-coated introducer sheaths have shown to significantly reduce RAS in selected patients. Several patient-related factors have been identified as predictors of RAS, such as female gender, younger age, diabetes mellitus, smaller wrist size, and smaller radial artery diameter causing sheath-artery mismatch. Extra precaution is required in this high-risk group of patients to minimize discomfort and radial artery injury.

Radial catheterization has shown to cause reversible endothelial dysfunction and vascular dysfunction, which could be further optimized by exercise prehabilitaion.

REFERENCES

1. Hildick-Smith DJR, Lowe MD, Walsh JT, et al. Coronary angiography from the radial artery—experience, complications and limitations. *Intern J Cardiol.* 1998;64:231–239.
2. Keimeneij F, Vajifdar BU, Eccleshall SC, et al. Evaluation of a spasmolytic cocktail to prevent radial artery spasm during coronary procedures. *Cathet Cardiovasc Intervent.* 2003;58:281–284.
3. Salmeron R, Mora R, Masotti M, et al. Assessment of the efficacy of phentolamine to prevent radial artery spasm during cardiac catheterisation procedures: a randomised study comparing phentolamine vs. verapamil. *Cathet Cardiovasc Intervent.* 2005;66:192–198.
4. Rathore S, Stables RH, Pauriah M, et al. Impact of length and hydrophilic coating of the introducer sheath on radial artery spasm during transradial coronary intervention: a randomised study. *J Am Coll Cardiol Intv.* 2010;3:475–483.
5. He G, Yang C. Characteristics of adrenoreceptors in the human radial artery: clinical implications. *J Thorac Cardiovasc Surg.* 1998;115:1136–1141.
6. Virchow RR. *Cellular Pathology.* London, UK: Churchill; 1860.
7. Van San JA, Smedts F, Vincent JG, et al. Comparative anatomic studies of various arterial conduits for myocardial revascularisation. *J Thorac Cardiovasc Surg.* 1990;99:703–707.
8. Acar C, Jebara VA, Portoghese M, et al. Comparative anatomy and histology of the radial artery and the internal thoracic artery. Implications for coronary artery bypass. *Surg Radiol Anat.* 1991;13:383–388.
9. Kaufer E, Factor SM, Frame R, et al. Pathology of the radial and internal thoracic arteries used as coronary artery bypass grafts. *Ann Thoracic Surg.* 1997;63:1118–1122.
10. He GW, Yang CQ. Comparison among arterial grafts and coronary artery: an attempt at functional classification. *J Thorac Cardiovasc Surg.* 1995;109:707–715.
11. Kiemeneij F, Vajifdar B, Eccleshall S, et al. Measurement of radial artery spasm using an automatic pull back device. *Cathet Cardiovasc Intervent.* 2001;54:437–441.
12. Saito S, Tanaka S, Hiroe Y, et al. Usefulness of hydrophilic coating on arterial sheath introducer in transradial coronary intervention. *Cathet Cardiovasc Intervent.* 2002;56:328–332.
13. He GW, Yang CQ. Characteristics of adrenoceptors in the human radial artery: clinical implications. *J Thorac Surg.* 1998;115:1136–1141.
14. Canon RO, III. Role of nitric oxide in cardiovascular disease: focus on the endothelium (published erratum appears in *Clin Chem.* 1998;44:2070). *Clin Chem.* 1998;44(8 pt2):1809–1819.
15. Greindling KK, Alexander RW. Endothelial control of the cardiovascular system: recent advances. *FASEB J.* 1996;10:283–292.
16. Channon KM, Gujik TJ. Mechanisms of superoxide production in human blood vessels: relationship to endothelial dysfunction, clinical and genetic risk factors. *L Physiol Pharmacol.* 2002;53(4 pt 1):515–524.
17. Aksungar FB, Moini H, Unai M, et al. Nitric oxide, enothelin-1, and superoxide production. *Tex Heart Inst J.* 2006;33:294–299.
18. Zhang Y, Tazzeo T, Chu V, et al. Membrane potassium currents in human artery and their regulation by nitric oxide donor. *Cardiovasc Res.* 2006;71:383–392.
19. Gaudino M, Tondi P, Serricchio M, et al. Atherosclerotic involvement of the radial artery in patients with coronary artery disease and its relation with midterm radial artery graft patency and endothelail function. *J Cardiovasc Surg.* 2003;126:1968–1971.
20. Stahli BE, Caduf RF, Greutert H, et al. Endothelial and smooth muscle cell dysfunction in human atherosclerotic radial artery: implications for coronary artery bypass grafting. *J Cardiovascul Pharmacol.* 2004;43:222–226.
21. Zhang Y, Jansen LJ, Chu FV. Atherosclerosis of radial arterial graft may increase the potential of vessel spasm in coronary artery bypass surgery. *J Thorac Cardiovasc Surg.* 2005;130:1477–1478.
22. He G. Verapamil plus nitroglycerine solution maximally preserves endothelial function of the radial artery: comparison with papaverine solution. *J Thorac Cardiovasc Surg.* 198;115:1321–1327.
23. Varenne O, Jegou A, Cohen R, et al. Prevention of arterial spasm during percutaneous coronary interventions through radial artery: the SPASM Study. *Cathet Cardiovasc Intervent.* 2006;68:231–235.
24. Filho JR, Assad JA, Zago AC, et al. Comparative study of the use of diltiazem as an antispasmodic drug in coronary angiography via the transradial approach. *Arq Bras Cardiol.* 2003;81(1):54–58.
25. Coppola J, Patel T, Kwan T, et al. Nitroglycerine, nitroprusside, or both in preventing radial artery spasm during transradial artery catheterisation. *J Invasive Cardiol.* 2006;18:155–158.
26. Chen CW, Lin CL, Lin TK, et al. A simple and effective regimen for prevention of radial artery spasm during coronary catheterisation. *Cardiology.* 2006;105:43–47.
27. Kim SH, Kim EJ, Cheon WS, et al. Comparative study of nicorandil and spasmolytic cocktail in preventing radial artery spasm during transradial coronary angiography. *Int J Cardiol.* 2007;3:325–330.
28. Fukuda N, Iwahara S, Harada A, et al. Vasospasms of the radial artery after the transradial approach for coronary angiography and angioplasty. *Jpn Heart J.* 2004;45(5):723–731.
29. Dery JP, Simard S, Barbeau, GR. Reduction of discomfort at sheath removal during transradial coronary procedures with the use of a hydrophilic coated sheath. *Cathet Cardiovasc Intervent.* 2001;54:289–294.
30. Keimeneij F, Fraser D, Slagboom T, et al. Hydrophilic coating aids radial sheath withdrawal and reduces patient discomfort following transradial coronary interventions: a randomised double-blind comparison of coated and uncoated sheath. *Cathet Cardiovasc Interv.* 2003;59:161–164.
31. Koga S, Ikeda S, Futugawa K, et al. The use of hydrophilic coated catheter during transradial cardiac catheterisation is associated with a low incidence of radial artery spasm. *Int J Cardiol.* 2004;96:255–258.
32. Suzuki H, Kawai S, Aizawa T, et al. Histological evaluation of coronary plaque in patients with variant angina: relationship between vasospasm and neointimal hyperplasia in primary coronary lesions. *J Am Coll Cardiol.* 1999;33:198–205.
33. Kamiya H, Ushijima T, Kanamori T, et al. Use of the radial artery graft after transradial catheterisation: is it suitable as a bypass conduit? *Ann Thorac Surg.* 2003;76:1505–1509.
34. Burstein JM, Gidrewicz D, Hutchinson SJ, et al. Impact of radial artery cannulation for coronary angiography and angioplasty on radial artery function. *Am J Cardiol.* 2007;99:457–459.

35. Dawson EA, Rathore S, Cable T, et al. Impact of catheter insertion using the radial approach on vasodilatation in humans. *Clin Sci.* 2010;118:633–640.

36. Acar C, Jebara VA, Portoghese M, et al. Revival of the radial artery for coronary artery bypass grafting. *Ann Thorac Surg.* 1992;54:652–660.

37. Parolari A, Rubini P, Alamanni F, et al. The radial artery: which place in coronary operation? *Ann Thorac Surg.* 2000;69:1288–1294.

38. Oshima A, Takeshita S, Kozuma K, et al. Intravascular ultrasound analysis of the radial artery for coronary artery bypass grafting. *Ann Thorac Surg.* 2005;79:99–103.

39. Heiss C, Blazer J, Hauffe T, et al. Vascular dysfunction of brachial artery after transradial access for coronary catheterisation: impact of smoking and catheter changes. *JACC Cardiovasc Interv.* 2009;2:1067–1073.

40. Park KH, Park WJ, Kim MK, et al. Effects of trimetazidine on endothelial dysfunction after sheath injury of radial artery. *Am J Cardiol.* 2010;105:1723–1727.

41. Lei H, Dong WY, Song J, et al. Comparative study of 4Fr catheters using the ACIST variable rate injector system versus 6Fr catheters using hand manifold in diagnostic coronary angiography via transradial approach. *Chin Med J.* 2010;123:1373–1376.

42. Dawson EA, Rathore S, Cable T, et al. Impact of introducer sheath coating on endothelial function in humans after transradial coronary procedures. *Circ Cardiovasc Interv.* 2010;3:148–156.

43. Desai MD, Naylor CD, Kiss A, et al. Impact of patient and target-vessel characteristics on arterial and venous bypass graft patency: insight from a randomised trial. *Circulation.* 2007;115:684–691.

44. Gokce N, Vita JA, Bader DS, et al. Effect of exercise on upper and lower extremity endothelial function in patients with coronary artery disease. *Am J Cardiol.* 2002;90(2):124–127.

45. Hambrecht R, Hilbrich L, Erbs S, et al. Correction of endothelial dysfunction in chronic heart failure: additional effects of exercise training and oral L-arginine supplementation. *J Am Coll Cardiol.* 2000;35:706–713.

46. Hornig B, Maier V, Drexler H. Physical training improves endothelial function in patients with chronic heart failure. *Circulation.* 1996;93:210–214.

47. Tinken TM, Thijssen DH, Black MA, et al. Time course of change in vasodilator function and capacity in response to exercise training in humans. *J Physiol.* 2008;586:5003–5012.

48. Green DJ, Maiorana A, O'Driscoll G, et al. Effect of exercise training on endothelium-derived nitric oxide function in humans. *J Physiol.* 2004;561:1–25.

49. Dawson EA, Alkarmi A, Thijssen DH, et al. Low-flow mediated constriction is endothelium-dependent: effects of exercise training after radial artery catheterization. *Circ Cardiovasc Interv.* 2012;5:713–719.

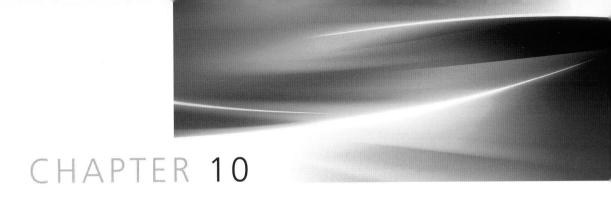

CHAPTER 10

Hemostasis and Radial Artery Occlusion

Eltigani Abdelaal, Ivo Bernat, and Samir B. Pancholy

Introduction

Radial artery occlusion (RAO) is the Achilles' heel of transradial catheterization. In this chapter, we review the incidence, pathophysiology, predictors, treatment, and prevention of RAO. Moreover, as suggested by recent evidence, we also emphasize key aspects of hemostasis that might directly have an impact on the risks of RAO. The anatomical characteristics of hand vasculature have been reviewed in Chapter 4 and are not discussed here. It is also important to mention that issues discussed with hemostasis and occlusion of the radial artery can apply to the ulnar artery (Chapter 6).

Radial Artery Occlusion: Definition and Incidence

To date, there have been more than 88 studies (involving >1,000 patients) that have directly or indirectly reported on the incidence of RAO following transradial approach (TRA) for cardiac catheterization, or in the setting of anesthetic practice (radial cannulation).[1] Despite this, and owing to the lack of consensus on how or when to assess for RAO, and diverse methods reported in the literature, there is currently no standardized definition of RAO. Well before the first introduction of TRA as an alternative route for cardiac catheterization by Campeau,[2] RAO following cannulation in anesthesia and intensive care practice was reported by several investigators. The incidence of RAO reported in the literature by various investigators differs greatly according to the population studied, type of procedure undertaken, size and length of sheaths, adjuvant pharmacotherapy, hemostatic technique and method, and time of assessment for radial artery (RA) patency.

In the context of prolonged RA cannulation for perioperative monitoring, rates of RAO have been reported to be as high as 25% to 40% using a combination of Allen test and Doppler flow,[3-5] with a small percentage of spontaneous recanalization over time. Albeit observational, some of these early studies also highlighted the findings of higher risk of RAO in females and those with small wrist circumference.[5,6]

The incidence of RAO following TRA cardiac catheterization, however, has been lower, with most series reporting between 3% and 10%.[7-14] More recently, however, Uhlemann[15] reported an incidence of 30% of RAO with 6F sheaths, as assessed by Duplex sonography prior to hospital discharge. (Fig. 10-1) shows the incidence of RAO over time and according to the method of detection.

Assessment of Radial Artery Patency

It is worth mentioning that according to a recent international survey, about 50% of radial operators do not assess RAO prior to hospital discharge, although a significant number assume that RAO might be >10%.[16] Owing to collateral circulation from the palmar arches, the radial pulse may still

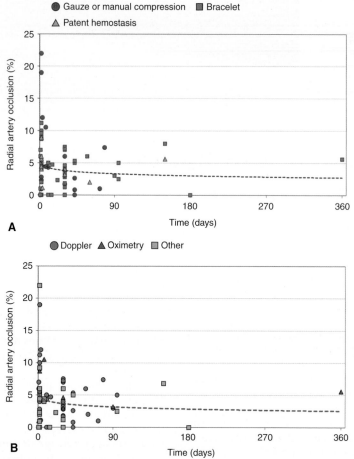

FIGURE 10-1   Incidence of RAO according to time (**A**) and the method of detection (**B**).

be palpable even in the presence of RAO on ultrasound.[15,17] It is therefore well understood that clinical radial pulse checks in establishing RA patency might be inaccurate and insensitive in detecting the true incidence of RAO.[18,19] Although this is a well-known and relatively old observation, radial pulse check is still the most frequent method used to detect RAO prior to hospital discharge.[16]

Although not feasible routinely because of costs and logistic constraints, the reference technique for RAO detection remains the visible obstruction in two-dimensional ultrasound and the absence of anterograde Doppler flow signal distal to access puncture site.[15,20] This must be differentiated from using a simple Doppler probe, which might detect a signal even if the RA is completely or partially obstructed due to reverse flow. Consequently, detection of RAO using Doppler probe only can grossly underestimate the true incidence of RAO. This might partially be improved if

one compresses the ulnar artery while assessing the radial flow.

More recently, we and others have used the modified oxymetry-plethysmography technique to assess the incidence of RAO postcatheterization. This technique was initially described by Cheng et al.[21] as a more sensitive technique than the Allen test, and Barbeau et al. used it as a semiquantitative method of assessment prior radial catheterization.[22]

Briefly, the pulse oximeter sensor is placed over the index finger and the plethysmographic signal observed. Both radial and ulnar arteries are simultaneously compressed to observe loss of plethysmographic signal. The RA is then released, and the return of plethysmographic signal is observed. Return of signal confirms RA flow and hence patency. The absence of return of signal implies RAO.

It should be emphasized that spontaneous recanalization of RA is relatively frequent, and consequently, the incidence of persistent RAO is lower over medium- to long-term follow-up.[15,17,20] The wide variation of reported incidence of RAO in the literature could therefore be explained not only by population and procedural variables, but also by the diverse methods and time of assessment for RA patency.

Pathophysiology of Radial Artery Occlusion

RAO is likely to be a multifactorial process due to the interplay of several factors, which in principle may relate to three main mechanisms: (a) arterial wall injury, endothelial denudation, and local vascular reactions induced by sheath insertion; (b) interruption of antegrade flow during procedure due to the presence of sheath or postprocedure due to the type and duration of compression; (c) "a" and "b" may facilitate local thrombus formation and occlusion, and/or chronic inflammatory process, leading to intimal hyperplasia and thickening of intima media, which may result in delayed luminal obliteration or reduction.

The RA is a primarily muscular vessel, with a dominant supply of α-1 adrenoceptors to its smooth muscle cells.[23] Shear stress at the time of sheath insertion evokes these receptors, leading to vasospasm due to local release of catecholamines, endothelin-I, and angiotensin-II.[23] In turn, this induces friction of the arterial wall in contact with the sheath, thereby further increasing shear stress, leading to itimal tear and medial dissection. In addition, the RA has a mean internal diameter of 2.69 ± 0.4 mm in men and 2.43 ± 0.38 mm in women (range, 1.15–3.95 mm).[24] It is therefore closer to the outer diameter of the catheters being placed in its lumen. As a result of these factors, the constrained intraluminal environment due to limited clearance between the catheter and the arterial wall may result in reduced pericatheter antegrade blood flow, raising the risk of arterial thrombosis.[25]

RA injury has been well described by Yonetsu et al.[26] Through the use of optical coherence tomography (OCT) to assess acute RA injuries immediately following TRA catheterization, this recent study demonstrated acute RA injury in a substantial number of patients, with intimal tear in 67% of patients and medial dissection in 36%.[26] More direct evidence comes from Staniloae et al.,[27] who studied the early histological changes induced by TRA catheterization. Thirty-four subjects undergoing coronary artery bypass grafting

(CABG) had their left RA harvested to serve as conduits. Fifteen of these had undergone TRA catheterization via left RA immediately prior to CABG, while 19 noncatheterized right radial arteries served as controls. Five-millimeter biopsy sections were obtained from distal and proximal ends of the RA, and examined by a single pathologist blinded to the clinical data. The distal end of the left RA group had significantly more intimal hyperplasia (73% vs 21%), periarterial tissue necrosis (26% vs 0%), and adventitial inflammation (33% vs 0%) in close proximity to entry site, when compared to the noncatheterized distal right radial arteries. Of note, no significant difference was noted in the proximal parts of both arteries (albeit numerically more intimal proliferation in left radial arteries). While these findings are relevant and may have implications on the use of RA as a conduit, they also highlight the extent of injury induced by the introducer sheath.[27] The extensive damage associated with sheath insertion and denuded endothelium may initiate a cascade of events not only predisposing to thrombosis resulting in RAO, but also triggering intima-media hyperplasia with nonocclusive narrowing of the RA over long term.[26,28]

Thrombotic RAO following percutaneous cannulation for monitoring has long been described, with an incidence as high as 30% to 40%. In 100 consecutive patients requiring arterial monitoring for major elective operations, Bedford et al. demonstrated a 35% incidence of occlusive RA thrombi, by performing contrast arteriography prior to decannulation, and confirming using both Allen test and Doppler examination following decannulation.[29] In another series, Bedford et al. also demonstrated a 38% incidence of thrombotic RA occlusion in patients undergoing radial cannulation for perioperative management.[6] A postmortem specimen from a participant in the study showed an organized RA thrombus corresponding to the exact length of occlusion, which had been precisely determined antemortem by the absence of Doppler flow signal over the area.[6]

Similarly, Pancholy reported the finding of an occlusive "plug" successfully retrieved from 5 out of 12 reaccessed radial arteries, which had been occluded for less than 4 weeks.[30] Histopathological examination of aspirated material was consistent with an organizing thrombus, with signs of neovascular microchannel formation.[30] Therefore, it is reasonable to assume thrombus formation as the main mechanistic process for early RAO. Kim et al. reported an occlusive RA thrombus in a male patient as visualized with an ultrasound examination the day following transradial cardiac diagnostic procedure.[31] Their patient had a "normal Allen" test prior to the procedure, and RAO was asymptomatic. A month later, and while on antiplatelet therapy, the RA recanalized with a normal appearance on ultrasound.[31] Similarly, Zankl et al.[32] assessed RA patency the day after the procedure by using duplex ultrasonography over in 488 patients who underwent either diagnostic procedures (with 4F) or PCI (5–6F). The study demonstrated partial or complete thrombotic RAO in 11% of patients.[32]

Therefore, existing evidence from histopathological as well as clinical studies with echoduplex examinations indicates that RAO in the acute to subacute phase is often due to thrombus formation, with various degrees of spontaneous recanalization on medium to long term.

A separate potential mechanism of "gradual" RAO relates to progressive intimal hyperplasia following unique or repeat RA cannulation. The resultant endothelial damage following radial cannulation and sheath insertion may trigger a cascade of events leading to intimal hyperplasia and vascular remodeling. Using intravascular ultrasound imaging of the RA following cardiac catheterization in 100 subjects, Wakeyam et al.[28] demonstrated significantly smaller mean distal radial arterial diameter in those who had repeat TRA compared to first TRA procedure. Similarly, and using OCT, Yonetsu et al.[26] demonstrated significant intimal tear as well as chronic intimal thickening of RA following repeat TRA.

Factors Associated with Increased Risk of Radial Artery Occlusion/ Predictors of Radial Artery Occlusion

Multiple patient- and procedural-related factors have been shown to influence or predict the occurrence of RAO (Table 10-1). These come from observational studies, registries, as well as randomized studies.

TABLE 10-1 **Predictors of RAO**		
Factors		**Comments**
Patient related	Diabetes	Diabetes predisposes to RAO as shown in a large study of predictors of RAO, using a regression model
	Female gender	RAO is more frequent in females as shown in a large study of predictors of RAO, using a regression model
	Low body mass index	Low-body-weight patients are at significantly higher risk of RAO
Procedural related	Anticoagulation	Heparin was shown to be crucial in reducing the incidence of RAO, with a dose-dependent beneficial effect. No difference in magnitude of effect between IV and IA route of administration
	Size of sheath and catheters	Ratio of sheath outer diameter to inner diameter of RA is indirectly proportional to incidence of RAO. The lower the ratio (i.e., the bigger the sheath), the higher the incidence of RAO
	Successive cannulation	Incidence of TRA dropouts increases as successive punctures are performed due to narrowing and occlusion of the RA, probably as a function of repeated punctures
	Occlusive hemostasis	The use of occlusive hemostasis and duration of RA compression postprocedure are an independent predictor of RAO. Patent hemostasis reduces the incidence of RAO

Patient-Related Factors: Gender, Age, Body Mass Index, Peripheral Arterial Occlusive Disease, and Diabetes

In a large series of >7,215 patients who underwent TRA coronary intervention, Zhou et al.[33] described an incidence of 0.94% of RAO. The study analyzed risk factors associated with RAO by using a logistic regression model, and as compared with those who did not develop RAO, there were more female and diabetic patients in the RAO group.[33] In the same study, the size of introducer sheath, heparin dose, and duration of compression were independent risk factors of RAO.[33] More recently, in a prospective vascular ultrasound registry of 455 patients undergoing TRA angiography and interventions, Uhlemann et al.[15] demonstrated by a multivariate analysis that, besides the use of 6F sheaths, female gender (OR: 2.36, 95% CI: 1.50-3.73, $P < 0.001$), younger age (OR: per year 0.96, 95% CI: 0.94-0.98, $P = 0.001$), and the presence of peripheral arterial occlusive disease (OR: 2.04, 95% CI: 1.02-4.22, $P = 0.04$) independently predicted RAO in all patients.[15] It should be noted that in both studies, RA was compressed, hence probably maintained occluded during hemostasis.

Procedural Factors

Radial Artery Diameter: Ratio of Internal Radial Artery Diameter to Outer Sheath Diameter

The relationship between sheath size and RAO has long been established. Occlusion is directly related to the size of the introducer sheath and is influenced by the ratio of the inner radial arterial diameter to the outer sheath diameter, as demonstrated by Saito et al.[11] In a series of 250 patients who underwent ultrasound examinations before and after TRA catheterization, they reported an incidence of RAO of 4% in patients with an RA internal diameter greater than the outer diameter of the sheath (ratio > 1) versus 13% in those with a ratio <1.[11] These findings have been confirmed in a study by Dahm et al.[12] on 171 subjects undergoing TRA PCI randomized to 5F versus 6F sheath. The study revealed that the radial diameter to catheter ratio was <1.0 for all 6F patients in whom profound radial spasm occurred. In addition, RAO occurred in 1.1% of the 5F group versus 5.9% of the 6F group at 1 month ($P = 0.05$).[12] More recently, Uhlemann et al.[15] showed in their observational analysis of 455 patients that the risk of RAO was significantly higher with 6F (30.5%)

than with 5F sheaths ($P < 0.001$). Using both Allen test and Doppler, Bedford demonstrated a negative linear relationship between the size of the cannulated radial arteries and the incidence of thrombotic occlusions.[6] Hence, in accordance with the relationship between vessel trauma and risks of RAO, it can be concluded that the smaller the sheaths/catheters are, the lesser the risks of RAO.

Anticoagulation: Type, Dose, and Route of Administration

For the purpose of cardiac catheterization, once the radial puncture has been successfully performed, and after sheath insertion, unfractionated heparin is administered intravenously at a dose of 5,000 units for diagnostic procedures, for it has been shown to greatly reduce the incidence of thrombotic RAO associated with RA cannulation.

Dosing of Heparin. Anticoagulation during TRA procedures is paramount, as it has been shown to significantly reduce the incidence of RAO.[34] As described by Lefevre et al. in the original report of the role of heparin in TRA, the effect of heparin in the prevention of RAO appears to be dose dependent, with a substantial reduction in the incidence of RAO by increasing the dose of heparin from 2,000 to 3,000 and further to 5,000 IU.[34] This has been substantiated further in a recent study of the incidence and predictors of RAO in a large cohort of >7,000 patients who underwent TRA coronary intervention.[33] In a more recent study, Bernat et al.[35] compared the echo-duplex incidence of RAO with a single intravenous heparin bolus of 2,000 IU versus 5,000 IU. Using patent hemostasis (see below), he and his colleagues demonstrated that immediate posthemostasis RAO rate was higher in the 2,000 IU group compared to the 5,000 IU group (5.9% vs 2.9%, $P = 0.17$).[35] The authors also described a nonpharmacological technique of 1-hour ulnar compression to treat RAO, with again higher efficacy with higher heparin dose (final incidence of RAO was 4.1% in the 2000 IU group vs 0.8% in the 5000 IU group, $P = 0.03$). Thus, it seems prudent to recommend a minimal fixed dose of 5,000 IU or 70 IU/kg heparin after radial sheath insertion, even for simple diagnostic angiography.

The role of new anticoagulants, such as bivalirudin, a direct thrombin inhibitor, in conjunction with radial access remains to be discussed. Plante et al. performed a study comparing a single 70 IU/kg heparin bolus administered at the completion of the diagnostic angiography to bivalirudin administration in the case of ad hoc PCI.[36] Overall, the incidence of RAO at 30 days in the heparin-only group was 7% compared with 3.5% in the bivalirudin-only group. Although numerically lower in the bivalirudin group, the difference did not reach statistical significance ($P = 0.18$). It should be emphasized that the incidence of RAO remained quite high in both groups, perhaps due to the fact that the authors did not use patent hemostasis and used a classic compressive bracelet to obtain hemostasis. At this point, it seems that the incidence of RAO is independent of the type of anticoagulant. Some groups in Europe routinely use low-molecular-weight heparin (LMWH). No study directly comparing LMWH to heparin on the incidence of RAO has been reported yet. Conversely, given the low risk of access-site-related bleeding, some authors have advocated the initiation of the diagnostic procedure with a reduced heparin bolus and simply complementing with bivalirudin in the case of ad hoc PCI. The time to obtain hemostasis after radial sheath removal is also independent of the type of intravenous anticoagulant. It should be emphasized, however, that patients on warfarin still require intravenous anticoagulant therapy after radial sheath insertion to prevent RAO.[37] However, we recently reported that if RA patency can be demonstrated during hemostasis, intravenous anticoagulation could be safely omitted.[38] This might lead to the hypothesis that with patent hemostasis, the role of intravenous anticoagulation could be less critical (see below).

Route of Administration. Although the original report on the beneficial effect of heparin on the prevention of RAO used the intravenous route of administration, some operators prefer to administer heparin intraradially together with the spasmolytic cocktail. However, a recent randomized study demonstrated that intravenous heparin is equivalent to intra-arterial heparin in reducing the incidence of RAO, suggesting that the systemic rather than the local effect of heparin is the most important factor.[39] As such, and given its low pH, which causes patients to experience local burning sensation in the hand when given intra-arterially (similar to verapamil administration), heparin may preferentially be administered routinely intravenously.

Occlusive Hold versus Patent Hemostasis

Despite the use of heparin during cardiac catheterization, RAO was noted in 7% to 10%, presumably related to occlusive pressure applied postprocedurally for hemostasis, and local thrombus formation as the initial catalyst for early occlusion.

In a prospective observational study of 275 patients who underwent transradial catheterization, Sanmartin et al.[40] first demonstrated that flow interruption or occlusive compression of the radial puncture site was a strong and independent predictor of RAO at follow-up. Then, two randomized trials have demonstrated that maintaining antegrade blood flow through RA during compression hemostasis, the so-called patent hemostasis, significantly reduces both early and late RAO.[17,41] Pancholy et al. in the PROPHET study randomized 436 patients undergoing elective cardiac catheterization to patent hemostasis versus conventional compression for hemostasis to determine its effect on the incidence of RAO as assessed by oxymetry-plethysmography.[17] Following successful transradial cardiac catheterization, 219 patients were randomized to conventional compression for hemostasis, and 218 to patent hemostasis. Briefly, in the patent hemostasis group, once Hemoband™ plastic band was applied following sheath removal, and with a pulse oximeter placed over the index finger, manual ipsilateral ulnar occlusion was performed, and the hemoband was loosened until radial patency was confirmed with the return of plethysmographic signal, or until bleeding occurred. The hemoband was left on for 2 hours, with hourly checks on patency. In the conventional compression group, the hemoband was applied as usual following sheath removal, and those who had flow-limiting compression were recorded to have "occlusive hold." At 24-hour follow-up, 27 patients (12%) in the occlusive hold group developed plethysmographic evidence of RAO, compared with 11 patients (5%) in the patent hemostasis group (59% reduction in occlusion, $P < 0.05$). At 30-day follow-up, the incidence was 7% versus 1.8%, respectively (with 75% reduction in radial occlusion with the patent hemostasis, $P < 0.05$). In the RACOMAP study, Cubero et al. randomized 351 patients to a mean pressure-guided hemostasis with the TR band or standard inflation with 15 cm³ of air.[41] Using inverse Allen and bidirectional Doppler, RAO was 1.1% in the group with patent hemostasis and 12% in the standard hold ($P = 0.0001$). This low incidence of RAO is similar to the one obtained with patent hemostasis using the TR band and echo-duplex assessment in the randomized study performed by Bernat et al. Today, studies using patent hemostasis have reported the lowest incidence of RAO whichever was the hemostasis device and the technique to assess RAO. Hence, it seems that patent hemostasis technique should be strongly recommended to minimize the risks of postprocedural RAO (Box 10-1).

BOX 10-1   **Patent Hemostasis Technique**

Patent hemostasis, as the name implies, aims at obtaining RA hemostasis, with maintenance of RA patency. This can be achieved in the following manner.

Step 1: Apply the radial hemostasis device to the RA puncture site (Fig. 10-2).

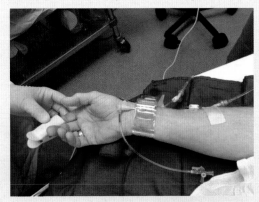

FIGURE 10-2   Patent hemostasis technique: step 1.

Step 2: Tighten or inflate the device to apply pressure at the arterial puncture site. Of note, it is important to center the device at the point of arterial entry, and not skin entry, to prevent subcutaneous hemorrhage (Fig. 10-3)

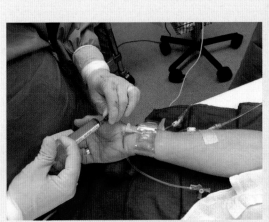 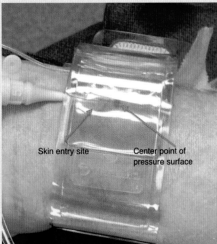

Skin entry site   Center point of pressure surface

FIGURE 10-3   Patent hemostasis technique: step 2.

Step 3: Remove the introducer sheath from under the compression device. It is optimal to open the stopcock and let the side arm of the introducer "bleed" in order to remove the prethrombotic material and thrombi from the RA lumen (Fig. 10-4).

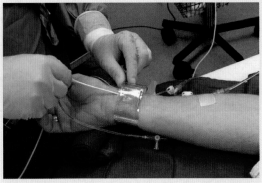

FIGURE 10-4   Patent hemostasis technique: step 3.

(continued)

BOX 10-1   Patent Hemostasis Technique (continued)

Step 4: Loosen or deflate the compression device till visible and continuous leakage of blood from the access site is noted. Once "bleeding" is seen, gently tighten or reinflate the device till complete cessation of bleeding occurs. Apply the least necessary pressure to eliminate active bleeding (Fig. 10-5).

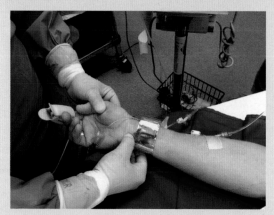

FIGURE 10-5   Patent hemostasis technique: step 4.

Step 5: Perform reverse Barbeau's test, by using oxymetry-plethysmography, to assess RA flow. If RA flow is present, you have achieved both end points, and periodic monitoring of adequacy of hemostasis and RA patency is recommended (evaluations every 15 minutes) (Fig. 10-6).

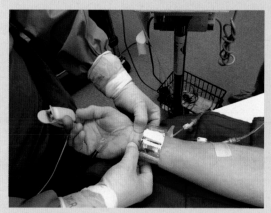

FIGURE 10-6   Patent hemostasis technique: step 5.

Step 6: If RA patency is not observed, repeat the process of decreasing hemostatic compression pressure maintaining hemostasis. In the first 15 minutes of compression, the balance of radial patency and hemostasis changes frequently, in view of changes in the patient's blood pressure, and hence frequently even if patency is not achieved on the initial attempt, it could be established with subsequent attempts.

Please note that the first 15 minutes are the most critical to ensure RA patency. It is important to note that in 25% to 30% patent hemostasis is not obtainable.

Duration of Hemostatic Compression

Shorter duration of haemostatic compression has been shown to significantly influence the incidence of both early (within 24 hours) and late (at 30 days) RAO following TRA catheterization, without adversely affecting bleeding complications.[42] However, on multivariate analysis, the adverse effect of longer duration of RA compression was eliminated when patent hemostasis was adopted.[42] In fact, it has been routinely observed that patent hemostasis can lead to faster hemostasis than occlusive hemostasis. Nevertheless, it should also be reminded that after sheath removal, patent hemostasis is not feasible in 25% to 33% of the cases.

Clinical Sequelae of Radial Artery Occlusion

Ischemia

RAO usually follows a "benign" and clinically quiescent course and seldom leads to clinical events due to the protective effect of dual hand blood supply, and this may be one of many reasons for its underestimated incidence. To this date, there is no proof that RAO per se may produce distal ischemia. Indeed, despite the fact that radial approach has been practiced for more than 20 years, there has been no case of amputation following transradial catheterization. However, there have been documented reports of digital and hand ischemia with necrosis following prolonged cannulation in the setting of anesthetic practice and hemodynamic monitoring of critically ill patients.[43] Several factors come into play in these settings, which may explain the occurrence of ischemia, including hemodynamic instability, use of vasopressor agents, and infrequency of anticoagulation use in these patients, increasing the chance of in situ thrombus formation and, most importantly, distal embolization.

For example, Mangar et al.[44] reported a case of delayed hand ischemia necessitating amputation after RA cannulation in a diabetic male patient with end-stage renal failure and advanced atherosclerotic vascular disease. Following uneventful general anesthetic for his peripheral vascular surgery, the left radial arterial line was accidentally pulled out, and 10 days later, the patient developed symptoms and signs of hand ischemia.[44] The authors documented intraoperative findings of advanced atherosclerotic disease affecting both radial and ulnar arteries with severe calcification and 95% stenosis, and local thrombi, which

clearly acted as a catalyst in this unfortunate case. The case was a further evidence of poor reliability of Allen test (equivocal in this case) in predicting poor collateral hand circulation.[44,45]

To date, there have been only three case reports of distal ischemia following TRA coronary procedures. The first, by Rhyne and Mann,[46] was of a 72-year-old male patient with a multitude of cardiovascular risk factors who underwent TRA catheterization and ad hoc PCI to right coronary artery (RCA), received 7,000 IU of unfractionated heparin, and was discharged on dual antiplatelet therapy. The patient developed symptoms of right-hand ischemia 2 weeks following the procedure, and RAO was confirmed on Doppler examination. Owing to persistent symptoms, selective angiography was performed 4 months later, which demonstrated not only RAO but also diffusely diseased ulnar artery tapering down to a complete occlusion. RAO was successfully treated with antegrade angioplasty, resulting in immediate symptomatic relief. de Bucourt and Teichgraber[47] also described a case of prolonged hand ischemia following TRA PCI in a patient who presented with a biomarker positive cardiac event and required intubation for cardiogenic shock. The patient reportedly continued to have hand ischemic symptoms for 2 months postprocedure, and digital necrosis requiring amputation.[47] More recently, Rademakers and Laarman[48] described a case of a female smoker who developed hand ischemia 5 days following TRA procedure, manifesting as right-hand numbness, paresthesia, and sensitivity to touch. RAO was confirmed by Doppler evaluation, and selective angiography of the distal brachial artery showed patent ulnar artery, occluded RA, and distal embolization in the digital arteries. Attempted treatment with LMWH and thrombolysis with urokinase was of no avail; therefore, the patient underwent vascular surgery with thrombectomy and patch angioplasty.[48]

Treatment of Radial Artery Occlusion: What Is Proven, and What Is Hypothesis-Generating

Pharmacologic Treatment

Low-Molecular-Weight Heparin

Although there is scanty evidence from some observational single-center studies of the role of LMWH to treat "symptomatic" RAO, there is still no compelling evidence-based pharmacological treatment for RAO from randomized data that includes a control group.

In a single-center prospective observational study of 488 patients undergoing TRA procedures, Zankl et al.[32] examined the efficacy of LMWH for 4 weeks in improving the patency rate of the RA in patients with symptomatic RAO. The authors identified 51 cases (10.5%) of postprocedural RAO using systematic Doppler sonography in all patients. Of these, 30 (58.8%) presented with various symptoms, whereas 21 (41.2%) were asymptomatic. After 4 weeks of LMWH therapy in symptomatic patients, recanalization rate was shown to be complete in 21 (70%) and partial in 6 (20%) versus 0 (0%) and 4 (19%) in asymptomatic patients who did not receive LMWH.[32] Using a similar strategy, Uhlemann et al.[15] recently reported a recanalization rate of 31.5% (17 of 54) in those treated with either weight-adjusted or lower-dose LMWH for a mean of 6 days versus 5.4% (2 of 37) among those who did not receive anticoagulant therapy for RAO. As this was not a truly randomized study with lack of a control group, several confounding factors would stand in the face of recommending LMWH as a blanket therapy for RAO, until this is tested in a future randomized study.[49]

Thrombolysis

In their recent case report of critical hand ischemia due to RAO five days after TRA procedure, Rademakers and Laarman[48] attempted treatment with both LMWH and streptokinase. However, patient remained symptomatic with persistent RAO, and ultimately required emergency vascular surgery and patch angioplasty. Failure of extensive thrombolytic regimen in this case probably highlights the fact that anticoagulant or thrombolytic therapy is unlikely to have an effect once occlusion is established. There have been several anecdotal attempts of intravenous thrombolysis for RAO but none have lead to significant angiographic or clinical improvement.

Nonpharmacologic Treatment

Ipsilateral Ulnar Compression

In a randomized study, Bernat et al.[35] compared the incidence of RAO with very low-dose heparin (2,000 IU) versus low dose (5,000 IU) during TRA procedures. Using patent hemostasis, they demonstrated that immediate posthemostasis RAO rate was higher in the 2,000-IU group compared to the 5,000-IU group (5.9% vs 2.9%, $P = 0.17$). For the first time, they also described a nonpharmacological technique of 1-hour ulnar compression

to treat acute RAO, with again higher efficacy with higher heparin dose (final incidence of RAO was 4.1% in the 2,000-IU group, vs 0.8% in the 5,000-IU group, $P = 0.03$). The authors postulated that the potential mechanism is that ulnar artery compression results in a steep increase in antegrade flow through the RA, thus promoting local fibrinolysis and acute recanalization of the RA. Initially, manual ulnar compression had been described by Dr. Tian Jun in China as a preventive method against RAO during hemostasis (unpublished data). Whether mechanical ulnar compression might be applicable routinely deserves further investigation and is currently tested in the PROPHET II trial (ClinicalTrials.gov identifier: NCT01564888).

Mechanical Recanalization of Occluded Radial Artery

Several authors have described small series of anterograde or retrograde mechanical recanalization or angioplasty, thereby successfully treating isolated cases of RAO.[30,50,51] Overall, there have been more than 50 attempts to early recanalization of RAO. It should be emphasized that those cases have been performed by radial operators with long-standing experience in radial approach, and although acute results were encouraging, retrograde recanalization of RAO cannot be recommended at this time. Furthermore, late patency of those cases remains unknown. Recently, Jaradat et al. reported on a series of five women with symptomatic RAO who underwent anterograde recanalization by femoral approach of right RAO within 6 days of index procedure.[52] Interestingly, in four patients, balloon angioplasty was followed by local delivery of abciximab using a clearway balloon, whereas in one case, only balloon angioplasty was used. Late patency was documented by echo-duplex in all four except the one with balloon angioplasty alone.

Medicated Sheaths

With the expected surge in uptake of TRA for coronary angiography and intervention procedures worldwide, it is incompact on the interventional community to adhere to proven RAO avoidance strategies, and adopt quality assurance measures in any transradial program to safe guard against this complication, which is preventable to a large extent. Whether the true impact of RAO on possible distal ischemia will likely remain a hot topic, one should not forget that the first consequence of chronic RAO is that it prevents repeated use of the RA for catheterization and possible intervention.[53]

Therefore, it seems prudent to continue to explore other options to further mitigate or completely abolish the risk of RAO. In this regard, Hemetsberger et al.[54] evaluated the concept of using a drug-eluting introducer sheath to prevent local vascular complications. In a randomized preclinical study, the authors inserted nitric oxide (NO)-coated sheaths into juvenile porcine femoral arteries (similar diameter to human radial arteries), and compared these to control uncoated sheaths. There was less spasm and significantly higher vessel diameter at the time of sheath insertion, and less luminal thrombosis immediately, and significantly less intimal hyperplasia and luminal thrombosis 1 week after PCI, respectively. Although the concept of employing spasmolytic, anti-inflammatory, and antithrombotic properties of NO is captivating, future studies would be required to test clinical and cost effectiveness of NO-coated sheath in standard clinical practice.

Sheathless Guides

Saito et al. demonstrated that the RA lumen is smaller than a 7F sheath in 29% of men and 60% of women, and smaller than a 6F sheath in 15% of men and 28% of women. Although using 5F instead of 6F catheters can reduce the incidence of RAO, in real life this restricts guide catheter selection and the use of adjunctive devices for complex interventions. This limitation could largely be overcome by the use of sheathless guide catheters[55] (see chapter by D Fraser). Sheathless guide catheters have an inner lumen equivalent to, but an external diameter ~2F sizes less than, that of the corresponding standard catheter. As no introducer sheath is required, these could potentially retain the advantages of a larger Fr sheath, while keeping the low RAO rates observed with conventional 5F systems. However, at this time, there is no convincing evidence that sheathless techniques reduce RAO.

Conclusion

Despite its marked safety, cost effectiveness, increased patient preference, and mortality reduction in high-risk patients compared with femoral access, TRA has its own limitations. RAO should be recognized as an adverse consequence and avoided by adopting evidence-based practice to reduce its incidence. Currently, this includes working with the lowest-sized hardwares, using intravenous anticoagulation, and adopting patent hemostasis technique. The routine checks for postprocedural RAO should be an integral part of catheterization laboratory quality improvement program.

REFERENCES

1. Brzezinski M, Luisetti T, London MJ. Radial artery cannulation: a comprehensive review of recent anatomic and physiologic investigations. *Anesth Analg.* 2009;109(6):1763–1781.
2. Campeau L. Percutaneous radial artery approach for coronary angiography. *Cathet Cardiovasc Diagn.* 1989;16(1):3–7.
3. Bedford RF, Wollman H. Complications of percutaneous radial-artery cannulation: an objective prospective study in man. *Anesthesiology.* 1973;38(3):228–236.
4. Davis FM, Stewart JM. Radial artery cannulation: a prospective study in patients undergoing cardiothoracic surgery. *Br J Anaesth.* 1980;52(1):41–47.
5. Slogoff S, Keats AS, Arlund C. On the safety of radial artery cannulation. *Anesthesiology.* 1983;59(1):42–47.
6. Bedford RF. Wrist circumference predicts the risk of radial-arterial occlusion after cannulation. *Anesthesiology.* 1978;48(5):377–378.
7. Agostoni P, Biondi-Zoccai GG, de Benedictis ML, et al. Radial versus femoral approach for percutaneous coronary diagnostic and interventional procedures: systematic overview and meta-analysis of randomized trials. *J Am Coll Cardiol.* 2004;44(2):349–356.
8. Rao SV, Ou FS, Wang TY, et al. Trends in the prevalence and outcomes of radial and femoral approaches to percutaneous coronary intervention: a report from the National Cardiovascular Data Registry. *JACC Cardiovasc Interv.* 2008;1(4):379–386.
9. Rathore S, Stables RH, Pauriah M, et al. Impact of length and hydrophilic coating of the introducer sheath on radial artery spasm during transradial coronary intervention: a randomized study. *JACC Cardiovasc Interv.* 2010;3(5):475–483.
10. Spaulding C, Lefèvre T, Funck F, et al. Left radial approach for coronary angiography: results of a prospective study. *Cathet Cardiovasc Diagn.* 1996;39(4):365–370.
11. Saito S, Ikei H, Hosokawa G, et al. Influence of the ratio between radial artery inner diameter and sheath outer diameter on radial artery flow after transradial coronary intervention. *Catheter Cardiovasc Interv.* 1999;46(2):173–178.
12. Dahm JB, Vogelgesang D, Hummel A, et al. A randomized trial of 5 vs. 6 French transradial percutaneous coronary interventions. *Catheter Cardiovasc Interv.* 2002;57(2):172–176.
13. Rathore S, Stables RH, Pauriah M, et al. A randomized comparison of TR band and radistop hemostatic compression devices after transradial coronary intervention. *Catheter Cardiovasc Interv.* 2010;76(5):660–667.
14. Kiemeneij F, Laarman GJ, Odekerken D, et al. A randomized comparison of percutaneous transluminal coronary angioplasty by the radial, brachial and femoral approaches: the access study. *J Am Coll Cardiol.* 1997;29(6):1269–1275.
15. Uhlemann M, Möbius-Winkler, S, Mende, M, et al. The Leipzig prospective vascular ultrasound registry in radial artery catheterization: impact of sheath size on vascular complications. *JACC Cardiovasc Interv.* 2012;5(1):36–43.
16. Bertrand OF, Rao SV, Pancholy S, et al. Transradial approach for coronary angiography and interventions: results of the first international transradial practice survey. *JACC Cardiovasc Interv.* 2010;3(10):1022–1031.
17. Pancholy S, Coppola J, Patel T, et al. Prevention of radial artery occlusion-patent hemostasis evaluation trial (PROPHET study): a randomized comparison of

traditional versus patency documented hemostasis after transradial catheterization. *Catheter Cardiovasc Interv.* 2008;72(3):335–340.

18. Kerawala CJ, Martin IC. Palmar arch backflow following radial forearm free flap harvest. *Br J Oral Maxillofacial Surg.* 2003;41(3):157–160.

19. Greenwood MJ, Della-Siega AJ, Fretz EB, et al. Vascular communications of the hand in patients being considered for transradial coronary angiography: is the Allen's test accurate? *J Am Coll Cardiol.* 2005;46(11):2013–2017.

20. Stella PR, Kiemeneij F, Laarman GJ, et al. Incidence and outcome of radial artery occlusion following transradial artery coronary angioplasty. *Cathet Cardiovasc Diagn.* 1997;40(2):156–158.

21. Cheng EY, Lauer KK, Stommel KA, et al. Evaluation of the palmar circulation by pulse oximetry. *J Clin Monit.* 1989;5(1):1–3.

22. Barbeau GR, Arsenault F, Dugas L, et al. Evaluation of the ulnopalmar arterial arches with pulse oximetry and plethysmography: comparison with the Allen's test in 1010 patients. *Am Heart J.* 2004;147(3):489–493.

23. He GW, Yang CQ. Characteristics of adrenoceptors in the human radial artery: clinical implications. *J Thorac Cardiovasc Surg.* 1998;115(5):1136–1141.

24. Loh YJ, Nakao M, Tan WD, et al. Factors influencing radial artery size. *Asian Cardiovasc Thorac Ann.* 2007;15(4):324–326.

25. Caputo RP, Tremmel JA, Rao S, et al. Transradial arterial access for coronary and peripheral procedures: executive summary by the transradial committee of the SCAI. *Catheter Cardiovasc Interv.* 2011;78:823–839.

26. Yonetsu T, Kakuta T, Lee T, et al. Assessment of acute injuries and chronic intimal thickening of the radial artery after transradial coronary intervention by optical coherence tomography. *Eur Heart J.* 2010;31(13):1608–1615.

27. Staniloae CS, Mody KP, Sanghvi K, et al. Histopathologic changes of the radial artery wall secondary to transradial catheterization. *Vasc Health Risk Manag.* 2009;5:527–532.

28. Wakeyama T, Ogawa H, Iida H, et al. Intima-media thickening of the radial artery after transradial intervention. An intravascular ultrasound study. *J Am Coll Cardiol.* 2003;41(7):1109–1114.

29. Bedford RF. Radial arterial function following percutaneous cannulation with 18- and 20-gauge catheters. *Anesthesiology.* 1977;47(1):37–39.

30. Pancholy SB. Transradial access in an occluded radial artery: new technique. *J Invasive Cardiol.* 2007;19(12):541–544.

31. Kim KS, Park HS, Jang WI, et al. Thrombotic occlusion of the radial artery as a complication of the transradial coronary intervention. *J Cardiovasc Ultrasound.* 2010;18(1):31.

32. Zankl AR, Andrassy M, Volz C, et al. Radial artery thrombosis following transradial coronary angiography: incidence and rationale for treatment of symptomatic patients with low-molecular-weight heparins. *Clin Res Cardiol.* 2010;99(12):841–847.

33. Zhou YJ, Zhao YX, Cao Z, et al. Incidence and risk factors of acute radial artery occlusion following transradial percutaneous coronary intervention. *Zhonghua Yi Xue Za Zhi* 2007;87(22):1531–1534.

34. Lefevre T, Thebault B, Spaulding C, et al. Radial artery patency after percutaneous left radial artery approach for coronary angiography. The role of heparin. *Eur Heart J.* 1995;16:293.

35. Bernat I, Bertrand OF, Rokyta R, et al. Efficacy and safety of transient ulnar artery compression to recanalize acute radial artery occlusion after transradial catheterization. *Am J Cardiol.* 2011;107(11):1698–1701.

36. Plante S, Cantor WJ, Goldman L, et al. Comparison of bivalirudin versus heparin on radial artery occlusion after transradial catheterization. *Catheter Cardiovasc Interv.* 2010;76(5):654–658.

37. Pancholy SB, Ahmed I, Bertrand OF, et al. Frequency of radial artery occlusion after transradial access in patients receiving warfarin therapy and undergoing coronary angiography. *Am J Cardiol.* 2014;113(2):211–214.

38. Pancholy SB, Bertrand OF, Patel T. Comparison of a priori versus provisional heparin therapy on radial artery occlusion after transradial coronary angiography and patent hemostasis (from the PHARAOH Study). *Am J Cardiol.* 2012;110(2):173–176.

39. Pancholy SB. Comparison of the effect of intra-arterial versus intravenous heparin on radial artery occlusion after transradial catheterization. *Am J Cardiol.* 2009;104(8):1083–1085.

40. Sanmartin M, Gomez M, Rumoroso JR, et al. Interruption of blood flow during compression and radial artery occlusion after transradial catheterization. *Catheter Cardiovasc Interv.* 2007;70(2):185–189.

41. Cubero JM, Lombardo J, Pedrosa C, et al. Radial compression guided by mean artery pressure versus standard compression with a pneumatic device (RACOMAP). *Catheter Cardiovasc Interv.* 2009;73(4):467–472.

42. Pancholy SB, Patel TM. Effect of duration of hemostatic compression on radial artery occlusion after transradial access. *Catheter Cardiovasc Interv.* 2012;79(1):78–81.

43. Baker RJ, Chunprapaph B, Nyhus LM. Severe ischemia of the hand following radial artery catheterization. *Surgery.* 1976;80(4):449–457.

44. Mangar D, Laborde RS, Vu DN. Delayed ischaemia of the hand necessitating amputation after radial artery cannulation. *Canad J Anaesth.* 1993;40(3):247–250.

45. Bertrand OF, Carey PC, Gilchrist IC. Allen or no Allen: that is the question! *J Am Coll Cardiol.* 2014;63(18):1842–1844.

46. Rhyne, D, Mann T. Hand ischemia resulting from a transradial intervention: successful management with radial artery angioplasty. *Catheter Cardiovasc Interv.* 2010;76(3):383–386.

47. de Bucourt M, Teichgraber U. Digital ischemia and consecutive amputation after emergency transradial cardiac catheter examination. *Cardiovasc Intervent Radiol.* 2012;35(5):1242–1244.

48. Rademakers LM, Laarman GJ. Critical hand ischaemia after transradial cardiac catheterisation: an uncommon complication of a common procedure. *Neth Heart J.* 2012;20(9):372–375.

49. Rao SV. Observations from a transradial registry: our remedies oft in ourselves do lie. *JACC Cardiovasc Interv.* 2012;5(1):44–46.

50. Babunashvili AM, Chase AJ, Dundua DP. Recanalization of late radial artery occlusion after transradial coronary interventions: a new technique for interventionalists practising radial artery approach. *Catheter Cardiovasc Interv.* 2006;67(5):828.

51. Skvaril J, Kockova R, Danickova K, et al. Chronic radial artery occlusion after transradial catheterization: recanalization via an ipsilateral ulnar artery. *Acta Cardiol.* 2012;67(3):367–370.

52. Jaradat Z, Basir B, Revtyak G. Treatment of radial artery occlusions using balloon angioplasty and localized intra-arterial abciximab. *J Interv Cardiol.* 2014;27(2):217–222.

53. Abdelaal E, Molin P, Plourde G, et al. Successive transradial access for coronary procedures: experience of Quebec Heart-Lung Institute. *Am Heart journal.* 2013;165(3):325–331.

54. Hemetsberger R, Posa A, Farhan S, et al. Drug-eluting introducer sheath prevents local peripheral complications: pre-clinical evaluation of nitric oxide-coated sheath. *JACC Cardiovasc Interv.* 2011;4(1):98–106.

55. Mamas M, D'Souza S, Hendry C, et al. Use of the sheathless guide catheter during routine transradial percutaneous coronary intervention: a feasibility study. *Catheter Cardiovasc Interv.* 2010;75(4):596–602.

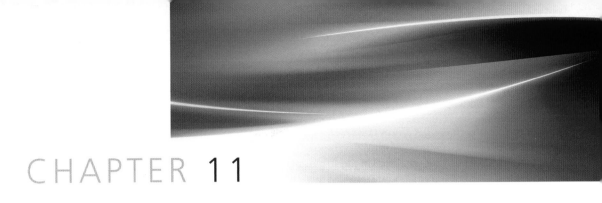

CHAPTER 11

The Learning Curve for Transradial Coronary Angiography and Intervention

Basem Elbarouni and Asim N. Cheema

Introduction

Despite the demonstrated benefits of transradial angiography and intervention, its adoption by physicians has been quite slow compared with the incorporation of other technological advances in interventional cardiology such as the use of drug-eluting stents. There are several potential reasons for poor uptake of transradial approach for coronary diagnostic and intervention procedures by individual physicians. These range from inertia in changing established practice patterns to fear of technical difficulties encountered in complex and high-risk patients. However, the most commonly cited reason for not employing the transradial approach is the challenges encountered during the learning curve of transradial approach for coronary diagnostic and intervention procedures. Operators who are experienced or familiar with transfemoral approach are often intimidated by prospects of cannulation of a much smaller vessel, occurrence of radial arterial spasm, navigating tortuous subclavian vessels, and engaging coronary arteries with catheters designed mainly for femoral access. These are all new skills that must be mastered for competence in transradial coronary interventions. Furthermore, experienced femoral operators are comfortable with their technique and may find little reason to change practice in their specific patient population. This attitude is transferred to trainees who do not get exposure to transradial procedures and continue to practice

interventional cardiology after completion of training without incorporating new techniques and approaches. The lack of radial experts in training centers, therefore, is an important limiting factor for a wider adoption of the transradial approach. The role of procedural volume is also an important consideration for the uptake of transradial approach by an individual physician or institution. A high-volume transfemoral operator or institution might feel that adopting a new technique will slow down the coronary intervention procedures and interfere with proper patient flow. Similarly, low-volume operators or centers might feel that lower volumes are a hindrance for adequate skill development.

Clinical Outcomes and the Learning Curve of Transradial Coronary Intervention

Like many other technical skills, greater experience in performing coronary interventions has been shown to be associated with a lower risk of procedural complications since the early days of angioplasty.[1] The RIVAL study,[2] a multicenter trial comparing radial versus femoral percutaneous coronary intervention (PCI) in patients with acute coronary syndrome, is the largest study yet to evaluate the impact of vascular access site on patient outcomes. The study showed no difference in the rates of death, myocardial infarction, stroke, or major bleeding (primary outcome of trial) between the two access sites, but the rate of major vascular complications was significantly lower in the radial group (1.4% vs 3.7%, $P < 0.001$) than in the femoral group.[2] It is important to note, however, that operators in the RIVAL study were experienced radial operators and that the median annual volume was 300 radial procedures per operator. In addition, the radial access group had significantly lower events in centers with the highest radial PCI volume, compared with femoral access (1.6% vs 3.2%, $P = 0.015$), with lowest rates of access site crossover.[2] These findings confirmed that the benefits of radial access are strongly influenced by operator experience, and greater operator experience with radial procedures improves patient outcomes. Interestingly, the femoral access was not superior to radial access at high-volume femoral centers. This finding suggests that the radial learning curve has important implications for improving clinical outcomes in transradial coronary intervention procedures.

The Importance and Challenges of Characterizing Transradial Learning Curve

How many procedures should a novice radial operator perform to be considered proficient in transradial access? Quantifying the learning curve for transradial coronary procedures is a challenging prospect. Characterizing the learning curve would help transfemoral operators wishing to adopt this approach plan appropriately and designate adequate time and case load to develop the necessary skills. Furthermore, it would help training programs and credentialing bodies to standardize training and recognize competence in transradial access. In addition, it would help future research related to access site to categorize radial operator experience in a standardized and universally acceptable manner. Ideally, measuring patient and procedural outcomes would be the preferable way to quantify the learning curve. However, given the relatively low rates of complications with coronary angiography and angioplasty in general,[3,4] such studies would require an excessively large number of patients and might not be feasible. Surrogate outcomes such as procedure success rates, procedure time,

fluoroscopy time, and contrast media usage have been investigated in prior studies. Researchers have either compared these parameters between transradial and transfemoral approaches or examined the relationship between various markers of procedural safety and efficacy and an operator's transradial experience. While these indices are reasonable and acceptable measures of efficiency, whether or not they correlate with patient outcomes has not been demonstrated. For example, some reports have suggested an association between fluoroscopy time and transradial procedural complications and used fluoroscopy time as a parameter reflecting operator experience with transradial procedures.[5] However, it is likely that higher fluoroscopy times are related to technical complexity of the coronary intervention procedure rather than to operator experience or lack thereof.[6]

The Learning Curve of Transradial Coronary Angiography

Operators new to the radial approach will face most of the challenges unique to this approach when starting with diagnostic transradial coronary angiography. New skills such as radial access, avoiding and managing radial artery spasm, navigating tortuous subclavian arteries, and engaging the coronary arteries with catheters designed for the femoral approach must be acquired to become efficient in transradial coronary angiography. A few studies have attempted to quantify the learning curve for transradial diagnostic angiography. In one of the earlier reports, Spaulding et al.[7] prospectively studied 415 patients undergoing left transradial coronary angiography between March 1994 and June 1995. All procedures were performed by four experienced cardiologists; the authors did not report on their prior familiarity with the radial approach. They reported a clear improvement in indices of procedural success with greater experience. The procedure failure rates, sheath insertion time, and procedure duration decreased from 14%, 10.2 min, 25.7 min in the first 80 patients to 2%, 2.85 min, and 17.5 min in the last 100 patients, respectively.[7] However, when compared to the femoral approach, the last 100 patients still had longer sheath insertion time and procedure duration. Louvard et al.[8] reported on his early experience with 800 transradial coronary catheterizations, performed between 1994 and 1997. The overall procedural success rate was 97.6% for the entire cohort. However, when patients were divided into three volume cohorts, failure rates decreased significantly from 10% for first 50 patients to 4% for the 50–500 group and to 1% after the first 500 patients. In a Spanish study, the first 200 patients were compared with the subsequent 326 patients undergoing coronary angiography, and the authors reported decreasing procedural failure rates, reduced procedure time, and less fluoroscopy time with increasing experience.[9]

In a contemporary study from New Zealand published in 2011, Looi et al.[10] examined the transradial coronary angiography learning experience of several operators at their center that encompassed a 12-month initial radial learning period. All operators were femoral experts. Radial experts were defined as having performed at least 100 angiographies using the radial approach. During the study period, nonradial experts performed an average of 63 radial angiographies each. Radial angiographies performed by nonradial experts had longer procedure time, fluoroscopy time, and contrast use when compared to femoral procedures, while radial experts demonstrated no difference in procedure or fluoroscopy time between the transradial and the transfemoral approaches except for contrast use, which was higher with transradial angiographic procedures. To assess the learning curve, procedures were categorized into quartiles (three months per quartile). The results of this analysis showed a significant difference in the first two quartiles between expert and nonexpert radial operators in all examined indices of procedural outcomes, while no significant difference was observed for the procedure performed during the third and fourth quartiles. An interesting finding was that the number of radial procedures performed by the nonexperts during the first half of the year was much less compared to the number of procedures performed in the second half of the year, 82 and 164 angiographies, respectively, suggesting that with increasing experience, operators became more confident in selecting patients for transradial access. An interesting finding was reported from the TALENT study[11] that compared fluoroscopy time and cannulation time between right and left radial accesses for coronary procedures. The results showed that the learning curve for diagnostic angiography was shorter for left radial approach than for right radial artery access. These findings suggest that coronary engagement from left radial artery access is easier due to the favorable angle for assessing the ascending aorta and coronary cannulation from left subclavian compared to right subclavian artery.

The Learning Curve of Transradial Coronary Interventions

There are limited data on the learning curve for transradial coronary PCI. The first study looking at this question was published by Goldberg et al.[12] in 1998. Goldberg described his own transradial PCI experience in 27 patients, with a procedural success rate of 84%. The main reason for failure in his experience was radial artery spasm. In a more contemporary study of >1,600 patients from our institution, Ball et al.[13] examined the transradial learning curve for simple single-vessel PCI procedures. Operators included both interventional trainees and staff physicians who started performing transradial PCI at our institution with no prior transradial experience. Procedures by each operator were chronologically classified into the first 50 procedures, subsequent 51–100, 101–150, and 150–300 procedures. The control group consisted of procedures performed by operators with more than 300 transradial PCI career volume. With increasing experience, there was a clear decline seen for procedure failure rates, contrast volume, and fluoroscopy times. Although there was continued benefit of higher experience, the magnitude of benefit tapered significantly after the first 50 cases, with only modest improvements with more procedures (Fig. 11-1). There was no difference in the procedural failure rates, number of guides used, fluoroscopy times, and contrast media usage in the 150–300 group compared to the control group (Table 11-1). These findings suggest that, for simple transradial PCI, the majority of skill development is acquired in the first 50 cases, and operators are highly proficient after 150 cases.

In a study by Gummadi et al.,[14] the learning curve was prospectively examined for three interventional cardiologists with varying transfemoral PCI expertise who started transradial PCI procedures. The procedural parameters of this group were compared with those of 50 consecutive cases performed by a radial expert (>500 transradial PCI career volume). Transradial proficiency was defined as contrast volume usage and procedure and fluoroscopy times at 90th centile of those

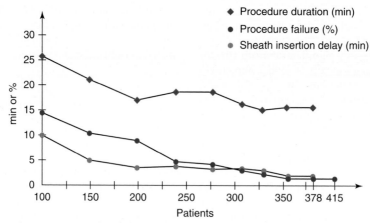

FIGURE 11-1   Learning curve: procedure failure rate, sheath insertion delay, and procedure duration. (From Spaulding C, Lefevre T, Funck F, et al. Left radial approach for coronary angiography: results of a prospective study. *Cathet Cardiovasc Diagn*. 1996;39(4):365–370.)

TABLE 11-1	**Procedural Outcomes**				
	TR-PCI Operator Experience				
	1–50 *(N = 655)*	*51–100* *(N = 344)*	*101–150* *(N = 213)*	*151–300* *(N = 141)*	**Control (N = 319)**
TR-PCI failure[a]	43 (7)	10 (3)	5 (2)	5 (3)	6 (2)
No. guides[b]	1.4 ± 1	1.4 ± 1	1.3 ± 1	1.3 ± 1	1.3 ± 1
Contrast volume[c]	180 ± 79	174 ± 79	170 ± 79	157 ± 75	168 ± 79
Fluoroscopy time (min)[d]	15 ± 10	14 ± 10	13 ± 10	11 ± 8	12 ± 9

All values are mean ± SD or *N* (%).
TR-PCI, transradial percutaneous coronary intervention.
[a]Analyzed by repeated-measures logistic regression model (*P* = 0.007 [1–50 vs 51–100], *P* = 0.01 [1–50 vs control]).
[b]Analyzed by the Poisson regression model (*P* = 0.90).
[c]Analyzed by repeated-measures linear regression model on log-transformed contrast volume with Tukey adjustment for multiple comparisons (*P* = 0.007 [overall], *P* = 0.02 [1–50 vs 151–300], *P* = 0.05 [1–50 vs control]).
[d]Analyzed by repeated-measures linear regression model on log-transformed fluoroscopy time with Tukey adjustment for multiple comparisons (*P* = 0.003 [overall], *P* = 0.04 [1–50 vs 101–150], *P* = 0.02 [1–50 vs control]).
From Ball WT, Sharieff W, Jolly SS, et al. Characterization of operator learning curve for transradial coronary interventions. *Circ Cardiovasc Interv*. 2011;4(4):336–341.

determined for the cases performed by the expert transradial PCI operator. The results showed that the most experienced operator (>10 years' practice) achieved >75% of target proficiency within 50 cases, while the other two operators needed 150 cases to achieve similar proficiency. More importantly, even at 150 cases, none of the operators were as proficient at transradial PCI as the radial expert. This study suggests that the learning curve may be continuous, with greater improvement with higher volumes.

The Learning Curve of Transradial Angiography and Intervention for Novice Operators

The previously discussed studies mostly dealt with the learning curve of radial access among experienced femoral operators. The preferable method for training new interventional fellows in radial access is not well studied. Should they initially focus on femoral access and once comfortable with this approach, move on to radial procedures? Or is it preferable to train in both access routes in a parallel manner? A study presented at TCT 2011 by Javed et al.[15] looked at procedure performance indices of interventional cardiology fellows during their first year of training. A total of 1,777 coronary catheterizations were performed (34% of procedures were PCI). Of these, 19% were done via the radial route. The authors reported high procedure success rates (95.6% for radial access and 99.9% for femoral access). There was no difference in procedure time, fluoroscopy time, or contrast use between radial and femoral routes. On comparing the radial procedures performed in the first six months versus the second six months, there was a significant reduction in all measured indices.

The Implication of Transradial Learning Curve for Training and Competency Guidelines

There are no clear recommendations or consensus on the period of training or the number of cases required to be proficient in transradial coronary procedures, although recommendations from Society for Cardiovascular Angiography and Interventions (SCAI) and ESC have been published recently (Fig. 11-2). In the United States, to be eligible for certification by the American Board of Internal Medicine, each trainee needs to perform a minimum of 250 PCI procedures during training, but no specific recommendations are provided in terms of radial access.[16]

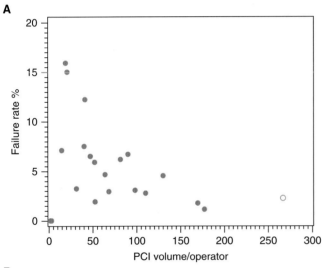

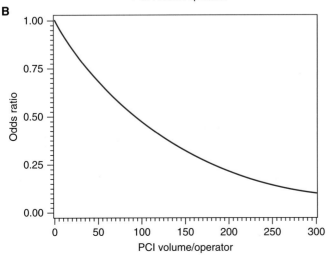

FIGURE 11-2 Relationship between TR-PCI volume and failure rate. **A:** Data for individual operators are shown. Solid circles represent individual TR-PCI operators for four experience groups and the open circle represents the control group shown as a reference. Case volume was defined as total cases performed by individual operators in the four experience groups and total cases performed by all operators in the control group. **B:** Data illustrated as odds ratios of failure to total TR-PCI volume. The results of logistic regression analysis showed that the relative odds of TR-PCI failure decline substantially up to 50 cases, and further decline after 100 cases is small. PCI, percutaneous coronary intervention; TR-PCI, transradial percutaneous coronary intervention. (From Ball WT, Sharieff W, Jolly SS, et al. Characterization of operator learning curve for transradial coronary interventions. *Circ Cardiovasc Interv.* 2011;4(4):336–341.)

The ACC Core Cardiology Training Symposium (COCATS) guidelines recommend that trainees need to be able to "perform vascular access from the femoral, radial, or brachial route," but do not provide criteria or guidelines for competency in transradial procedures. The curriculum and syllabus for interventional cardiology subspecialty training in Europe recommends trainees learn "vascular access, including principles of femoral, radial and brachial procedures," with no further recommendations on recognizing competence in transradial procedures. The SCAI has recognized and called for the need of formalizing transradial PCI training. The SCAI has also proposed a three-tiered competency classification[17] as follows:

- *Level 1 competency:* Able to perform simple diagnostic cases on patients with favorable upper limb anatomy (large men).
- *Level 2 competency:* Able to perform simple diagnostic and interventional procedures on patients with more challenging upper limb anatomy (elective single-vessel PCI, bypass grafts, small women, and radial and subclavian loops).
- *Level 3 competency:* Able to perform complex interventional procedures even with challenging limb anatomy (CTOs, multivessel, and AMI).

These three levels have been recently updated (Fig. 11-2).

The Learning Curve of Transradial Angiography and Intervention: Future Research

A few questions remain in categorizing the learning curve and require further investigation. There is mounting evidence that using the radial route in primary PCI improves patient outcomes.[2,18] However, long procedure times in novice radial interventionists might prolong the door-to-balloon time, potentially causing harm. However, equivalent procedure and fluoroscopy times can be achieved by radial experts using either access route. Further studies are required to identify the number of elective radial procedures an operator should perform before attempting radial access in primary PCI, although SCAI has recently provided some guidance.[19] Furthermore, there is limited information for the learning curve in complex PCI procedures. The issue of poor guide support with transradial access might add to the complexity and challenge of these procedures with potential for increased exposure to radiation and contrast media. Finally, the best approach for introducing interventional cardiology trainees to transradial procedures needs to be determined by characterizing the learning curve of these novice operators. This will allow increased utilization of transradial approach in a safe manner for the wider patient population.

Conclusion

Despite the slow adoption of radial access over the last decade, it is likely that patient benefits and health-care savings will drive increased demand and wider application of transradial procedures over the next decade. Radial access should be available as an option for patients at most PCI centers, especially for those at high risk of vascular complications. Interventional cardiologists, both novice and experienced, will need to learn this technique to remain competitive, and PCI training programs need to offer this skill to attract the top candidates. Expert interventional cardiologists wishing to adopt this approach should plan accordingly keeping in mind the learning period. The current data suggest that a minimum of 50 procedures are required to deliver transradial PCI in a safe and effective manner. However, greater experience with a transradial volume of >150 procedures provides similar results as seen for expert transradial operators. These numbers should be considered as a general recommendation, as the learning curve is probably variable for individual operators, and seems to be shorter in more experienced operators. When starting initially, it is advisable to use a stepwise approach, starting with diagnostic angiography and simple PCI in patients with favorable anatomy, before proceeding to more complex procedures and patients with less favorable anatomy. Radial skills can probably be developed in a relatively short period by utilizing radial access in all eligible patients during the learning period. For training programs, trainees should be exposed to radial access early on and trained in both radial and femoral accesses in a parallel manner. Recruiting primarily radial operators to training programs can result in early and consistent radial exposure and make the program more attractive to potential candidates.

REFERENCES

1. Ammann P, Brunner-La Rocca HP, Angehrn W, et al. Procedural complications following diagnostic coronary angiography are related to the operator's experience and the catheter size. *Catheter Cardiovasc Interv.* 2003;59:13–18.

2. Jolly SS, Yusuf S, Cairns J, et al. Radial versus femoral access for coronary angiography and intervention in patients with acute coronary syndromes (RIVAL): a randomised, parallel group, multicentre trial. *Lancet.* 2011;377:1409–1420.

3. Chandrasekar B, Doucet S, Bilodeau L, et al. Complications of cardiac catheterization in the current era: a single-center experience. *Catheter Cardiovasc Interv.* 2001; 52:289–295.

4. Jamal SM, Shrive FM, Ghali WA, et al. In-hospital outcomes after percutaneous coronary intervention in Canada: 1992/93 to 2000/01. *Can J Cardiol.* 2003;19:782–789.

5. Jensen UJ, Lagerquist B, Jensen J, et al. The use of fluoroscopy to construct learning curves for coronary angiography. *Catheter Cardiovasc Interv.* 2012;80:564–569.

6. Nikolsky E, Pucelikova T, Mehran R, et al. An evaluation of fluoroscopy time and correlation with outcomes after percutaneous coronary intervention. *J Invasive Cardiol.* 2007;19:208–213.

7. Spaulding C, Lefevre T, Funck F, et al. Left radial approach for coronary angiography: results of a prospective study. *Cathet Cardiovasc Diagn.* 1996;39:365–370.

8. Louvard Y, Krol M, Pezzano M, et al. Feasibility of routine transradial coronary angiography: a single operator's experience. *J Invasive Cardiol.* 1999;11:543–548.

9. Salgado Fernandez J, Calvino Santos R, Vazquez Rodriguez JM, et al. Transradial approach to coronary angiography and angioplasty: initial experience and learning curve [in Spanish]. *Rev Esp Cardiol.* 2003;56:152–159.

10. Looi JL, Cave A, El-Jack S. Learning curve in transradial coronary angiography. *Am J Cardiol.* 2011;108:1092–1095.

11. Sciahbasi A, Romagnoli E, Trani C, et al. Evaluation of the "learning curve" for left and right radial approach during percutaneous coronary procedures. *Am J Cardiol.* 2011;108:185–188.

12. Goldberg SL, Renslo R, Sinow R, et al. Learning curve in the use of the radial artery as vascular access in the performance of percutaneous transluminal coronary angioplasty. *Cathet Cardiovasc Diagn.* 1998;44:147–152.

13. Ball WT, Sharieff W, Jolly SS, et al. Characterization of operator learning curve for transradial coronary interventions. *Circ Cardiovasc Interv.* 2011;4:336–341.

14. Gummadi B, Blackburn J, Percy R, et al. Transradial approach to coronary interventions: how steep is the learning curve for trained interventional cardiologists? *J Am Coll Cardiol.* 2011;58:B141.

15. Javed U, Armstrong E, Southard J, et al. Procedural trends associated with successful initiation of a transradial program at an academic training institution. *J Am Coll Cardiol.* 2011;58:B147.

16. American Board of Internal Medicine. *Interventional Cardiology Policies.* 2012. http://www.abim.org/specialty/interventional-cardiology.aspx

17. Caputo RP, Tremmel JA, Rao S, et al. Transradial arterial access for coronary and peripheral procedures: executive summary by the transradial committee of the scai. *Catheter Cardiovasc Interv.* 2011;78:823–839.

18. Romagnoli E, Biondi-Zoccai G, Sciahbasi A, et al. Radial versus femoral randomized investigation in st-segment elevation acute coronary syndrome: the rifle-steacs (Radial versus Femoral Randomized Investigation in ST-Elevation Acute Coronary Syndrome) study. *J Am Coll Cardiol.* 2012;60:2481–2489.

19. Rao SV, et al. Best practices for transradial angiography and intervention: a consensus statement from the society for cardiovascular angiography and intervention's transradial working group. *Catheter Cardiovasc Interv.* 2014;83(2):228–236.

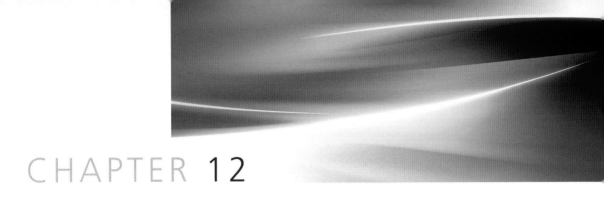

CHAPTER 12

Complications of Transradial Catheterization

Olivier F. Bertrand, Gérald Barbeau, and Ferdinand Kiemeneij

Introduction

Since the early days of cardiac catheterization, vascular access for diagnostic coronary angiography and interventions was either by the upper limb or by the femoral artery. The brachial artery as an access site by a cut-down technique for selective coronary angiography was initially described by Dr. Mason Sones in 1962 at the Cleveland Clinic.[1] Interestingly enough, cannulation for the left and right coronary ostia was done with a single catheter. Other investigators soon promoted a percutaneous femoral artery approach. Dr. Melvin Judkins developed separate preshaped catheters designed specifically for left and right coronary injections.[2] Arterial access and rapid exchange with a wire using the Seldinger technique resulted in the preferential adoption of the femoral approach due to its relative simplicity as well as the reduction in local complications associated with the brachial cut-down technique. Following the first coronary balloon angioplasty performed by Dr. Andreas Gruentzig in 1977 using the percutaneous femoral approach (9F), this access site definitely achieved the status of default access site around the world. Thus, from the beginning of percutaneous coronary interventions (PCI), consideration for reduction in access-site complications was a main driver for access-site selection.

Early pioneers, for example, Dr. Bruce Radner in Sweden, proposed using the distal radial artery as an access site to perform aortography as early as 1948.[3] In this early experience, no vascular complication was noted. The first description of a radial technique for selective coronary angiography was reported in 1974 in France. Concerned about potential trauma to surrounding veins and nerve in close proximity to the brachial artery, Dr. Michel Bertrand developed a cut-down technique for the proximal radial artery, a few centimeters distal to the usual surgical site for accessing the brachial artery.[4] It is worth noting that at the conclusion of these procedures, the radial artery was always sutured, hence creating iatrogenic proximal radial artery occlusion (RAO). In his experience of more than 100 cases, distal ischemia never occurred and radial pulse remained present presumably due to the recruitment of collaterals originating from the ulnar artery and both the deep and superficial vascular palmar arches (Dr. M Bertrand, personal communication, November 2010). Despite anticoagulation, both Dr. Lucien Campeau and Dr. Masaki Otaki in their initial experience reported cases of asymptomatic RAO but no other complications.

With the advent of coronary stenting and required intensive antiplatelet and anticoagulation therapy, vascular complications and periprocedural bleeding became a major issue.[5] In the ACCESS study, the first randomized study comparing the three access sites—femoral, brachial, and radial—for percutaneous transluminal coronary angioplasty, Kiemeneij et al. demonstrated similar procedural success, but significantly less vascular complications with radial access were noted.[6] Yet it is worth noting that in the femoral group ($n = 300$), four patients had major bleeding, with two requiring transfusion and two requiring surgery. Furthermore, three others developed pseudoaneurysm, with one requiring surgery. In the brachial group ($n = 300$), three patients developed a large hematoma, with one requiring transfusion, and four developed pseudoaneurysm, with three requiring surgery. In contrast, in the radial group ($n = 300$), no major bleeding, no surgery, and no transfusion were required, yet RAO was found in 5% at discharge and in 3% 1 month later. So from this very first comparison, radial approach was clearly associated with lesser risks of bleeding and vascular complications than other access site, yet RAO was identified as a radial access–specific complication. For a detailed review on bleeding and RAO, see Chapters 2 and 10, respectively.

In this chapter, we review the incidence and types of vascular complications associated with femoral and radial access sites as well as discussing radial-specific complications and methods to prevent and treat them.

Femoral Artery Access and Complications

For many years, there was little focus on optimizing femoral access puncture and management to reduce periprocedural bleeding and complications. To ensure puncture of the common femoral artery (CFA) and to limit risks of vascular complications, two techniques have been recently proposed. The first is to use fluoroscopy, while the second relies on ultrasound to guide the puncture. Although using fluoroscopy was proposed as early as 1978 by Dr. Charles Dotter, there have been surprisingly few randomized studies afterward.[7]

Fitts et al. reviewed the impact of fluoroscopic guidance in 2,651 consecutive patients.[8] Overall, the use of fluoroscopy was associated with a lower incidence of pseudoaneurysms (0.3% vs 1.1%, $P = 0.017$) and any arterial injury, defined by hematoma >8 cm, pseudoaneurysm, arteriovenous (A/V) fistula, retroperitoneal bleeding (RPB), or any vascular complication requiring intervention (0.7% vs 1.9%, $P < 0.01$). Of note, there was no difference in bleeding requiring transfusion (1.6% vs 1.8%, $P = 0.69$). To date, there has been only a single randomized trial comparing fluoroscopy-guided puncture to puncturing below the inguinal ligament.[9] Overall, the mean time to successfully insert an arterial sheath in the CFA was similar in both groups. Furthermore, in this study involving a large majority of diagnostic procedures (~70%), the rate of vascular complications, albeit numerically lower in the fluoroscopy-guided group, did not reach statistical significance. Two other randomized studies comparing CFA puncture with and without fluoroscopic guidance found similar results, with a potential benefit only in morbidly obese patients.[10,11]

A randomized study compared the use of ultrasound guidance to femoral pulse to guide CFA puncture in 112 patients referred for diagnostic angiography.[12] In this population at low risk of vascular complications, ultrasound guidance was helpful in cannulating the CFA successfully only in patients with weak pulsation or with a leg circumference ≥60 cm. No benefit in reducing vascular complications was found.

Seto et al.[13] reported the results of the large FAUST (Femoral Arterial Access with Ultrasound Trial), which randomized 1,004 patients to ultrasound or fluoroscopic guidance in several US centers. Vascular complications (hematoma >5 cm, pseudoaneurysm, RPB, arterial dissection or thrombosis, or major bleeding as defined by REPLACE-2 criteria) were significantly reduced with ultrasound guidance than with fluoroscopic guidance (1.4% vs 3.4%, $P = 0.04$). Of note, while the success rate for CFA cannulation under fluoroscopic guidance was 83.3%, the authors observed a significant learning curve with ultrasound guidance as the success rate improved from 82.4% with <6 ultrasound-guided procedures to 87.6% with ≥15 ultrasound-guided procedures. The same group did a similar study with radial access, but no clear benefit for ultrasound guidance was noted.[14]

On the basis of these studies, despite some benefit in using fluoroscopy or ultrasound guidance to cannulate the CFA in selected groups of patients has been noted, the incidence of bleeding and vascular complications remains close to 5%, a rate that appears much larger than after radial access.

Over the last two decades, several factors and independent predictors of vascular complications after diagnostic and interventional procedures using femoral approach have been identified. Some are nonmodifiable, such as gender, age, or chronic kidney failure, and some are modifiable, such as the sheath size and the anticoagulation regimen. Overall, the incidence of vascular complications with severe bleeding, especially in the last 5 years, has decreased mainly due to catheter downsizing and lower periprocedural levels of anticoagulation. However, the clinical impact of vascular closure devices (VCDs) remains highly controversial. Although they seem clearly associated with earlier ambulation, there is no compelling evidence for a significant reduction of vascular complications.

Studies in the early days of percutaneous balloon angioplasty and other devices reported femoral access-site complications between 2% and >15% in patients undergoing diagnostic or interventional procedures. A single-center study in the late nineties reported an incidence of vascular complications of 1.8% for diagnostic and 4% for interventional procedures.[15] More recently, data from another high-volume center reported an incidence of 0.9% for diagnostic procedures and 3.6% post-PCI.[16] A recent study from the Mayo Clinic on 300 patients with femoral angiography showed that in 13% the access site was located outside the optimal landing zone of CFA.[17] Overall, vascular complications occurred in 5.7%, with a significantly higher incidence when the puncture site was outside the optimal landing zone (18% vs 4%, $P < 0.001$).

The most common complication of percutaneous arterial puncture remains puncture site oozing, bruising, and hematoma.[18] Although hematomas per se have not been correlated with impaired long-term outcomes, they remain a significant nuisance associated with prolonged bed rest, significant morbidity, and costs, often prolonging hospitalization duration. As definitions have evolved, the true incidence of hematoma is difficult to evaluate throughout the different PCI periods.[19] In the nineties, definitions encompassed large hematoma with a significant hematocrit drop and requirement of surgical repair or transfusion. Using those definitions, rates of 2% to 5% were reported. More recently, hematoma have been defined as >5 to 10 cm, and their prevalence in large series or in randomized trials evaluating closure devices or antithrombotic agents has dropped.[20] Most important risk factors associated with hematoma formation are female gender, the type and duration of antithrombotic regimen, and the sheath size.

The prevalence of femoral artery pseudoaneurysm has ranged from 0.7% to 5.3%, with recent studies suggesting a contemporary incidence of <1%. It should be noted, however, that in a recent study including 400 consecutive patients using systematic duplex ultrasound, the incidence of pseudoaneurysm was found to be 3.7%.[21] Initially, such complications often required surgical intervention following the failure of echo-guided compression. In current practice, direct thrombin injection is the preferred technique, although this should be performed by expert operators as thrombin passage to the main circulation may have catastrophic consequences.[22]

Arteriovenous fistulae are rare complications (0.1%–0.4%) and have been associated with the inadvertent puncture of the femoral vein while searching for the femoral artery or during the placement of a venous sheath. In most instances, surgical repair is required. Femoral artery dissection leading to thrombosis and limb ischemia is a life-threatening event, which has been reported in 0.2% to 0.4% of cases. It requires immediate recognition and urgent surgical intervention. VCDs have also been associated with examples of femoral artery thrombosis or limb ischemia due to embolization of foreign material. Infection, although described without the use of VCDs (0.6%), has more recently been associated predominantly with different types of VCDs.

One of the most feared complications of femoral artery access remains RPB. Predictors of RPB include high puncture site, female gender, and low body surface area. The incidence of RPB has ranged from 0.2% to 6%. In one large series involving 3,508 patients undergoing PCI and reported in 2005, its incidence was 0.74%. This was concurred in a very recent series involving 11,129 patients post-PCI where the incidence remained at 0.7%.[23,24] Mortality rates ranging from 4% to 12% have been reported. Nearly all patients suffer significant blood loss and require blood transfusions (73.5%–100%).[25] Doyle et al. reviewed the incidence of major femoral bleeding at the Mayo Clinic in 17,901 patients divided into three groups: group 1 (1994–1995), group 2 (1996–1999), and group 3 (2000–2005). Overall, the incidence of major femoral bleeding (hematoma >4 cm or any femoral bleeding requiring transfusion, surgery, or prolonged stay or RPB) decreased from 8.4% in group 1 to 5.3% in group 2 and 3.5% in group 3.[26] Reductions in sheath size, intensity and duration of anticoagulation with heparin, and procedural time were identified as independent predictors of major femoral bleeding. A large observational study including 103,070 patients undergoing femoral PCI has also shown that larger-caliber sheaths (7F and 8F) were associated with more vascular access complications, bleeding and transfusions, as well as mortality and major cardiac adverse events than with 6F sheaths.[27] In addition to sheath size reduction, the use of the direct antithrombin bivalirudin has been associated with a significant reduction of access-site bleeding following femoral PCI.[20]

In conclusion, despite better techniques for CFA puncture, downsizing of equipments, and less-stringent anticoagulation protocols, bleeding and vascular complications after femoral approach remain a concern in everyday practice. Furthermore, it should be emphasized that in contrast to radial approach, a significant proportion of those vascular complications involving femoral artery access require either blood transfusions or surgical repair.

Radial Artery Access and Complications

The major anatomical advantage of the radial artery as compared to femoral artery resides in its relative superficiality, which makes it more easily palpable and facilitates compression to obtain hemostasis. The risks of access-site bleeding thus appear limited. In contrast to femoral or brachial arteries, there are no major nerves or veins in close proximity to the radial artery. Obviously, the radial artery is smaller ($\leq$3 mm) than the CFA, which is in the 6-mm range. The ulnar artery, which is sometimes used as an alternate to the radial artery, has a diameter similar to that of the radial artery, but it is deeper and the ulnar nerve lies in close proximity (see Chapter 6).

Several micropuncture kits have been developed for radial or ulnar artery puncture. Radial artery puncture can be performed in two ways. With the first technique, the operator can use a modified Seldinger technique with a single anterior wall puncture with 19G to 21G needle, and a short wire (0.018"-0.035") is introduced once back flow is visible. With the angiocath technique, once the operator observes back flow in the reservoir, he advances the needle through the posterior wall until back flow stops. The needle is then removed and the cannula is slowly pulled back until back flow is observed. At this stage, a small wire may safely be inserted as the cannula is positioned in the right lumen. There has been only one study comparing the two techniques.[28] Although faster access was obtained with through and through technique, no differences in vascular complication or RAO were noted. Therefore, the selection of either one technique remains a matter of operator preference. Of note, the use of micropuncture kits (21G needle) with femoral approach did not reduce the incidence of vascular complications.[29]

Sheath diameters from 4F to 8F have been used with radial access, although most diagnostic cases can be performed in 4F to 5F and most PCI are currently performed in 5F and 6F. In contrast to femoral approach, wherein 5F to 6F PCI have been associated with less bleeding and vascular complications, larger devices have not been associated with more vascular complications with radial approach, except for spasm and RAO (see Chapter 10).[30,31] More recently, sheathless techniques with home-made standard catheters or specially designed hydrophilic large lumen guiding catheters (Eucath, ASAHI, Japan) have been described with radial or ulnar access.[32] The true clinical benefit of this approach remains to be clarified. Clinically, sheathless techniques are associated with frequent oozing and no clear reduction in RAO, especially with home-made sheathless techniques. Hydrophilic-coated sheaths have become popular with transradial techniques as they reduce the force required to remove them and prevent the occurrence of spasm, improving patient comfort (see Chapter 9). Although spasm and vasomotor dysfunction are discussed elsewhere, it is important to mention that in case of severe spasm, there have been reports of segments of radial artery avulsion (Fig. 12-1). Although impressive, those extremely rare complications have not led to clinical sequelae.[33] A more recent case related, in fact, to the advancement of long sheath in small recurrent artery instead of main vessel.[34] This must remind that "brachial" spasm does not exist, and pain at the arm level must make the operator suspect that the wire, long sheath, or catheter entered a recurrent and smaller branch at the elbow level (see Chapters 4 and 7).

Like any other vessel, puncture, sheath insertion, and catheter manipulation of the radial (or ulnar) artery may still lead to injury, bleeding, and vascular complications.[35,36] However, a small diameter, combined with its superficial location, makes the incidence of vascular complications after transradial catheterization quite limited compared with the femoral artery approach, and more importantly clinical consequences remain relatively benign. Nevertheless, it should be emphasized that the radial is not a small femoral artery and that although a number of vascular complications are common between the radial and the femoral approaches, some complications are specific to the transradial approach (Table 12-1). In Table 12-2, we compare reported incidence of most vascular complications associated with femoral or transradial catheterization as reported in the literature.

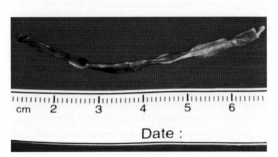

FIGURE 12-1 Radial artery avulsion with 8F guiding catheter. (Courtesy of G. Barbeau.)

TABLE 12-1 Complete List of Published Vascular Complications with Radial/Ulnar Access

- Accelerated atherosclerosis
- Arteriovenous fistula
- Cardiovocal syndrome
- Compartment syndrome
- Distal finger ischemia/necrosis
- Pseudoaneurysm
- Radial/ulnar occlusion
- Reflex sympathetic dystrophy
- Retrograde perforation/dissection
- Retropleural hematoma
- Severe spasm
- Wrist, forehand, arm, pectoral hematoma

A recent meta-analysis of randomized studies reported an incidence of major vascular complications of 1.4% (49/3507 cases) with transradial approach (TRA) compared to 3.7% (131/3514 cases) with the femoral approach, a relative reduction of 63% (OR 0.37, 95% CI 0.27–0.52, $P < 0.0001$).[37] Initial and more recent data have generally reported a frequency of radial access-site failure of less than 5%.[38] Reasons associated with access-site failure include puncture failure, spasm and radial, brachio-cephalic trunk abnormalities, or excessive loops, and can be additionally related to lack of experience, small artery size, or transient or permanent reduction in vessel diameter. In a large series of all-comers undergoing transradial PCI in an experienced radial center, Abdelaal et al. reported a primary failure rate of 2.7% and a crossover rate to femoral approach

of 1.8%. Independent predictors of radial failure included female sex, prior coronary artery bypass grafting (CABG), and cardiogenic shock.[39] Importantly, patients who had radial access failure had more ischemic, bleeding, and vascular complications.

Access-site failure may also result from anatomical variations, severe tortuosities, or loops in radial or brachial arteries. The incidence of these variations in vessel anatomy is close to 5%.[40,41] Most of the time, operators manage to negotiate them using hydrophilic wires, 0.014-inch angioplasty wires, or hydrophilic catheters (see Chapter 7). It is advised to perform an angiography of the arm in case of difficulty of wire or catheter advancement, as failure to identify the problem may lead to vessel perforation or dissection. Radial or brachial artery dissections can produce marked angiographic images, but it should be emphasized that they represent retrograde dissections. Therefore, it is worth attempting to carefully recross them with a soft 0.014-inch angioplasty wire. If this attempt is successful, the catheter will usually seal the dissection or perforation, and there will be no clinical consequence for the patient. In some cases, operators have proceeded with placement of long sheath, long balloon inflation, or even covered stent implantation for refractory bleeding. Failure to recognize these perforations might be dramatic as slow and delayed intramuscular bleeding may potentially lead to compartment syndrome.

The incidence of compartment syndrome after intramuscular bleeding or vascular damage is extremely low but should be promptly recognized, as it may lead to devastating consequences (Fig. 12-2). One series reported acute compartment syndrome in five cases out of 250 patients treated (2%), while a

TABLE 12-2 Comparison of Femoral and Radial Complications

	Femoral (%)		Radial (%)
Type	*Before year 2000*	*After year 2000*	
Hematoma (>5–10 cm)	5–10	<5	1
RPB	<2	0.2–1.5	–
Pseudoaneurysm	Up to 2	Up to 1.5	<0.1
Arteriovenous fistula	<0.5	<1.5	<0.1
Thrombosis/embolism with limb ischemia	<0.5	<0.1	<0.001
Infection	<1	<5	<0.1
Dissection/perforation	–	<0.5	<1
Surgical repair	Up to 20	<5	<0.01

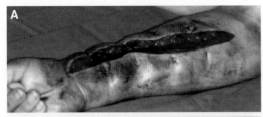

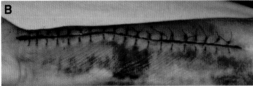

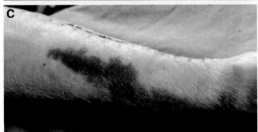

FIGURE 12-2 Compartment syndrome. **A:** Long surgical cut to relieve the pressure. **B:** The wound is closed during a second surgery. **C:** With prompt diagnosis and treatment, the outlook is excellent for recovery of the muscles and nerves inside the compartment. (Courtesy of G. Barbeau.)

more recent study reported two cases in 51,296 procedures (<0.01%).[42] Open surgical fasciotomy can be avoided if effective preventative measures are employed as soon as local bleeding is suspected. These include (1) stopping intravenous anticoagulant therapy, (2) controlling the pain and blood pressure, and (3) using transient external compression with a blood pressure cuff.[43]

Several large meta-analyses have found a relative reduction >75% of bleeding with TRA compared with the femoral approach.[44–46] The benefit for TRA remains even if closure devices are used with femoral access.[47,48] Access-site bleeding represents 60%–80% of bleeding episodes with the femoral approach, and the major benefit of TRA is the marked reduction of major bleeding related to access site (see Chapter 2). It should also be recognized that some blood loss has long been associated with femoral PCI. In the eighties, patients after percutaneous transluminal coronary angioplasty and heparin anticoagulation suffered hemoglobin (Hb) drops of 1–2 g/dL within 24 hours, with 6% of patients presenting with a fall in Hb of >3 g/dL.[49,50] In contrast, in a recent study with transradial PCI and maximal

antiplatelet therapy, the mean Hb fall was 0.6 ± 1.0 g/dL, with only 1.3% of patients presenting Hb drop > 3 g/dL within 24 hours.[51]

Most initial studies comparing bleeding with radial and femoral approaches did not use standardized bleeding classifications. Investigators in the EASY trial developed a hematoma classification adapted to TRA and this can be compared to recent hematoma scale proposed with femoral approach[52,53] (Fig. 12-3). In this trial performed with maximal antiplatelet therapy, the incidence of hematoma <5 cm (grade I) was 5.3%, <10 cm (grade II) was 2.5%, distal to the elbow (grade III) was 1.6%, and proximal to elbow (grade IV) was 0.1%. Grade V is reserved for hematoma inducing compartment syndrome. It should be noted that while grade I and II hematomas are directly related to the puncture site, higher grades usually result from wire damages to vessels and small perforations. These may induce very unusual and rare hematomas such as hematoma of the pectoral muscle, of the neck, or even of the mediastinum.[54] Ilhan et al.[55] recently reported a first case of retropleural right hematoma which required transfusion and drainage with right radial diagnostic angiography complicated by difficult advancement of wire at the subclavian artery level. Following difficulty with wire advancement at the left subclavian artery, Parikh et al. described a patient who developed a large neck hematoma following post-PCI.[56] A CT scan revealed diffuse hematoma infiltration with displacement of the trachea. Conservative management was performed without any sequelae. Following similar difficulty at the brachio-cephalic level, Arsanjani et al.[57] reported bleeding following damage to a pericardio-phrenic artery, which required coil embolization to seal the perforation. Romagnoli et al.[58] reported a transient cardiovocal syndrome in a patient where they had also faced difficulties with crossing the right subclavian artery but no clear hematoma was found with CT scan.

Complications resulting from vessel trauma such as pseudoaneurysm or arteriovenous fistula are rare (<0.1%), presumably due to the small caliber of these vessels. Pseudoaneurysms are easily diagnosed as they present with or without pain as a pulsating swelling. Most of the time there are signs of inflammation, which may let fear bacterial infection, but this is exceedingly rare.[59,60] They are usually managed by repeat and prolonged compression after ultrasound confirmation, and extremely rarely require surgical interventions (ligation or patch).[61] Several reports of successful thrombin injection have also been published[62,63] (Fig. 12-4). Risks factors for

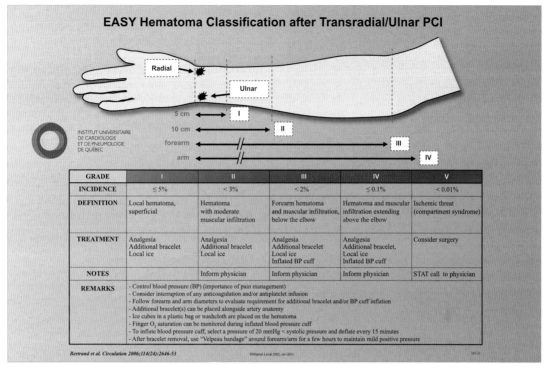

FIGURE 12-3   EASY hematoma classification after transradial/ulnar intervention. (From Bertrand OF. Acute forearm muscle swelling post transradial catheterization and compartment syndrome: prevention is better than treatment! *Catheter Cardiovasc Interv*. 2010; 75(3):366–368.)

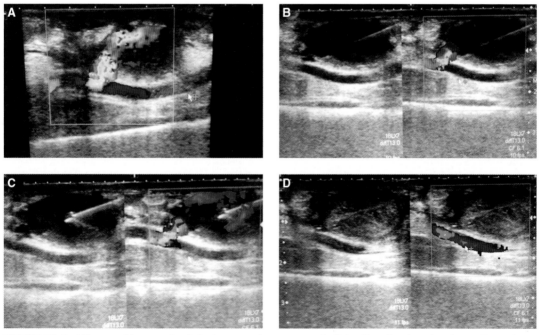

FIGURE 12-4   Ultrasound image of radial artery pseudoaneurysm. **A:** Color Doppler view showing pattern of turbulent blood flow between radial artery and pseudoaneurysm. **B:** Needle is positioned inside pseudoaneurysm. **C:** During thrombin injection. **D:** After thrombin injection, observe occlusion of pseudoaneurysm and closure of connection between radial artery and pseudoaneurysm.

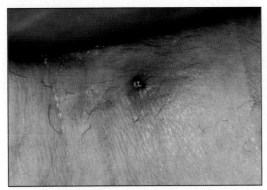

FIGURE 12-5 Adverse local reaction to the use of hydrophilic sheaths (Cook) after radial artery cannulation.

pseudoaneurysm include female gender, hypertension, and chronic anticoagulation.

Arteriovenous fistula posttransradial catheterization can also present with pain but often is found by chance when the patient presents for repeat catheterization sometimes many months after the index procedure. There are three ways of managing those rare complications: first, abstention if the patient is asymptomatic; second, surgical management if the patient is asymptomatic and there are multiple channels; and third, percutaneous sealing using covered stent.[64-66]

In the large RIVAL trial involving >7,000 patients, the incidence of pseudoaneurysm requiring closure and arteriovenous fistula was 0.2% and 0% in the radial group compared to 0.6% and 0.1% in the femoral group, respectively.[37]

The use of certain types of hydrophilic-coated sheaths (Cook Medical Inc., Bloomington, IN) has been associated with severe granulomatous reactions of the skin, which were attributed to foreign-body reaction but could resemble cutaneous infection (Fig. 12-5).[67] No similar reaction has been reported with other brands of hydrophilic sheaths or catheters. Lastly, with and without associated RAO, some authors have described regional pain syndrome following uncomplicated transradial catheterization.[68-70]

Although there is no evidence of more coronary dissections with radial approach compared to femoral approach,[37] cases of sinus of valsalva and aortic valve perforations have been reported with guide-catheter manipulation by radial approach.[71,72]

Conclusion

In conclusion, vascular complications after TRA for diagnostic angiography or interventions are rare and almost always can be managed conservatively.

The reduction of these complications when compared to those resulting from the femoral approach is also associated with a marked reduction in health-care costs. It should be emphasized that experience accumulated over the last 15 years with TRA has demonstrated that rapid recognition of these complications is vital in order to prevent severe complications, that is, hand ischemia or surgical repair.

REFERENCES

1. Sones FM Jr, Shirey EK. Cine coronary arteriography. *Mod Concepts Cardiovasc Dis.* 1962;31:735–738.
2. Judkins MP. Selective coronary arteriography, I: a percutaneous transfemoral technic. *Radiology.* 1967;89(5):815–824.
3. Radner S. Thoracal aortography by catheterization from the radial artery: preliminary report of a new technique. *Acta Radiol.* 1948;29(2):178–180.
4. Bertrand ME, Ketelers JY, Carré A, et al. A new approach in the hemodynamic exploration of the left cardiac cavities via the radial artery below the elbow. *Coeur Med Interne.* 1974;13(2):345–346.
5. Serruys PW, de Jaegere P, Kiemeneij F, et al. A comparison of balloon-expandable-stent implantation with balloon angioplasty in patients with coronary artery disease. Benestent Study Group. *N Engl J Med.* 1994;331(8):489–495.
6. Kiemeneij F, Laarman GJ, Odekerken D, et al. A randomized comparison of percutaneous transluminal coronary angioplasty by the radial, brachial and femoral approaches: the access study. *J Am Coll Cardiol.* 1997;29(6):1269–1275.
7. Dotter CT, Rosch J, Robinson M. Fluoroscopic guidance in femoral artery puncture. *Radiology.* 1978;127(1):266–267.
8. Fitts J, Ver Lee P, Hofmaster P, et al. Fluoroscopy-guided femoral artery puncture reduces the risk of PCI-related vascular complications. *J Interv Cardiol.* 2008;21(3):273–278.
9. Abu-Fadel MS, Sparling JM, Zacharias SJ, et al. Fluoroscopy vs. traditional guided femoral arterial access and the use of closure devices: a randomized controlled trial. *Catheter Cardiovasc Interv.* 2009;74(4):533–539.
10. Huggins CE, Gillespie MJ, Tan WA, et al. A prospective randomized clinical trial of the use of fluoroscopy in obtaining femoral arterial access. *J Invasive Cardiol.* 2009;21(3):105–109.
11. Jacobi JA, Schussler JM, Johnson KB. Routine femoral head fluoroscopy to reduce complications in coronary catheterization. *Proc (Bayl Univ Med Cent.)* 2009;22(1):7–8.
12. Dudeck O, Teichgraeber U, Podrabsky P, et al. A randomized trial assessing the value of ultrasound-guided puncture of the femoral artery for interventional investigations. *Int J Cardiovasc Imaging.* 2004;20(5):363–368.
13. Seto AH, Abu-Fadel MS, Sparling JM, et al. Real-time ultrasound guidance facilitates femoral arterial access and reduces vascular complications: FAUST (Femoral Arterial Access with Ultrasound Trial). *JACC Cardiovasc Interv.* 2010;3(7):751–758.
14. Seto A, Roberts JS, Lasic, Z. The radial artery access with ultrasound trial (RAUST). Late-breaking Clinical Trial presentation conducted at the Aim-RADIAL 2013 Meeting, New York, NY, 2013. Retrieved from http://www.slideshare.net/theradialist/seto-a-aimradial-2013-raust-final-minimal-animation.
15. Chandrasekar B, Doucet S, Bilodeau L, et al. Complications of cardiac catheterization in the current era: a single-center experience. *Catheter Cardiovasc Interv.* 2001;52(3):289–295.

16. Sherev DA, Shaw RE, Brent BN. Angiographic predictors of femoral access site complications: implication for planned percutaneous coronary intervention. *Catheter Cardiovasc Interv.* 2005;65(2):196–202.

17. Pitta SR, Prasad A, Kumar G, et al. Location of femoral artery access and correlation with vascular complications. *Catheter Cardiovasc Interv.* 2011;78(2):294–299.

18. Cosman TL, Arthur HM, Natarajan MK. Prevalence of bruising at the vascular access site one week after elective cardiac catheterisation or percutaneous coronary intervention. *J Clin Nurs.* 2011;20(9–10):1349–1356.

19. Nikolsky E, Mehran R, Halkin A, et al. Vascular complications associated with arteriotomy closure devices in patients undergoing percutaneous coronary procedures: a meta-analysis. *J Am Coll Cardiol.* 2004;44(6):1200–1209.

20. Hamon M, Rasmussen LH, Manoukian SV, et al. Choice of arterial access site and outcomes in patients with acute coronary syndromes managed with an early invasive strategy: the ACUITY trial. *EuroIntervention.* 2009;5(1):115–120.

21. Kacila M, Vranic H, Hadzimehmedagic A, et al. The frequency of complications of pseudo aneurysms after cardiac interventional diagnostic and therapeutic interventions. *Med Arh.* 2011;65(2):78–81.

22. Gabrielli R, Rosati MS, Vitale S, et al. Fatal complication after thrombin injection for post-catheterization femoral pseudoaneurysm. *Thorac Cardiovasc Surg.* 2011;59(6):372–375.

23. Farouque HM, Tremmel JA, Raissi Shabari F, et al. Risk factors for the development of retroperitoneal hematoma after percutaneous coronary intervention in the era of glycoprotein IIb/IIIa inhibitors and vascular closure devices. *J Am Coll Cardiol.* 2005;45(3):363–368.

24. Maluenda G, Delhaye C, Gonzalez, MA, et al. Conservative versus invasive management strategy for retroperitoneal hemorrhage after percutaneous coronary intervention. *J Am Coll Cardiol.* 2010;55(10A):A215:E2039 (abstract).

25. Chan YC, Morales JP, Reidy JF, et al. Management of spontaneous and iatrogenic retroperitoneal haemorrhage: conservative management, endovascular intervention or open surgery? *Int J Clin Pract.* 2008;62(10):1604–1613.

26. Doyle BJ, Ting HH, Bell MR, et al. Major femoral bleeding complications after percutaneous coronary intervention: incidence, predictors, and impact on long-term survival among 17,901 patients treated at the Mayo Clinic from 1994 to 2005. *JACC Cardiovasc Interv.* 2008;1(2):202–209.

27. Grossman PM, Gurm HS, McNamara R, et al. Percutaneous coronary intervention complications and guide catheter size: bigger is not better. *JACC Cardiovasc Interv.* 2009;2:636–44.

28. Pancholy SB, Sanghvi KA, Patel TM. Radial artery access technique evaluation trial: randomized comparison of Seldinger versus modified Seldinger technique for arterial access for transradial catheterization. *Catheter Cardiovasc Interv.* 2012;80:288–91.

29. Ben-Dor I, Maluenda G, Mahmoudi M, et al. A novel, minimally invasive access technique versus standard 18-gauge needle set for femoral access. *Catheter Cardiovasc Interv.* 2012;79:1180–1185.

30. Metz D, Meyer P, Touati C, et al. Comparison of 6F with 7F and 8F guiding catheters for elective coronary angioplasty: results of a prospective, multicenter, randomized trial. *Am Heart J.* 1997;134:131–137.

31. Buchler JR, Ribeiro EE, Falcão JL, et al. A randomized trial of 5 versus 7 French guiding catheters for transfemoral percutaneous coronary stent implantation. *J Interv Cardiol.* 2008;21:50–55.

32. Mamas M, D'Souza S, Hendry C, et al. Use of the sheathless guide catheter during routine transradial percutaneous

coronary intervention: a feasibility study. *Catheter Cardiovasc Interv.* 2010;75:596–602.

33. Dieter RS, Akef A, Wolf M. Eversion endarterectomy complicating radial artery access for left heart catheterization. *Catheter Cardiovasc Interv.* 2003;58:478–480.

34. Alkhouli M, Cohen HA, Bashir R. Radial artery avulsion—a rare complication of transradial catheterization. *Catheter Cardiovasc Interv.* 2014. DOI: 10.1002/ccd.25528.

35. Caputo RP, Tremmel JA, Rao S, et al. Transradial arterial access for coronary and peripheral procedures: executive summary by the transradial committee of the SCAI. *Catheter Cardiovasc Interv.* 2011;78(6):823–839.

36. Kanei Y, Kwan T, Nakara NC, et al. Transradial cardiac catheterization: a review of access site complications. *Catheter Cardiovasc Interv.* 2011;78(6):840–846.

37. Jolly SS, Yusuf S, Cairns J, et al. Radial versus femoral access for coronary angiography and intervention in patients with acute coronary syndromes (RIVAL): a randomised, parallel group, multicentre trial. *Lancet.* 2011;377(9775):1409–1420.

38. Guedes A, Dangoisse V, Gabriel L, et al. Low rate of conversion to transfemoral approach when attempting both radial arteries for coronary angiography and percutaneous coronary intervention: a study of 1,826 consecutive procedures. *J Invasive Cardiol.* 2010;22(9):391–397.

39. Abdelaal E, Brousseau-Provencher C, Montminy S, et al. Risk score, causes, and clinical impact of failure of transradial approach for percutaneous coronary interventions. *JACC Cardiovasc Interv.* 2013;6(11):1129–1137.

40. Marque N, Jegou A, Varenne O, et al. Impact of an extension tube on operator radiation exposure during coronary procedures performed through the radial approach. *Arch Cardiovasc Dis.* 2009;102(11):749–754.

41. Burzotta F, Trani C, Devita M, et al. A new operative classification of both anatomic vascular variants and physiopathologic conditions affecting transradial cardiovascular procedures. *Int J Cardiol.* 2010;145(1):120–122.

42. Tizon-Marcos H, Barbeau GR. Incidence of compartment syndrome of the arm in a large series of transradial approach for coronary procedures. *J Interv Cardiol.* 2008;21(5):380–384.

43. Bertrand OF. Acute forearm muscle swelling post transradial catheterization and compartment syndrome: prevention is better than treatment!" *Catheter Cardiovasc Interv.* 2010;75(3):366–368.

44. Agostoni P, Biondi-Zoccai GG, de Benedictis ML, et al. Radial versus femoral approach for percutaneous coronary diagnostic and interventional procedures: systematic overview and meta-analysis of randomized trials. *J Am Coll Cardiol.* 2004;44(2):349–356.

45. Jolly SS, Amlani S, Hamon M, et al. Radial versus femoral access for coronary angiography or intervention and the impact on major bleeding and ischemic events: a systematic review and meta-analysis of randomized trials. *Am Heart J.* 2009;157(1):132–140.

46. Bertrand OF, Belisle P, Joyal D, et al. Comparison of transradial and femoral approaches for percutaneous coronary interventions: a systematic review and hierarchical Bayesian meta-analysis. *Am Heart J.* 2012;163(4):632–648.

47. Morice MC, Dumas P, Lefèvre T, et al. Systematic use of transradial approach or suture of the femoral artery after angioplasty: attempt at achieving zero access site complications. *Catheter Cardiovasc Interv.* 2000;51(4):417–421.

48. Sciahbasi A, Fischetti D, Picciolo A, et al. Transradial access compared with femoral puncture closure devices in percutaneous coronary procedures. *Int J Cardiol.* 2009;137(3):199–205.

49. Ellis SG, Roubin GS, Wilentz J, et al. Effect of 18- to 24-hour heparin administration for prevention of restenosis

after uncomplicated coronary angioplasty. *Am Heart J.* 1989;117(4):777–782.

50. Jauch W, Kurnik PB, Hanlon SJ, et al. Expected hemoglobin decrease following percutaneous transluminal coronary angioplasty. *Am J Cardiol.* 1997;80(1):71–74.

51. Bertrand OF, Larose E, Rodés-Cabau J, et al. Incidence, range, and clinical effect of hemoglobin changes within 24 hours after transradial coronary stenting. *Am J Cardiol.* 2010;106(2):155–161.

52. Bertrand OF, Larose E, Rodés-Cabau J, et al. Incidence, predictors, and clinical impact of bleeding after transradial coronary stenting and maximal antiplatelet therapy. *Am Heart J.* 2009;157(1):164–169.

53. Bertrand OF, Rao SV, Pancholy S, et al. Transradial approach for coronary angiography and interventions: results of the first international transradial practice survey. *JACC Cardiovasc Interv.* 2010;3(10):1022–1031.

54. Park KW, Chung JW, Chang SA, et al. Two cases of mediastinal hematoma after cardiac catheterization: a rare but real complication of the transradial approach. *Int J Cardiol.* 2008;130(3):e89–e92.

55. Ilhan E, Ozgen A, Gürsürer M. Retroperitoneal hematoma counterpart of transradial coronary angiography; retropleural hematoma. *Int J Cardiol.* 2013;169:e43–e44.

56. Parikh P, Staniloae C, Coppola J. Pain in the neck: a rare complication of transradial cardiac catheterization. *J Invas Cardiol.* 2013;25(4):198–200.

57. Arsanjani R, Echeverri J, Movahed MR. Successful coil embolization of pericardiacophrenic artery perforation occurring during transradial cardiac catheterization via right radial artery. *J Invas Cardiol.* 2012;24(12):671–674.

58. Romagnoli E, Nasso G, Angelino G, et al. Cardiovocal syndrome after transradial cardiac catheterization: an unusual complication. *Int J Cardiol.* 2008;124(3):e39–e41.

59. Burzotta F, Trani C, Mazzari MA, et al. Vascular complications and access crossover in 10,676 transradial percutaneous coronary procedures. *Am Heart J.* 2012;163(2):230–238.

60. Collins N, Wainstein R, Ward M, et al. Pseudoaneurysm after transradial cardiac catheterization: case series and review of the literature. *Catheter Cardiovasc Interv.* 2012;80(2):283–287.

61. Hyde TA, Ramcharitar S, Singh-Ranger R. A right radial artery false aneurysm. *Eurointervention.* 2010;5(8):995.

62. D'Achille A, Sebben RA, Davies RP. Percutaneous ultrasound-guided thrombin injection for coagulation of post-traumatic pseudoaneurysms. *Aus Radiol.* 2001;45(2):218–221.

63. Komorowska-Timek E, Teruya TH, Abou-Zamzam AM Jr, et al. Treatment of radial and ulnar artery pseudoaneurysms using percutaneous thrombin injection. *J Hand Surg.* 2004;29(5):936–942.

64. Na KJ, Kim MA, Moon HJ, et al. Radial arteriovenous fistula developed late after coronary angiography: a case report. *Korean J Thorac Cardiovasc Surg.* 2012;45(6):421–423.

65. Summaria F, Romagnoli E, Preziosi P. Percutaneous antegrade transarterial treatment of iatrogenic radial arteriovenous fistula. *J Cardiovasc Med.* 2012;13(1):50–52.

66. Dehghani P, Culig J, Patel D, et al. Arteriovenous fistula as a complication of transradial coronary angiography: a case report. *J Medical Case Rep.* 2013;7(1):21.

67. Zellner C, Ports TA, Yeghiazarians Y, et al. Sterile radial artery granuloma after transradial procedures: a unique and avoidable complication. *Catheter Cardiovasc Interv.* 2010;76(5):673–676.

68. Papadimos TJ, Hofmann JP. Radial artery thrombosis, palmar arch systolic blood velocities, and chronic regional pain syndrome 1 following transradial cardiac catheterization. *Catheter Cardiovasc Interv.* 2002;57(4):537–540.

69. Sasano N, Tsuda T, Sasano H, et al. A case of complex regional pain syndrome type II after transradial coronary intervention. *J Anesth.* 2004;18(4):310–312.

70. Silviu B, Mark WJ, Reuben I, et al. Complex regional pain syndrome type I following radial artery cardiac catheterization. *Int J Cardiol.* 2005;101(1):167–168.

71. Ong G, Bagur R, Barbeau G, et al. Severe aortic regurgitation after transradial percutaneous coronary intervention. *Circ Cardiovasc Interv.* 2011;4(2):e8–e11.

72. Tomassini F, Gagnor A, Varbella F. Perforation of the sinus of Valsalva by guiding catheter during the percutaneous coronary intervention via the right transradial approach: a very unusual complication." *Catheter Cardiovasc Interv.* 2011;78(6):888–891.

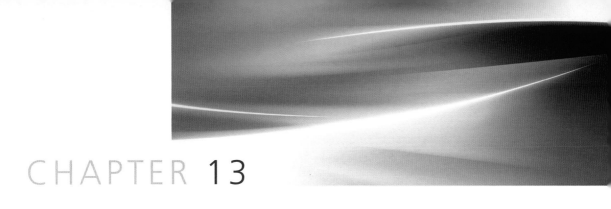

CHAPTER 13

Right Heart Catheterization Using the Arm: Total Wrist Approach for Diagnosis and Intervention

Ian C. Gilchrist

Introduction

Utilization of right heart catheterization during cardiac catheterization has declined over the last several decades from almost 100% at some institutions to less than 2% nationwide in the United States.[1] Less invasive techniques such as echocardiography have evolved to reliably define right heart anatomy and derive hemodynamics. In addition, the use of pulmonary artery catheters in critical care units has been demonized by some factions involved in intensive care medicine as clinical trials have failed to show improved outcomes when these devices are used.[2] Despite the reduced reliance on invasive monitoring and diagnosis, right heart catheterization and central venous access still plays a role in present-day medicine.

The appropriate use criteria for diagnostic catheterization[3] list a broad range of clinical scenarios where invasive right heart catheterization appeared appropriate (Table 13-1). Beyond diagnostic catheterization, needs for central venous access extend from temporary pacemakers to vena cava filters. Integrating access to the central venous system within the practice of transradial catheterization furthers the potential of the transradial approach.

History

Central venous access from the forearm is not a new concept. In 1905, Drs. Bleichroder, Unger, and Loeb reportedly passed catheters up the basilic vein of Dr. Bleichroder into the central system,[4] but they failed to document the accomplishment at the time. The first well-documented venous route to the heart was demonstrated by Forssmann[5] in 1929, with self-passage of a uretic catheter up his arm into the heart. Bilateral cardiac catheterization from the arm with arterial access from the ulnar artery was reported by Zimmerman et al.[6] in 1950 when describing the ulnar artery as a route for cardiac catheterization (Fig. 13-1). The subsequent evolution of arterial techniques, and a better understanding of the anatomy of large neck veins and how to access them, resulted in a migration away from forearm vascular access to alternative routes. By the 1990s, techniques developed decades earlier to access the forearm veins to reach the central venous system had been all but forgotten.

Initially, this shift was a logical progression as earlier access techniques often involved surgical cut-downs and the vein was tied off at the end of the procedure. This rendered the vein useless for future use. Subsequently developed percutaneous Seldinger techniques in the larger central veins of the neck and femoral regions allowed removal of access without a loss of long-term venous function and represented advancement in technique. There was a price to pay for this advance. The entry site locations for central vein access provided little room for geographic error, and complications such as pneumothorax and retroperitoneal hematoma occurred even in expert hands. While life-threatening complications from central venous access are less frequent than

TABLE 13-1 Appropriate Use Criteria for Right Heart Catheterization as Defined in 2012[a]

Indication	Appropriate Use Score[b]
Define better a known or suspected shunt	A
Diagnosis of Pulmonary HTN	
When ECHO is equivocal or borderline	A
Confirm elevated RV pressure by ECHO	A
Determine response to vasodilators	
Acutely administered in cath lab	A
Follow-up after oral therapy	A
Post–heart transplant ± biopsy	A
Clarify indeterminate volume status	A
Clarify degree of valve disease if conflicting data exist	A
Pericardial evaluation	
Suspected pericardial tamponade	A
Clarify constrictive vs restrictive physiology	A
Cardiomyopathy	
Initial evaluation of cardiomyopathy	A
Reevaluation of known cardiomyopathy	A
Define change in clinical status	A
Evaluate or guide therapy	A

[a]See ref. 3.
[b]Score of "A" indicates an appropriate test for specific indication.
HTN, hypertension; RV, right ventricular; ECHO, echocardiogram.

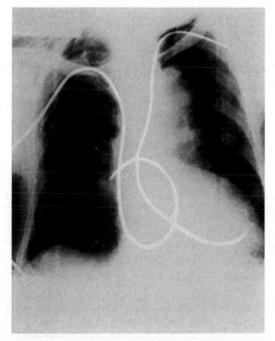

FIGURE 13-1 Early X-ray of bilateral cardiac catheterization using left ulnar arterial access and forearm central venous access from the right arm. (From Zimmerman HA, Scott RW, Becker NO. Catheterization of the left side of the heart in man. *Circulation.* 1950;1:357–359.)

those seen in arterial access, they still exist and represent a modifiable risk. Using the forearm veins for central venous access can essentially eliminate these risks.

Modern Era

During the 1990s, transradial arterial access techniques expanded as catheterization equipment improved with both a reduction in size and an improvement in performance. Lost in this enthusiasm for transradial cardiac catheterization was the stagnation in central venous techniques. Patients could undergo eloquent transradial procedures only to have their femoral vein also punctured so a right heart catheterization could be accomplished. The presumed inability to provide a central venous access to match the newer arterial technique was often used by doubters of the transradial approach to stick to their historic methods. Even among transradial converts, the need for right heart catheterization was used as an indication to revert to legacy techniques in the femoral artery and vein along with its concomitant risks and comorbidities.

Central access from forearm veins was redeveloped in the mid-1970s with the evolution of flexible polymer catheters that avoided many of the sequelae of long-term venous access.[7] These peripherally inserted central catheters (PICC or PIC lines) became, and continue to be, popular in oncology, nutritional support, and other specialties, but the potential for use by the cardiology community was not generally recognized. As a medical resident in 1984, I passed an 8F-balloon-tipped, thermodilution catheter up the forearm of a young, highly anticoagulated patient with a prosthetic valve dehiscence in the middle of the night to help manage the hemodynamics prior to an emergency surgery planned for the following morning. The catheter passed without problems and entered the pulmonary artery and wedge position without X-ray support. My supervising cardiology fellow was less sanguine about this procedure and demanded the removal of the catheter before the attending's arrival in the morning. According to her, it just did not seem right.

Extending the pilot experience as a resident almost 20 years before, Gilchrist et al.,[8] in 2002, published a report reintroducing the utility of forearm venous access in the setting of radial artery access. This early work attempted to use veins that were very distal in the arm using special-order 125-cm-length 6F catheters provided by Arrow, Inc. (Teleflex USA, Reading, PA). Access was obtained at the time of catheterization by the physician with a tourniquet. This technique was limited by an inability to find veins at

times on the distal forearm and occasional failure at blind cannulation of the deep veins that tend to course close to the radial artery. Otherwise, once venous access was obtained, the placement of vascular sheaths and 6F diagnostic balloon-tipped catheters was relatively unremarkable.

Subsequently, a slightly different approach was adapted with the access obtained anywhere along the forearm. In addition, initial intravenous puncture was done outside of the catheterization laboratory by the precatheterization technical staff who would establish a heparin-well venous access. This access site was then exchanged for a vascular sheath in the catheterization laboratory large enough to accept the right heart catheter or other indicated transvenous device. This markedly improved the efficiency of the procedure and demonstrated almost universal success.[9]

Table 13-2 lists the comparison of the procedural times and arterial times and X-ray exposure between bilateral heart catheterizations done via the forearm/transradial versus the traditional transfemoral route.[9] While observational and single site, the data support that the shift to a forearm approach can be associated with procedural efficiency similar to that of the traditional techniques. A similar result was seen in a study done at a high-volume British center.[10] While the outcomes were analogous to those listed in Table 13-2, the procedure times were slightly longer in the transradial groups (radial: 48 $\pm$ 15 minutes, vs femoral: 32 $\pm$ 9 minutes, $P < 0.05$).

TABLE 13-2 Characteristics of Patients, Procedural Times, and Complications in Those Undergoing Either Femoral or Radial Right and Left Heart Catheterization

	Access Site		
	Femoral (n = 175)	Radial (n = 105)	P
Age $\pm$ 95% CI	64 $\pm$ 1.8 y	62 $\pm$ 2.8 y	NS
All Procedures			
Procedural time $\pm$ 95% CI	75 $\pm$ 5.4 min	70 $\pm$ 5.0 min	$P < 0.01$
Arterial time[a] $\pm$ 95% CI	45 $\pm$ 6.4 min	35 $\pm$ 4.2 min	$P < 0.01$
Diagnostic Procedures Only	n = 143	n = 98	
Procedural time $\pm$ 95% CI	70 $\pm$ 4.1 min	70 $\pm$ 5.0 min	NS
Arterial time[a] $\pm$ 95% CI	40 $\pm$ 5.1 min	35 $\pm$ 4.2 min	$P < 0.04$
Complications	12	0	
AV fistula	2	0	
Pseudoaneurysm	4	0	
Hematoma	6	0	

[a]Arterial time starts with arterial puncture and ends at the conclusion of the procedure in the cardiac catheterization laboratory. The femoral arterial sheath is removed later in a recovery area. Radial sheaths are removed at the end of arterial time while the patient is in the laboratory.
From Gilchrist IC, Moyer CD, Gascho JA. Transradial right and left heart catheterization: a comparison to traditional femoral approach. *Cathet Cardiovasc Interv.* 2006;67:585–588.

This difference in results can probably be accounted for by differences in practices. Lo et al. obtained venous access in the catheterization laboratory versus the practice of using precatheterization venous access sites as done by Gilchrist et al. Since this publication, the institution is now utilizing prelaboratory venous access (J. Nolan, personal communication, September 2012). Several groups have now reported analogous reports of transvenous forearm access, confirming the successful application of this approach to central venous access.[11,12]

Practical Aspects of Venous Catheterization

Vein Physiology

Veins are distinctly different from arteries due to their different physiologic roles. The vessels of the arterial system are muscular and capable of controlling the high-pressure arterial system and redirect blood flow away from the heart to the end organs. The venous system is a low-pressure collecting system that delivers blood back to the heart. It serves a capacitance role. Veins are eight times more distensible than similar-sized arteries. Arterial vessels are composed of significantly more smooth muscle constitutions, resulting in far less compliance and distensibility than are seen in veins. In addition, the veins tend to respond to mechanical contact by catheter surfaces with far less tendency toward spasm than is commonly seen in the arterial system.

Vasoreactivity

While a growing body of literature concerning arterial vasoreactivity and prescriptions for cocktails to prevent arterial spasm exists, publications concerning the venous system are almost nonexistent. The venous system has less of a tendency for vasospasm, although there are older case reports from the era of large-sized, stiff catheters being passed up peripheral veins that confirm the potential for vigorous venospasm under some circumstances. From a pharmacologic viewpoint, veins are not responsive to calcium channel blockers[13] but are readily responsive to nitrates. Since veins are often relatively superficial, nitrates can be applied topically in addition to being given in the usual intravenous, intra-arterial, or sublingual form to treat spasm. Application of warmth is another technique to release venous spasm. Raising the local extremity temperature to 42°C results in maximal vasodilatation.[14]

Venous Anatomy of Arm

Veins of the forearm and hand coalesce toward the antecubital fossa on the palmar side of the forearm into the basilic vein, which passes up the medial aspect of the upper arm or the cephalic vein of the lateral upper arm. In general, while individual variability is the rule with potential arrays of collaterals and alternative channels at all levels of the arm, forearm veins on the ulnar side drain up the basilic vein, while the veins from the radial side of the forearm show equal tendency toward cephalic or basilic drainage.[15]

The basilic vein offers the most direct passage to the central system as it forms the axillary vein at the junction with the cephalic vein, and then the subclavian vein as it passes into the chest cavity under the clavicle. The cephalic vein takes a more circuitous route up the lateral aspect of the upper arm, finally joining the axillary vein. This junction often forms a right angle and is described as a T-junction where the smaller cephalic enters the main venous channel. In older cardiology literature, this region was known for difficulties in permitting large, stiff catheters from completing successful passage. With modern soft and flexible catheters, this is not a barrier to catheter passage, but its presence must be considered as specific techniques and precautions may be needed to transit this region.

Localizing Veins

The primary task in central venous catheterization from the periphery is finding suitable access. Veins that appear very large and superficial in young healthy people tend to be lacking in those who are older and in less-than-ideal health awaiting cardiac catheterization. Once venous access is established, the actual passage of sheaths and catheters is relatively simple compared with the challenges found at times passing up the arterial system.

The most efficient use of catheterization laboratory time involves having preprocedure staff obtain venous access via a heparin-well site with a standard angiocath under sterile conditions. This facilitates the procedure by ensuring venous access at a time when the patient is in a warmer environment and in a more relaxed situation that encourages reduced venous tone. In general, if a 20G or larger line can be placed in the vein, it will usually accept a larger vascular sheath passed over a wire in exchange without difficulties.

The most common mode of obtaining venous access is via direct visualization. Inspection for superficial veins should encompass both arms, and consideration of any vein, in either arm, that is geographically within the equipment's reach of the central venous goal. If superficial veins are not evident, there will be deep veins unless the patient has evidence of gross lymphedema. The location of these deep veins can be found using ultrasound techniques applying technology readily available in most catheterization laboratories. Likewise, in the catheterization laboratory, one can use angiographic inspection by injecting a contrast into the arterial system and awaiting the levophase to occur and outline the venous course.[16] Between attempting venous access in the precatheterization holding area and backup techniques such as ultrasound or levophase angiographic techniques in the catheterization laboratory, the need for venous access via the neck or femoral region can be kept to a minimum.

The location of entry into the venous system can be anywhere on the arm, limited only by the length of the equipment being adequate to reach the wedge position or its working position. The antecubital fossa offers some large and easily visible veins that are geographically close to the central system. The downside of these veins is that they are also near the brachial artery and its branches along with nerve bundles that potentially could be injured during access. More distal venous locations along the forearm below the antecubital fossa lack similar potential for collateral damage due to greater physical separation from arterial and nervous system counterparts. Ultimately, one may be limited by the distance from the wedge position, as present commercially available right heart catheters are only in the order of 110 cm in length. Since these devices can be obtained as small as 4F, the size of the vein is less of a limitation than the distance from the heart.

Entering the Venous System

Once venous access is obtained, the introducing sheath's guidewire can be placed via an indwelling angiocath or a needle. The skin may need some local anesthetic to reduce pain from the sheath stretching the skin, while tough skin may need a slight laceration with a surgical blade if resistance to sheath passage is encountered. The use of a blade needs to be tempered by the superficial position of the vein, which could be easily lacerated with the skin. Passage of the sheath over the introducing wire should be pain-free and just as prior wire passage should have been without resistance. Pain and resistance may indicate perforation, which is possible with inherently thinner walls of the venous system, as seen in

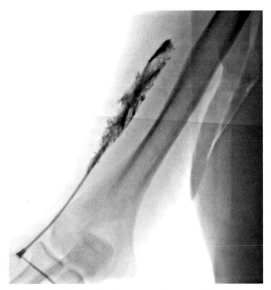

FIGURE 13-2 Cephalic vein perforation after the placement of sheath resulted in perforation of the vein.

Figure 13-2. Once the internal dilator and introducing wire are removed from the vascular entry sheath, the sheath should be flushed, but no vasoactive cocktail is needed. It is quite common for blood drawback to be minimal or impossible as the vein is so compliant that it easily collapses on the end of the sheath. As long as flush passes into the sheath without pain and the procedure has otherwise been unremarkable, one can be confident that the venous sheath is truly in the correct intraluminal position. If in doubt, a small bolus of contrast can quickly confirm the location.

Passage of the Central Venous Catheter or Device

Once the sheath is in the proper position in the vein, the right heart catheter or device can be passed up the vein. This passage should be smooth and without resistance. The operator needs to determine whether passage is up the cephalic or basilic vein using fluoroscopy over the shoulder. Basilic passage is so straightforward that it can often be done under pressure wave form control without the use of fluoroscopy. The cephalic approach requires supervision of the catheter as it passes from the cephalic into the axillary vein at the T-junction. One does not want to puncture the contralateral wall of the axillary vein by applying too much force. If the catheter cannot be tracked into the proximal venous system, a wire may be passed through the central lumen of the catheter to help direct the catheter.

A deep breath that draws venous return centrally and alters the geometry may also facilitate central passage. Once the subclavian vein is reached, passage further into the heart is identical to that of other central venous approach.

While routine right heart catheterization can be done using either the cephalic or the basilic routes, the same may not be possible with other technologies. The basilic vein is usually several times larger than the cephalic vein and can permit just about any vascular device that is used in a femoral vein. The cephalic vein may not be large enough for all devices and the T-junction may be problematic if the device is not flexible enough. Temporary pacemakers without central lumens may be difficult to get around the T-junction and endomyocardial biopsy catheters may also be too stiff to easily navigate this area without risking venous trauma. Assuming enough shaft length is available, vena cava filters and other similar devices should all pass easily up the basilic approach.

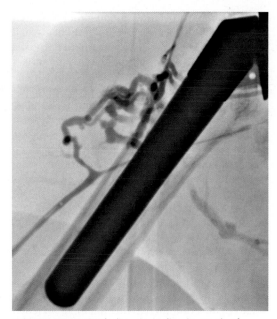

FIGURE 13-3 Cephalic vein ending in a web of collaterals years after a traumatic shoulder fracture with orthopedic repair.

Anatomic Challenges

The venous system itself tends to be very accepting of catheters and their passage. Challenges arise when the patient has experienced trauma, medical conditions, or prior medical procedures that have modified the venous system. Forearm, humerus, or shoulder fractures (Fig. 13-3) may have resulted in damage to the venous drainage and resulted in extensive collateral systems that may or may not be transversible by usual catheters. Trauma such as motor vehicle accidents sufficient to fracture bones in this region should raise one's suspicion of possible venous abnormalities. Soft tissue injury from overuse, such as rotator cuff tears, is usually not associated with venous damage and is less of a concern.

Medical conditions such as breast cancer are another complicating concern. Radial lymph node dissections may involve damage to the deep venous structures along with accompanying radiation therapy. Many survivors of breast cancer will often warn health-care providers of the fact that their affected arm should not be used for procedures, and this is best respected both on medical grounds and for emotional purposes in these patients. Use the other arm instead. Likewise, preexisting lymphedema associated with any disorder that can cause central venous thrombosis should be a deterrent against using that particular arm for venous access.

Another challenge that is commonly encountered is in patients with electrophysiologic devices implanted. All of these devices with leads in the central venous system have some form of obstruction to venous drainage. This does not necessarily preclude ipsilateral central access, but it does raise the possibility of occlusion (Fig. 13-4) and may require contrast injection or

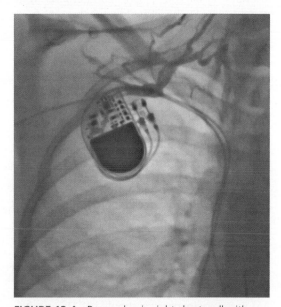

FIGURE 13-4 Pacemaker in right chest wall with leads entering the subclavian vein and producing vein occlusion. Collaterals noted via the external/internal jugular venous system.

wire manipulation to permit passage successfully into the right heart. In total central venous occlusion, collaterals may be sufficient in size to allow passage of catheters, but this may also result in the need for a contralateral approach to the central venous system.

Practical Suggestions

Once venous access is obtained, be it in the pre-procedure area or cardiac catheterization laboratory, passage to the central system is usually a reality. Obstruction to catheter passage should quickly prompt a limited venogram to gain an understanding of the problem. Many times it is a normal finding such as a valve or an unusual turn of the vein that can be easily overcome with the use of a wire through the lumen similar to techniques used in the arterial system. Less likely, one will discover an obstruction or other problem that prevent standard passage and may result in a change of course. Regardless of the outcome, the limited venogram is important as it prevents excessive manipulation and the potential for perforation or damage to the venous system, and it facilitates problem solving and completion of the case.

Finishing the Procedure

Central venous access through a peripheral vein is essentially a venous puncture not unlike that of an intravenous catheter. Hemostasis is very similar to that afforded intravenous access and is primary a superficial pressure dressing. While it might be tempting to maintain the central venous catheter or pacemaker placed from the peripheral vein for longer term monitoring or back up, this must be tempered by the understanding that venous thrombosis is a function of the dwell time of the line. There may be situations where the risk of venous thrombosis is reasonable considering the benefit, but in general the practice of removing central venous access obtained peripherally promptly results in the lowest risk of thrombosis.

Potential Extensions for Peripheral Access to Central Venous System

The ability to access the central venous system from the peripheral arm veins opens up a number of options for the operator beyond just the right heart catheterization from the brachial vein.

With appropriate-length catheters, right heart access from the level of the wrist is possible. Likewise, analogous techniques can be used to pass right ventricular biopsy equipment to the heart[17] and can provide an alternative to more traditional approaches. Temporary pacing catheters can also be placed via the forearm veins. Typically these would be 4F to 6F balloon-tipped pacing catheters. Some care in their passage is necessary as these have no central lumen, but instilling a small amount of contrast into the sheath side arm results in outlining of the vascular pathway up the arm to the central system the pacing catheter needs to follow.

Small and flexible devices can be passed via either the medial coursing brachial vein or the lateral laying cephalic vein. For devices that are stiff or large in diameter, the brachial vein is the vein of choice. This vein is a straight path to the heart and is large enough to accommodate percutaneous device of any size. Vena cava filters and other devices have potential use via this approach, with the primary limitations at present offered not by the device's diameter but rather the workable lengths provided by the manufacturers.

Conclusion

Central venous access originating from a peripheral arm vein is an old technique that can be readily adapted and improved with modern technology and catheter design. Basic right heart catheterization techniques can be provided by this route and complete the overall eloquence of the transradial approach and avoid the use of central neck or femoral veins with their associated risks. Moving further, the use of the arm may be viewed as an access site not only for right heart catheterization, but also a route for right ventricular biopsy, venous interventions, and vena cava filters. In effect, the peripheral vessels can be considered potential access for any technology that can be used within the femoral vein without the risks inherent in femoral access. The veins are large enough and their potential is only limited by the lack of appropriately designed devices.

REFERENCES

1. Agency for Healthcare Research and Quality. *Inpatient Quality Indicator Comparative Data: Based on the 2009 Nationwide Inpatient Sample (NIS) Version 4.4.* August 2012. http://www.qualityindicators.ahrq.gov.
2. Shah MR, Hasselblad V, Stevenson LW, et al. Impact of the pulmonary artery catheter in critically ill patients: meta-analysis of randomized clinical trials. *JAMA.* 2005;294(13):1664–1670.

3. Patel MR, Bailey SR, Bonow RO, et al. ACCF/SCAI/AATS/AHA/ASE/ASNC/HFSA/HRS/SCCM/SCCT/SCMR/STS 2012 appropriate use criteria for diagnostic catheterization. *J Am Coll Cardiol*. 2012;59(22):1-33.

4. Cournand AF. Cardiac catheterization: development of the technique, its contributions to experimental medicine, and its initial applications in man. *Acta Med Scand*. 1975;579(suppl):3-32.

5. Forssmann W. Die Sondierung des rechten Herzens. *Klin Wochenschr*. 1929;8:2085-2087.

6. Zimmerman HA, Scott RW, Becker NO. Catheterization of the left side of the heart in man. *Circulation*. 1950;1:357-359.

7. Hoshal VL Jr. Total intravenous nutrition with peripherally inserted silicone elastomer central venous catheters. *Arch Surg*. 1975;110(5):644-646.

8. Gilchrist IC, Kharabsheh S, Nickolaus MJ, et al. Radial approach to right heart catheterization: early experience with a promising technique. *Catheter Cardiovasc Interv*. 2002;55:20-22.

9. Gilchrist IC, Moyer CD, Gascho JA. Trans-radial right and left heart catheterization: a comparison to traditional femoral approach. *Catheter Cardiovasc Interv*. 2006;67:585-588.

10. Lo TSN, Buch AN, Hall IR, et al. Percutaneous left and right heart catheterization in fully anticoagulated patients

11. Cheng NJ, Ho WC, Ko YH, et al. Percutaneous cardiac catheterization combining direct venipuncture of superficial forearm veins and transradial arterial approach—a feasible approach. *Acta Cardiol Sin*. 2003;19:159-164.

12. Yang C-H, Guo B-F, Yip H-K, et al. Bilateral cardiac catheterization: the safety and feasibility of a superficial forearm venous and transradial arterial approach. *Int Heart J*. 2006;47:21-27.

13. Low RI, Takeda P, Mason DT, et al. The effects of calcium channel blocking agents on cardiovascular function. *Am J Cardiol*. 1982;49:547-553.

14. Taylor WF, Johnson JM, O'Leary DS, et al. Effect of high local temperature on reflex cutaneous vasodilatation. *J Appl Physiol*. 1984;57:191-196.

15. Chun HJ, Byun JY, Yoo S-S, et al. Tourniquet application to facilitate axillary venous access in percutaneous central venous catheterization. *Radiology*. 2003;226:918-920.

16. Pancholy SB, Sweeney J. A technique to access difficult to find upper extremity veins for right heart catheterization: the levogram technique. *Catheter Cardiovasc Interv*. 2011;78(5):809-812.

17. Moyer CD, Gilchrist IC. Transradial bilateral-cardiac catheterization with endomyocardial biopsy: a feasibility study. *Catheter Cardiovasc Interv*. 2005;64:134-137.

utilizing the radial artery and forearm vein: a two-center experience. *J Interv Cardiol*. 2006;19:258-263.

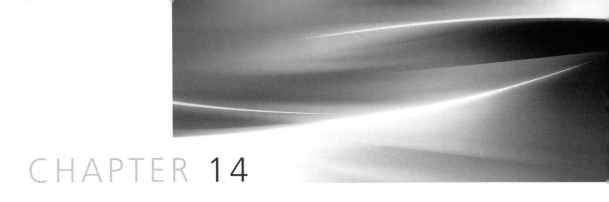

CHAPTER 14

Coronary Interventions: 5F versus 6F to 7F

Gioel Gabrio Secco and Pierfrancesco Agostoni

Introduction

Since the first human cardiac catheterization performed by Forssman in 1929, access site approach as well as angioplasty equipment have undergone considerable evolution and technical improvement. Miniaturization and refinement of the materials has been one of the most important goals, allowing interventionalists to perform more complex procedures and solving most of the percutaneous limitations. The size of sheath, catheter, balloon, and stent delivery system have been markedly reduced in the last few years. From 9F devices used by Gruntzig[1] in the late 1970s, the size has gradually decreased and now most of the percutaneous coronary interventions (PCI) can be safely performed with a 6F guiding catheter. Even more, new smaller guiding catheters with enough large lumen have been developed and are now wildly used.[2] (See also Chapter 8 on slender techniques.) These new smaller catheters appear to be of particular interest in the *"transradial era,"* where transradial PCI has emerged as a gold standard in many centers, replacing the transfemoral route in daily practice. In fact, there is a strong evidence that transradial intervention reduces vascular complication and shortens hospital stay while improving the patients' comfort,[3,4] paying the price for a slight increase in risk of crossover to femoral puncture, procedural duration, and radiation exposure with a variable incidence (up to 7% at 30 days) of loss of radial pulse, mostly asymptomatic.[5]

Size of the Radial Artery and Artery Diameter/ Sheath Size Ratio

A traditional limitation of the transradial approach is the caliber of the radial artery, much smaller than the femoral one, so the manipulation of the arterial sheath and catheter can result in discomfort or pain in the forearm. Previous studies showed that the artery diameter to sheath size ratio is an independent predictor of postprocedural radial thrombosis and occlusions, especially when the value is lower than 1.0[6,7] (see also Chapter 10 on radial artery occlusion). Therefore, the diameter of the radial artery may be an important parameter to consider when it comes to choose instruments in view of its small size. Preprocedural evaluation of the radial artery diameter appears to be crucial since the correct size of the arterial sheath must be chosen according to the radial diameter and lesion characteristics, which may require adjunctive tools for a successful treatment.[8] Using two-dimensional ultrasonography in vivo, the mean diameter of the radial artery is 2.60 ± 0.41 mm.[9] In a study using cadavers, the average diameters of the radial artery in the proximal portion and distal portion were 2.3 and 2.2 mm, respectively[10]; the smaller diameters found in this study were probably due to the possibility that measurements were made after the artery was constricted since it was fixed in cadavers. The radial artery diameter is usually larger in males than in females and is weakly correlated with the height and weight of the patients. Moreover, it has been reported that the ratio of the sheath outer diameter to the internal arterial diameter (S/A ratio) is significantly correlated with pain during sheath insertion and removal.[11] In a study testing the feasibility of using ≥7F guiding catheters in transradial coronary intervention, it has been shown that the inner diameter of the radial artery was smaller than a 6F sheath in 14% of male and 27% of female patients[7]; however, sheath insertion into these small arteries was possible without serious complications. This means that the radial artery can be expanded over the resting diameter during sheath insertion. These data suggest that the use of a guiding catheter ≥6F to 7F from the radial artery is feasible at least in selected cases when the ratio of the radial artery inner diameter/sheath outer diameter is ≥1.0. Moreover, the introduction of the hydrophilic coating has solved most of the discomfort and complications related to transradial cannulation.

Backup Support and Vascular Tortuosity

Whatever the size of the artery is, the advantage of using smaller catheters appears obvious; however, as of today, 5F guiding catheters have not replaced 6F ones in transradial interventions. The real reason must be searched in practical considerations. In fact, not all percutaneous interventions can be performed through a 5F large-lumen guiding catheter because of less strength, less backup support, and poorer angiographic visualization offered by its small inner lumen. Another potential issue in using routinely smaller guiding catheters can be related to anatomic variations of the vasculature of the arm, which can occur in about 15% to 20% of the patients. The most common anatomic variations are radial loops and radial artery hypoplasia (2%), high origin of the radial artery (7%), and tortuous radial artery or subclavian system (10%).[12,13] The higher flexibility of the 5F guiding catheters may be an advantage in these situations; however, more delicate manipulation is necessary to avoid kinking of the catheter.

The lack of backup support can be partially compensated by extra stiff wires for the cannulation of the ostium and extra support or Wiggle (Abbott Vascular, Santa Clara, CA) guidewire during the intervention. However, guide support can be insufficient to advance long stents or bulky devices across tortuous and calcific arteries. Two main strategies are usually adopted in order to achieve greater backup support: the use of large rigid guiding catheters well seated at the ostium of the coronary artery

(passive support, not compatible with the 5F interventions) or the use of small flexible guiding catheters that can be successfully advanced to deeply intubate the epicardial arteries (active support).[14] The capability for deep intubation of a 5F guiding catheter can represent a crucial feature and, due to its smaller and more flexible texture, can afford additional safety than do larger catheters. However, this technique presents several relative limitations. First, the obstruction of flow during deep cannulation may induce severe ischemia that cannot always be prevented by the presence of side holes.[14] Moreover, there is a potential risk of air embolism because of aspiration of air through the Y-connector while the catheter is damped inside the artery with a low back pressure. In any case, if the guide catheter is advanced coaxial with gentle rotation over the rail offered by a previously inserted wire and balloon, the risk of vessel damage is low even if the deep intubation is performed with a 6F catheter. A balloon can also be inflated at low pressure in the artery to stabilize the system while pushing the guiding catheter. Besides, the active support offered by the deep intubation technique may be insufficient in the most challenging situations. The most complex cases need alternative techniques that require the use of adjunctive interventional devices inserted into the coronary vasculature in order to provide increased support. A 5F guiding catheter is compatible with the "buddy-wire technique," an adjunctive wire advanced in a branch proximal or distal to the lesion in order to provide a rail facilitating the advancement of balloons and stents across calcific and tortuous segments or inside a recently deployed stent. If the support achieved is insufficient and requires an additional inflation of an adequately-sized balloon at low pressure (the so-called anchor balloon technique), the use of a 6F or larger guiding catheter is required. Another trick is to use Rotaglide (Boston Scientific, Natick, MA) as a lubricant, either applied directly on the balloon or stent or preferably injected (3–4 mL) directly into the coronary artery.

5F versus 6F Guiding Catheters for Coronary Intervention

Today 6F guiding catheters are the most wildly used size in the daily practice during PCI through both femoral and radial approaches. The diameter of the radial artery is much narrower than the femoral one, and the use of smaller sheath and guiding catheter can reduce arterial spasm, improve success rate, and reduce access site bleeding complications. However, 5F-lumen guiding catheters afford less strength and their 0.056- to 0.058-inch lumen diameter cannot be enough to advance the materials required during the intervention (Table 14-1). Several studies have evaluated the efficacy of using a mini-invasive 5F strategy in daily practice. In one study, using a 5F strategy via the radial approach in 125 patients presenting with acute coronary syndrome, it was possible to perform successful stenting of the culprit lesion in majority of the cases, with a 3% rate of crossover to a 6F guiding catheter because of lack of backup support.[15] In another study, the transradial 5F guiding catheter approach was compared with the 6F approach in 171 consecutive patients with coronary lesions considered eligible for balloon angioplasty. Procedural success was achieved in the vast majority of cases without any significant difference. A tendency toward a lower vascular access site complication rate was observed in the 5F group, especially in patients with small radial diameter detected by duplex/Doppler ultrasound.[16] Similar findings were reported in another study in which the use of a 5F or 6F catheter via the radial approach did not differ in terms of success rate or local complications,

with only a slightly more unsatisfactory support in the 5F group.[11] These findings were not completely confirmed by another study in which 216 patients were randomized to a 5F or a 6F transradial strategy. The procedural success was found to be nonsignificantly higher in the 6F group (90% vs 95%, $P = 0.25$), with a higher tendency of crossover in the 5F group (5F–6F = 6.8% vs 6F–5F = 0.9%, $P = 0.05$).[2] At this time, although most procedures can be performed using 5F guiding catheters with procedural success similar to those obtained with 6F catheters, the potential benefit of using 5F catheters for lowering risks of radial occlusion remains to be better explored. Moreover, we must keep in mind that in case of dreadful complications such as vessel perforation, the use of covered stents requires larger catheter sizes ($\geq$6F).

The Slender Catheters for Percutaneous Intervention

As mentioned before, one of the major limitations in the daily utilization of 5F guiding catheters is that their smaller lumen does not accept

TABLE 14-1 Guiding Catheters for Coronary Intervention

Catheter Size	Brand (Internal Diameter)	Devices	Comments
5F	Cordis (0.056") Medtronic (0.057") Boston Scientific Asahi	Balloon up to 5 mm Cutting balloon up to 2.5 mm Drug-eluting balloon up to 5 mm Stent up to 4.5 mm BVS-absorb up to 3.0 mm Rotablator blurr 1.25 mm IVUS (volcano-phased array)	For bifurcation, two wires allowed for provisional technique (kissing balloons only with slender devices)
6F	Cordis (0.070") Medtronic (0.0701") Boston Scientific (0.066"–0.071") Asahi	Any balloon size Any stent sizes Any cutting balloon size Rotablator ≤1.5 mm Thrombectomy and protection devices IVUS (Boston-Scientific and Volcano mechanical) OCT Thrombectomy devices SVG protection devices Mother-in-child Guideliner	Kissing balloon
7F		Rotablator > 1.75 mm	Kissing stents

Data from Machaalany J, Abdelaal E, Bertrand OF. Guide catheter selection for transradial PCI. *Cardiac Interv Today*. July/August 2013;1–5.

more than one balloon or stent delivery system at the same time. Moreover, frictions or crisscross of the devices inside the guiding catheter can make the intervention harder due to the difficulties in advancing the materials. In order to overcome this limitation, a 0.010-inch guidewire and a compatible balloon catheter system were developed (Ikazuchi-X, Kaneka Medix Corporation, Osaka, Japan). We refer to these devices as the "slender system," and previous studies suggest that complex procedures requiring kissing balloon dilatation can be performed without the need for a large guiding catheter.[17,18] Recently, another study reported the outcomes of a registry in which the "slender" technique was routinely used for PCI.[19] Most of the patients were treated by a transradial approach (79.7%) with an 5F guiding catheter (77.4%). The lesions treated included chronic total occlusions (CTOs) and true bifurcations. In the registry, the operators were able to perform interventions in almost all the cases without a significant need for crossover to a larger-lumen catheter and conventional devices. The few lesions that required 0.014-inch conventional guidewires were always related to the need for noncompliant balloons (there are no slender noncompliant balloons available on the market) or to the inability to deliver a stent into the lesion. However, we must take into account that, at present, the stent delivery systems are designed to achieve the best performance with a 0.014-inch guidewire; despite this, the stent delivery success rate with 0.010-inch guidewires was over 90%. Finally, they hypothesized that, thanks to its smaller cross-sectional area, the 0.010-inch guidewire, together with the smaller outer diameter of the balloon, can easily pass through microchannels, highlighting its usefulness in the setting of recanalization of CTOs. Even though these devices appear interesting, on one hand, they need further evaluation, and on the other, they require a greater widespread and careful evaluation. Moreover, they definitely require a specific learning curve and dedicated training.

Bifurcational Lesions

Another potential limitation in the routine use of the 5F guiding catheters can occur when complex coronary bifurcations are encountered. Bifurcation disease accounts for about 15% to 20% of all coronary artery disease treated by percutaneous intervention[20] (see Chapter 18 on bifurcations). Whatever technique is used, bifurcation interventions present a lower procedural success, with poorer outcome and higher restenosis rate, than does nonbifurcation PCI. These findings have prompted, in the last few years, an intense research activity with the development of new dedicated devices such as side-branch dilatation balloons[21] or especially designed stents that require a 6F or even larger guiding catheters.[22] There are many accepted techniques currently used in the treatment of bifurcation lesions. The recommended treatment remains provisional stenting of the side branch as the gold standard with eventual kissing balloon dilatation as the final step. This requires the simultaneous advancement of two monorail balloons, which cannot be performed in a 5F guiding catheter unless the 0.010-inch guidewires and compatible balloon catheters are available.[19] However, most recent data, while recommending the provisional approach, have shown no improvement of routine kissing balloon postdilatation on the patient's outcome.[23] Hence, it should be recognized that using 5F for bifurcation allows for protecting the side branch with a guidewire, but if a more complex procedure is contemplated, the operator might prefer to upscale catheter size from the start.

Debulking Procedures

The mechanical properties of the arterial wall are critically dependent on the thickness of the wall and the characteristics of the intimal plaque[24]; consequently, the balloon pressure necessary to achieve circumferential overstretch and a satisfactory lumen expansion is intrinsically dependent on the tissue property and wall thickness. Thick neointimal hyperplasia and severe coronary calcification contribute to the increase of the hoop stress to the point that even high-pressure noncompliant balloons might be insufficient to overcome the hoop stress and induct a satisfactory dilatation. Additional devices have been developed to overcome this limitation. Cutting balloons have been designed to relieve the vessel hoop stress by creating controlled small incisions in the vessel wall and present the practical advantage that they do not move during inflation due to the stabilizing effect of the blades. Cutting balloons present several advantages for the treatment of severe calcified lesions, allowing a larger luminal gain at lower pressure compared to balloon angioplasty alone and preventing the late recoil due to the incisions created by the blades.[25] The lack of clinical benefit observed in the early studies of cutting balloon versus conventional balloon angioplasty in de novo lesions has created skepticism on the potential mechanical usefulness offered by a focal concentration of force on the intimal plaque. However, cutting balloon may present advantages during the treatment of severe in-stent restenosis when thick neointimal hyperplasia and the stent itself contribute to increase the hoop stress.[26] Mehran et al.[27] demonstrated that when treating in-stent restenosis with balloon angioplasty, luminal gain is achieved by a combination of additional stent expansion and neointimal tissue compression through the stent, resulting in a displacement through the stent struts and compression of neointimal tissue. Although satisfactory initial clinical and angiographic results were obtained with balloon angioplasty, a significant early lumen loss was also observed shortly after in-stent restenosis treatment due to recoil and reintrusion of neointimal tissue in the lumen.[28] This early phenomenon possibly influences the long-term outcome after balloon angioplasty for in-stent restenosis, affected by a high re-restenosis rate.[29,30] Cutting balloons, compared with conventional balloons, present a significant advantage that the incisions of the microblades reduce the recoil of neointimal tissue into the lumen and allow greater stent expansion by reducing the hoop stress in the neointimal tissue and subsequent better extrusion of the neointima outside the stent and direct transmission of the expanding force of the balloon to the stent struts. Another potentially useful tool during treatment of severe calcified lesions is atherectomy. The most common atherectomy technologies are Excimer laser therapy and Rotablator. The Excimer laser therapy is based on the principle of photoablation converting occlusive material into microbubbles being immediately dissolved in the blood.[31] The Excimer laser coronary ablation catheter is 6F compatible and its use has been successfully described both during the treatment of severe calcified lesions and in the acute ST-elevation myocardial infarction setting when a significant amount of thrombus burden is present.[32,33] Rotational atherectomy is a technique in which a small grinder is inserted into the coronary arteries to ablate the plaque. It is specifically effective in the treatment of calcified lesions because of its differential cutting mechanism. Differential cutting is a phenomenon by which soft tissues (such as the normal arterial wall) are deflected so that the grinder will not contact them during high-speed rotation, while hard calcified plaques are not deflected and can be ablated by the grinder.[34] The currently available rotational atherectomy device is the Rotablator (Boston Scientific-Scimed Corporation, Natick, MA), equipped with a diamond particulate-coated, spinning burr available in various sizes for coronary use (from 1.25 up to 2.50 mm diameter). At this time, only the smallest burr (1.25 mm) can be used with 5F guiding catheters. Series using rotablator successfully to debulk

lesions prior to stenting in 5F catheters have been reported, but most operators probably still prefer to use 6F guiding catheters in case of very calcified lesions and rotablator use. Alternatively, only smaller-sized cutting balloons can be used in 5F guiding catheters.

Chronic Total Occlusion

CTO affect almost 30% of the patients with coronary artery disease undergoing angiography,[35,36] and it remains a challenge for interventional cardiologists. Recent advancement in materials such as guidewires, microcathers, and crossing devices have increased the success rate of CTO percutaneous recanalization from 50%–60%[37,38] to 70%–80%,[39–41] with peaks above 90% for a few highly specialized centers.[42,43] The lack of a general consensus regarding the usefulness of CTO recanalization, together with the hardness of the procedure, has partially affected the development of CTO PCI in daily practice. Two large registries in the United States addressed the real benefit of CTO recanalization procedure on long-term survival, leading to conflicting results: negative the first[44] and positive only for left anterior descending artery recanalization the other.[45] However, they both included patients treated with plain old balloon angioplasty alone suffering from a high percentage of reocclusion. More recent studies, including only patients treated with stent implantation, showed that successful recanalization is associated with improved long-term survival and reduced need for surgical revascularization at follow-up compared to failed CTO procedure. Moreover, it has been recently shown that successful recanalization provided a significant improvement in quality of life, with less physical activity limitation, rarer angina episodes, and higher treatment satisfaction when compared to patients with failed procedure.[46] For these complex interventions, the selection of the correct guiding catheter is pivotal. In fact, along with the importance of having a good backup support, these procedures usually require adjunctive tools such as intravascular ultrasound, microcatheters, or reentry systems that require at least 6F or commonly 7F to 8F large-lumen guiding catheters. In conclusion, if an attempt of percutaneous CTO recanalization is approached, we believe that a minimum of 6F large-lumen guiding catheter is required. However, Japanese operators using slender techniques have started to use smaller guiding catheter sizes for CTO PCI.[19]

Feasibility of 7F Radial Approach for Complex Percutaneous Coronary Interventions

Nowadays, complex interventions that might still require the use of adjunctive devices can be performed using 6F guiding catheters. Yet, in some cases, even devoted radial operators might choose to upscale to 7F or 8F guiding catheters to maximize passive support. The use of the radial artery may appear of particular interest especially in these cases where the use of larger sheath may result in a higher access site bleeding complication rate. Moreover, a few reports have tested the safety and feasibility of transradial intervention performed with larger guiding catheters.[47-49] In a retrospective study in which patients were treated with a 7F strategy via radial artery,[50] the radial cannulation was successfully performed in all cases, with a total of 77 procedures, including left main interventions, bifurcations treated with two-stent strategy, and complex interventions that required the use of bulky devices such as rotablator or Excimer laser therapy. No major vascular complications were reported, although the presence of radial pulse postprocedure was tested only by physical examination in few patients, without the use of duplex scan to confirm the presence of antegrade flow. These findings were confirmed in another recent retrospective study[51] in which 60 complex coronary and peripheral interventions were radially approached with large-lumen catheters (87% 7F, and the rest 8F guiding catheters). All the interventions were successfully performed, the rate of occlusion of the radial artery being 10% (always asymptomatic). Interestingly, in both studies, the preprocedural evaluation of the radial artery was performed only by physical examination. The vast majority of the patients were males who are known to have a larger-lumen artery when compared to females. Thus, it must be emphasized that the choice of using the radial artery with large-bore catheters must be balanced with the higher risks of radial artery occlusion. Newer options exist with specially designed hydrophilic sheathless catheters (see Chapter 20 about sheathless catheters) which offer large internal diameter still with the outside diameter of ≤6F catheters.

Conclusion

It is undeniable that there is a general trend for downsizing catheters to perform elective and urgent, simple and complex PCIs by radial or femoral approach. Although 6F is now routine around the world, 5F equipment has become available and allows to perform a large number of everyday interventions. Lately, industry has put more efforts toward device miniaturization such that, for example, intravascular ultrasound can be easily performed in 5F guiding catheters. The prerequisite of using 5F versus ≥6F relies on the assumption that smaller-sized catheters will reduce the risks of radial artery occlusion while still allowing similar procedural success. At this time, further research is still required to validate this postulate.

REFERENCES

1. Gruntzig A. Transluminal dilatation of coronary-artery stenosis. *Lancet*. 1978;1:263.
2. Gobeil F, Bruck M, Louvard Y, et al. Comparison of 5 French versus 6 French guiding catheters for transradial coronary intervention: a prospective, randomized study. *J Invasive Cardiol*. 2004;16:353-355.
3. Hamon M, Mehta S, Steg PG, et al. Impact of transradial and transfemoral coronary interventions on bleeding and net adverse clinical events in acute coronary syndromes. *EuroIntervention*. 2011;7:91-97.
4. Jolly SS, Yusuf S, Cairns J, et al. Radial versus femoral access for coronary angiography and intervention in patients with acute coronary syndromes (rival): a randomised, parallel group, multicentre trial. *Lancet*. 2011;377:1409-1420.
5. Di Mario C, Viceconte N. Radial angioplasty: worthy rival, not undisputed winner. *Lancet*. 2011;377:1381-1383.
6. Barbeau GR, Bilodeau S, Carrier G, et al. Predictors of radial artery thrombosis after transradial approach: a multivariate analysis of a large series. *Can J Cardiol*. 1999;15:222D.
7. Saito S, Ikei H, Hosokawa G, et al. Influence of the ratio between radial artery inner diameter and sheath outer diameter on radial artery flow after transradial coronary intervention. *Catheter Cardiovasc Interv*. 1999;46:173-178.
8. Nagai S, Abe S, Sato T, et al. Ultrasonic assessment of vascular complications in coronary angiography and angioplasty after transradial approach. *Am J Cardiol*. 1999;83:180-186.
9. Yoo BS, Yoon J, Ko JY, et al. Anatomical consideration of the radial artery for transradial coronary procedures: arterial diameter, branching anomaly and vessel tortuosity. *Int J Cardiol*. 2005;101:421-427.
10. Shima H, Ohno K, Michi K, et al. An anatomical study on the forearm vascular system. *J Craniomaxillofac Surg*. 1996;24:293-299.
11. Gwon HC, Doh JH, Choi JH, et al. A 5Fr catheter approach reduces patient discomfort during transradial coronary intervention compared with a 6Fr approach: a prospective randomized study. *J Interv Cardiol*. 2006;19:141-147.
12. Rognoni A, Lupi A, Sansa M, et al. Radial approach for percutaneous coronary intervention. *Rev Recent Clin Trials*. 2012;7:127-132.
13. Valsecchi O, Vassileva A, Musumeci G, et al. Failure of transradial approach during coronary interventions: anatomic considerations. *Catheter Cardiovasc Interv*. 2006;67:870-878.
14. Di Mario C, Ramasami N. Techniques to enhance guide catheter support. *Catheter Cardiovasc Interv*. 2008;72:505-512.

15. Hamon M, Sabatier R, Zhao Q, et al. Mini-invasive strategy in acute coronary syndromes: direct coronary stenting using 5 Fr guiding catheters and transradial approach. *Catheter Cardiovasc Interv.* 2002;55:340-343.

16. Dahm JB, Vogelgesang D, Hummel A, et al. A randomized trial of 5 vs. 6 French transradial percutaneous coronary interventions. *Catheter Cardiovasc Interv.* 2002;57:172-176.

17. Matsukage T, Masuda N, Ikari Y. Simultaneous triple-balloon inflation technique within a 6 Fr guiding catheter for a trifurcation lesion. *J Invasive Cardiol.* 2008;20:E210-E214.

18. Yoshimachi F, Masutani M, Matsukage T, et al. Kissing balloon technique within a 5 Fr guiding catheter using 0.010 inch guidewires and 0.010 inch guidewire-compatible balloons. *J Invasive Cardiol.* 2007;19:519-524.

19. Matsukage T, Yoshimachi F, Masutani M, et al. A new 0.010-inch guidewire and compatible balloon catheter system: the IKATEN registry. *Catheter Cardiovasc Interv.* 2009;73:605-610.

20. Hildick-Smith D, Lassen JF, Albiero R, et al. Consensus from the 5th European bifurcation club meeting. *EuroIntervention.* 2010;6:34-38.

21. Secco GG, Di Mario C. A new dedicated ultrashort steerable balloon for side branch ostial dilatation. *Catheter Cardiovasc Interv.* 2011;77:363-366.

22. Agostoni P, Foley D, Lesiak M, et al. A prospective multicentre registry, evaluating real-world usage of the tryton side branch stent: results of the e-tryton 150/benelux registry. *EuroIntervention.* 2012;7:1293-1300.

23. Niemela M, Kervinen K, Erglis A, et al. Randomized comparison of final kissing balloon dilatation versus no final kissing balloon dilatation in patients with coronary bifurcation lesions treated with main vessel stenting: the nordic-baltic bifurcation study III. *Circulation.* 2011;123:79-86.

24. Vito RP, Dixon SA. Blood vessel constitutive models-1995-2002. *Annu Rev Biomed Eng.* 2003;5:413-439.

25. Lee MS, Singh V, Nero TJ, et al. Cutting balloon angioplasty. *J Invasive Cardiol.* 2002;14:552-556.

26. Secco GG, Foin N, Viceconte N, et al. Optical coherence tomography for guidance of treatment of in-stent restenosis with cutting balloons. *EuroIntervention.* 2011;7:828-834.

27. Mehran R, Mintz GS, Popma JJ, et al. Mechanisms and results of balloon angioplasty for the treatment of in-stent restenosis. *Am J Cardiol.* 1996;78:618-622.

28. Shiran A, Mintz GS, Waksman R, et al. Early lumen loss after treatment of in-stent restenosis: an intravascular ultrasound study. *Circulation.* 1998;98:200-203.

29. Alfonso F, Cequier A, Angel J, et al. Value of the American College of Cardiology/American Heart Association angiographic classification of coronary lesion morphology in patients with in-stent restenosis: insights from the restenosis intra-stent balloon angioplasty versus elective stenting (ribs) randomized trial. *Am Heart J.* 2006;151:681.e1-681.e9.

30. Mehran R, Dangas G, Abizaid AS, et al. Angiographic patterns of in-stent restenosis: classification and implications for long-term outcome. *Circulation.* 1999;100:1872-1878.

31. Schwarzwalder U, Zeller T. Debulking procedures: potential device specific indications. *Tech Vasc Interv Radiol.* 2010;13:43-53.

32. Ben-Dor I, Maluenda G, Pichard AD, et al. The use of excimer laser for complex coronary artery lesions. *Cardiovasc Revasc Med.* 2011;12:69.e1-69.e8.

33. Dorr M, Vogelgesang D, Hummel A, et al. Excimer laser thrombus elimination for prevention of distal embolization and no-reflow in patients with acute ST elevation myocardial infarction: results from the randomized laser-ami study. *Int J Cardiol.* 2007;116:20-26.

34. Kim MH, Kim HJ, Kim NN, et al. A rotational ablation tool for calcified atherosclerotic plaque removal. *Biomed Microdevices.* 2011;13:963-971.

35. Aziz S, Ramsdale DR. Chronic total occlusions—a stiff challenge requiring a major breakthrough: is there light at the end of the tunnel? *Heart.* 2005;91(suppl 3):iii42-iii48.

36. Puma JA, Sketch MH Jr, Tcheng JE, et al. Percutaneous revascularization of chronic coronary occlusions: an overview. *J Am Coll Cardiol.* 1995;26:1-11.

37. Di Mario C, Barlis P, Tanigawa J, et al. Retrograde approach to coronary chronic total occlusions: preliminary single European centre experience. *EuroIntervention.* 2007;3:181-187.

38. Tsujita K, Maehara A, Mintz GS, et al. Intravascular ultrasound comparison of the retrograde versus antegrade approach to percutaneous intervention for chronic total coronary occlusions. *JACC Cardiovasc Interv.* 2009;2:846-854.

39. Aziz S, Stables RH, Grayson AD, et al. Percutaneous coronary intervention for chronic total occlusions: improved survival for patients with successful revascularization compared to a failed procedure. *Catheter Cardiovasc Interv.* 2007;70:15-20.

40. De Felice F, Fiorilli R, Parma A, et al. 3-Year clinical outcome of patients with chronic total occlusion treated with drug-eluting stents. *JACC Cardiovasc Interv.* 2009;2:1260-1265.

41. Lee NH, Seo HS, Choi JH, et al. Recanalization strategy of retrograde angioplasty in patients with coronary chronic total occlusion—analysis of 24 cases, focusing on technical aspects and complications. *Int J Cardiol.* 2010;144:219-229.

42. Kimura M, Katoh O, Tsuchikane E, et al. The efficacy of a bilateral approach for treating lesions with chronic total occlusions the cart (controlled antegrade and retrograde subintimal tracking) registry. *JACC Cardiovasc Interv.* 2009;2:1135-1141.

43. Morino Y, Kimura T, Hayashi Y, et al. In-hospital outcomes of contemporary percutaneous coronary intervention in patients with chronic total occlusion insights from the J-CTO registry (multicenter CTO registry in Japan). *JACC Cardiovasc Interv.* 2010;3:143-151.

44. Prasad A, Rihal CS, Lennon RJ, et al. Trends in outcomes after percutaneous coronary intervention for chronic total occlusions: a 25-year experience from the mayo clinic. *J Am Coll Cardiol.* 2007;49:1611-1618.

45. Suero JA, Marso SP, Jones PG, et al. Procedural outcomes and long-term survival among patients undergoing percutaneous coronary intervention of a chronic total occlusion in native coronary arteries: a 20-year experience. *J Am Coll Cardiol.* 2001;38:409-414.

46. Borgia F, Viceconte N, Ali O, et al. Improved cardiac survival, freedom from mace and angina-related quality of life after successful percutaneous recanalization of coronary artery chronic total occlusions. *Int J Cardiol.* 2012;161:31-38.

47. Ho PC. Transradial complex coronary interventions: expanding the comfort zone. *J Invasive Cardiol.* 2008;20:222.

48. Kim JY, Lee SH, Choe HM, et al. The feasibility of percutaneous transradial coronary intervention for chronic total occlusion. *Yonsei Med J.* 2006;47:680-687.

49. Ziakas A, Klinke P, Mildenberger R, et al. Comparison of the radial and femoral approaches in left main PCI: a retrospective study. *J Invasive Cardiol.* 2004;16:129-132.

50. Egred M. Feasibility and safety of 7-Fr radial approach for complex PCI. *J Interv Cardiol.* 2011;24:383-388.

51. Coroleu SF, Burzotta F, Fernandez-Gomez C, et al. Feasibility of complex coronary and peripheral interventions by trans-radial approach using large sheaths. *Catheter Cardiovasc Interv.* 2012;79:597-600.

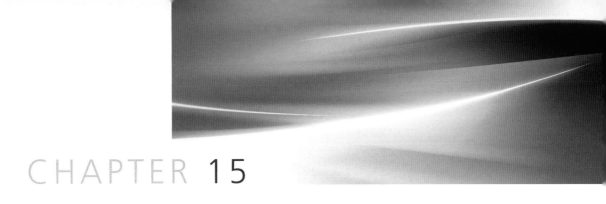

CHAPTER 15

Primary and Rescue Percutaneous Coronary Intervention

Sanjit S. Jolly and Ashok Gangasandra Basavaraj

Introduction

Acute ST-elevation myocardial infarction (STEMI) remains a major cause of morbidity and mortality. It is estimated that approximately 500,000 STEMI events occur annually in the United States alone.[1]

Reperfusion therapies have reduced mortality in patients with STEMI.[2,3] While fibrinolysis has been shown to reduce mortality compared to placebo, meta-analyses of randomized trials suggest that primary percutaneous coronary intervention (PCI) reduces mortality, reinfarction, and stroke compared to fibrinolysis.[4]

However, even with primary PCI, 4% to 10% of patients with STEMI do not survive their hospital stay, and 7% to 15% die during the first year.[5,6] Of those who do survive, another 7% to 9% develop complications such as severe heart failure, cardiogenic shock, and recurrent infarction.[5,6] Across the spectrum of acute coronary syndromes from unstable angina to non-STEMI to STEMI, STEMI has the highest risk of death (Fig. 15-1).[7]

Importance of Bleeding

In the Global Registry of Acute Coronary Events (GRACE), the incidence of major bleeding in patients presenting with STEMI was 4.8% (Fig. 15-2)[8] and the mortality of patients with STEMI who had a major bleeding event was 22.8% versus 7.0% those without bleeding ($P < 0.001$, Fig. 15-3).[8] Multiple studies have demonstrated a relationship with bleeding and mortality in acute coronary syndromes and STEMI.[8-11] However, what remains uncertain is whether bleeding is a marker of risk or causal for mortality.

Access Site versus Non–access Site Bleeding

In the RIVAL trial, only a third of non-CABG (noncoronary artery bypass grafting) major bleeding was access site related.[12] The incidence of access-site and non–access site bleeding may vary according to clinical scenarios (see Chapter 2). In a combined analysis from the REPLACE 2, ACUITY, and HORIZONS AMI trials ($N = 17,393$), the rate of access site bleeding in ACS and STEMI patients undergoing PCI was 2.1% and that of non–access site bleeding was 3.3%.[13] The mortality of patients with no bleeding was 2.5%, with access site bleeding was 6.2%, and with non–access site bleeding was 14.4%. After adjustment, the risk of death with non–access

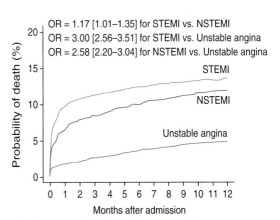

FIGURE 15-1 Kaplan–Meier curves of 1-year mortality among patients with acute STEMI, NSTEMI, and unstable angina. (From Ndrepepa G, Mehilli J, Schulz S, et al. Patterns of presentation and outcomes of patients with acute coronary syndromes. *Cardiology.* 2009;113(3):198–206.)

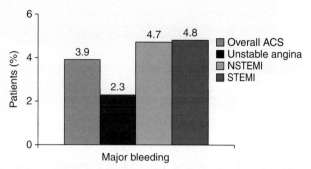

FIGURE 15-2 In-hospital major bleeding rates in unstable angina, NSTEMI, and STEMI. (From Moscucci M, Fox KA, Cannon CP, et al. Predictors of major bleeding in acute coronary syndromes: the Global Registry of Acute Coronary Events (GRACE). *Eur Heart J.* 2003;24(20):1815–1823.)

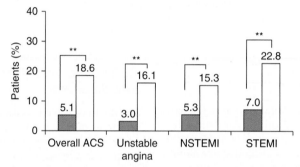

FIGURE 15-3 In-hospital death rate in patients who developed (*open bars*) or did not develop major bleeding (*closed bars*). (From Moscucci M, Fox KA, Cannon CP, et al. Predictors of major bleeding in acute coronary syndromes: the Global Registry of Acute Coronary Events (GRACE). *Eur Heart J.* 2003;24(20):1815–1823.) **P <0.001 for differences in unadjusted death rates.

site bleeds was nearly twice that of access site bleeds (HR 3.94; 95% CI 3.07–51.15 vs HR 1.82; 95% CI 1.17–2.83), but both were associated with increased mortality.[13] It is clear that both access-site and non–access site bleeding are associated with worst prognosis.

Time Is Important in ST-Elevation Myocardial Infarction

Following the occlusion of the coronary artery, myocardial damage starts soon (Fig. 15-4). Re-initiating coronary perfusion at the earliest is the cornerstone in the management of STEMI.[14]

There is a relationship between a delay of more than 120 minutes in door-to-balloon times and mortality in STEMI; it has been proposed to consider door-to-balloon times as a valid quality-of-care indicator, and improved door-to-balloon times have been suggested to physicians and the health system.[15]

There have been concerns that the use of radial access could lead to delays in door-to-balloon times compared to that with femoral access. In RIVAL trial, there was a 5-minute delay with radial access primary PCI, compared with femoral access, from the time of randomization to the completion of primary PCI (58 minutes vs 53 minutes; $P = 0.0009$).[16] Recent sensitivity analysis using the mortality benefit demonstrated in large randomized clinical trials has suggested that the extra time associated with radial approach is unlikely to affect the clinical benefit, compared to femoral access.[17]

Potential Advantages of Radial Access in ST-Elevation Myocardial Infarction

Radial access can prevent femoral vascular bleeding complications such as retroperitoneal hemorrhage, pseudoaneurysms, and large

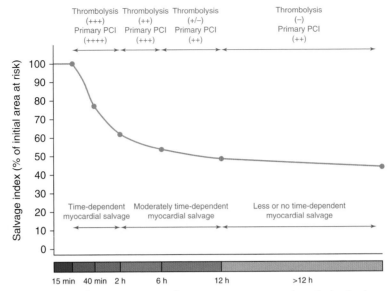

| Thrombolysis (+++) | Thrombolysis (++) | Thrombolysis (+/–) | | Thrombolysis (–) |
| Primary PCI (++++) | Primary PCI (+++) | Primary PCI (++) | | Primary PCI (++) |

Time-dependent myocardial salvage   Moderately time-dependent myocardial salvage   Less or no time-dependent myocardial salvage

15 min   40 min   2 h   6 h   12 h   >12 h

FIGURE 15-4 The initial parts of the curve up to 2 hours were reconstructed on the basis of experimental studies. For the first 15 minutes (15 m) after coronary occlusion, myocardial necrosis is not observed. At 40 minutes (40 m) after coronary occlusion, myocardial cell death develops rapidly, and the myocardial necrosis is confluent. After this point, progression to necrosis is slowed considerably. The other part of the curve showing myocardial salvage from 2 to more than 12 hours from symptom onset is reconstructed on the basis of data from scintigraphic studies in patients with acute myocardial infarction. Efficacy of reperfusion is expressed as follows: (++++), very effective; (+++), effective; (++), moderately effective; (±), uncertainly effective; and (–), not effective. (From Schomig A, Ndrepepa G, Kastrati A. Late myocardial salvage: time to recognize its reality in the reperfusion therapy of acute myocardial infarction. *Eur Heart J.* 2006;27(16):1900–1907.)

hematomas. This advantage may be particularly important in patients with STEMI as they receive more potent forms of antiplatelet and anticoagulant therapies. Bleeding has been linked to mortality in multiple observational analyses, and so by reducing bleeding, radial access may have the potential to reduce mortality.[9-11]

After radial access in patients with STEMI with severe congestive heart failure, patients can sit up immediately and can potentially avoid intubation and nosocomial pulmonary infections. Finally, patients prefer radial to femoral access on the basis of published literature.[12]

Potential Disadvantages of Radial Access in ST-Elevation Myocardial Infarction

Owing to technical challenges with radial access (e.g., subclavian tortuosity and radial loops), there have been concerns of longer door-to-balloon times with radial access than with femoral access.

There have also been concerns that owing to anatomic abnormalities, radial access could be associated with reduced guide support and differential PCI success rates. The rates of PCI success were the same and very high with both radial and femoral accesses in the RIVAL trial (95.4% vs 95.2%, $P = 0.83$). Similar and very high procedural success rates were also found in RIFLE-STEACS (Radial versus Femoral Randomized Investigation in ST-Elevation Acute Coronary Syndrome) and STEMI-RADIAL randomized trials.[18,19]

In smaller, particularly elderly, individuals, the radial artery may only be able to accommodate 5F sheaths. This may be a potential problem if thrombectomy is needed because most available thrombectomy devices are 6F compatible. However, the use of hydrophilic sheathless guiding catheter might be particularly helpful in such complex situations (see Chapter 20).

Finally, another potential disadvantage is radial artery occlusion. Most radial artery occlusions are silent but may preclude future radial access. Radial artery occlusion is discussed in further detail in Chapter 10.

Evidence Regarding the Use of Radial versus Femoral Access in ST-Elevation Myocardial Infarction

There have been at least 11 randomized trials of radial versus femoral access for STEMI PCI. The characteristics and results of these trials are listed in Tables 15-1 and 15-2. But the majority of these trials have been small single-center trials not powered for hard clinical outcomes. However, recently three large randomized trials have been published.

The first was the RIVAL trial, an international multicenter randomized trial of 7,021 patients with acute coronary syndromes that included STEMI ($n = 1,958$). The overall trial showed no difference in primary outcome of death, MI, stroke, or non-CABG major bleeding (Fig. 15-5).

TABLE 15-1	**Characteristics of Randomized Trials of Radial versus Femoral Access**			
Study (year)	Sample Size (*N*)	Single- or Multicenter Trial	Radial Experience of the Operator	Primary Outcome
TEMPURA (2003)[20]	149	Single-center	NA	Cardiac death, MI, target lesion revascularization
RADIAL-AMI (2005)[21]	50	Multicenter	At least 100 transradial PCIs before study	Primary efficacy end point: reperfusion time. Primary safety end point: major bleeding
FARMI (2007)[22]	114	Single-center	Minimum 100 successful transradial PCIs before study	Peripheral vascular complication and PCI efficiency and tolerance of the procedure
Vazquez-Rodriguez et al. (2007)[23]	439	Multicenter	NA	Death, MI, unplanned revascularization, and major vascular complication
Yan et al. (2008)[24]	103	Single-center	All had done more than 500 transradial PCIs before the study	Vascular access site complications, including minor bleeding, major bleeding, recurrent AMI, and repeat TVR
RADIAMI (2009)[25]	100	Single-center	Done 50–100 transradial PCIs before the study	Procedural efficacy and access site complications
Gan et al. (2009)[26]	195	Multicenter	NA	Death, MI, CABG, and target lesion revascularization
Hou et al. (2010)[27]	200	Single-center	Had done at least 200 transradial PCIs	Death, recurrent MI, and target vessel revascularization
RIVAL STEMI subgroup (2011)[16]	1,958	Multicenter	At least 50 radial angiographies or PCIs within past year	Composite of death, MI, stroke, and non-CABG-related major bleed

(continued)

TABLE 15-1   Characteristics of Randomized Trials of Radial versus Femoral Access (Continued)

Study (year)	Sample Size (N)	Single- or Multicenter Trial	Radial Experience of the Operator	Primary Outcome
RADIAMI II (2011)[28]	108	Single-center	All operators were well experienced	Death, MI, repeat revascularization in infarct-related artery, and new CABG
STEMI-RADIAL[19]	707	Multicenter	All operators were well experienced with >200 PCIs/year and >80% radial	Primary end point cumulative of major bleed and vascular complication

There was no difference in the rate of major bleeding utilizing RIVAL definition, but there was a 50% reduction in ACUITY major bleeding and more than 60% reduction in major vascular access site complications favoring radial access.[12]

However, in the STEMI subgroup, radial access reduced the primary outcome (3.1% vs 5.2%, HR 0.60, 95% CI 0.38–0.94, $P = 0.026$) as well as mortality (1.3% vs 3.2%, HR 0.39, 95% CI 0.20–0.76, $P = 0.006$) compared with femoral access (Figs. 15-6 and 15-7).[16]

The second large trial was the RIFLE-STEACS study, which enrolled 1,001 patients with STEMI undergoing PCI who were randomized to either radial or femoral access.[18] The primary composite end point was the net adverse clinical event (NACE) rate, which included bleeding and major adverse cardiac and cerebrovascular events at 30 days. Patients were enrolled at four high-volume radial centers in Italy. The primary outcome of NACE was 13.6% in the radial group and 21.0% in the femoral group ($P = 0.003$) (Fig. 15-8).[18] Of note, there were lower rates of cardiac death with radial access than with femoral access (5.2% vs 9.2%; $P = 0.020$). In terms of bleeding complications, the bleeding rates in RIFLE-STEACS were also significantly reduced in the radial access group than in the femoral access group: 7.8% versus 12.2%, respectively ($P = 0.026$). The reduction in bleeding complications was driven almost entirely by a 47% reduction in access site bleeding.[18] Symptom-to-balloon times for radial versus femoral access were 328 ± 301 minutes versus 322 ± 292 minutes ($P = 0.752$). There was a 60% reduction in access

site bleeding in the radial arm when compared with that in the femoral arm.[18]

The most recent randomized trial of radial versus femoral access in STEMI was the STEMI RADIAL trial ($N = 707$), a multicenter trial performed in four high-volume radial centers in Czech Republic, with 359 patients in the femoral group and 348 patients in the radial group.[19] The rate of major bleeding using HORIZONS AMI trial definition and local vascular complications were reduced by 80% with radial access (1.4% vs 7.2% in femoral group; $P = 0.0001$). The rate of MACE plus major bleeding was 58% lower (4.6% vs 11.0%, $P = 0.0028$). There was no difference in mortality (2.3% vs 3.1%, $P = NS$); however, this trial was not powered for mortality. Importantly, in this trial, operators had a large experience both with radial and with femoral access for primary PCI prior to initiation of the trial.

A meta-analysis of 11 published randomized trials of radial versus femoral access ($N = 4,417$) for STEMI (Fig. 15-9) demonstrated that the radial access was associated with a lower mortality than was the femoral access (OR 0.56; 95% CI 0.40–0.76, $P = 0.0003$, $I^2 = 0$).[29] Despite the finding of the meta-analysis, no single randomized trial has been powered for mortality to compare radial versus femoral access. As a result, large-scale randomized trials are still needed to determine whether radial instead of femoral access can reduce mortality during primary PCI. It should also be noted that there has been no large randomized study comparing radial and femoral approaches in patients referred for rescue PCI after failed

TABLE 15-2 Event Rates in Randomized Trials of Radial versus Femoral Access

Study (year)	Mortality		Major Bleeding		Access Site Bleeding	
	Radial	Femoral	Radial	Femoral	Radial	Femoral
TEMPURA (2003)[20]	4/77 (5.2%)	6/72 (8.3%)	0/77 (0%)	2/72 (3%)	NA	NA
RADIAL-AMI (2005)[21]	0/25 (0%)	1/25 (4%)	0/25 (0%)	0/25 (0%)	2/25 (8%)	5/25 (20%)
FARMI (2007)[22]	3/57 (5.3%)	3/57 (5.3%)	3/57 (5.3%)	3/57 (5.3%)	8/57 (14%)	20/57 (35.1%)
Vazquez-Rodriguez et al. (2007)[23]	8/217 (3.7%)	9/222 (4.1%)	1/217 (0.5%)	5/222 (2.3%)	6/217 (2.8%)	15/222 (6.8%)
Yan et al. (2008)[24]	3/57 (5.3%)	3/46 (6.5%)	0/57 (0%)	1/46 (2.2%)	1/57 (1.8%)	6/46 (13.1%)
RADIAMI (2009)[25]	0/50 (0%)	1/50 (2%)	3/50 (6%)	7/50 (14%)	NA	NA
Gan et al. (2009)[26]	2/90 (2.2%)	3/105 (2.9%)	0/90 (0%)	2/105 (1.9%)	2/90 (2.2%)	12/105 (11.4%)
Hou et al. (2010)[27]	4/100 (4%)	5/100 (5%)	0/100 (0%)	3/100 (3%)	NA	NA
RIVAL STEMI subgroup (2011)[16]	12/955 (1.3%)	32/1003 (3.2%)	8/955 (0.8%)	9/1003 (0.9%)	12/955 (1.3%)	35/1003 (3.5%)
RADIAMI II (2011)[28]	0/49 (0%)	0/59 (0%)	4/49 (8.2%)	6/59 (10.2%)	NA	NA
STEMI-RADIAL[a] (2012)[19]	2.3%	3.1%	1.4%	7.2%	NA	NA

[a]Presented as abstract only, absolute numbers not available.

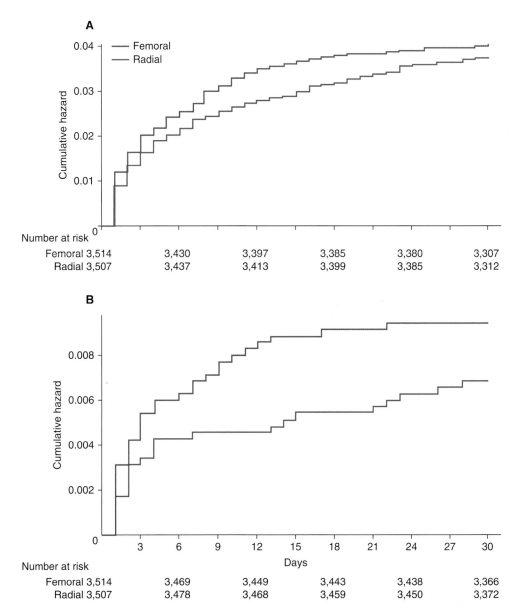

FIGURE 15-5   Kaplan–Meier event curves for the primary outcome and a key secondary outcome for the RIVAL trial. **A:** Composite primary outcome of death, myocardial infarction, stroke, or noncoronary artery bypass graft–related major bleeding. **B:** Secondary outcome of noncoronary artery bypass graft–related major bleeding. (From Jolly SS, Yusuf S, Cairns J, et al. Radial versus femoral access for coronary angiography and intervention in patients with acute coronary syndromes (RIVAL): a randomised, parallel group, multicentre trial. *Lancet.* 2011;377(9775):1409–1420.)

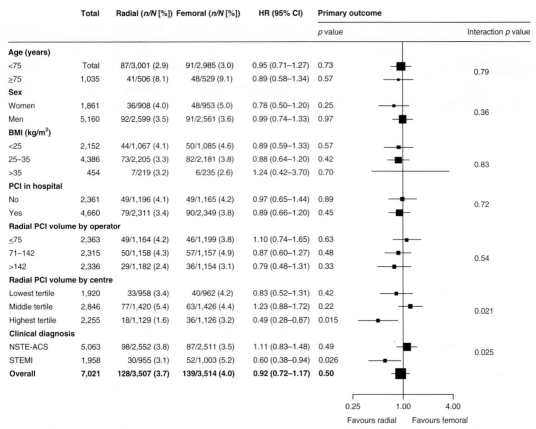

	Total	Radial (n/N [%])	Femoral (n/N [%])	HR (95% CI)	p value	Interaction p value
Age (years)						
<75	Total	87/3,001 (2.9)	91/2,985 (3.0)	0.95 (0.71–1.27)	0.73	0.79
≥75	1,035	41/506 (8.1)	48/529 (9.1)	0.89 (0.58–1.34)	0.57	
Sex						
Women	1,861	36/908 (4.0)	48/953 (5.0)	0.78 (0.50–1.20)	0.25	0.36
Men	5,160	92/2,599 (3.5)	91/2,561 (3.6)	0.99 (0.74–1.33)	0.97	
BMI (kg/m²)						
<25	2,152	44/1,067 (4.1)	50/1,085 (4.6)	0.89 (0.59–1.33)	0.57	
25–35	4,386	73/2,205 (3.3)	82/2,181 (3.8)	0.88 (0.64–1.20)	0.42	0.83
>35	454	7/219 (3.2)	6/235 (2.6)	1.24 (0.42–3.70)	0.70	
PCI in hospital						
No	2,361	49/1,196 (4.1)	49/1,165 (4.2)	0.97 (0.65–1.44)	0.89	0.72
Yes	4,660	79/2,311 (3.4)	90/2,349 (3.8)	0.89 (0.66–1.20)	0.45	
Radial PCI volume by operator						
≤75	2,363	49/1,164 (4.2)	46/1,199 (3.8)	1.10 (0.74–1.65)	0.63	
71–142	2,315	50/1,158 (4.3)	57/1,157 (4.9)	0.87 (0.60–1.27)	0.48	0.54
>142	2,336	29/1,182 (2.4)	36/1,154 (3.1)	0.79 (0.48–1.31)	0.33	
Radial PCI volume by centre						
Lowest tertile	1,920	33/958 (3.4)	40/962 (4.2)	0.83 (0.52–1.31)	0.42	
Middle tertile	2,846	77/1,420 (5.4)	63/1,426 (4.4)	1.23 (0.88–1.72)	0.22	0.021
Highest tertile	2,255	18/1,129 (1.6)	36/1,126 (3.2)	0.49 (0.28–0.87)	0.015	
Clinical diagnosis						
NSTE-ACS	5,063	98/2,552 (3.8)	87/2,511 (3.5)	1.11 (0.83–1.48)	0.49	0.025
STEMI	1,958	30/955 (3.1)	52/1,003 (5.2)	0.60 (0.38–0.94)	0.026	
Overall	**7,021**	**128/3,507 (3.7)**	**139/3,514 (4.0)**	**0.92 (0.72–1.17)**	**0.50**	

FIGURE 15-6 Forest plot of prespecified subgroup analyses of the composite primary outcome in RIVAL trial. (From Jolly SS, Yusuf S, Cairns J, et al. Radial versus femoral access for coronary angiography and intervention in patients with acute coronary syndromes (RIVAL): a randomised, parallel group, multicentre trial. *Lancet.* 2011;377(9775):1409–1420.)

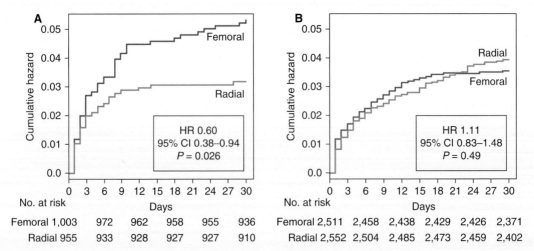

FIGURE 15-7 Primary outcome in patients with STEMI and NSTEMI in RIVAL trial. For the primary outcome, there was a significant interaction between access site allocation (radial or femoral) and acute coronary syndrome type (STEMI or NSTEACS) with an interaction *P*-value of 0.025. In patients with STEMI (**A**), radial artery access reduced the primary outcome compared with femoral artery access, whereas in patients with NSTEACS (**B**), there was no significant difference between radial and femoral artery access. (From Mehta SR, Jolly SS, Cairns J, et al. Effects of radial versus femoral artery access in patients with acute coronary syndromes with or without ST-segment elevation. *J Am Coll Cardiol.* 2012;60(24):2490–2499.)

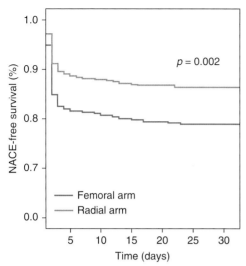

FIGURE 15-8 Time-to-event curves for net adverse cardiac events in RIFLE study (composite of cardiac death, myocardial infarction, target lesion revascularization, stroke, and bleeding). (From Romagnoli E, Biondi-Zoccai G, Sciahbasi A, et al. Radial versus femoral randomized investigation in ST-segment elevation acute coronary syndrome: the RIFLE-STEACS (Radial versus Femoral Randomized Investigation in ST-elevation Acute Coronary Syndrome) Study. *J Am Coll Cardiol.* 2012;27:27.)

thrombolysis. In a pilot randomized study with 50 patients (two-third after failed thrombolysis), Cantor et al.[30] found a trend for less hematoma and less hemoglobin drop (>30 g/L) in the radial group. In a large observational study performed in Scotland over 9 years and including 4,534 patients, the radial approach was associated with similar and striking reduction (≥50%) in 1-year mortality and access site complications/bleeding after primary or rescue PCI.[31]

Guidelines

The 2012 European Society of Cardiology guidelines state that "[i]f performed by an experienced operator, radial access should be preferred over femoral access" for primary PCI. A class IIa indication with a level of evidence of B is assigned.[32] This is the first time that a guideline has specifically specified radial access for primary PCI.

Growth in the Use of Radial Access during Primary Percutaneous Coronary Intervention

In the United States, data from the American College of Cardiology National Cardiovascular data registry have shown that radial access during primary PCI has grown more than sixfold from 0.9% to 6.4% between 2007 and 2011 (Fig. 15-10).[33] In Sweden, data from the SCAAR registry have shown that radial access has grown sixfold as well, from less than 10% to approximately 60% for PCI for STEMI between 2003 and 2011.[34] Similarly in the United Kingdom, the rate of radial access during PPCI has risen from 12.5% to 55.9% from 2006 to 2011.[35]

Recommendations

Radial access should be adopted in a stepwise approach, starting with diagnostic procedures and then simple PCI procedures. STEMI PCI via radial access should be performed by operators with proficiency in radial access and who have performed more than 250 radial PCI based on the guidance document from the European Society of Cardiology (Fig. 15-11).[29]

In addition, the first STEMI patients who are chosen by an operator for radial access should be those with a large radial artery who are not in shock. Less experienced operators should have a low threshold to switch to an alternative access site if facing difficulties because of the importance of door-to-balloon time.[29]

Conclusion

- Radial, compared to femoral, access reduces vascular complications during STEMI PCI and may reduce mortality; however, future randomized trials are needed to confirm this finding.
- Both access site and non–access site bleeding are associated with increased mortality.
- Radial access should be the default approach for primary PCI in experienced radial operators based on the available evidence.
- Operators adopting radial access should wait until minimum proficiency is obtained before attempting STEMI PCI via radial access.

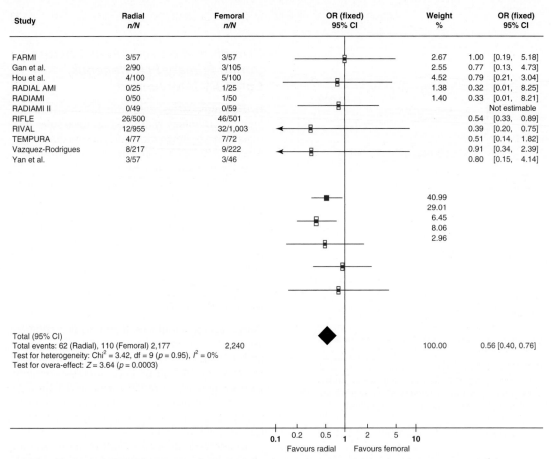

Study	Radial n/N	Femoral n/N	OR (fixed) 95% CI	Weight %	OR (fixed) 95% CI
FARMI	3/57	3/57		2.67	1.00 [0.19, 5.18]
Gan et al.	2/90	3/105		2.55	0.77 [0.13, 4.73]
Hou et al.	4/100	5/100		4.52	0.79 [0.21, 3.04]
RADIAL AMI	0/25	1/25		1.38	0.32 [0.01, 8.25]
RADIAMI	0/50	1/50		1.40	0.33 [0.01, 8.21]
RADIAMI II	0/49	0/59			Not estimable
RIFLE	26/500	46/501			0.54 [0.33, 0.89]
RIVAL	12/955	32/1,003			0.39 [0.20, 0.75]
TEMPURA	4/77	7/72			0.51 [0.14, 1.82]
Vazquez-Rodrigues	8/217	9/222			0.91 [0.34, 2.39]
Yan et al.	3/57	3/46			0.80 [0.15, 4.14]
				40.99	
				29.01	
				6.45	
				8.06	
				2.96	
Total (95% CI)				100.00	0.56 [0.40, 0.76]

Total events: 62 (Radial), 110 (Femoral) 2,177   2,240
Test for heterogeneity: Chi^2 = 3.42, df = 9 (p = 0.95), I^2 = 0%
Test for overa-effect: Z = 3.64 (p = 0.0003)

0.1   0.2   0.5   1   2   5   10
Favours radial   Favours femoral

FIGURE 15-9 Forest plot depicting the meta-analysis of mortality of randomized trials comparing radial versus femoral access for primary PCI. (From Hamon M, Pristipino C, Di Mario C, et al. Consensus document on the radial approach in percutaneous cardiovascular interventions: position paper by the European Association of Percutaneous Cardiovascular Interventions and Working Groups on Acute Cardiac Care** and Thrombosis of the European Society of Cardiology. *Eurointervention*. 2013;8(11):1242–1251.)

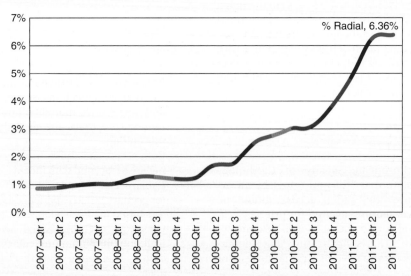

FIGURE 15-10 The use of transradial access in the United States for primary PCI. (From Baklanov DV, Kaltenbach LA, Marso SP, et al. The prevalence and outcomes of transradial percutaneous coronary intervention for ST-segment elevation myocardial infarction: analysis from the National Cardiovascular Data Registry (2007 to 2011). *J Am Coll Cardiol*. 2013;61(4):420–426.)

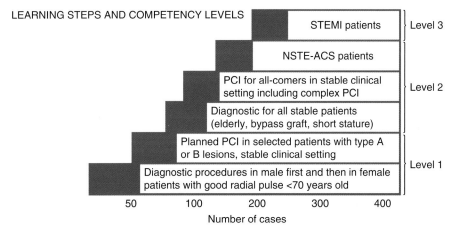

FIGURE 15-11 Stepwise approach and competency levels for radial access. (From Hamon M, Pristipino C, Di Mario C, et al. Consensus document on the radial approach in percutaneous cardiovascular interventions: position paper by the European Association of Percutaneous Cardiovascular Interventions and Working Groups on Acute Cardiac Care** and Thrombosis of the European Society of Cardiology. *Eurointervention*. 2013; 8(11):1242–1251.)

REFERENCES

1. American Heart Association. *Heart Disease and Stroke Statistics—2009 Update*. Dallas, TX: American Heart Association, 2009.
2. Effectiveness of intravenous thrombolytic treatment in acute myocardial infarction. Gruppo Italiano per lo Studio della Streptochinasi nell'Infarto Miocardico (GISSI). *Lancet*. 1986;1(8478):397–402.
3. Randomised trial of intravenous streptokinase, oral aspirin, both, or neither among 17,187 cases of suspected acute myocardial infarction: ISIS-2. ISIS-2 (Second International Study of Infarct Survival) Collaborative Group. *Lancet*. 1988;2(8607):349–360.
4. Keeley EC, Boura JA, Grines CL. Primary angioplasty versus intravenous thrombolytic therapy for acute myocardial infarction: a quantitative review of 23 randomised trials. *Lancet*. 2003;361(9351):13–20.
5. Armstrong PW, Granger CB, Adams PX, et al. Pexelizumab for acute ST-elevation myocardial infarction in patients undergoing primary percutaneous coronary intervention: a randomized controlled trial. *JAMA*. 2007;297(1):43–51.
6. Yusuf S, Mehta SR, Chrolavicius S, et al. Effects of fondaparinux on mortality and reinfarction in patients with acute ST-segment elevation myocardial infarction: the OASIS-6 randomized trial. *JAMA*. 2006;295(13):1519–1530.
7. Ndrepepa G, Mehilli J, Schulz S, et al. Patterns of presentation and outcomes of patients with acute coronary syndromes. *Cardiology*. 2009;113(3):198–206.
8. Moscucci M, Fox KA, Cannon CP, et al. Predictors of major bleeding in acute coronary syndromes: the Global Registry of Acute Coronary Events (GRACE). *Eur Heart J*. 2003;24(20):1815–1823.
9. Eikelboom JW, Mehta SR, Anand SS, et al. Adverse impact of bleeding on prognosis in patients with acute coronary syndromes. *Circulation*. 2006;114(8):774–782.
10. Budaj A, Eikelboom JW, Mehta SR, et al. Improving clinical outcomes by reducing bleeding in patients with non-ST-elevation acute coronary syndromes. *Eur Heart J*. 2008;30(6):655–661
11. Rao SV, O'Grady K, Pieper KS, et al. Impact of bleeding severity on clinical outcomes among patients with acute coronary syndromes. *Am J Cardiol*. 2005;96(9):1200–1206.
12. Jolly SS, Yusuf S, Cairns J, et al. Radial versus femoral access for coronary angiography and intervention in patients with acute coronary syndromes (RIVAL): a randomised, parallel group, multicentre trial. *Lancet*. 2011;377(9775):1409–1420.
13. Verheugt FW, Steinhubl SR, Hamon M, et al. Incidence, prognostic impact, and influence of antithrombotic therapy on access and nonaccess site bleeding in percutaneous coronary intervention. *JACC Cardiovasc Interv*. 2011;4(2):191–197.
14. Schomig A, Ndrepepa G, Kastrati A. Late myocardial salvage: time to recognize its reality in the reperfusion therapy of acute myocardial infarction. *Eur Heart J*. 2006;27(16):1900–1907.
15. Cannon CP, Gibson CM, Lambrew CT, et al. Relationship of symptom-onset-to-balloon time and door-to-balloon time with mortality in patients undergoing angioplasty for acute myocardial infarction. *JAMA*. 2000;283(22):2941–2947.
16. Mehta SR, Jolly SS, Cairns J, et al. Effects of radial versus femoral artery access in patients with acute coronary syndromes with or without ST-segment elevation. *J Am Coll Cardiol*. 2012;60(24):2490–2499.
17. Cohen AT, Harrington R, Goldhaber SZ, et al. The design and rationale for the acute medically ill venous thromboembolism prevention with extended duration betrixaban (APEX) study. *Am Heart J*. 2014;167(3):335–341.
18. Romagnoli E, Biondi-Zoccai G, Sciahbasi A, et al. Radial versus femoral randomized investigation in ST-segment elevation acute coronary syndrome: the RIFLE-STEACS (Radial Versus Femoral Randomized Investigation in ST-Elevation Acute Coronary Syndrome) study. *J Am Coll Cardiol*. 2012;27:27.
19. Bernat I, Horak D, Stasek J, et al. A prospective randomized trial of radial vs. femoral access in patients with ST-Segment elevation myocardial infarction. 2012. http://www.cardiosource.org/Science-And-Quality/Clinical-Images/_TCT12/STEMI-RADIAL-Presentation-Slides.aspx?w_nav=Search&WT.oss=STEMI%20radial&WT.oss_r=159&
20. Saito S, Tanaka S, Hiroe Y, et al. Comparative study on transradial approach vs. transfemoral approach in primary stent implantation for patients with acute myocardial infarction: results of the test for myocardial infarction by prospective unicenter randomization for

access sites (TEMPURA) trial. *Catheter Cardiovasc Interv.* 2003;59(1):26–33.

21. Cantor WJ, Puley G, Natarajan MK, et al. Radial versus femoral access for emergent percutaneous coronary intervention with adjunct glycoprotein IIb/IIIa inhibition in acute myocardial infarction—the RADIAL-AMI pilot randomized trial. *Am Heart J.* 2005;150(3):543–549.

22. Brasselet C, Tassan S, Nazeyrollas P, et al. Randomised comparison of femoral versus radial approach for percutaneous coronary intervention using abciximab in acute myocardial infarction: results of the FARMI trial. *Heart.* 2007;93(12):1556–1561.

23. Vazquez-Rodriguez JM, Calvino Santos R, Baz-Alonso JA, et al. Radial vs. femoral arterial access in emergent coronary interventions for acute myocardial infarction with ST segment elevation. *J Am Coll Cardiol.* 2007;49(9, Suppl 2):12B.

24. Yan ZX, Zhou YJ, Zhao YX, et al. Safety and feasibility of transradial approach for primary percutaneous coronary intervention in elderly patients with acute myocardial infarction. *Chinese Med J.* 2008 ;121(9):782–786.

25. Chodor PKT, Sokal A, Krupa H, et al. Radial vs femoral approaches for PCI for patients with acute myocardial infarction. The RADIAMI prospective, randomized, single center trial. *Eur Heart J.* 2007;28:663.

26. Gan L, Qingxian L, Rong L, et al. Effectiveness and feasibility of transradial approaches for primary percutaneous coronary intervention in patients with acute myocardial infarction. *J Nanjing Med Univ.* 2009;23:270–274.

27. Hou L, Wei YD, Li WM, et al. Comparative study on transradial versus transfemoral approach for primary percutaneous coronary intervention in Chinese patients with acute myocardial infarction. *Saudi Med J.* 2010;31(2):158–162.

28. Chodor P, Kurek T, Kowalczuk A, et al. Radial vs femoral approach with StarClose clip placement for primary percutaneous coronary intervention in patients with ST-elevation myocardial infarction. RADIAMI II: a prospective, randomised, single centre trial. *Kardiologia Polska.* 2011;69(8):763–771.

29. Hamon M, Pristipino C, Di Mario C, et al. Consensus document on the radial approach in percutaneous cardiovascular interventions: position paper by the European Association of Percutaneous Cardiovascular Interventions and Working Groups on Acute Cardiac Care** and Thrombosis of the European Society of Cardiology. *Eurointervention.* 2013;8(11):1242–1251.

30. Cantor WJ, Puley G, Natarajan MK, et al. Radial versus femoral access for emergent percutaneous coronary intervention with adjunct glycoprotein IIb/IIIa inhibition in acute myocardial infarction—the RADIAL-AMI pilot randomized trial. *Am Heart J.* 2005;150(3):543–549.

31. Johnman C, Pell JP, Mackay DF, et al. Clinical outcomes following radial versus femoral artery access in primary or rescue percutaneous coronary intervention in Scotland: retrospective cohort study of 4534 patients. *Heart.* 2012;98(7):552–557.

32. Task Force on the management of STseamiotESoC, Steg PG, James SK, Atar D, et al. ESC Guidelines for the management of acute myocardial infarction in patients presenting with ST-segment elevation. *Eur Heart J.* 2012;33(20):2569–2619.

33. Baklanov DV, Kaltenbach LA, Marso SP, et al. The prevalence and outcomes of transradial percutaneous coronary intervention for ST-segment elevation myocardial infarction: analysis from the National Cardiovascular Data Registry (2007 to 2011). *J Am Coll Cardiol.* 2013;61(4):420–426.

34. *SWEDEHEART 2011 Annual Report.* 2011. www.ucr.uu.se/swedeheart/index.php/arsrapporter.

35. Ratib K, Mamas M, Large A, et al. Radial vs. femoral access for primary PCI, observational data from the British Cardiovascular Intervention Society Database. *J Am Coll Cardiol.* 2012;60(17S):TCT26.

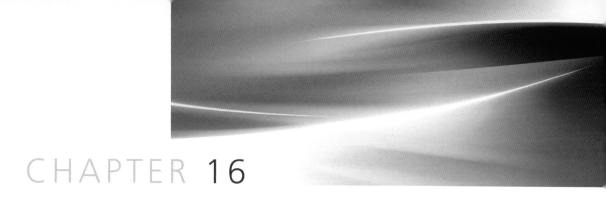

CHAPTER 16

Transradial Approach for Diagnostic and Interventional Procedures in Patients with Coronary Bypass Grafts

Francesco Burzotta, Marta F. Brancati, and Carlo Trani

Introduction

The use of transradial approach is achieving more and more popularity worldwide due to its clinical and economic benefits. Radial route can also be safely and successfully used for the engagement of coronary bypass grafts in order to perform diagnostic or interventional procedures. Left radial approach is usually preferred, owing to its major effectiveness in selective cannulation of grafts compared to the right one. However, right radial route in patients with double mammary artery grafts has been described and is often feasible. A variety of catheters are available to successfully perform selective angiography and percutaneous interventions involving coronary bypass grafts.

Transradial approach (TRA), initially introduced by Campeau for coronary angiography[1] and then developed by Kiemeneij for percutaneous coronary interventions (PCI),[2–4] has demonstrated its technical feasibility after a dedicated learning curve and has been growing worldwide, in order to reduce entry site and hemorrhagic complications, to allow postprocedural comfort and early ambulation, and to offer more cost effectiveness compared to transfemoral approach (TFA).[5–10] A consensus document on TRA in percutaneous cardiovascular interventions has been recently elaborated by the European Association of Percutaneous Cardiovascular Interventions and Working Groups on Acute Cardiac Care and Thrombosis of the European Society of Cardiology.[11]

Patients with previous coronary artery bypass grafting (CABG) represent a high-risk subset with long-lasting atherosclerosis and often complex target coronary lesions (left main stem stenoses, chronic total occlusions, degenerated saphenous vein grafts [SVGs], etc.). Visualization of both saphenous veins and arterial grafts can be successfully achieved by TRA and, indeed, in CABG patients TRA has been shown to be associated with similar total procedural times compared to TFA.[12,13]

Here, we discuss the technical aspects to be taken into account for cardiac catheterization in patients with previous CABG, suggesting some tips and tricks to overcome possible troubles and to routinely adopt TRA in this particular setting.

Procedure Planning

History Evaluation

Diagnostic angiography in patients with coronary grafts is anticipated to be longer compared to procedures performed in patients without grafts, and poses specific challenges. A careful report of the CABG procedure, detailing the exact number of previously implanted conduits, type of grafts, presence of Y-graft, or other surgical constructions, is advisable to guide the selection of access site and catheter curves.

Radial Artery Evaluation

Since the radial artery (RA) is routinely used for the invasive arterial pressure monitoring during the perioperative phase, before catheterization particular attention must be paid to the assessment of blood supply to the hand and, specifically, of the patency of RA. Its integrity should be confirmed through palpation throughout its course and not only at the very distal site of arterial puncture (radial injury/occlusion is usually more proximal and distal radial pulsation may be maintained by collateral circulation). The "reverse" Allen test (compression of both the radial and ulnar arteries followed by the release of radial pressure and checking of color return to the hand in 7 seconds) or plethysmographic evaluation of palmar circulation with Barbeau's test should be used to assess the presence of patent RA.[14] If the test is negative (no reversion of ischemia after radial compression release), proximal radial occlusion is highly probable; when a delayed response to the "reverse" Allen test is observed, suspicion of RA occlusion should still rise, since the slow response is often due to collateral circulation via radial side branches.

In Situ Internal Mammary Artery Grafts

Internal mammary artery (IMA) grafting for revascularization of the left anterior descending artery constitutes the gold standard for contemporary surgical revascularization, in view of its proven long-term benefit. Accordingly, selective cannulation of IMA represents a critical step for the angiographic evaluation of graft patency; moreover, IMA failures, sometimes encountered, can nowadays be successfully managed by percutaneous interventions with last-generation drug-eluting stent implantation.

Homolateral Transradial Approach in Patients with Internal Mammary Graft

Preliminary Remarks

The direct, homolateral, TRA can facilitate the IMA cannulation compared to TFA, with better achievement of selective vessel cannulation. A study showed that the time for IMA cannulation and for IMA study (interval between attempt to cannulate the IMA and last projection) is respectively 39% and 46% lower with TRA than with TFA, with a trend toward reduction of the number of projections needed to study the IMA graft (2.6 ± 1.1 vs 3.0 ± 1.2, $P = 0.10$).[13]

Techniques for Cannulation

The key point for successful left or right IMA cannulation is recognition of take-off angle between the subclavian artery and the IMA, which is highly variable, thus influencing catheter selection. Generally, coming from the homolateral arm, the angle between the distal subclavian and the IMA is acute ($<90°$), while coming from the femoral artery, the angle between the proximal subclavian and the IMA is usually square or obtuse ($\geq90°$) (Fig. 16-1). As a consequence of the combination of asymmetric IMA take-off angle and different approach axis, the standard IM curve, designed for TFA, is not ideal in a relevant subgroup of homolateral TRA cases. Accordingly, a wide choice of curves for diagnostic and guiding catheters for PCI, including some dedicated curves for TRA, may be considered. Among these, in our practice, the first choice is the William's three-dimensional right catheter (Cordis, Bridgewater, NJ) (Fig. 16-1), which is highly effective in the majority of cases and often provides a very good backup in the case of need for PCI. An example of selective left IMA angiography performed by left TRA using three-dimensional right catheter is shown in Figure 16-2.

However, sometimes, the take-off angle is extremely sharp or located immediately before an acute angulation of the subclavian artery (a conformation more often faced in the case of right IMA cannulation from right TRA). In such conditions, the IM-VB1 curve (Cordis)[15] can be used to facilitate selective cannulation (Fig. 16-3). Finally, Mann et al.[16] have designed a dedicated, 90-cm-long guiding catheter for transradial IMA interventions.

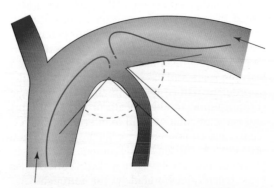

FIGURE 16-1 Different angles between distal subclavian and internal mammary arteries and different catheter selection according to the access route (three-dimensional right catheter for radial one vs IM catheter for femoral one).

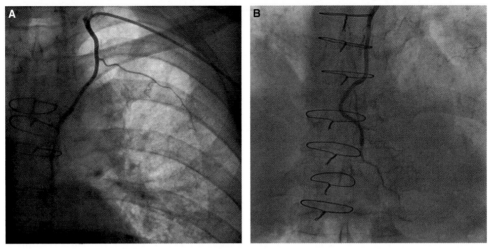

FIGURE 16-2 Selective angiography of left internal mammary artery graft to left anterior descending performed by left radial approach using three-dimensional right catheter **(A, B)**.

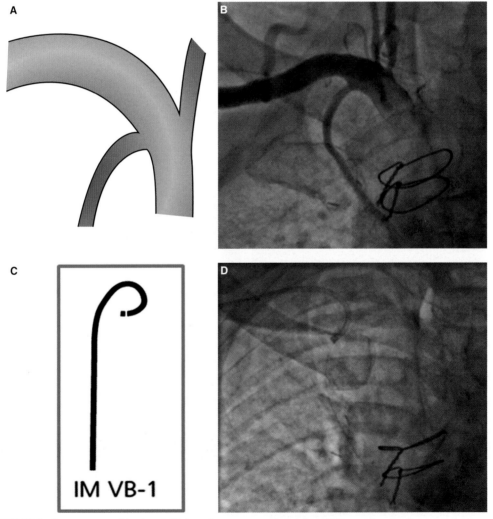

IM VB-1

FIGURE 16-3 In rare cases of horizontal internal mammary artery take-off from a "vertical" segment of subclavian artery (more frequent for right mammary artery) **(A, B)**, IM-VB1 catheter may be useful from homolateral radial approach **(C, D)**.

Contralateral Transradial Approach in Patients with Internal Mammary Graft

Preliminary Remarks

In patients with double IMA conduit usage during surgical revascularization, selective angiography of grafts is usually performed by TFA. Indeed, while selection of bilateral radial arterial access is poorly desirable, selective cannulation of IMA from contralateral TRA brings about technical troubles due to high frictions and multiple angulations—without adequate support—which often hamper catheter advancement into the contralateral subclavian artery.

While selecting contralateral TRA in patients with double IMA grafts, it should be taken into account that, even in skilled hands, unselective IMA angiography is sometimes the best achievable result.[17]

Techniques for Cannulation

If TRA is selected, bilateral radial arterial access or single radial approach may be used; in the latter case, it is preferable to select the right radial approach, as left IMA cannulation by the contralateral radial access has been previously described.[18–25] The first step is the achievement of subclavian artery cannulation; aortic arch and/or subclavian artery angiography are sometimes useful to choose the appropriate catheters. Different catheters are often necessary to cannulate the opposite subclavian artery and then (after 0.25-inch-long wire catheter exchange) the IMA. The Judkins left, left coronary bypass (LCB), or Tiger (Terumo, Tokyo, Japan) diagnostic catheters can be used to pass the exchange-length wire through the aortic arch to gain the contralateral subclavian artery; after advancement of the wire as far as possible down to the arm, the Judkins left catheter is exchanged for

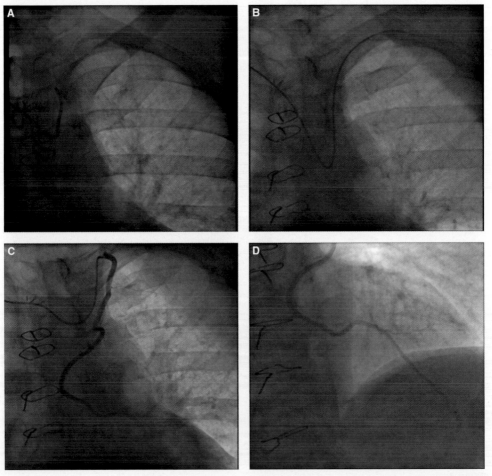

FIGURE 16-4 Cannulation of left IMA graft to left anterior descending from right radial approach. The Judkins left diagnostic catheter is used to pass the exchange-length wire through the aortic arch, gaining the contralateral subclavian artery **(A, B)**; then, the Judkins left catheter is exchanged for a JR4 catheter for selective engagement of left IMA **(C, D)**.

an IM or JR4 catheter[22] (Fig. 16-4). The Simmons catheter has been specifically used for left IMA cannulation by right radial approach, with 89% of selective cannulation rate[18]; moreover, a dedicated catheter curve—Yumiko catheter (Goodman, Japan), a modified version of Simmons catheter with an atraumatic soft tip—has been realized.[19]

When catheter advancement is particularly challenging, support and stabilization of the wire in the contralateral brachial artery may be obtained by trapping the exchange-length wire in the arm by external compression (either manually or by using an inflated blood pressure cuff) or by elbow flexion.[25]

Aorto-coronary Grafts

Aorto-coronary grafts have been for years the only type of graft performed during surgical revascularizations and are still contemporarily used. The vast majority of aorto-coronary grafts are SVGs. The reason for referral to coronary angiography is often due to the accelerated degenerative process involving SVGs, so that the clinical suspicion of their failure is high[26]; when this suspicion is confirmed, in many cases PCI of the degenerated graft is necessary. Thus, obtaining a very high backup support by selecting the appropriate guiding catheter shape may be a key factor for a successful transradial PCI in patients with complex SVG lesions.

Transradial Approach in Patients with Saphenous Vein Grafts

Preliminary Remarks

Owing to the highly variable location within the supra-bulbar ascending aorta of proximal aortic anastomoses of SVGs (according to the technique and the preference of the surgeons), the variability of catheter curves needed to engage the SVG ostium is probably higher was coming from the RA than from the femoral one. In the above-mentioned comparative study between TRA and TFA for CABG patients, the higher the number of SVGs to be assessed, the higher was the additional time needed for their cannulation by TRA.[13] According to our experience, ascending aorta angiography may be advisable when more than two SVGs have to be studied and whenever difficulties are encountered for their localization.

Techniques for Cannulation

The multipurpose or the Judkins right catheters are usually selected to cannulate SVGs originating from the right side of the ascending aorta (generally SVG to the right coronary artery) (Figs. 16-5 and 16-6); the efficacy of their curves is smaller from right than from left TRA. Moreover, the right side of the aorta immediately proximal to the anonymous trunk origin is a "black zone" difficult to be explored by right TRA. Such area, represented in black in Figure 16-5, is an infrequent but troublesome location for proximal SVG anastomosis, and should be taken into account while selecting the radial approach side. When this "black zone" is explored by right TRA, unusual guiding catheter curve selections and manipulations may be useful (e.g., Hockey Stick catheter or Voda left 3 rotated with a 0.35-inch wire inside).

Out of the right side of the ascending aorta SVG engagement is usually achieved by the Amplatz left curves (Figs. 16-5 and 16-6). Moreover, pullback of the Judkins left may be successfully used for the cannulation of SVGs located in the left side of the ascending aorta.

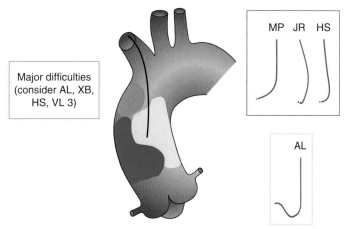

Major difficulties
(consider AL, XB, HS, VL 3)

MP JR HS

AL

FIGURE 16-5 Catheters for SVG cannulation from right radial approach according to the origin of proximal graft anastomosis from ascending aorta; the troublesome "black zone" is represented in red (AL, Amplatz left; HS, Hockey Stick; JR, Judkins right; MP, multipurpose; VL 3, Voda left 3; XB, eXtra backup).

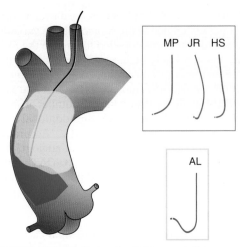

FIGURE 16-6 Catheters for SVG cannulation from left radial approach according to the origin of proximal graft anastomosis from ascending aorta (AL, Amplatz left; HS, Hockey Stick; JR, Judkins right; MP, multipurpose).

Recently, technical feasibility of coronary and bypass graft angiography including left IMA angiography by right TRA using a single catheter (Tiger catheter) has been reported.[27]

Some studies compared outcomes in patients undergoing SVG PCI from TRA and TFA, showing that the use of TRA is technically feasible and advantageous in terms of clinical (decreased vascular access complications, even with high use of platelet inhibitors) and economical (decreased hospital stay) benefits, with similar fluoroscopy time.[28,29]

In the case of a need to proceed with PCI on degenerated SVG, the issue of compatibility between guiding catheter and adjunctive, antiembolic, devices is pivotal. In Table 16-1, the guiding catheter size requirement for the main antiembolic devices needed in SVG interventions is provided.

Examples of complex SVG PCI successfully performed by TRA at our catheterization laboratory are shown in Figures. 16-7 and 16-8.

TABLE 16-1 Compatibility between Guiding Catheter and Antiembolic Devices in Percutaneous Interventions on Degenerated SVGs

Protection System	Vessel Size	Minimum Guiding Catheter Size
Distal protection with filter	–	6F
Distal protection with balloon occlusion (PercuSurge)	–	6F
Proximal protection with Proxis	2.5–4.5 mm	6F
	2.5–5.0 mm	7F

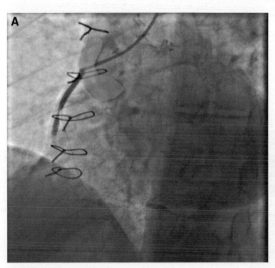

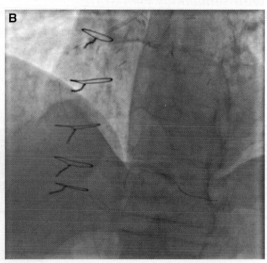

FIGURE 16-7 PCI on an occluded SVG to right coronary artery performed by left radial approach at our catheterization laboratory. Multipurpose 1 guiding catheter is used to engage the graft, which arises from the right side of the ascending aorta (violet zone) and shows thrombotic occlusion **(A)**; after thromboaspiration **(B,** *yellow arrow*), multiple stents are implanted and overlapped after positioning of distal filter for embolic protection **(C)**; and the final angiographic result is excellent **(D)**.

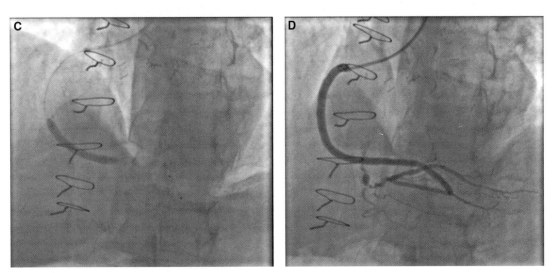

FIGURE 16-7 *(continued)*

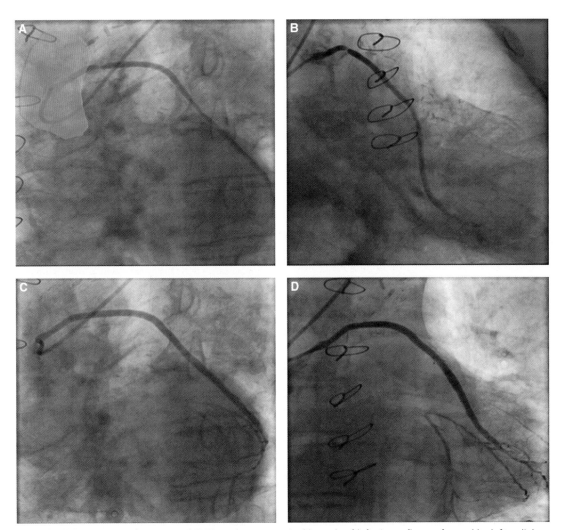

FIGURE 16-8 PCI on a degenerated SVG to obtuse marginal branch of left circumflex performed by left radial approach at our catheterization laboratory. Amplatz left 1 guiding catheter is used to engage the graft, which arises from left side of ascending aorta ("yellow zone") and shows two critical stenosis along its body **(A, B)**; after stenting with embolic protection, the final angiographic result is excellent **(C, D)**.

Radial Artery Grafts and Grafts Rising from Descending Aorta

Even if the majority of patients treated by CABG receive IMA graft(s) and SVGs, two other arterial conduits are sometimes used as arterial conduits: the RA and the right gastroepiploic artery (GEA). The aorto-coronary RA grafting has been reported to warrant lower rate of graft occlusion compared to SVGs, with similar patency to left IMA,[30] although the increased incidence of string sign is of potential clinical concern.[31] Cannulation techniques are similar to those described for SVG.

Finally, some surgeons use the GEA to perform distal anastomosis to the right coronary territory. The selective angiography of GEA graft requires selective engagement of celiac tripod, hepatic artery, and gastroduodenal artery from the descending aorta. Thus, in these conditions, TRA requires the availability of long catheters (e.g.,125-cm-long MP). Indeed, Yamashita and colleagues[32] recently described the use of a novel 130- or 150-cm-long 4F catheter to achieve cannulation of arterial vessels stemming from the descending aorta.

Conclusion

TRA can be successfully adopted for coronary angiography and interventions in patients with previous CABG operation, facilitating cannulation of the IMA conduits and allowing, with an appropriate catheter curve selection and manipulation, SVG engagement for angiography and interventions.

REFERENCES

1. Campeau L. Percutaneous radial artery approach for coronary angiography. *Cathet Cardiovasc Diagn.* 1989;16:3–7.
2. Kiemeneij F, Laarman GJ, de Melker E. Transradial coronary artery angioplasty [abstract]. *Circulation.* 1993;88:I-251.
3. Kiemeneij F, Laarman GJ. Percutaneous transradial artery approach for coronary Palmaz-Shatz stent implantation. *Am Heart J.* 1994;128:167–174.
4. Kiemeneij F, Laarman GJ, de Melker E. Transradial coronary artery angioplasty. *Am Heart J.* 1995;129:1–7.
5. Agostoni P, Biondi-Zoccai GG, de Benedictis ML, et al. Radial versus femoral approach for percutaneous coronary diagnostic and interventional procedures; systematic overview and meta-analysis of randomized trials. *J Am Coll Cardiol.* 2004;44:349–356.
6. Jolly SS, Amlani S, Hamon M, et al. Radial versus femoral access for coronary angiography or intervention and the impact on major bleeding and ischemic events: a systematic review and meta-analysis of randomized trials. *Am Heart J.* 2009;157:132–140.
7. Pristipino C, Trani C, Nazzaro Ms, et al; Prospective Registry of Vascular Access in Interventions in Lazio Region Study

Group. Major improvement of percutaneous cardiovascular procedure outcomes with radial artery catheterisation: results from the PREVAIL study. *Heart.* 2009;95:476–482.
8. Hamon M, Mehta S, Steg PG, et al. Impact of transradial and transfemoral coronary interventions on bleeding and adverse clinical events in acute coronary syndromes. *EuroIntervention.* 2011;7:91–97.
9. Mamas MA, Ratib K, Routledge H, et al. Influence of access site on PCI-related adverse events in patients with STEMI: meta-analysis of randomized controlled trials. *Heart.* 2012;98:303–311.
10. Jolly SS, Yusuf S, Cairns J, et al; RIVAL Trial Group. Radial versus femoral access for coronary angiography and intervention in patients with acute coronary syndromes (RIVAL): a randomized, parallel group, multicenter trial. *Lancet.* 2011;377:1409–1420.
11. Hamon M, Pristipino C, Di Mario C, et al. Consensus document on the radial approach in percutaneous cardiovascular interventions: position paper by the European Association of Percutaneous Cardiovascular Interventions and Working Groups on Acute Cardiac Care and Thrombosis of the European Society of Cardiology. *EuroIntervention.* 2013;8:1242–1251.
12. Sanmartin M, Cuevas D, Moxica J, et al. Transradial cardiac catheterization in patients with coronary bypass grafts: feasibility analysis and comparison with transfemoral approach. *Catheter Cardiovasc Interv.* 2006;67:580–584.
13. Burzotta F, Trani C, Todaro D, et al. Comparison of the transradial and transfemoral approaches for coronary angiographic evaluation in patients with internal mammary artery grafts. *J Cardiovasc Med.* 2008;9:263–266.
14. Barbeau GR, Arsenault F, Dugas L, et al. Evaluation of the ulnopalmar arterial arches with pulse oximetry and plethysmography: comparison with the Allen's test in 1010 patients. *Am Heart J.* 2004;147:489–493.
15. Warner JJ, Gehrig TR, Behar VS. The VB-1 catheter: an improved catheter for difficult-to-engage internal mammary artery grafts. *Catheter Cardiovasc Interv.* 2003;59:361–365.
16. Mann T, Cubeddu G, Schneider J, et al. Left internal mammary artery intervention: the left radial approach with a new guide catheter. *J Invasive Cardiol.* 2000;12:298–302.
17. Cha KS, Kim MH, Woo JS, et al. Nonselective left internal mammary artery angiography during right transradial coronary angiography: a simple, rapid, and safe technique. *Angiology.* 2001;52:773–779.
18. Cha KS, Kim MH. Feasibility and safety of concomitant left internal mammary arteriography at the setting of the right transradial coronary angiography. *Catheter Cardiovasc Interv.* 2002;56:188–195.
19. Kim MH, Cha KS, Kim HJ, et al. Bilateral selective internal mammary artery angiography via right radial approach: clinical experience with newly designed Yumiko catheter. *Catheter Cardiovasc Interv.* 2001;54:19–24.
20. Louvard Y, Krol M, Pezzano M, et al. Feasibility of routine transradial coronary angiography: a single operator's experience. *J Invasive Cardiol.* 1999;11:543–548.
21. Valsecchi O, Vassileva A. Safety and feasibility of selective angiography of left internal mammary artery grafts via right transradial approach. *Indian Heart J.* 2010;62:255–257.
22. Burzotta F, Trani C, Hamon M, et al. Transradial approach for coronary angiography and interventions in patients with coronary bypass grafts: tips and tricks. *Catheter Cardiovasc Interv.* 2008;72:263–272.
23. Zheng H, Pentousis D, Corcos T, et al. Bilateral internal mammary angiography through a right radial approach: a case report. *Cathet Cardiovasc Diagn.* 1998;45:188–190.
24. Tai Z. Selective LIMA injection via the right radial approach. *Cardiac Interventions Today.* January/February 2011:31–32.

25. Patel T, Shah S, Patel T. Cannulating LIMA graft using right transradial approach: two simple and innovative techniques. *Catheter Cardiovasc Interv.* 2012;80:316–320.

26. Fitzgibbon GM, Kafka HP, Leach AJ, et al. Coronary bypass graft fate and patient outcome: angiographic follow-up of 5,065 grafts related to survival and reoperation in 1,388 patients during 25 years. *J Am Coll Cardiol.* 1996;28: 616–626.

27. Suh WM, Kern MJ. Coronary and bypass graft angiography via the right radial approach using a single catheter. *J Invasive Cardiol.* 2012;24:295–297.

28. Rathore S, Roberts E, Hakeem AR, et al. The feasibility of percutaneous transradial coronary intervention for saphenous vein graft lesions and comparison with transfemoral route. *J Interv Cardiol.* 2009;22:336–340.

29. Bundhoo SS, Earp E, Ivanauskiene T, et al. Saphenous vein graft percutaneous coronary intervention via radial artery access: safe and effective with reduced hospital length of stay. *Am Heart J.* 2012;164:468–472.

30. Tranbaugh RF, Dimitrova KR, Friedmann P, et al. Coronary artery bypass grafting using the radial artery: clinical outcomes, patency, and need for reintervention. *Circulation.* 2012;126(11)(suppl 1):S170–S175.

31. Cao C, Manganas C, Horton M, et al. Angiographic outcomes of radial artery versus saphenous vein in coronary artery bypass graft surgery: a meta-analysis of randomized controlled trials. *J Thorac Cardiovasc Surg.* 2013;146(2):255–261.

32. Yamashita T, Imai S, Tamada T, et al. Transradial approach for noncoronary angiography and interventions. *Catheter Cardiovasc Interv.* 2007;70:303–308.

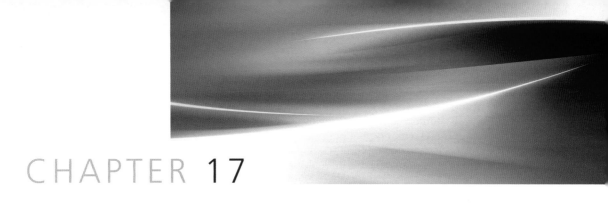

CHAPTER 17

Radial and Complex Coronary Interventions: Chronic Occlusion

Yves Louvard, Thomas Hovasse, Philippe Garot, Thierry Unterseeh, Hakim Benamer, and Thierry Lefèvre

Toward the end of World War II, Stephen Radner, a member of the prestigious Swedish school of vascular radiology, carried out the first nonselective coronary angiography by proximal denudation and subsequent ligation of the radial artery.[1]

The transradial approach was discarded following the advent of the percutaneous femoral technique developed by Seldinger, another member of the Swedish school.[2]

In 1964, Lucien Campeau revived the radial approach for coronary angiography by proximal denudation followed by suturing.[3] The denudation technique was abandoned when the first introducers became available.[4] In 1989, Campeau reported a series of coronary angiographies performed via the transradial percutaneous approach using Potts–Cournand needles and 6F catheters.[5]

The revolution engendered by the radial approach in the field of interventional cardiology began in 1992, thanks to the miniaturization of angioplasty devices (6F) and to Ferdinand Kiemeneij and Gertjian Laarman, who successively performed the first transradial angioplasties, the first stenting implantations, and the first outpatient angioplasty procedures.[6-9] Since then the transradial approach in interventional cardiology has been increasingly adopted worldwide as a result of multiple supportive scientifically validated publications. The feasibility of this vascular route has been demonstrated in a variety of clinical settings and lesion subsets, and the technique is currently implemented in up to 90% of angioplasty procedures in numerous centers all over the world.

The percutaneous treatment of chronic total coronary occlusions (CTOs) was carried out relatively early in the history of coronary angioplasty.[10] The definition of CTO varied with time (functional occlusion) until 2007, when the European CTO club proposed the following definition: the presence of thrombolysis in myocardial infarction (TIMI) 0 flow within the occluded segment with an estimated occlusion duration of >3 months.[11] CTO revascularization constitutes the most complex procedural setting for interventional cardiologists, given that it is associated with a lower success rate, longer procedure duration, higher volume of contrast media, specific complications, and increased X-ray exposure for both the patient and the operator.

A number of reasons for selecting the radial route for percutaneous coronary intervention (PCI) have been approved by the relevant medical societies, namely, improvement in patient comfort and earlier patient ambulation, reduction in vascular complications and procedural cost, and even reduction in the mortality rate in the setting of acute myocardial infarction.[12] The benefit of treating chronically occluded coronary arteries has been demonstrated in multiple instances by the outcome of patients in whom procedural success was associated with improvement in symptoms, ventricular function related to myocardial viability, and survival rates.[13-15]

The presence of a CTO is a predictive factor of mortality in patients with ST-elevation myocardial infarction (STEMI)[16-26] (possibly also in those with non-STEMI) and is associated with a higher number of defibrillating shocks in patients who have been implanted with a defibrillator.[27] Several randomized studies comparing percutaneous treatment of CTO with optimal medical treatment (OMT) are currently being conducted.

Transradial PCI of CTO poses specific difficulties, which are addressed in this chapter.

PCI of CTOs: Techniques, Strategies, and Devices

There are currently three strategies for CTO treatment. These approaches are implemented using a variety of techniques with dedicated or nonspecific equipment.

- The anterograde approach under contralateral angiographic guidance
- The retrograde (bilateral) approach
- The creation of a subintimal dissection followed by distal reentry, which may be applied to both approaches

Numerous techniques have been developed in order to cross, dilate, and stent CTOs. North American and Japanese operators advocate the use of large-diameter guiding catheters with distal lateral holes, which are often occlusive and provide optimal support.

Another reason for selecting large guiding catheters is the use of anterograde echographic guidance for distal reentry or penetration with a guidewire and a microcatheter. Specific guiding-catheter shapes, such as left Amplatz (0.75–2), are recommended for the right coronary artery.

Almost all CTO procedures are currently carried out with microcatheters. They facilitate visualization of the occlusion site (selective injection proximal to the occluded segment and distal to the branches, rapid guidewire exchange, guidewire reshaping, covering of the most proximal shape, and crossing of the occlusion with the wire). In addition to crossing the occluded segment, these microcatheters allow retrograde penetration of the CTO and even in the anterograde guiding catheter in order to externalize a dedicated guidewire and complete the procedure rapidly and elegantly. In such instances, short guiding catheter or very long microcatheters (or both) may be required.

Terumo's Finecross microcatheter encompasses the features of a typical CTO guiding catheter: good pushability, low risk of kinking, tapered tip, flexibility, and distal hydrophilic segment. It has the ability to adapt to the passage of the wire across sinuous segments without causing the wire to exit, as would be the case with a coaxial balloon in a loop. Asahi's Corsair microcatheter (channel crosser) is hydrophilic, tapered, and extremely soft, albeit with strong axial support. It was designed to cross both collateral channels, septal and even more epicardial ones. Once it reaches the distal cap, the microcatheter transmits the axial strength provided by the wire.[28,29] Although used less often, other dedicated microcatheters are available, such as the Tornus (2.1F or 2.6F) manufactured by Asahi (Asahi-Intecc, Aichi, Japan).[30,31] This device is maneuvered by counterclockwise rotation and was designed to traverse "uncrossable occlusions" following wire insertion or even to ensure guiding catheter stability before complete crossing of the occluded segment.[32] The Venture (Saint-Jude, Vascular Solutions, Minneapolis, USA) microcatheter[33,34] has a distally deflectable tip, enabling the coaxial crossing of an occlusion located in an angle, penetration of a side branch, or reentry from a dissection.

Guidewires for CTO PCI may be selected regardless of the vascular route except for the catheter length, which should be longer for right transradial procedures.

After using increasingly stiff guidewires, operators have gradually returned to very soft wires, with subsequent use of very stiff wires in cases of failed attempts and no more gradual progression from soft to stiff wires.

The most recently developed wires combine hydrophilic segments, tapered tips, excellent torque, and moderately increased stiffness. The parallel wire technique, which was very popular when stiff wires were used, can be implemented with two microcatheters in the same guiding catheter, thus providing extra backup support (Seesaw technique).

Balloons are mainly used for pre- and post-stent dilation. However, they are also useful for performing kissing inflation in bifurcations, which are frequent in the setting of CTO. They can also serve the following purposes: wire immobilization in the guiding catheter for coaxial device exchange; wire entrapment in the distal part of the occlusion retrogradely in order to facilitate the passage of a balloon or microcatheter across the occluded segment, or in the proximal part of a CTO or anterograde guiding after retrograde crossing to allow retrograde microcatheter advancement, or inflation in a side branch to ensure guiding catheter stability (anchoring balloon technique) (Fig. 17-1).[35]

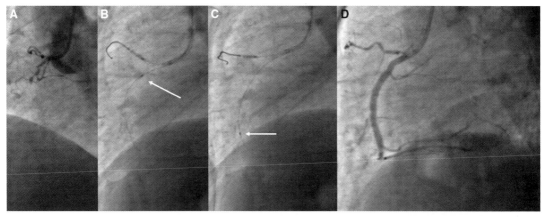

FIGURE 17-1   Anchoring balloon technique for proximal RCA CTO. **A:** Proximal tapered occlusion, JR4 6F guiding catheter (right radial approach). **B:** Anchoring 1.5-mm monorail balloon in an infundibular branch after CTO wire crossing. **C:** A monorail balloon is crossing the occlusion (*white arrows*). **D:** Final result.

Specific Issues of Transradial PCI for CTO

The pitfalls of transradial PCI in the setting of CTO have been described as follows:

- Higher degree of technical difficulty compared with the transfemoral route.
- The size of the radial artery does not allow utilization of large-diameter guiding catheter to accommodate the equipment required and apply appropriate technical strategies.
- The small-diameter guiding catheters used via the transradial route do not provide adequate support.
- Difficulty in using a bilateral route.

Radial puncture undoubtedly poses more difficulties than does femoral puncture. However, the rate of success is closely related to operator experience.[36] Although unpredictable, congenital anatomical variations (antebrachial loops, retrooesophageal right subclavian artery, etc.)[37,38] can be crossed using appropriate techniques. Acquired difficulties[39-41] such as stenosis or occlusion are less frequent compared with the femoral route. Antebrachial, brachial, and especially subclavian loops (less frequent on the left side) are associated with long-standing hypertension, older age, and obesity, all of which increase the risk of complications related to the transfemoral approach.[42]

The mean diameter of the radial artery has been assessed and reported in a few previous series. In a series involving 120 male and female patients published by our group, the diameter was 2.9 + 0.6 mm by ultrasound assessment. In a

Korean series involving 1,191 cases, the mean angiographic diameter was 2.66 ± 0.44 mm (2.69 ± 0.40 mm in males and 2.43 ± 0.38 mm in females) (Dr. B. S. Yoo, personal communication, October 10, 2002). In a Japanese population of 250 male and female patients, the median diameter measured by ultrasound was 3.15 mm in males and 2.85 mm in females.[43] In this Japanese series, the radial arteries accommodated a 6F introducer in 92% of male patients and 82% of female patients, a 7F introducer in 76% of male patients and 57% of female patients, and an 8F introducer in 45% of male patients and 25% of female patients. In our European series, 6F, 7F, and 8F introducers were used in 86.9%, 76.9%, and 64.7% of a mixed group of male and female patients, respectively.

Table 17-1 lists the compatibility between the equipment and the technical strategies applied in the treatment of CTO, the size of guiding catheter and introducers, and their compatibility with the transradial approach in a French population. The use of a 6F catheter with an introducer enables the implementation of strategies such as the anchoring balloon technique with a monorail balloon inserted simultaneously with another monorail balloon or a microcatheter (Finecross, Terumo, Terumo Corp., Tokyo, Japan) (Fig. 17-2). However, a 7F catheter is required for the penetration of the proximal cap with a wire and a microcatheter under IVUS (intravascular ultrasound) guidance (Fig. 17-3).

There is a difference in the diameter between an introducer and a guiding catheter of similar nominal size (around 2F). Measurements assessing the compatibility between an introducer and a radial artery only involve the segment of the introducer inserted in the most distal and the

TABLE 17-1   **Compatibility of Materials and Techniques with 5F to 8F Guiding Catheters and Sheath Size in a French Population**

Catheter Size	Devices	Techniques	CTO	Radial Sheath Compatibility
5F	Balloons ≤ 5 mm	No kissing balloon	Microcatheter	100%
	Stents ≤ 4.5 mm		Coaxial balloon	
	IVUS		Parallel wire	
	Rota 1.25 mm		Tornus	
6F	All coronary balloons	Kissing balloon	Anchoring + microcatheter	86.9%
	All coronary stents	(Compliants or non compliant (NC))	Anchoring + monorail bal.	
	Cutting balloon		Seesaw (2 microcath.)	
	Rotablator ≤ 1.75 mm			
	Protection device			
7F	Angioguard	Kissing stent	IVUS + microcatheter	76.9%
	Rota 2 mm			
8F	Percusurge			64.7%
	Simpson			
	Rota >2 mm			

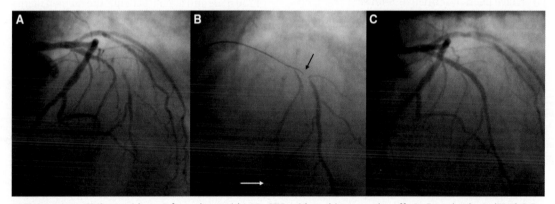

FIGURE 17-2 "Micro guidance" for a short mid-LAD CTO with ambiguous take-off. **A:** Extra back-up (EBU) 3.5 guiding-catheter injection (right radial approach). **B:** Finecross microcatheter injection deeply in the second septal branch (*white arrow*) while a Fielder XT wire, Asahi-Intecc, Aichi, Japan is crossing the occlusion (*black arrow*). **C:** Final result.

narrowest segment of the radial artery. Attempts at decreasing the sheath diameter by reducing the thickness of the wall are ongoing. Sheathless guiding catheters (Asahi) (Fig. 17-4)[44] may allow the use of larger-diameter catheters via the radial approach. Their efficiency is largely dependent on their hydrophilic nature enabling the crossing of, for instance, the proximal segment of brachio-radial arteries (high take-off radial artery),[45] which can be very narrow, in the absence of any connection with the brachial artery at the elbow level.

Even in settings other than CTO treatment, radial operators have long been developing technical strategies to make up for the weakness of guiding catheter passive support in the coronary ostium (sensitivity to respiratory movements, use of guiding catheter shapes adapted to transfemoral procedures, etc.). Certain catheter shapes provide better backup support at the level of the coronary ostium in the setting of complex CTO angioplasty. Left Amplatz shapes are very useful for lesions located in the circumflex artery and sometimes in the left anterior descending (LAD) artery (AL2 or AL3 left Amplatz) or the right coronary artery (RCA) (AL1 or AL2) (Fig. 17-5). However, active support techniques using 6F guiding catheter are widely applied by experienced transradial

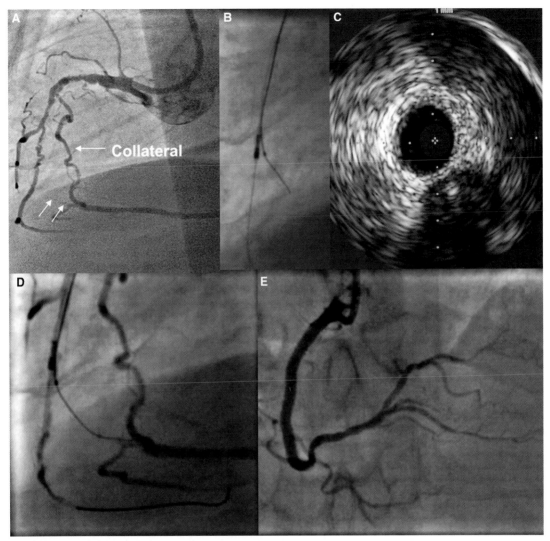

FIGURE 17-3 IVUS-guided penetration for a very old CTO (20 years) initially on the RCA first segment. Reperfusing channels on first and second segments (sinuosities). The patient is symptomatic despite a big homolateral collateral channel. The occlusion site is not clearly visible but the end is (*white arrows*). **A:** The guiding catheter is an AL2 7F from right radial. **B, C:** After proximal and mid-RCA balloon angioplasty, an IVUS catheter is pushed on a wire in a right inferior ventricular branch, and a Finecross microcatheter is pushed slightly proximal to the occlusion cap clearly visible on IVUS. **D:** An XT wire is pushed in the occlusion to the distal bed. **E:** Final result.

operators (Fig. 17-6). Certain guiding catheter shapes facilitate deep-seating intubation (three-dimensional right catheter) (Fig. 17-7). The mother-and-child technique (child-in-mother technique) was first described by Saito as follows: a 5F catheter (Heartrail, Terumo), longer than the guiding catheter by 15 cm, is inserted into a nonspecific 6F guiding catheter and advanced over a wire inside the target artery. This enhances guiding catheter support in direct proportion to the length of the intubated segment and may provide the same backup as would an 8F guiding catheter positioned at the ostium (Figs. 17-8 and 17-9).[46–48]

The Guideliner guiding catheter extension (Vascular Solutions, Minneapolis, USA) was designed according to the same principle in order to provide enhanced support for stent or balloon delivery.[49,50]

Other guiding catheter stabilization techniques are available, such as the anchoring balloon strategy.[35,51–55] This technique may be implemented in a side branch proximal to the occlusion or an arterial segment distal to the occlusion by retrograde insertion of a balloon, in the anterograde guiding catheter following retrograde crossing of the occluded segment, or in

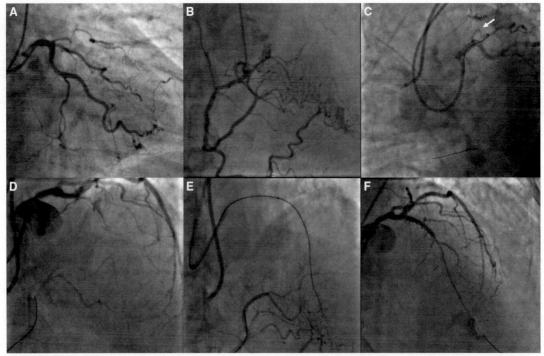

FIGURE 17-4   Bilateral radial approach for a short proximal LAD CTO. **A:** RAO view from coronary angiography. **B:** Collateral filling from RCA with some good channels. **C:** Bilateral injection in the RCA with a 6F JR4 guiding catheter (and a BMW wire to stabilize it), and an SPB4 (EBU-like) sheathless (from right radial) in the LCA (a potential take-off is shown by the *white arrow*). **D:** A Fielder XT wire supported by a Finecross microcatheter is reaching the distal bed. **E:** XT wire deeply in the LAD (controlateral injection). **F:** Final result.

the guiding catheter before wire externalization (Fig. 17-10). The use of a Proxis catheter designed for proximal thromboaspiration may help to stabilize the guiding catheter and to allow stent delivery.[56] A conventional thromboaspiration catheter may serve the same purpose.[57]

Although considered an acrobatic maneuver, simultaneous injection in both coronary arteries via the two radial arteries is frequently performed. However, certain catheterization laboratory setups were designed to allow operators to carry out bilateral transradial procedures in comfortable conditions both for the operator and for the patient (arm support, inflatable or shapeable cushion) (Fig. 17-11), as in the setting of transfemoral procedures.

Transradial PCI Treatment of CTO: Experience and Results

The use of the transradial route in the percutaneous treatment of CTO has been reported in a few case reports and short series. In 2006, Kim et al.[58] achieved a 65.5% success rate in 85 patients. In 2010, Yang et al. published a series of 419 CTO procedures, of which 400 were carried out via the radial approach, with a 69.25% success rate.[59] In 2011, Liu et al. reported a consecutive series of 120 patients treated through the transradial approach, with an 80% success rate, demonstrating the feasibility of this vascular route.[60] In 2011, Wu et al.[62] described bilateral transradial techniques whereby 7F catheters of 85 cm length were positioned 10–15 cm above the radial styloid; 71.8% of CTOs were treated via the retrograde route and the operators achieved a remarkable global success rate of 87.7%.[61] In 2011, Rinfret et al.[62] published a single-operator series of 42 patients treated via the retrograde approach, with an 88% success rate.

All the above-mentioned series demonstrated in a more or less convincing manner the feasibility of transradial angioplasty, including the bilateral radial approach and retrograde routes, in the treatment of CTOs.

To date, there are no randomized studies comparing the radial and femoral routes in the PCI of CTOs. However, a comparison between the two

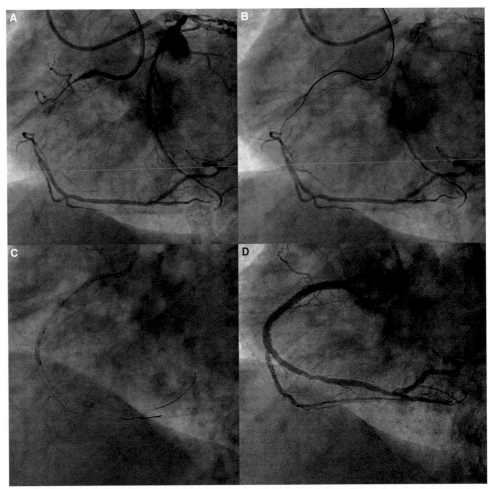

FIGURE 17-5 Bilateral radial approach for a long tapered proximal RCA CTO. **A:** Double injection: EBU 4F 6F guiding catheter from left radial artery for LCA, AL2 6F guiding catheter from the right radial artery for RCA. **B:** CTO crossing with a Fielder XT wire without support. **C:** Balloon angioplasty. **D:** Final result.

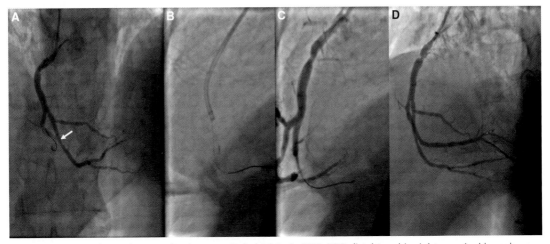

FIGURE 17-6 Catheter deep seating in an occluded RCA. **A:** RCA CTO distal to a big right marginal branch (*white arrow*, JR4 6F guiding). **B:** Increased support with deep seating of the guiding obtained with simple clockwise rotation. **C:** Wire crossing with an Asahi Medium wire (3g). **D:** Final result.

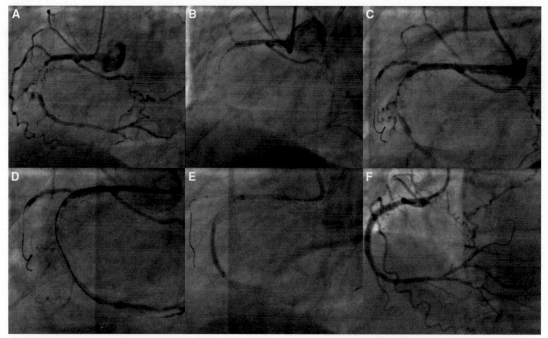

FIGURE 17-7   An old bridged and collateralized mid-RCA CTO. **A:** RCA CTO on diagnostic angiography (JR 5F). **B:** AL2 guiding catheter from right radial approach with poor support. The Fielder XT wire supported by a Finecross microcatheter is not crossing. **C:** Three-dimensional right guiding catheter (Medtronic) intubated deeply by clockwise rotation (*white arrows*) and supported by a 2-mm monorail anchoring balloon; the XT wire is in the distal part of the CTO. **D:** Asahi Confianza pro 12 wire and microcatheter crossing with the anchoring balloon. **E:** Predilatation with a monorail balloon. **F:** Final result after stenting (anchoring balloon removed).

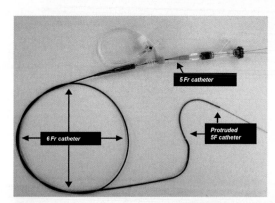

FIGURE 17-8   "5 in 6" ("mother and child") Heartrail catheter from Terumo. Very soft long 5F internal catheter, protruding up to 15 cm distal to the 6F guiding catheter. The system can be used with only the 5F Y connector without valve on the 6F.

strategies was carried out in two single-center registries.

In 2009, Rathore et al. compared 318 transradial procedures (68%) with 150 transfemoral procedures in similar populations with comparable vessels and lesions.[63] Table 17-2 lists identical success rates, similar procedure durations, X-ray exposure, and volumes of contrast.

The purpose of the ongoing Institut Cardiovasculaire Paris Sud (ICPS) CTO registry study (initiated in 2004) is to collect prospectively all attempted CTO interventions in three centers of the Greater Paris area where interventional cardiology procedures are carried out by the same group. A total of 14 interventional cardiologists took part in this study, with an individual volume of procedures ranging from a few cases to several hundreds. All coronary angiograms were reviewed by the same operator. The success rate was reported for each procedure regardless of any repeat intervention or further attempts. Table 17-3 lists the comparison between 848 transradial procedures and 544 transfemoral procedures.

Although the baseline characteristics of patients were similar in each study group, the lesion and vessel characteristics were clearly different. More circumflex coronary arteries were treated in the radial group and there were longer lesions with a higher J-CTO score, and a higher percentage of procedures performed via the controlateral route in the femoral group.

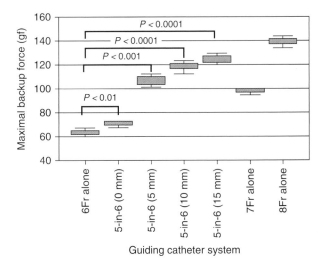

FIGURE 17-9 Additional guiding-catheter support from "5 in 6" Heartrail catheter with different protrusion lengths compared with, respectively, 6F, 7F, and 8F guiding catheters alone. (From Saito S, Ikei H, Hosokawa G, et al. Influence of the ratio between radial artery inner diameter and sheath outer diameter on radial artery flow after transradial coronary intervention. *Catheter Cardiovasc Interv*. 1999;46(2):173–178.)

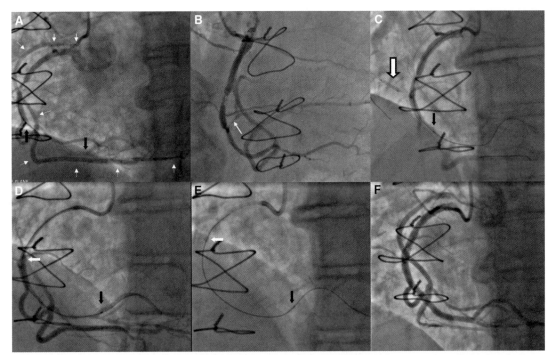

FIGURE 17-10 Distal RCA CTO in a patient with previous CABG. **A:** Subselective injection (AL2 6F) of both native RCA and radial graft implanted on PDA distal to a tight stenosis (*hashed white arrows*). A stent is positioned in a proximal graft stenosis (*white arrows*). The native vessel is stenosed on the second segment and occluded on the third immediately after the marginal branch, the occlusion end at the crux level (*black arrows*). **B:** Crossing the occlusion with a Fielder XT wire. **C:** Finecross microcatheter failure to cross after anchoring balloon in the marginal branch (*white arrow*). **D:** Finecross crossing after deep intubation (*white arrow*) of "5 in 6" Heartrail catheter after anchoring balloon removal. **E:** Distal small 1.2-mm balloon inflation. **F:** Final result after stenting.

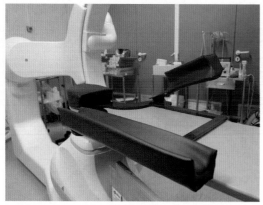

FIGURE 17-11 ICPS Massy dedicated transradial setup ("Cazaconfort"). The right arm is lying along the body or pushed away for radial artery puncture by a left-handed operator. The same support can be used on the left side along the body for a left-handed operator or pushed away for right-handed ones. Then a "pusher" maintains the left arm on the patient's abdomen.

Multivariate analysis showed a similar success rate in both groups (radial: odds ratio 1.14, 95% CI: 0.88–1.48, $P = 0.33$). In 2012, we reported a series of 85 CTO procedures carried out via a double radial approach for lesions of a 21-mm median length, with a 74.1% success rate. The current number of double transradial interventions in our CTO registry is in excess of 200. Such an increase was made possible by a specific catheterization laboratory setup, coupled with operator experience, which enabled the implementation of the retrograde techniques through the transradial approach.

Conclusion

The use of the transradial route in interventional cardiology procedures is by no means a recently developed strategy. CTO treatment techniques have become more and more sophisticated, resulting in a steady improvement in the success rate achieved in increasingly complex lesions.

Experienced large-volume operators have adapted the transradial route to a wide variety of clinical settings and complex lesions. Enhanced transradial strategies in the percutaneous treatment of CTO are being constantly developed as a result of broadening operator experience and following the advent of new devices and techniques, dedicated or not.

Certain Japanese operators are currently working on the possibility of treating CTOs with 5F sheathless catheters.[64]

TABLE 17-2   Comparison of the Transradial and the Transfemoral Approaches in CTO PCI

Variables	Transradial (N = 318)	Transfemoral (N = 150)	P Value
Procedural success (%)	82	86	0.28
Total fluoroscopy time (min ± SD)	24.49 + 13.18	24.07 + 14.12	0.36
Total contrast volume (mL ± SD)	395.54 + 180.25	406.15 + 173.98	0.27
Total procedure time (min ± SD)	54.22 + 25.35	60.23 + 28.15	0.23
In-hospital MI CK >5 times (%)	3.8	3.5	0.40
In-hospital mortality (%)	0	0.7	NS
Urgent CABG (%)	0.62	0.7	NS
Access site complication (%)	3.5	11.3	<0.001
Large access site hematoma (%)	0	2.6	<0.001

From Rathore S, Hakeem A, Pauriah M, et al. A comparison of the transradial and the transfemoral approach in chronic total occlusion percutaneous coronary intervention. *Catheter Cardiovasc Interv.* 2009;73(7):883–887.

TABLE 17-3   **Nonrandomized Comparison of Radial and Femoral Approaches in ICPS CTO Database**

	Transradial ($n = 848$)	Transfemoral ($n = 544$)	P
J-CTO score $\geq$ 2(%)	39.4	48.4	0.001
Target vessel (%)			<0.001
LAD	30.1	29.1	
Left circonflex artery (LCX)	28.7	15.5	
RCA	41.3	55.4	
CTO length, mm (25%–75% percentiles)	14.7 (8.4–24.4)	17.1 (10.6–28.6)	<0.001
Retrograde approach (%)	5.7	17.1	<0.001
Success rate (%)	72.6	68.4	0.09

REFERENCES

1. Radner S. Thoracal aortography by catheterization from the radial artery; preliminary report of a new technique. *Acta radiol.* 1948;29(2):178–180.
2. Seldinger SI. Catheter replacement of the needle in percutaneous arteriography; a new technique. *Acta Radiol.* 1953;39(5):368–376.
3. Campeau L. Entry sites for coronary angiography and therapeutic interventions: from the proximal to the distalradial artery [Review]. *Can J Cardiol.* 2001;17(3):319–325.
4. Desilets DT, Hoffman R. A new method of percutaneous catheterization. *Radiology.* 1965;85:147–148.
5. Campeau L. Percutaneous radial artery approach for coronary angiography. *Cathet Cardiovasc Diagn.* 1989;16(1):3–7.
6. Kiemeneij F, Laarman GJ. Percutaneous transradial artery approach for coronary stent implantation. *Cathet Cardiovasc Diagn.* 1993;30(2):173–178.
7. Kiemeneij F, Laarman GJ. Percutaneous transradial artery approach for coronary Palmaz-Schatz stent implantation. *Am Heart J.* 1994;128(1):167–174.
8. Kiemeneij F, Laarman GJ. Bailout techniques for failed coronary angioplasty using 6 French guiding catheters. *Cathet Cardiovasc Diagn.* 1994;32(4):359–366.
9. Kiemeneij F, Laarman GJ, Slagboom T, et al. Transradial Palmaz-Schatz coronary stenting on an outpatient basis: results of a prospective pilot study. *J Invasive Cardiol.* 1995;7 (suppl A):5A–11A.
10. Serruys PW, Umans V, Heyndrickx GR, et al. Elective PTCA of totally occluded coronary arteries not associated with acute myocardial infarction; short-term and long-term results. *Eur Heart J.* 1985;6(1):2–12.
11. Di Mario C, Werner GS, Sianos G, et al. European perspective in the recanalisation of chronic total occlusions (CTO): consensus document from the EuroCTO Club. *Eurointervention.* 2007;3(1):30–43.
12. Hamon M, Pristipino C, Di Mario C, et al. Consensus document on the radial approach in percutaneous cardiovascular interventions: position paper by the European Association of Percutaneous Cardiovascular Interventions and Working Groups on Acute Cardiac Care and Thrombosis of the European Society of Cardiology. *Eurointervention.* 2013;8(11):1242–1251.
13. Grantham JA, Jones PG, Cannon L, et al. Quantifying the early health status benefits of successful chronic total occlusion recanalization: results from the Flow Cardia's Approach to Chronic Total Occlusion Recanalization (FACTOR) trial. *Circ Cardiovasc Qual Outcomes.* 2010;3(3):284–290.
14. Kirschbaum SW, Baks T, van den Ent M, et al. Evaluation of left ventricular function three years after percutaneous recanalization of chronic total coronary occlusions. *Am J Cardiol.* 2008;101(2):179–185.
15. Joyal D, Afilalo J, Rinfret S. Effectiveness of recanalization of chronic total occlusions: a systematic review and meta-analysis. *Am Heart J.* 2010;160(1):179–187.
16. Moreno R, Conde C, Perez-Vizcayno MJ, et al. Prognostic impact of a chronic occlusion in a noninfarct vessel in patients with acute myocardial infarction and multivessel disease undergoing primary percutaneous coronary intervention. *J Invasive Cardiol.* 2006;18(1):16–19.
17. Claessen BE, van der Schaaf RJ, Verouden NJ, et al. Evaluation of the effect of a concurrent chronic total occlusion on long-term mortality and left ventricular function in patients after primary percutaneous coronary intervention. *JACC Cardiovasc Interv.* 2009;2(11):1128–1134.
18. van der Schaaf RJ, Claessen BE, Vis MM, et al. Effect of multivessel coronary disease with or without concurrent chronic total occlusion on one-year mortality in patients treated with primary percutaneous coronary intervention for cardiogenic shock. *Am J Cardiol.* 2010;105(7):955–959.
19. Claessen BE, Hoebers LP, van der Schaaf RJ, et al. Prevalence and impact of a chronic total occlusion in a non-infarct-related artery on long-term mortality in diabetic patients with ST elevation myocardial infarction. *Heart.* 2010;96(24):1968–1972.
20. Lexis CP, van der Horst IC, Rahel BM, et al. Impact of chronic total occlusions on markers of reperfusion, infarct size, and long-term mortality: a substudy from the TAPAS-trial. *Catheter Cardiovasc Interv.* 2011;77:484–491.
21. Claessen BE, Dangas GD, Weisz G, et al. Prognostic impact of a chronic total occlusion in a non-infarct-related artery in patients with ST-segment elevation myocardial infarction: 3-year results from the HORIZONS-AMI trial. *Eur Heart J.* 2012;33(6):768–775.
22. Tajstra M, Gasior M, Gierlotka M, et al. Comparison of five-year outcomes of patients with and without chronic total occlusion of noninfarct coronary artery after primary coronary intervention for ST-segment elevation acute myocardial infarction. *Am J Cardiol.* 2012;109(2):208–213.

23. Hoebers LP, Vis MM, Claessen BE, et al. The impact of multivessel disease with and without a co-existing chronic total occlusion on short- and long-term mortality in ST-elevation myocardial infarction patients with and without cardiogenic shock. *Eur J Heart Fail.* 2013;15(4):425–432.

24. Bataille Y, Déry JP, Larose E, et al. Incidence and clinical impact of concurrent chronic total occlusion according to gender in ST-elevation myocardial infarction. *Catheter Cardiovasc Interv.* 2013;82(1):19–26.

25. Lee JH, Park HS, Ryu HM, et al. Impact of multivessel coronary disease with chronic total occlusion on one-year mortality in patients with acute myocardial infarction. *Korean Circ J.* 2012;42(2):95–99.

26. De Felice F, Fiorilli F, Parma A, et al. Effect of multivessel coronary artery disease with or without a concomitant chronic total occlusion on 1-year survival of patients treated with rescue angioplasty. *J Invasive Cardiol.* 2013;25(2):64–68.

27. Nombela-Franco L, Mitroi CD, Fernández-Lozano I, et al. Ventricular arrhythmias among implantable cardioverter-defibrillator recipients for primary prevention: impact of chronic total coronary occlusion (VACTO Primary Study). *Circ Arrhythm Electrophysiol.* 2012;5(1):147–154.

28. Obata JE, Nakamura T, Kitta Y, et al. Usefulness of a collateral channel dilator for antegrade treatment of chronic total occlusion of a coronary artery. *J Interv Cardiol.* 2012;25(6):533–539.

29. Otsuka Y, Nakamura K, Saito T. Usefulness of the Corsair microcatheter for treatment of complex chronic total occlusion. *J Invasive Cardiol.* 2012;24(2):E35–E38.

30. Reifart N, Enayat D, Giokoglu K. A novel penetration catheter (Tornus) as bail-out device after balloon failure to recanalise long, old calcified chronic occlusions. *Eurointervention.* 2008;3(5):617–621.

31. Brilakis ES, Banerjee S. Crossing the "balloon uncrossable" chronic total occlusion: Tornus to the rescue. *Catheter Cardiovasc Interv.* 2011 ;78(3):363–365.

32. Kirtane AJ, Stone GW. The Anchor-Tornus technique: a novel approach to "uncrossable" chronic total occlusions. *Catheter Cardiovasc Interv.* 2007;70(4):554–557.

33. Iturbe JM, Abdel-Karim AR, Raja VN, et al. Use of the venture wire control catheter for the treatment of coronary artery chronic total occlusions. *Catheter Cardiovasc Interv.* 2010;76(7):936–941.

34. Badhey N, Lombardi WL, Thompson CA, et al. Use of the venture wire control catheter for subintimal coronary dissection and reentry in chronic total occlusions. *J Invasive Cardiol.* 2010;22(9):445–448.

35. Hirokami M, Saito S, Muto H. Anchoring technique to improve guiding catheter support in coronary angioplasty of chronic total occlusions. *Catheter Cardiovasc Interv.* 2006;67(3):366–371.

36. Louvard Y, Kumar S, Lefèvre T. Percentage of transradial approach for interventional cardiology in the world and learning the technique. *Ann Cardiol Angeiol (Paris).* 2009;58(6):327–332.

37. Louvard Y, Lefèvre T. Loops and transradial approach in coronary diagnosis and intervention. *Catheter Cardiovasc Interv.* 2000;51(2):250–252.

38. Abhaichand RK, Louvard Y, Gobeil JF, et al. The problem of arteria lusoria in right transradial coronary angiography and angioplasty. *Catheter Cardiovasc Interv.* 2001;54(2):196–201.

39. Lo TS, Nolan J, Fountzopoulos E, et al. Radial artery anomaly and its influence on transradial coronary procedural outcome. *Heart.* 2009;95(5):410–415.

40. Burzotta F, Trani C, De Vita M, et al. A new operative classification of both anatomic vascular variants and physiopathologic conditions affecting transradial cardiovascular procedures. *Int J Cardiol.* 2010;145(1):120–122.

41. Burzotta F, Brancati MF, Trani C, et al. Impact of radial-to-aorta vascular anatomical variants on risk of failure in trans-radial coronary procedures. *Catheter Cardiovasc Interv.* 2012;80(2):298–303.

42. Louvard Y, Benamer H, Garot P, et al; OCTOPLUS Study Group. Comparison of transradial and transfemoral approaches for coronary angiography and angioplasty in octogenarians (the OCTOPLUS study). *Am J Cardiol.* 2004;94(9):1177–1180.

43. Saito S, Ikei H, Hosokawa G, et al. Influence of the ratio between radial artery inner diameter and sheath outer diameter on radial artery flow after transradial coronary intervention. *Catheter Cardiovasc Interv.* 1999;46(2):173–178.

44. Lin CJ, Fang HY, Chen TH, et al. Transradial percutaneous coronary intervention for chronic total occlusion using sheathless technique and retrograde approach. *Catheter Cardiovasc Interv.* 2013;82(3):E206–E210.

45. Rodríguez-Niedenführ M, Vázquez T, Nearn L, et al. Variations of the arterial pattern in the upper limb revisited: a morphological and statistical study, with a review of the literature. *J Anat.* 2001;199(pt 5):547–566.

46. Takahashi S, Saito S, Tanaka S, et al. New method to increase a backup support of a 6 French guiding coronary catheter. *Catheter Cardiovasc Interv.* 2004;63(4):452–456.

47. Hayashida K, Louvard Y, Lefèvre T. Transradial complex coronary interventions using a five-in-six system. *Catheter Cardiovasc Interv.* 2011;77(1):63–68.

48. Zhang Q, Zhang RY, Kirtane AJ, et al. The utility of a 5-in-6 double catheter technique in treating complex coronary lesions via transradial approach: the DOCA-TRI study. *Eurointervention.* 2012;8(7):848–854.

49. Kumar S, Gorog DA, Secco GG, et al. The GuideLiner "child" catheter for percutaneous coronary intervention—early clinical experience. *J Invasive Cardiol.* 2010;22(10): 495–498.

50. Pershad A, Sein V, Laufer N. GuideLiner catheter facilitated PCI—a novel device with multiple applications. *J Invasive Cardiol.* 2011;23(11):E254–E259.

51. Lee NH, Suh J, Seo HS. Double anchoring balloon technique for recanalization of coronary chronic total occlusion by retrograde approach. *Catheter Cardiovasc Interv.* 2009;73(6):791–794.

52. Fang HY, Wu CC, Wu CJ. Successful transradial antegrade coronary intervention of a rare right coronary artery high anterior downward takeoff anomalous chronic total occlusion by double-anchoring technique and retrograde guidance. *Int Heart J.* 2009;50(4):531–538.

53. Aeby G, Surmely JF, Togni M, et al. A modified technique of balloon anchoring for tricky stent delivery. *Eurointervention.* 2013;8(9):1099–1102.

54. Pervaiz MH, Laham RJ. Distal anchoring technique: yet another weapon for successful intervention. *J Invasive Cardiol.* 2011;23(7):295–296.

55. Mahmood A, Banerjee S, Brilakis ES. Applications of the distal anchoring technique in coronary and peripheral interventions. *J Invasive Cardiol.* 2011;23(7):291–294.

56. Banerjee S, Brilakis ES. Use of the Proxis embolic protection device for guide anchoring and stent delivery during complex saphenous vein graft interventions. *Cardiovasc Revasc Med.* 2009;10(3):183–187.

57. Ashikaga T, Nishizaki M, Yamawake N. Difficult stent delivery: use of an aspiration catheter as a "sheath." *Catheter Cardiovasc Interv.* 2008;71(7):909–912.

58. Kim JY, Lee SH, Choe HM, et al. The feasibility of percutaneous transradial coronary intervention for chronic total occlusion. *Yonsei Med J.* 2006;47(5):680–687.

59. Yang CH, Guo GB, Chen SM, et al. Feasibility and safety of a transradial approach in intervention for chronic total

occlusion of coronary arteries: a single-center experience. *Chang Gung Med J*. 2010;33(6):639–645.

60. Liu W, Wagatsuma K, Toda M, et al. Short- and long-term follow-up of percutaneous coronary intervention for chronic total occlusion through transradial approach: tips for successful procedure from a single-center experience. *J Interv Cardiol*. 2011;24(2):137–143.

61. Wu CJ, Fang HY, Cheng CI, et al. The safety and feasibility of bilateral radial approach in chronic total occlusion percutaneous coronary intervention. *Int Heart J*. 2011; 52(3):131–138.

62. Rinfret S, Joyal D, Nguyen CM, et al. Retrograde recanalization of chronic total occlusions from the transradial approach; early Canadian experience. *Catheter Cardiovasc Interv*. 2011;78(3):366–374.

63. Rathore S, Hakeem A, Pauriah M, et al. A comparison of the transradial and the transfemoral approach in chronic total occlusion percutaneous coronary intervention. *Catheter Cardiovasc Interv*. 2009;73(7):883–887.

64. Masutani M, Yoshimachi F, Matsukage T, et al. Use of slender catheters for transradial angiography and interventions [Review]. *Indian Heart J*. 2008;60(1 suppl A):A22–A26.

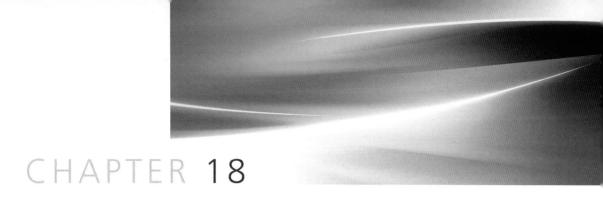

CHAPTER 18

Radial Approach and Complex Coronary Interventions: Bifurcations

Vladimír Džavík and Nicholas Collins

Introduction

Intervention of bifurcation lesions occurs in up to 20% of all percutaneous coronary intervention (PCI) procedures.[1,2] Bifurcation lesions continue to pose a challenge to the interventional cardiologist. In this chapter, we briefly review the history of bifurcation PCI, and describe the techniques that have been devised in an effort to optimize patient outcomes, current trends, and issues specific to the transradial approach.

The difficulty that side-branch involvement posed to the safety of PCI was recognized soon after the advent of the procedure. Meier et al.[3] reported the potential for compromise of a side branch in more than half of the patients undergoing balloon angioplasty. Attempts to reduce periprocedural side-branch occlusion by protecting the side branch with a guidewire, and later, by the use of sequential balloon inflations, reduced this risk; however, abrupt closure continued to occur not infrequently and restenosis rates remained high.[4,5]

The introduction of bare-metal stents brought the risk of postprocedural abrupt closure to an acceptable level. Colombo et al.[6] were the first to report the use of two stents with a kissing or modified T-stent approach to treat a coronary bifurcation lesion. A true T-stenting technique using the Wiktor tantalum stent was reported in a rescue procedure to treat a severe dissection of the main vessel and side branch.[7] A Y-stenting technique was developed in which stents were deployed in both branches and then a third stent in the proximal main vessel.[8,9] Other variations included the V-stent technique[10] and trouser technique in which a stent was bent at the hinge point and the two stent segments were then deployed on two balloons into the two branch vessels.[11] The trouser configuration was then completed by deploying a third stent in the proximal vessel. The culotte technique, also developed in the bare-metal stent era,[12] was subsequently found to be associated with a very high major adverse cardiac event (MACE) rate[13] and was abandoned, only to be rediscovered in the drug-eluting stent era. The specific procedural aspects of this technique and relevance to the radial approach are outlined in further detail later in this chapter.

Outcomes after bare-metal bifurcation stenting were underwhelming, with reported MACE rates as high as 53% after stenting of both the main vessel as well as the side branch, and 38% following stenting of the main vessel only.[14] Slightly better outcomes were reported by Lefevre et al.[15] after systematic adoption of the final kissing balloon inflation. Utilizing primarily 6F guiding catheters and the radial approach, these investigators deployed a stent in the side branch in 59.5% of cases by means of T-stenting techniques. MACE and target vessel revascularization (TVR) rates at 7 months, 29.2% and 20.6%, respectively, in a group of patients treated in the first period from January 1996 to August 1997 decreased to 17.1% and 13.8% from September 1997 to November 1998 when final kissing balloon inflation was utilized routinely.

The main challenge in achieving satisfactory long-term clinical outcomes was to reduce the very high rates of restenosis observed after bifurcation treatment with bare-metal stents, especially when two-stent techniques were utilized. The excitement generated by the results of the first drug-eluting stent trials over a decade ago[16] resulted in rapid adoption of this new technology to the treatment of patients with bifurcation disease. The problem with T-stenting rested on the fact that the majority of nonleft main bifurcation lesions are acute-angle bifurcations when measured along an axis that follows the proximal main vessel and the take-off of the side branch (Fig. 18-1). In an acute-angle or Y-bifurcation, a stent positioned at the os-tium of the side branch in a T-stenting procedure would either fail to cover the proximal segment of the ostium or protrude into the main vessel.

As a solution to the problem, Colombo et al.[17] devised the crush technique. The necessity of per-forming the final kissing balloon inflation was em-phasized in a subsequent report of the San Rafaele Hospital crush-stenting registry experience, in which 25 of 65 (38.5%) patients without a final kiss-ing balloon inflation suffered a MACE compared to 23 of 116 (19.8%) patients in whom a final kiss-ing balloon inflation was performed.[18] Similarly, in a nonrandomized comparison of crush versus T-stenting, the group reported better 1-year tar-get lesion revascularization (TLR)-free survival in patients treated with the crush technique (86.0% vs 68.9%, $P = 0.005$); however, crush-treated pa-tients who did not undergo a kissing balloon inflation had poor outcomes, with 34.1% experi-encing angiographic restenosis in the side branch at 6 months compared to 8.6% of those treated with a final kissing balloon inflation ($P < 0.001$).[19]

While the crush technique seemed to ensure full coverage of the side-branch ostium, it was apparent from the data that in order to optimize clinical success, a final kissing balloon inflation was indeed necessary, and this task was far from simple. Predilation of the crushed stent mass with the smallest, lowest-profile balloons was often re-quired before the stent could be recrossed with the larger-caliber balloon needed to adequately appose the struts against the side-branch ostium. Most certainly, the use of this technique markedly increased procedural and fluoroscopic times, and contrast volume compared with the simpler single main vessel stent or provisional approach.[1,20,21]

Other groups have subsequently modified the crush technique to reduce the complexity of the side-branch recrossing and to ensure a better stent apposition result from the final kissing bal-loon inflation.[22,23] These techniques evolved, in part, from the need to modify bifurcation PCI to allow for radial artery access and are elaborated on further subsequently.

Another approach to stenting both the main vessel and the side branch, described by Sharma et al.,[24] involved the simultaneous deployment of two stents in the main vessel and the side branch, with the creation of a metal "neocarina" in the proximal main vessel. Owing to persisting high rates of MACE during mid- and long-term follow-up, this technique has generally fallen out of favor as a default strategy in the treatment of bifurcation lesions; however, as it is quite easy to perform, it may be a reasonable strategy for some

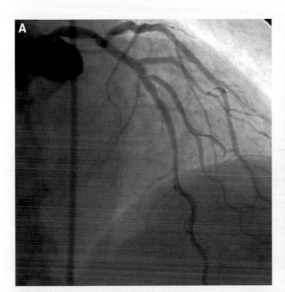
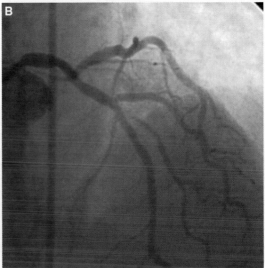

FIGURE 18-1 Angiography demonstrating acute bifurcation angle between left anterior descending and diagonal branch arteries; this anatomy is unlikely to be adequately treated with T-stent technique, with a provisional stent technique preferred, given the small caliber of the side branch and the minimal extent of disease into the side-branch vessel.

high-risk patients, particularly those with left main bifurcations.

A technique that in the drug-eluting stent era has found much better success is the culotte technique. The technique has been validated in the Nordic-2 trial, a randomized comparison of the culotte and crush techniques.[25] Of 424 patients enrolled in the trial, 209 patients were randomized to crush and 215 to culotte. MACE occurred in 4.3% of the patients in the crush group and 3.7% of those in the culotte group ($P = 0.87$). In-stent restenosis in the side branch occurred less frequently in the culotte group (9.8% vs 3.8%, $P = 0.04$).

Given the complexities acknowledged with the use of standard stent therapies in the treatment of bifurcation lesions, interest in novel, dedicated stent platforms to treat both main vessel and side branch subsequently emerged. The initially available platforms were designed to treat the main vessel and to simultaneously allow ongoing access to the side branch through an aperture in the main vessel stent, thus maintaining access to the side branch without the need to rewire through stent struts. The first dedicated stent platform using this approach was the Frontier stent (Guidant Medical, Indianapolis, IN), which, although initially demonstrated to be safe and feasible in clinical trials,[26] including from the radial approach,[27] was limited by difficulties with device delivery and complexity of use. Although several dedicated bifurcation stents have been evaluated in clinical trials, none has clearly demonstrated superiority. The AXXESS self-expanding biolimus-coated stent (Biosensors International, Switzerland) is specifically designed to be placed in the proximal main vessel precisely at the carina before implanting a further two stents into each of the main vessel and side branch. The concept of this device is for the AXXESS stent to conform to the proximal vessel, ensuring stent coverage to the point of the bifurcation carina, with stents then placed in the side branch to cover the ongoing vessels. These dedicated bifurcation stents can be used from the radial approach, as the majority of those in development may be used through a 6F or 7F guide catheter. An inherent limitation in the development of such technology is the variability in bifurcation anatomy, with differences in vessel caliber, extent of disease, and bifurcation angle, meaning a single device type is unlikely to be able to meet the requirements of every anatomical variant.

As the two-stent techniques proliferated, many operators questioned the two-stent approach as a default strategy for patients needing intervention of bifurcation lesions. The Nordic Bifurcation Study randomized 413 patients to the simple or two-stent approach.[21] The crush and culotte techniques were utilized in the majority of patients randomized to the two-stent approach. No difference between the groups was observed in the occurrence of MACE at 6 months, while the two-stent technique was associated with significantly longer procedural and fluoroscopy times, as well as larger volumes of contrast used. The authors concluded that the provisional strategy should remain the preferred method for the majority of patients undergoing bifurcation stenting. In 2010, the British Bifurcation Coronary (BBC) Study investigators reported similar results.[20] In a patient-level pooled analysis that included all 910 patients enrolled in these two studies, Behan et al.[28] found a highly significant difference between the simple and complex approaches in the occurrence of MACE at 9 months (10.1% vs 17.3%, $P = 0.001$). Subgroup analyses of patients with true bifurcations only, those with large side branches, at least 2.75 mm in diameter, side-branch lesions at least 5 mm long, similarly revealed better outcomes with the simple, provisional stenting technique. While Nordic and BBC-1 thus appear to provide strong support for the preferential use of the provisional approach in most bifurcation procedures, the techniques utilized in the complex group of both studies resulted in suboptimal treatment in that treatment group. The final kissing balloon inflation, the key final step in any two-stent bifurcation technique, was performed in only 75% of patients, undoubtedly as a result of the inherent difficulty in performing this step with the original single-step crush technique, noting the subsequent advent of techniques designed to optimize the likelihood of final kissing inflation.

Nonetheless, the preferred approach for the majority of bifurcation interventions remains the provisional approach.[29,30] Considerable research has been done to optimize the results of the provisional or planned one-stent approach. As a result, outcomes associated with this simple approach have improved considerably over the years. These refinements are discussed in subsequent sections.

Adaptation of Bifurcation Techniques to the Transradial Approach

Greater operator familiarity with the radial artery approach now allows for the performance of complex bifurcation PCI. It is now possible to perform bifurcation PCI from the radial artery access site using provisional strategy, as well as the various complex, two-stent procedures. The radial artery approach is ideally suited for complex bifurcation PCI, given the need to balance the risks of bleeding complications and associated deleterious effects on outcome and the need for aggressive antiplatelet therapy, often using glycoprotein IIb/IIIa inhibitors, especially when employing a two-stent strategy.[31] Today, it is imperative that the bifurcation strategy be planned in advance considering all details of the anatomy of the bifurcation lesions.

Bifurcation PCI, particularly when utilizing a complex, two-stent strategy, is associated with longer procedural duration, higher volumes of contrast, and prolonged radiation exposure.[21,32-34] As previous data have demonstrated that radial artery access may be associated with similar adverse characteristics in terms of procedural duration, contrast dose, and radiation exposure,[33,35] the cumulative effects of these issues should be an important consideration before proceeding to bifurcation PCI from the radial access site. Consideration of a staged procedure is appropriate when a complex intervention is planned after diagnostic angiography, given the potential for contrast nephropathy.

An important limitation of the radial artery approach is the radial artery size, which is more problematic in the older, female population.[36] While the use of smaller-caliber guide catheters, such as 5F guides (see Chapter 8), has improved the feasibility of PCI from the radial approach, the use of smaller-caliber guide catheters may have important implications in terms of procedural ease and success. The smaller internal diameter precludes simultaneous delivery of intravascular devices when performing complex bifurcation PCI. This may involve delivery of multiple stents or balloons to both the main vessel and the side branch, with final kissing inflation imperative when using complex techniques such as the crush or culotte technique. Rewiring of the side branch in order to complete final kissing inflation may be problematic in any bifurcation strategy and result in excess contrast exposure; the use of dedicated microcatheters designed to facilitate side-branch access, such as the Crusade microcatheter (Kaneka Medical Products, Osaka, Japan), may be beneficial in these situations.[37] When using a simple strategy of main vessel stenting alone, the presence of disease within the side branch may also require final kissing balloon inflation in order to optimize results and reduce the risk of restenosis at the side-branch ostium.[38] With current guiding catheters available outside

Japan, if the operator considers performing kissing techniques, then a $\geq$6F is required.

The use of smaller-caliber guide catheters may also result in inadequate backup, which may be critical in terms of the ability to deliver devices to the target lesion. Such difficulties may be minimized by the use of guide catheters that provide optimal support, such as Amplatz curve and extra backup (e.g., XB [Cordis, Bridgewater, NJ], EBU [Medtronic, Minneapolis, MN]) guides. Additional support may be provided by the use of larger-caliber guides, noting the importance of guide caliber in providing adequate support. Standard large-caliber guide catheters, such as 7F and 8F guides, may be used from the radial approach in selected patients in centers with considerable radial artery access experience.[39] The development of sheathless guide catheters (such as the Eaucath [Asahi Intecc, Tokyo, Japan]) has further improved the ability of operators to utilize large-caliber guide catheters[40] (see Chapter 20). These devices may improve procedural success, without increasing the risk of radial artery injury; however, larger-caliber guides may predispose to ostial vessel dissection and increased contrast volumes.[41] The use of traditional guide catheters without a standard introducing vascular sheath has recently been described and may also overcome the limitations of radial artery size in allowing larger-caliber guides.[42] Additional techniques to improve backup and ensure delivery of devices in complex procedures include the use of anchor balloons, buddy wires, and internal guide catheter extension tools such as the Guideliner (Vascular Solutions, Minneapolis, MN) and Heartrail (Terumo, Somerset, NJ) systems.[43-45]

Complex strategies in bifurcation PCI amplify the limitations seen in PCI from the radial approach. Randomized data have confirmed the additional contrast load, radiation exposure, and increased periprocedural complications in complex strategies compared to main vessel stenting alone[21,34] without offering clinical advantages.[46,47] As outlined, the extent of disease in, and the vessel caliber of, the side branch may, however, necessitate a two-stent strategy. The decision as to which complex approach to utilize may depend on the relative size of the side branch compared to the proximal and distal main vessel. An important caveat when considering a two-stent strategy is the inferior results seen when performing left main PCI. While left main PCI is feasible from the radial approach, complex strategies when applied to left main lesions are consistently disappointing.[9,48,49] Additional factors influencing the technique used will include appreciation of the bifurcation angle, which is an important predictor of outcome when using complex bifurcation PCI techniques; this may influence the type of approach should a two-stent strategy be considered.[1,50]

The Single-Stent or Provisional Approach

As we discussed earlier, the single or provisional approach is widely regarded as the preferred approach for the majority of bifurcation lesions. The provisional stenting approach is ideally suited to the transradial approach. In terms of guide catheter size, it is possible to perform a simple bifurcation intervention with a 5F guide catheter, deploying devices with a second wire in the side branch. Smaller guide catheters, however, may not be suitable in cases requiring more complex side-branch management should this vessel become compromised. This should be kept in mind if the operator plans to use a 5F guide catheter.

In general, a side branch that we would consider as supplying significant myocardial territory should be protected with a wire. The exception to this recommendation might be a side branch without ostial disease in a T-bifurcation (bifurcation angle >70°) that is very unlikely to be occluded after main vessel stenting and may be problematic to wire, exposing the risk of ostial vessel dissection. There is little downside to protecting any other type of side branch and much to be gained in case of significant narrowing after deployment of the main vessel stent that could result in occlusion of the branch. In such cases, the wire will serve two important purposes. First, it will serve as a directional guide to recrossing with another wire. Second, it will serve as a scaffold to maintain some degree of patency in the side-branch origin. If the side-branch ostium is compromised, the side branch should be recrossed and dilated, expanding the struts to open the cell and thus side-branch ostium. The recrossing of the side branch is facilitated by first performing the proximal optimization technique (POT).[51] This is accomplished by inflating a balloon in the proximal main vessel with a balloon, the distal tip of which is positioned at the bifurcation. Inflation of this larger balloon in this position results in an angled approach to the side branch that will facilitate reentry through the struts into the side branch (Fig. 18-2) and will minimize the possibility of the new guidewire advancing underneath the proximal stent struts. The recrossing of the side branch should be at the level of the distal-most struts overlying the side-branch ostium. Distal recrossing results in the least stent

distortion in the main vessel, and creates a "flap" of stent material that can serve as a scaffold for the proximal wall of the side-branch ostium (Fig. 18-3). Once the side branch is recrossed, a noncompliant balloon of a diameter appropriate for the branch should be positioned covering the diseased ostial tissue and into a normal segment. A second noncompliant balloon should be positioned in the main vessel, and the proximal markers of the two balloons should then be aligned, ensuring that they are within the stented segment. The side branch should be dilated first to ensure optimal opening of the stent struts at the side-branch ostium. A kissing balloon inflation should then be performed. If the flow is TIMI 3 and no significant dissection is observed, the procedure is then completed. Interestingly, Sgueglia et al.[52] have recently shown that kissing balloon techniques could be performed with drug-eluting balloons using the transradial approach.

If side-branch compromise persists, a suitable two-stent technique should then be performed. The techniques that can be utilized are T-stent, TAP (T and protrude), or culotte, depending on the bifurcation angle and size of the side branch relative to the proximal main vessel.[29] All of these techniques are easily suited to the transradial approach utilizing 6F guides. We will discuss them further with respect to considerations specific to this access in upcoming sections.

The Culotte Technique

The culotte technique is an elegant bifurcation strategy when the side branch is considered to require stent implantation, with documented superiority when compared to the crush and other two-stent techniques.[1,25] This technique ensures that complete coverage of the side-branch ostium, however, is limited by two layers of stent in the proximal main vessel. As this technique requires sequential delivery of (drug-eluting) stents, it is ideally suited to the radial approach, with the final kissing balloon inflation the only component requiring simultaneous delivery of multiple devices. In terms of preprocedural evaluation, the culotte technique may be considered when the side branch is similar in caliber to the proximal and distal main vessel with significant disease in the side branch beyond the ostium. A low bifurcation angle and moderate distal vessel size (>3 mm diameter) will favor an optimal outcome in terms of subsequent events.[1]

Following predilatation of the main vessel and side branch, the first stent is positioned, typically

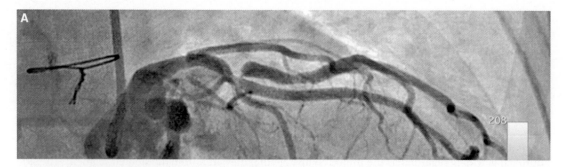

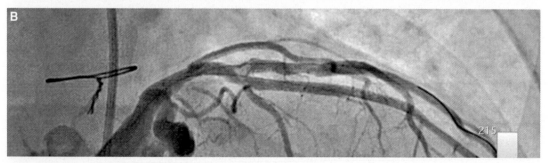

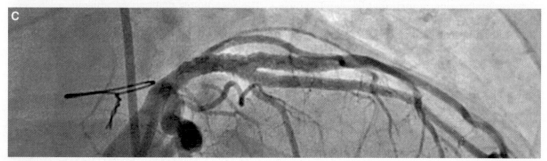

FIGURE 18-2 **A:** Complex percutaneous intervention of bifurcation stenosis involving origin of large-caliber diagonal branch using the POT. **B:** Following deployment of main vessel stent, the stented segment immediately proximal to the diagonal branch ostium is postdilated; note the increased caliber of the main vessel stent immediately before the diagonal ostium. This technique facilitates wire passage into the diagonal branch. **C:** Final angiographic result following final kissing inflation.

in the distal vessel with the greatest angulation (usually the side branch). As difficulty is usually encountered when positioning the second stent through the stent struts of the previously deployed stent, reducing the degree of angulation may facilitate the delivery of the second stent. After the first stent is deployed, jailing the main vessel wire (which may act as a guide for subsequent rewiring through the struts of the first stent into the distal vessel), the side-branch wire is removed. After opening the stent struts using a small-diameter compliant balloon following rewiring, the second stent is placed distally in the main vessel and deployed after removal of both the jailed and side-branch wire, resulting in the two layers of stent in the proximal, main vessel. The side branch is then

rewired with the aim of completing the procedure with a final kissing balloon inflation.

The Crush Technique Modifications

While the crush technique was devised to allow ongoing access to the main vessel after stent delivery in the side branch, it is now acknowledged to not offer any advantage in bifurcation PCI when compared to either a simple, provisional strategy or indeed the culotte technique when complex approaches are considered.[21,25,34,47] The predominant limitation of this technique relates to the consequences of excess stent material at

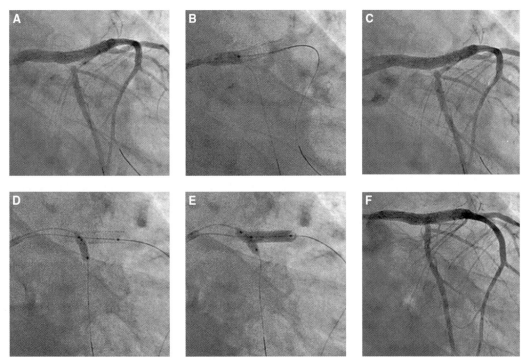

FIGURE 18-3   **A:** Suboptimal result in side-branch ostium following main vessel stent deployment. **B:** POT with postdilation in the main vessel immediately proximal to the side-branch ostium to facilitate rewiring of the side branch. **C:** Side branch is successfully rewired, aiming to pass the wire through the most distal stent strut to optimize side-branch coverage when a single-stent strategy is used. **D:** Initial dilatation of side branch using appropriate caliber noncompliant balloon. **E:** Final kissing balloon inflation. **F:** Final angiographic result.

the side-branch ostium, which acts as a nidus for stent thrombosis and in-stent restenosis.[53]

As originally described, the crush technique required positioning of a stent in both the main vessel and side branch following appropriate predilatation. The proximal side-branch stent is left protruding into the main vessel and then deployed; after ensuring there is no distal edge dissection, the side-branch wire is removed and the main vessel stent deployed, "crushing" the component of the side-branch stent protruding into the main vessel. Subsequent iterations of this technique have focused on leaving a minimal amount of side-branch stent material in the main vessel, which limits the amount of stent material at the carina (the so-called modified mini crush).[54] After main vessel stent deployment, the side branch is rewired and the procedure completed with a final kissing balloon inflation. It was quickly recognized that the propensity to side-branch ostium restenosis could be limited by high-pressure inflation in the side branch (16 atm), followed by final kissing balloon inflation.[55,56] In order to achieve optimal results with this complex technique, adequate final kissing balloon inflation is critical.

The original technique required large-caliber guide catheters to permit simultaneous delivery of two stents; the crush technique was then modified to allow radial access by employing a "balloon crush" technique, whereby the side-branch stent was "crushed" using a balloon (rather than a stent) positioned in the main vessel after the removal of the side-branch wire, followed by delivery of a stent in the main vessel. This technique has been further modified with a view to improving side-branch results and to facilitate rewiring of the side branch; wiring through both the main vessel stent and crushed component of the side-branch stent is potentially problematic, with implications in terms of contrast volume and procedural duration. Rewiring of the side branch after side-branch stent deployment and before main vessel stenting is typically more straightforward and allows for balloon dilation of the side-branch ostium, either alone or with a kissing balloon inflation (the so-called DK crush) to optimize the result at the carina.[23,57] The main vessel stent is then deployed after the removal of the side-branch wire; subsequent wiring into the side branch before completing the procedure with a final kissing inflation is more straight-forward through the single layer of main vessel stent struts. In our initial modified balloon crush technique, we did not perform a kissing balloon inflation (DK crush) prior to main vessel stent deployment[23]; however, as Chen et al.[22,58] pointed out, dilating the side-branch stent through the crushed struts alone can result in protrusion of the struts into the main vessel that may create difficulty in advancing the main vessel stent. The strut protrusion can be modified either by a kissing inflation or a second crush. Our own preference has been for the second crush, which ensures that the protruding struts are completely compressed against the main vessel wall. In performing this modification, the final kissing balloon success rate approaches 100%.[59]

While previous randomized data have suggested the crush technique to be inferior to single-stent strategies, Chen et al.[57] reported the results of a randomized trial comparing the DK crush with the provisional stenting approach in 370 patients undergoing bifurcation PCI. The final kissing balloon inflation rate in the DK-crush group was 100%. The DK-crush technique ensures success in performing the kissing balloon inflation, since the crushed side-branch stent is recrossed prior to the deployment of the main vessel stent, thus eliminating the need to cross three stent layers. When a high-pressure inflation is performed at the ostium prior to the kissing balloon inflation, the technique also ensures optimal apposition of the struts against the wall of the ostium of the side branch. Chen et al.[60] demonstrated a lower MACE rate compared to the classic crush technique at 2 years (11.4% vs 24.4%, $P = 0.03$) and better 1-year TLR-free survival in patients randomized to DK crush compared to the provisional side-branch stenting approach (95.7% vs 85.0%, $P = 0.003$).[57] While these modifications add additional steps in the procedure, they potentially limit difficulties associated with side-branch access by avoiding wiring into the side branch through multiple layers of stent.

The group from FuWai hospital has reported a large series of patients undergoing complex two-stent bifurcation PCI (mostly using crush techniques) by radial or femoral approach.[61] They reviewed their experience from 2004 to 2009 in 805 consecutive patients. Of note, 6F guiding catheters were used more often in the radial group. Bifurcation lesions involved quite large vessels as the mean stent size was >3.2 mm for the main branches and >2.8 mm for the side branches. Procedure and fluoroscopy times remained similar in both the groups, but the contrast volume was significantly less in the radial group. During hospitalization, there was significantly less BARC bleeding with the radial approach than with the femoral approach (3.9% vs 9.1%, $P < 0.01$), although BARC bleeding ≥3 were similar in both the groups. During late follow-up, MACE remained similar in both the groups, even after adjustment by propensity score.

T-stenting Techniques

The T-stent approach has been limited in the past due to an inability to adequately cover the side-branch ostium in cases of acute side-branch angulation. Indeed, optimal results for this technique as traditionally performed have been shown when the bifurcation angle approaches 90° (Fig. 18-4).[1] The T-stenting technique has since been adapted for acute-angle bifurcations in the TAP modification, which may be utilized from the radial access approach.[62] In this approach, the main vessel and side branch are predilated, and a stent is deployed in the main vessel, trapping the side-branch wire. The side branch is then recrossed with a third wire, and the jailed wire is removed. With a balloon positioned in the side branch through the main vessel stent struts and another in the main vessel, a kissing balloon inflation is then performed. A stent is then maneuvered into the side branch such that the proximal edge is positioned at the ostium, leaving the distal edge protruding into the main vessel. A balloon is also positioned in the main vessel to cover the side branch. The stent is deployed and a kissing balloon inflation is performed, leaving a neocarina consisting of the single layer of the proximal portion of the side-branch stent. Depending on the angle of the bifurcation, the length of this neocarina could approach the diameter of the side-branch stent. Timing of the deflation ending the kissing balloon inflation is critical. That is, deflation of the two balloons must occur simultaneously, or the neocarina will shift away from the balloon that is deflated last, potentially protruding excessively either into the main vessel or into the side branch, potentially creating a nidus for stent thrombosis.

Stent/Simultaneous Kissing Stent Techniques

Both the V-stent and the simultaneous kissing stent (SKS) techniques involve positioning of a stent in both the main vessel and the side branch before simultaneous stent deployment.[24,63] The key difference between the strategies involves the extent of proximal stent contact creating the neocarina. In the V-stent technique, there is minimal proximal stent contact, where the SKS approach

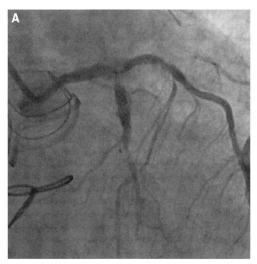
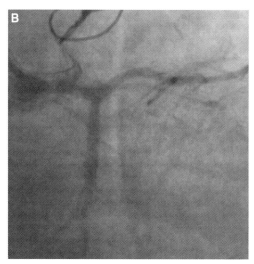

FIGURE 18-4 A: Complex distal left main stenosis (Medina classification 1,1,1) involving ostium of the left anterior and left circumflex coronary arteries in a patient with a background of previous coronary artery bypass surgery and biprosthetic aortic valve replacement; the left internal mammary bypass graft to the left anterior descending coronary artery was noted to be atretic with the saphenous graft to the obtuse marginal branch occluded. Given the large bifurcation angle, approaching 90°, a T-stent approach was used from the right radial artery approach. **B:** Final angiographic result after deployment of drug-eluting stents. Initial stent placed at the ostium of the left circumflex coronary artery before stent positioning from the left main into proximal left anterior descending coronary artery. The procedure was completed with a final kissing balloon inflation.

requires the proximal stent components extend into the proximal parent vessel.[64] Until the development of sheathless guide catheters, these bifurcation techniques were almost exclusively performed from the femoral approach due to the need for 7F and 8F guide catheters. These techniques have the advantage of relative simplicity, compared to other two-stent strategies, and can be considered when the caliber of the proximal vessel is larger than the ongoing main vessel and side branch (ideally, the proximal main vessel should be two-third the size of the combined diameter of the distal vessels; Fig. 18-5). This approach is therefore potentially suited to left main PCI in a potentially unstable patient or when surgery is not an option.

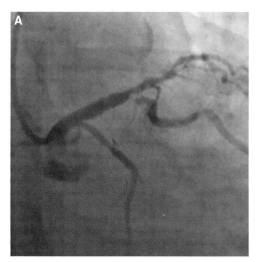
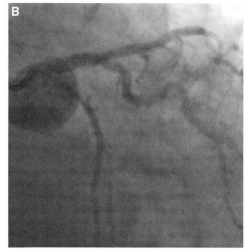

FIGURE 18-5 Bifurcation stenosis within proximal left anterior descending artery with severe stenosis at ostium of large-caliber diagonal branch (Medina classification 0,1,1). Given the disparate size of the proximal vessel compared to the distal left anterior descending and diagonal branch, a V-stent strategy was used, utilizing a sheathless guide (Eaucath, Asahi Intecc, Tokyo, Japan) to permit simultaneous delivery of two drug-eluting stents from the radial approach.

This procedure is limited due to the variable results as previously mentioned, which are certainly inferior to other two-stent strategies in some series.[1] Other difficulties relate to the approach in the event of proximal edge dissection, which may necessitate delivery of a further two stents in the proximal vessel, or a single large-caliber stent, which may not provide complete coverage of the vessel wall proximal to the neocarina. The formation of a neocarina may limit the long-term results as it may predispose to stent thrombosis and in-stent restenosis.

The technique requires wiring of both branches of the bifurcation and careful positioning of the two stents in each distal vessel, with care taken to ensure that the proximal stent edges are adjacent before stent employment to avoid unopposed proximal stent margins. After initial deployment to nominal pressures (8–10 atm), each stent is deployed sequentially to high pressure (up to 20 atm) before a final kissing inflation at nominal pressures once more. This sequence ensures optimal stent deployment and stent apposition at the neocarina.

While these techniques are now options from a radial approach perspective, they are limited in terms of long-term results, but may be suitable in certain clinical situations.[65]

The development of low-profile devices, advances in guide catheter technology, and improved understanding of the role of various bifurcation techniques now allow a radial artery approach to ven extremely complex anatomy. With increased operator experience, complex PCI, including bifurcation procedures, can be safely performed from the radial approach with excellent results.

More recently, the advent of bioresorbable vascular scaffolds (BVS; Abbot Vascular, Santa Clara, CA) has provided an alternate approach to contemporary PCI.[66,67] Given the potential advantages of the BVS restoration of vasomotor tone, no permanent metal in the vessel, and possibly duration of antiplatelet therapy, although currently one year is still recommended. These devices may have advantages in bifurcation PCI. While experience with the BVS in complex, two-stent strategies is limited, it appears that the BVS may be feasible in a variety of bifurcation PCI settings, including planned, complex two-stent procedures (Fig. 18-6), or as a "bail out" strategy in cases where the side-branch result is suboptimal.[66-68] While newer-generation

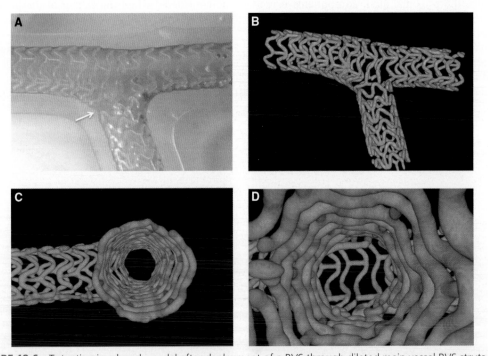

FIGURE 18-6 T-stenting in a bench model after deployment of a BVS through dilated main vessel BVS struts. **A:** After a final kissing balloon (FKB) with 3.0 × 20 and 2.5 × 20 mm balloons, inflated to at low pressures revealing optimal coverage without overlap and with scaffolding of the ostium of the side branch by the dilated main vessel BVS struts (*arrow*); **B:** a micro-CT image; **C:** optimal paving shown through the main vessel BVS lumen showing optimal paving; **D:** a well-scaffolded side-branch ostium shown through the side branch. (From Dzavik V, Colombo A. The absorb bioresorbable vascular scaffold in coronary bifurcations. *J Am Coll Cardiol Interv*. 2014;7(1):81–88.)

drug-eluting stents likely require shorter duration of dual antiplatelet therapy compared to earlier-generation devices,[69] information on duration in complex bifurcation procedures is lacking. As such, a shorter duration of dual antiplatelet therapy may be possible with BVS, reducing the inherent bleeding risks associated with prolonged treatment.

Conclusion

The evolution of bifurcation techniques has paralleled the rise in the transradial approach for PCI. While many operators continue to shy away from the transradial approach when planning intervention of complex bifurcation lesions due to the perceived need for large-caliber guiding catheters, most bifurcation interventions can be performed easily and effectively via the transradial approach, with the use of 6F guides. Thus, operators adopting the transradial approach do not need to revert to the transfemoral route, in this way retaining the benefits of the transradial approach for this considerable patient group undergoing complex coronary intervention.

REFERENCES

1. Collins N, et al. Long-term outcomes after percutaneous coronary intervention of bifurcation narrowings. *Am J Cardiol.* 2008;102(4):404–410.
2. Stankovic G, et al. Percutaneous coronary intervention for bifurcation lesions: 2008 consensus document from the fourth meeting of the European Bifurcation Club. *EuroIntervention.* 2009;5(1):39–49.
3. Meier B, et al. Risk of side branch occlusion during coronary angioplasty. *Am J Cardiol.* 1984;53(1):10–14.
4. Renkin J, et al. Angioplasty of coronary bifurcation stenoses: immediate and long-term results of the protecting branch technique. *Cathet Cardiovasc Diagn.* 1991;22(3):167–173.
5. Weinstein JS, et al. Salvage of branch vessels during bifurcation lesion angioplasty: acute and long-term follow-up. *Cathet Cardiovasc Diagn.* 1991;22(1):1–6.
6. Colombo A, et al., "Kissing" stents for bifurcational coronary lesion. *Cathet Cardiovasc Diagn.* 1993;30(4):327–330.
7. Mylotte D, et al. Non-compliant balloons for final kissing inflation in coronary bifurcation lesions treated with provisional side branch stenting: a pilot study. *EuroIntervention.* 2012;7(10):1162–1169.
8. Fort S, Lazzam C, Schwartz L. Coronary "Y" stenting: a technique for angioplasty of bifurcation stenoses. *Can J Cardiol.* 1996;12(7):678–682.
9. Lee MS, et al. Percutaneous coronary intervention of unprotected left main coronary artery disease: procedural strategies and technical considerations. *Catheter Cardiovasc Interv.* 2012;79(5):812–822.
10. Schampaert E, et al. The V-stent: a novel technique for coronary bifurcation stenting. *Cathet Cardiovasc Diagn.* 1996;39(3):320–326.
11. Khoja A, et al. Trouser-like stenting: a new technique for bifurcation lesions. *Cathet Cardiovasc Diagn.* 1997;41(2):192–196; discussion 197–199.
12. Chevalier B, et al. Placement of coronary stents in bifurcation lesions by the "culotte" technique. *Am J Cardiol.* 1998;82(8):943–949.
13. Al Suwaidi J, et al. Immediate and long-term outcome of intracoronary stent implantation for true bifurcation lesions. *J Am Coll Cardiol.* 2000;35(4):929–936.
14. Yamashita T, et al. Bifurcation lesions: two stents versus one stent—immediate and follow-up results. *J Am Coll Cardiol.* 2000;35(5):1145–1151.
15. Lefevre T, et al. Stenting of bifurcation lesions: classification, treatments, and results. *Catheter Cardiovasc Interv.* 2000;49(3):274–283.
16. Morice MC, et al. A randomized comparison of a sirolimus-eluting stent with a standard stent for coronary revascularization. *N Engl J Med.* 2002;346(23):1773–1780.
17. Colombo A, et al. Modified T-stenting technique with crushing for bifurcation lesions: immediate results and 30-day outcome. *Catheter Cardiovasc Interv.* 2003;60(2):145–151.
18. Ge L, et al. Clinical and angiographic outcome after implantation of drug-eluting stents in bifurcation lesions with the crush stent technique: importance of final kissing balloon post-dilation. *J Am Coll Cardiol.* 2005;46(4):613–620.
19. Ge L, et al. Treatment bifurcation lesions with two stents: crush versus T stenting—one year angiographic and clinical follow-up. *Heart.* 2006;92(3):371–376.
20. Hildick-Smith D, et al. Randomized trial of simple versus complex drug-eluting stenting for bifurcation lesions. The British bifurcation coronary study: old, new, and evolving strategies. *Circulation.* 2010;121:1235–1243.
21. Steigen TK, et al. Randomized study on simple versus complex stenting of coronary artery bifurcation lesions: the Nordic bifurcation study. *Circulation.* 2006;114(18):1955–1961.
22. Chen SL, et al. DK crush technique: modified treatment of bifurcation lesions in coronary artery. *Chin Med J* (Engl). 2005;118(20):1746–1750.
23. Collins N, Dzavik V. A modified balloon crush approach improves side branch access and side branch stent apposition during crush stenting of coronary bifurcation lesions. *Catheter Cardiovasc Interv.* 2006;68(3):365–371.
24. Sharma SK, et al. Simultaneous kissing stents (SKS) technique for treating bifurcation lesions in medium-to-large size coronary arteries. *Am J Cardiol.* 2004;94(7):913–917.
25. Erglis A, et al. Randomized comparison of coronary bifurcation stenting with the crush versus the culotte technique using sirolimus eluting stents: the Nordic stent technique study. *Circ Cardiovasc Interv.* 2009;2(1)27–34.
26. Lefevre T, et al. The Frontier stent registry: safety and feasibility of a novel dedicated stent for the treatment of bifurcation coronary artery lesions. *J Am Coll Cardiol.* 2005;46(4):592–598.
27. Aziz S, Morris JL. Transradial treatment of bifurcation coronary disease using the multi-link Frontier bifurcation stent system. *J Invasive Cardiol.* 2005;17(10):E1–E3.
28. Behan MW, et al. Simple or complex stenting for bifurcation coronary lesions: a patient-level pooled-analysis of the Nordic Bifurcation Study and the British Bifurcation Coronary Study. *Circ Cardiovasc Interv.* 2011;4(1):57–64.
29. Stankovic G, et al. Percutaneous coronary intervention for bifurcation lesions: 2008 consensus document from the fourth meeting of the European Bifurcation Club. *EuroIntervention.* 2009;5(1):39–49.
30. Nguyen T, et al. Editorial: at the bifurcation of the last frontiers. *J Interv Cardiol.* 2010;23(4):293–294.
31. Nathan S, Rao SV. Radial versus femoral access for percutaneous coronary intervention: implications for vascular complications and bleeding. *Curr Cardiol Rep.* 2012;14(4):502–509.
32. Tsapaki V, et al. Factors that influence radiation dose in percutaneous coronary intervention. *J Interv Cardiol.* 2006;19(3):237–244.

33. Mercuri M, et al. Predictors of increased radiation dose during percutaneous coronary intervention. *Am J Cardiol.* 2009;104(9):1241–1244.

34. Hildick-Smith D, et al. Randomized trial of simple versus complex drug-eluting stenting for bifurcation lesions: the British Bifurcation Coronary Study: old, new, and evolving strategies. *Circulation.* 2010;121(10):1235–1243.

35. Neill J, et al. Comparison of radiation dose and the effect of operator experience in femoral and radial arterial access for coronary procedures. *Am J Cardiol.* 2010;106(7):936–940.

36. Kotowycz MA, Dzavik V. Radial artery patency after transradial catheterization. *Circ Cardiovasc Interv.* 2012;5(1):127–133.

37. Abdou SM, Wu CJ. Stent malapposition caused by improper rewiring during left main intervention: the role of intravascular ultrasound in avoidance and management—a case report. *Catheter Cardiovasc Interv.* 2011;77(6):785–789.

38. Niemela M, et al. Randomized comparison of final kissing balloon dilatation versus no final kissing balloon dilatation in patients with coronary bifurcation lesions treated with main vessel stenting: the Nordic-Baltic Bifurcation Study III. *Circulation.* 2011;123(1):79–86.

39. Coroleu SF, et al. Feasibility of complex coronary and peripheral interventions by trans-radial approach using large sheaths. *Catheter Cardiovasc Interv.* 2012;79(4):597–600.

40. From AM, et al. Sheathless transradial intervention using standard guide catheters. *Catheter Cardiovasc Interv.* 2010;76(7):911–916.

41. Juergens CP, et al. Comparison of 6 and 7 French guiding catheters for percutaneous coronary intervention: results of a randomised trial with a vascular ultrasound endpoint. *Catheter Cardiovasc Interv.* 2005;66(4):528–534.

42. Kwan TW, et al. Feasibility and safety of 7F sheathless guiding catheter during transradial coronary intervention. *Catheter Cardiovasc Interv.* 2012;80(2):274–280.

43. Hynes B, et al. Enhancing back-up support during difficult coronary stent delivery: single-center case series of experience with the Heartrail II catheter. *J Invasive Cardiol.* 2011;23(3):E43–E46.

44. Hiwatashi A, et al. PCI using a 4-Fr "child" guide catheter in a "mother" guide catheter: Kyushu KIWAMI(R) ST registry. *Catheter Cardiovasc Interv.* 2010;76(7):919–923.

45. Takeshita S, Takagi A, Saito S. Backup support of the mother-child technique: technical considerations for the size of the mother guiding catheter. *Catheter Cardiovasc Interv.* 2012;80(2):292–297.

46. Pan M, et al. Rapamycin-eluting stents for the treatment of bifurcated coronary lesions: a randomized comparison of a simple versus complex strategy. *Am Heart J.* 2004;148(5):857–864.

47. Colombo A, et al. Randomized study of the crush technique versus provisional side-branch stenting in true coronary bifurcations: the CACTUS (Coronary Bifurcations: Application of the Crushing Technique Using Sirolimus-Eluting Stents) Study. *Circulation.* 2009;119(1):71–78.

48. Kim YH, et al. Comparison of simple and complex stenting techniques in the treatment of unprotected left main coronary artery bifurcation stenosis. *Am J Cardiol.* 2006;97(11):1597–1601.

49. Toyofuku M, et al. Comparison of target-lesion revascularisation between left main coronary artery bifurcations and left anterior descending coronary artery bifurcations using the one and two stent approach with sirolimus-eluting stents. *EuroIntervention.* 2011;7(7):796–804.

50. Dzavik V, et al. Predictors of long-term outcome after crush stenting of coronary bifurcation lesions: importance of the bifurcation angle. *Am Heart J.* 2006;152(4):762–769.

51. Hildick-Smith D, et al. Consensus from the 5th European Bifurcation Club meeting. *EuroIntervention.* 2010;6(1):34–38.

52. Sgueglia GA, et al. Kissing inflation is feasible with all second-generation drug-eluting balloons. *Cardiovasc Revasc Med.* 2011;12(5):280–285.

53. Costa RA, et al. Bifurcation coronary lesions treated with the "crush" technique: an intravascular ultrasound analysis. *J Am Coll Cardiol.* 2005;46(4):599–605.

54. Yang HM, et al. Long-term clinical and angiographic outcomes after implantation of sirolimus-eluting stents with a "modified mini-crush" technique in coronary bifurcation lesions. *Catheter Cardiovasc Interv.* 2009;74(1):76–84.

55. Ge L, et al. Clinical and angiographic outcome after implantation of drug-eluting stents in bifurcation lesions with the crush stent technique: importance of final kissing balloon post-dilation. *J Am Coll Cardiol.* 2005;46(4):613–620.

56. Colombo A. Bifurcational lesions and the "crush" technique: understanding why it works and why it doesn't—a kiss is not just a kiss. *Catheter Cardiovasc Interv.* 2004;63(3):337–338.

57. Chen SL, et al. A randomized clinical study comparing double kissing crush with provisional stenting for treatment of coronary bifurcation lesions results from the DKCRUSH-II (double kissing crush versus provisional stenting technique for treatment of coronary bifurcation lesions) trial. *J Am Coll Cardiol.* 2011;57(8):914–920.

58. Chen S, et al. More modified crush techniques for coronary bifurcation lesions: which one is better? *Catheter Cardiovasc Interv.* 2007;69(3):468–469; author reply 469–470.

59. Freixa X, et al. Long-term outcomes using a two-stent technique for the treatment of coronary bifurcations. *Int J Cardiol.* 2013;168(1):446–451.

60. Chen SL, Kwan TW. Twenty-four-month update on double-kissing crush stenting of bifurcation lesions. *J Interv Cardiol.* 2009;22(2):121–127.

61. Gao Z, et al. Transradial versus transfemoral method of two-stent implantation for true bifurcation lesions: comparison of immediate and long-term outcomes. *J Interv Cardiol.* 2014;27(2):99–107.

62. Burzotta F, et al. Modified T-stenting with intentional protrusion of the side-branch stent within the main vessel stent to ensure ostial coverage and facilitate final kissing balloon: the T-stenting and small protrusion technique (TAP-stenting). Report of bench testing and first clinical Italian-Korean two-centre experience. *Catheter Cardiovasc Interv.* 2007;70(1):75–82.

63. Sharma SK. Simultaneous kissing drug-eluting stent technique for percutaneous treatment of bifurcation lesions in large-size vessels. *Catheter Cardiovasc Interv.* 2005;65(1):10–16.

64. Iakovou I, Ge L, Colombo A. Contemporary stent treatment of coronary bifurcations. *J Am Coll Cardiol.* 2005;46(8):1446–1455.

65. Girasis C, et al. Long-term outcome after the V stenting technique in de novo bifurcation lesions using drug-eluting stents. *EuroIntervention.* 2009;5(2):197–205.

66. Dzavik V, Colombo A. The absorb bioresorbable vascular scaffold in coronary bifurcations: insights from bench testing. *JACC Cardiovasc Interv.* 2014;7(1):81–88.

67. Dzavik V, et al. Complex bifurcation percutaneous coronary intervention with the Absorb bioresorbable vascular scaffold. *EuroIntervention.* 2013;9(7):888.

68. Seth A, Sengottuvelu G, Ravisekar V. Salvage of Side branch by provisional "TAP Technique" using absorb bioresorbable vascular scaffolds for bifurcation lesions: first case reports with technical considerations. *Catheter Cardiovasc Interv.* 2014;84(1):55–61.

69. Pandit A, et al. Shorter ($</=$6 months) versus longer ($>/=$12 months) duration dual antiplatelet therapy after drug eluting stents: a meta-analysis of randomized clinical trials. *Catheter Cardiovasc Interv.* 2014.

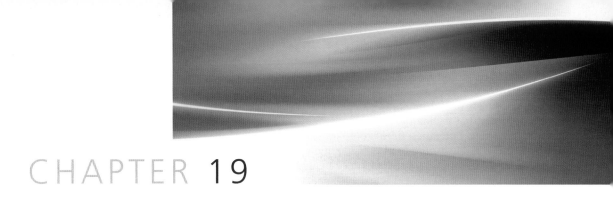

CHAPTER 19

Transradial Percutaneous Revascularization for Unprotected Left Main Coronary Artery Disease: An Evolution in Evidence and Technique

David E. Kandzari, Yue-Jin Yang, Bo Xu, and Run-Lin Gao

Introduction

Encouraged by randomized experience and comparisons from observational trials or subgroup analysis, enthusiasm for percutaneous unprotected (nonrevascularized) left main (ULM) coronary revascularization has increased, advancing in some geographies as an alternative treatment strategy to bypass surgery. Unlike many lesion subsets, however, left main coronary lesion complexity has clear procedural and clinical implications, underscoring not only the need for proper evaluation of the distribution and severity of disease but also technique. Specifically, percutaneous coronary intervention (PCI) for ULM disease can be technically challenging, requiring optimal strategies for the treatment of either complex distal bifurcation disease or ostial/shaft stenoses that jeopardize a large myocardial territory.

Considering the practical limitations associated with transradial (TR) percutaneous revascularization (e.g., guiding catheter support, equipment size limitations), ULM disease challenges the feasibility of a TR procedural strategy compared with a more traditional transfemoral (TF) approach. Although several trials have demonstrated the superiority of TR vascular access and bleeding complications,[1-13] expansion of TR PCI to more complex and high-risk anatomy has been limited by operator experience and lack of supportive evidence. Despite an increasing adoption of a TR access strategy worldwide, TR PCI is still challenged by an incomplete evidence basis, furthering perceptions that the practicality of TR PCI may be limited to less complex coronary anatomy and lower risk settings. This notion is especially relevant for ULM disease, considering the technical challenges of guiding catheter support, limitations of catheter size, oftentimes simultaneous need for multiple angioplasty catheters, and consequences of procedural failure.

Against this background, recent comparison between TR and TF methods of ULM PCI have demonstrated favorable procedural results, resource utilization, and clinical outcomes consistent with the larger evidence basis supporting TR PCI. The purpose of this chapter is to summarize the evidence supporting ULM PCI, describe procedural and technical challenges, and detail the results of studies comparing TR and TF methods of ULM PCI.

Contemporary Trials in ULM Percutaneous Revascularization

Coronary artery bypass grafting (CABG) has been considered the standard therapy for ULM coronary disease. However, increasing experience with ULM PCI has resulted in high procedural success and favorable early and late clinical outcomes. In particular, reduction in clinical restenosis with drug-eluting stents, evolution of procedural technique, and demonstration of favorable outcomes from comparative trials with CABG have promoted consideration of PCI as an alternative revascularization strategy in selected patients with ULM disease. Although varied in trial design, methods, and study population size, these trials suggest clinical equipoise for PCI and CABG, with consistently similar rates of combined safety outcomes of death, myocardial infarction, and stroke.[14,15] In selected instances, new insights from recent studies have identified patient characteristics for which PCI may represent an acceptable alternative or possibly even the preferred strategy. Accordingly, societal guidelines for ULM PCI have recently been revised.[16,17]

Recent trials and pooled analysis have provided important perspective to the safety and efficacy of ULM revascularization with drug-eluting stent (DES) compared with CABG.[14,15] The nonrandomized MAIN-COMPARE (Revascularization for Unprotected Left Main Coronary Artery Stenosis: Comparison of Percutaneous Coronary Angioplasty versus Surgical Revascularization from Multicenter Registry) trial involving 2,240 patients with ULM disease compared outcomes with PCI (DES 71%/ bare metal stent (BMS) 29%) or CABG.[18] At 5-year follow-up, according to propensity score adjustment including 542 matched patient pairs, ULM PCI was associated with similar mortality (hazard ratio [HR], 1.02; 95% CI, 0.74–1.39) and the composite outcome of death, Q-wave myocardial infarction, or stroke (HR, 1.10; 95% CI, 0.74–1.38).[19] However, repeat revascularization was significantly more common with PCI than with CABG (HR, 4.55; 95% CI, 2.88–7.20). Analysis following risk adjustment but limited to patients treated with CABG or DES (396 patient pairs) resulted in similar outcomes.

In the randomized SYNTAX (Synergy between Percutaneous Coronary Intervention with TAXUS and Cardiac Surgery) trial comparing CABG with PCI for left main and/or multivessel disease, patient treatment assignment was stratified according to the presence of significant ULM disease.[20,21] In the ULM subgroup ($N = 705$), despite significantly higher repeat revascularization for the PCI group at 5 years (26.7% PCI vs 15.5% CABG; $P < 0.001$), and lower incidence of stroke in the PCI group (1.5% PCI vs 4.3% CABG; $P = 0.03$), outcomes of death (12.8% PCI vs 14.6% CABG; $P = 0.53$), myocardial infarction (8.2% PCI vs 4.8% CABG; $P = 0.10$), and the composite end point of death/myocardial infarction/stroke (19.0% PCI vs

20.8% CABG; $P = 0.57$) remained similar between treatment groups.[22]

Two additional randomized trials have also reported similar outcomes. The PRECOMBAT trial ($N = 600$) compared ULM PCI with CABG, reporting no significant difference in the composite end point of death, myocardial infarction, or stroke (4.4% PCI vs 4.7% CABG, $P = 0.83$) despite higher repeat revascularization with PCI (9.0% PCI vs 4.2% CABG, $P = 0.02$).[23] In a smaller trial randomizing ULM patients to PCI with sirolimus-eluting stents or CABG ($N = 201$), 1-year repeat revascularization was more common with PCI, yet no differences in death and myocardial infarction were observed between treatment groups.[24] Altogether, these results are consistent with those from recent systematic overviews of comparative trials in ULM revascularization reporting similar composite safety outcomes between percutaneous and surgical revascularization strategies but a higher rate of repeat revascularization with PCI.[15,25] Larger ongoing trials are comparing newer-generation DES to CABG. The Nordic-Baltic-British Left Main Revascularization trial is randomizing 1,200 patients with ULM disease and a SYNTAX score less than 22 to CABG or DES with end points of major adverse cardiac events (MACEs) at 2 years and death at 5 years (clinicaltrials.gov identifier NCT01496651). The EXCEL (Evaluation of XIENCE PRIME versus Coronary Artery Bypass Surgery for Effectiveness of Left Main Revascularization) trial is a large international trial in which approximately 2,600 patients with ULM disease and a SYNTAX score ≤32 are randomized to revascularization with everolimus-eluting stents or CABG (clinicaltrials.gov identifier NCT01205776).

Procedural Strategy and Technique

At present, procedural strategy and technique are common practical considerations that are poorly addressed in clinical trials describing left main revascularization. In part related to this reason, optimal PCI strategies for ULM disease are yet to be clearly defined, especially those related to stent technique and bifurcation disease. Moreover, strategies may vary depending on different anatomic features of the entire coronary anatomy and lesion morphology. Treatment of distal bifurcation lesions is technically more challenging and is associated with higher rates of restenosis than isolated ostial or shaft disease, particularly when two stents are used. When angiographic restenosis does occur, it is most common at the ostium of the left circumflex artery,[26-28] a clinical observation that may depend on the bifurcation angle and carina shift rather than on the change in plaque geometry.[29] In accord with published results involving bifurcation stenting in nonleft main disease, uncontrolled studies of ULM bifurcation PCI favor a single-stent provisional approach compared with intentional two-stent techniques. Notably, one large study reported comparatively higher rates of cardiovascular death and target lesion revascularization with two-stent treatment of bifurcation disease, including instances of unsuccessful provisional approaches that required additional stent placement.[26] In addition, several recent observational studies have demonstrated nearly equivalent clinical outcomes with single-stent ULM bifurcation revascularization as compared with left main stenting for ostial or shaft disease.[30-33] Nevertheless, approximately 40% of ULM bifurcation treatment involves a two-stent method,[34] yet the optimal two-stent technique (e.g., crush, culotte, V- or T-stenting) has not been identified, and the procedure is instead determined more by operator and institutional preference. Novel dedicated bifurcation stent designs are in early clinical development,[35] yet evidence to support their procedural and clinical superiority over existing standards has not been sufficiently demonstrated.

Aside from stent technique, additional procedural uncertainties relate to the use of intravascular ultrasound (IVUS) and hemodynamic support. In many circumstances, the application of IVUS may be invaluable to optimally assess plaque distribution, bifurcation involvement, and vessel calcification that are characteristics often poorly defined by angiography alone. IVUS may also provide important information regarding stent sizing, postdeployment stent expansion, and stent-wall apposition. Nevertheless, the application of IVUS in ULM PCI trials has been inconsistent, with some studies reporting improved survival with IVUS-guided ULM PCI[36] and others describing favorable outcomes despite negligible use of IVUS.[34] Similarly, patient-specific angiographic- and procedural-related factors that predict the unplanned requirement for adjunctive hemodynamic support during ULM PCI are poorly characterized. In most instances, however, pharmacologic or mechanical circulatory support is not required; in the ISAR-LEFT MAIN (Intracoronary Stenting and Angiographic Results: Drug-Eluting Stents for Unprotected Coronary Left Main Lesions) trial, for example, intra-aortic balloon pump counterpulsation was used in less than 1% of the 607 patients undergoing ULM PCI.[34] Although procedural-related complications[37] or hemodynamic compromise[38] may be reduced with elective use of intra-aortic balloon pump counterpulsation or alternative methods of hemodynamic support,[39] a reduction in adverse clinical outcomes (e.g., myocardial infarction, death) compared with their provisional use has not been demonstrated.

Transradial ULM Percutaneous Revascularization

Despite the established clinical advantages of TR PCI, few studies have examined this method of percutaneous revascularization for ULM disease. Most published evidence is derived from isolated case reports or small, selected patient groups.[40,41] However, considering the complexity and risk associated with ULM PCI, there is a need to better characterize the feasibility of left main revascularization with a TR approach.

In the largest comparative study of TR and TF ULM PCI, procedural outcomes, resource use, in-hospital bleeding, and late clinical events were examined among 821 consecutive patients ($N = 353$ TR, 468 TF) (Table 19-1).[42] Overall, clinical and angiographic characteristics were similar between groups, except for a lower prevalence of unstable angina and bifurcation disease requiring two stents in the TR group. Procedural time was similar between cohorts, and there were no significant differences in procedural success (96% TR vs 97% TF, $P = 0.57$). However, consistent with previous comparative studies, hospital stay duration and thrombolysis in myocardial infarction (TIMI) major and minor bleeding (0.6% vs 2.8%, $P = 0.02$) were significantly lower with TR access (Table 19-1). In a propensity score model comparing 254 matched TR and TF patient pairs, clinical events were also reported over late term (Fig. 19-1). Over a mean follow-up period of 17 months, rates of cardiovascular death (1.2% vs 2.0%, $P = 0.28$), nonfatal myocardial infarction (4.7% vs 2.4%, $P = 0.16$), stent thrombosis (0.8% vs 2.8%, $P = 0.10$), and any target vessel revascularization (6.0% vs 6.7%, $P = 0.72$) did not statistically differ between TR and TF groups, respectively. Thus, in comparison with TF vascular access, ULM PCI using a TR strategy is feasible and associated with similar procedural success, shorter hospitalization, reduced bleeding, and comparable long-term safety and efficacy.

TABLE 19-1   Transradial versus Transfemoral Unprotected Left Main Percutaneous Revascularization Procedural, In-hospital, and Late Outcomes

	Tranradial (*N* = 353)	Transfemoral (*N* = 468)	*P* Value
Procedural and In-Hospital Outcomes			
Procedural success	97%	96%	0.57
MACE	4.0%	3.2%	0.57
TIMI major bleeding	0.6%	2.8%	0.02
Hospital stay	8.5 ± 5.9 days	9.9 ± 5.9 days	0.001
Late Clinical Outcomes (Mean 17 Months)			
Cardiac death	1.4%	1.7%	0.74
Nonfatal MI	4.0%	2.6%	0.26
LM-specific TLR	5.7%	5.8%	0.95
MACE	10.2%	9.2%	0.63

From Yang YJ, Kandzari DE, Gao Z, et al. Transradial versus transfemoral method of percutaneous coronary revascularization for unprotected left main coronary artery disease: comparison of procedural and late-term outcomes. *JACC Cardiovasc Interv.* 2010;3:1035–1042.

Among TR bifurcation cases treated with a two-stent technique (*N* = 67, 19%), bifurcation stent technique included stepped crush (72%), T-stenting (22%), and culotte (6%). In this study, all TR cases were performed using a 6F guiding catheter, an observation consistent with other nonleft main TR trials. In the RIVAL (RadIal Vs femorAL access for coronary intervention trial) study, for instance, PCI using a ≥7F guiding catheter occurred in only 1% (35/3,507) of cases.[43] Nevertheless, transradial PCI using ≥7F guiding catheters and larger-caliber sheathless guiding catheters that permit simultaneous two-stent techniques have also been described.[44,45] In contrast to a TR access method, the use of hemodynamic support and IVUS were more common with TF PCI. Despite such differences, left main-specific angiographic and procedural success rates were very high in each cohort and were similar between treatment strategies.

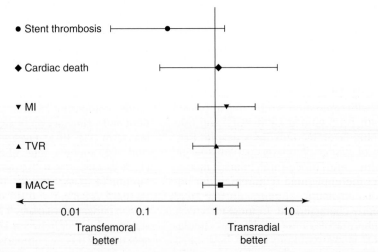

FIGURE 19-1   Multivariable matched propensity analysis of major adverse events following transradial or transfemoral unprotected left main PCI. (From Yang YJ, Kandzari DE, Gao Z, et al. Transradial versus transfemoral method of percutaneous coronary revascularization for unprotected left main coronary artery disease: comparison of procedural and late-term outcomes. *JACC Cardiovasc Interv.* 2010;3:1035–1042.)

Conclusion

Evidence from clinical trials of varied design and size consistently support the consideration of ULM PCI as an alternative revascularization strategy to CABG in selected patients. In particular, trials reporting late-term safety outcomes of cardiovascular death, myocardial infarction, and stroke comparable to CABG have fostered renewed enthusiasm for ULM PCI. Forthcoming trials designed with careful attention to patient selection, timing of end-point ascertainment, and relevance of safety and efficacy end points should inform clinical decision making and treatment guidelines.

In parallel, application of DES and advances in technique and strategy have enhanced the rates of early procedural and long-term clinical success of ULM PCI. However, although several studies have demonstrated the superiority of TR vascular access compared with a TF approach for reductions in vascular access and bleeding complications, expansion of TR PCI to more high-risk and complex coronary anatomy has been limited by lack of evidence and operator inexperience. Specific to ULM PCI, perceptions related to the challenges of guiding catheter support, equipment limitations, and consequences of procedural failure have challenged the advancement of TR vascular access in this indication.

More recently, our understanding of a TR strategy versus TF vascular access has advanced specifically in ULM PCI. Percutaneous ULM revascularization, including the treatment of distal bifurcation disease, is feasible by the TR method and is associated with high procedural success. Bleeding events are significantly less common with ULM TR PCI compared with TF, and hospital stay is abbreviated. Finally, TR PCI for ULM disease is associated with similar early and late outcomes of major cardiovascular events compared with TF access.

Altogether, these findings are consistent with other studies not only comparing vascular access methods for PCI but also ULM PCI in general. Altogether, favorable outcomes with ULM PCI reported in recent large observational studies may be attributed to technique, including high stent deployment pressure, kissing balloon postdilation, and the use of IVUS guidance, all of which are feasible with TR PCI. These results not only inform our understanding of TR PCI in more challenging and complex coronary anatomy, but also add to the evidence associating TR PCI with reduced bleeding events and yet similar procedural and clinical efficacy compared with TF vascular access.

REFERENCES

1. Mann T, Cubeddu G, Bowen J, et al. Stenting in acute coronary syndromes: a comparison of radial versus femoral access sites. *J Am Coll Cardiol.* 1998;32:572–576.
2. Kiemeneij F, Laarman GJ, Odekerken D, et al. A randomized comparison of percutaneous transluminal coronary angioplasty by the radial, brachial and femoral approaches: the access study. *J Am Coll Cardiol.* 1997;29:1269–1275.
3. Mann T, Cowper PA, Peterson ED, et al. Transradial coronary stenting: comparison with femoral access closed with an arterial suture device. *Catheter Cardiovasc Interv.* 2000;49:150–156.
4. Jolly SS, Amlani S, Hamon M, et al. Radial versus femoral access for coronary angiography or intervention and the impact on major bleeding and ischemic events: a systematic review and meta-analysis of randomized trials. *Am Heart J.* 2009;157:132–140.
5. Chase AJ, Fretz EB, Warburton WP, et al. Association of the arterial access site at angioplasty with transfusion and mortality: the M.O.R.T.A.L study (Mortality benefit Of Reduced Transfusion after percutaneous coronary intervention via the Arm or Leg). *Heart.* 2008;94:1019–1025.
6. Brueck M, Bandorski D, Kramer W, et al. A randomized comparison of transradial versus transfemoral approach for coronary angiography and angioplasty. *JACC Cardiovasc Interv.* 2009;2:1047–1054.
7. Rao SV, Ou F, Wang TY, et al. Trends in the prevalence and outcomes of radial and femoral approaches to percutaneous coronary intervention: a report from the National Cardiovascular Data Registry. *JACC Cardiovasc Interv.* 2008;1:379–386.
8. Agostoni P, Biondi-Zoccai GG, de Benedictis ML, et al. Radial versus femoral approach for percutaneous coronary diagnostic und interventional procedures; systematic overview and meta-analysis of randomized trials. *J Am Coll Cardiol.* 2004;44:349–356.
9. Cooper CJ, El-Shiekh RA, Cohen DJ, et al. Effect of transradial access on quality of life and cost of cardiac catheterization: a randomized comparison. *Am Heart J.* 1999;138:430–436.
10. Sciahbasi A, Pristipino C, Ambrosio G, et al. Arterial access-site-related outcomes of patients undergoing invasive coronary procedures for acute coronary syndromes (from the ComPaRison of Early Invasive and Conservative Treatment in Patients With Non-ST-ElevatiOn Acute Coronary Syndromes [PRESTO-ACS] Vascular Substudy). *Am J Cardiol.* 2009;103:796–800.
11. Hamon M, Rasmussen LH, Manoukian SV, et al. Choice of arterial access site and outcomes in patients with acute coronary syndromes managed with an early invasive strategy: the ACUITY trial. *Eurointervention.* 2009;5:115–120.
12. Louvard Y, Benamer H, Garot P, et al. Comparison of transradial and transfemoral approaches for coronary angiography and angioplasty in octogenarians (the OCTOPLUS study). *Am J Cardiol.* 2004;94:1177–1180.
13. Achenbach S, Ropers D, Kallert L, et al. Transradial versus transfemoral approach for coronary angiography and intervention in patients above 75 years of age. *Catheter Cardiovasc Interv.* 2008;72:629–635.
14. Kandzari DE, Colombo A, Park SJ, et al. Revascularization for unprotected left main disease: evolution of the evidence basis to redefine treatment standards. *J Am Coll Cardiol.* 2009;54:1576–1588.
15. Capodanno D, Stone GW, Morice MC, et al. Percutaneous coronary intervention versus coronary artery bypass graft surgery in left main coronary artery disease: a meta-analysis of randomized clinical data. *J Am Coll Cardiol.* 2011;58:1426–1432.
16. Wijns W, Kolh P, Danchin N, et al.; The Task Force on Myocardial Revascularization of the European Society of Cardiology (ESC) and the European Association for Cardio-Thoracic Surgery (EACTS). Guidelines on myocardial revascularization

(developed with the special contribution of the European Association for Percutaneous Cardiovascular Interventions (EAPCI)). *Eur Heart J.* 2010;31(10):2501–2555.

17. Levine GN, Bates ER, Blankenship JC, et al; American College of Cardiology Foundation; American Heart Association Task Force on Practice Guidelines; Society for Cardiovascular Angiography and Interventions. 2011 ACCF/AHA/SCAI guideline for percutaneous coronary intervention. A report of the American College of Cardiology Foundation/American Heart Association Task Force on Practice Guidelines and the Society for Cardiovascular Angiography and Interventions. *J Am Coll Cardiol.* 2011;58:e44–e122.

18. Seung KB, Park DW, Kim YH, et al. Stents versus coronary-artery bypass grafting for left main coronary artery disease. *N Engl J Med.* 2008;358:1781–1792.

19. Park DW, Seung KB, Kim YK, et al. Long-term safety and efficacy of stenting versus coronary artery bypass grafting for unprotected left main coronary artery disease: 5-year results from the MAIN-COMPARE (Revascularization for Unprotected Left Main Coronary Artery Stenosis: Comparison of Percutaneous Coronary Angioplasty Versus Surgical Revascularization) Registry. *J Am Coll Cardiol.* 2010;56:117–124.

20. Serruys PW, Morice MC, Kappetein AP, et al. Percutaneous coronary interventions versus coronary-artery bypass grafting for severe coronary artery disease. *N Engl J Med.* 2009;360:961–972.

21. Morice MC, Serruys PW, Kappetein AP, et al. Outcomes in patients with de novo left main disease treated with either percutaneous coronary intervention using paclitaxel-eluting stents or coronary artery bypass graft treatment in the Synergy between Percutaneous Coronary Intervention with TAXUS and Cardiac Surgery (SYNTAX) Trial. *Circulation.* 2010;121:2645–2653.

22. Serruys P. Five-year outcomes for unprotected left main subgroup in the SYNTAX Trial. Presented at *Transcatheter Therapeutics 2012 Scientific Sessions.* Miami, FL, October 23, 2012.

23. Park SJ, Kim YH, Park DW, et al. Randomized trial of stents versus bypass surgery for left main coronary artery disease. *N Engl J Med.* 2011;364:1718–1727.

24. Boudriot E, Thiele H, Walther T, et al. Randomized comparison of percutaneous coronary intervention with sirolimus-eluting stents versus coronary artery bypass grafting in unprotected left main stem stenosis. *J Am Coll Cardiol.* 2011;57:538–545.

25. Naik H, White AJ, Chakravarty T, et al. A meta-analysis of 3,773 patients treated with percutaneous coronary intervention or surgery for unprotected left main coronary artery stenosis. *JACC Cardiovasc Interv.* 2009;2:739–747.

26. Palmerini T, Marzocchi A, Tamburino C, et al. Impact of bifurcation technique on 2-year clinical outcomes in 773 patients with distal unprotected left main coronary artery stenosis treated with drug-eluting stents. *Circ Cardiovasc Interv.* 2008;1:185–192.

27. Kim YH, Park DW, Ahn JM, et al. Everolimus-eluting stent implantation for unprotected left main coronary artery stenosis: the PRECOMBAT-2 (Premier of Randomized Comparison of Bypass Surgery versus Angioplasty Using Sirolimus-Eluting Stent in Patients with Left Main Coronary Artery Disease) Study. *JACC Cardiovasc Interv.* 2012;5:708–717.

28. Kang SJ, Ahn JM, Song H, et al. Comprehensive intravascular ultrasound assessment of stent area and its impact on restenosis and adverse cardiac events in 403 patients with unprotected left main disease. *Circ Cardiovasc Interv.* 2011;4:562–569.

29. Kang SJ, Mintz GS, Kim WJ, et al. Changes in left main bifurcation geometry after a single-stent crossover technique: an intravascular ultrasound study using direct imaging of both the left anterior descending and the left circumflex coronary arteries before and after intervention. *Circ Cardiovasc Interv.* 2011;4:355–361.

30. Biondi-Zoccai GG, Lotrionte M, Moretti C, et al. A collaborative systematic review and meta-analysis on 1278 patients undergoing percutaneous drug-eluting stenting for unprotected left main coronary artery disease. *Am Heart J.* 2008;155:274–283.

31. Palmerini T, Marzocchi A, Tamburino C, et al. Impact of bifurcation technique on 2-year clinical outcomes in 773 patients with distal unprotected left main coronary artery stenosis treated with drug-eluting stents. *Circ Cardiovasc Interv.* 2008;1:185–192.

32. Park SJ, Kim YH, Lee BK, et al. Sirolimus-eluting stent implantation for unprotected left main coronary artery stenosis: comparison with bare metal stent implantation. *J Am Coll Cardiol.* 2005;45:351–356.

33. Kim YH, Park SW, Hong MK, et al. Comparison of simple and complex stenting techniques in the treatment of unprotected left main coronary artery bifurcation stenosis. *Am J Cardiol.* 2006;97:1597–1601.

34. Mehilli J, Kastrati A, Byrne R, et al. for the ISAR-LEFT MAIN (Intracoronary Stenting and Angiographic Results: Drug-Eluting Stents for Unprotected Coronary Left Main Lesions) Study Investigators. Paclitaxel- versus sirolimus-eluting stents for unprotected left main coronary artery disease. *J Am Coll Cardiol.* 2009;53:1760–1768.

35. Verheye S, Agostoni P, Dubois CL, et al. 9-Month clinical, angiographic, and intravascular ultrasound results of a prospective evaluation of the Axxess self-expanding biolimus A9-eluting stent in coronary bifurcation lesions: the DIVERGE (Drug-eluting Stent Intervention for Treating Side Branches Effectively) study. *J Am Coll Cardiol.* 2009;53:1031–1039.

36. Park SJ, Kim YH, Park DW, et al. Impact of intravascular ultrasound guidance on long-term mortality in stenting for unprotected left main coronary artery stenosis. *Circ Cardiovasc Interv.* 2009;2:167–177.

37. Perera D, Stables R, Thomas M, et al. Elective intra-aortic balloon counterpulsation during high-risk percutaneous coronary intervention: a randomized controlled trial. *JAMA.* 2010; 304:867–874.

38. Briguori C, Airoldi F, Chieffo A, et al. Elective versus provisional intraaortic balloon pumping in unprotected left main stenting. *Am Heart J.* 2006;152:565–572.

39. O'Neill WW, Kleiman NS, Moses J, et al. A prospective, randomized clinical trial of hemodynamic support with Impella 2.5 versus intra-aortic balloon pump in patients undergoing high-risk percutaneous coronary intervention: the PROTECT II study. *Circulation.* 2012;126:1717–1727.

40. Bertrand OF, Bagur R, Costerousse O, et al. Transradial versus femoral percutaneous coronary intervention for left main disease in octagenarians. *Indian Heart J.* 2010;62:234–237.

41. Prasad SB, Malaipan Y, Ahmar W, et al. Transradial left main stem rotational atherectomy and stenting: case report and literature review. *Cardiovasc Revasc Med.* 2009; 10:136–139.

42. Yang YJ, Kandzari DE, Gao Z, et al. Transradial versus transfemoral method of percutaneous coronary revascularization for unprotected left main coronary artery disease: comparison of procedural and late-term outcomes. *JACC Cardiovasc Interv.* 2010;3:1035–1042.

43. Jolly SS, Yusuf S, Cairns J, et al., for the RIVAL trial group. Radial versus femoral access for coronary angiography and intervention in patients with acute coronary syndromes (RIVAL): a randomised, parallel group, multicentre trial. *Lancet.* 2011;377:1409–1420.

44. Kwan TW, Cherukuri S, Huang Y, et al. Feasibility and safety of 7F sheathless guiding catheter during transradial coronary intervention. *Catheter Cardiovasc Interv.* 2012;80:274–280.

45. From AM, Bell MR, Rihal CS, et al. Minimally invasive transradial intervention using sheathless standard guiding catheters. *Catheter Cardiovasc Interv.* 2011;78:866–871.

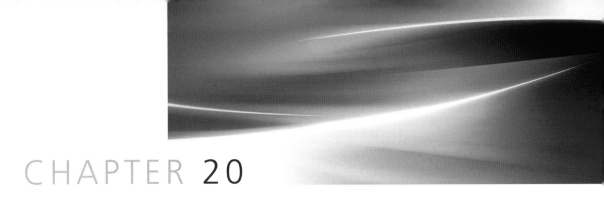

CHAPTER 20

Sheathless Guide Catheters

Douglas G. Fraser and Giovanni Amoroso

Background

Previous chapters have described the use of 5F, 6F, and 7F conventional transradial systems and the types of procedures that can be performed using these systems. In practice, most percutaneous coronary intervention (PCI) procedures, both radial and femoral, are performed using 6F guide catheters. For example, in the RIVAL trial of more than 7,000 ACS patients from 32 countries, 80% of procedures in both the radial and femoral arms were 6F procedures, with 7F and 5F used in 1% and 14% of radial procedures, respectively.[1] Similarly, in a recent worldwide practice survey of more than 1,000 radial operators, 60% of operators used 6F in the majority of cases (>75% cases) and 70% of operators used 6F in most cases (>50% cases).[2] This choice is for good reason, as several interventional techniques and types of equipment are 6F but not 5F compatible. Examples include kissing balloon, dedicated bifurcation stents, intravascular ultrasound (IVUS), thrombectomy catheters, rotablation, as described in the previous chapters. Furthermore, 6F sheath systems are well tolerated transradially— or so it seems.

In fact, owing to the routine use of vasodilators, anxiolytics, and analgesics during transradial procedures and failure by most operators to check for signs of radial occlusion, a significant degree of radial trauma goes undetected.[2] For example, in the absence of a vasodilator cocktail, during removal of a 6F sheath (defined as a pullback force >1 kg), spasm was detected in 22% of patients, and in a separate study pain score >3 (painful, very painful, or unbearable) was detected in 38% of patients.[3,4] Optical coherence tomography (OCT) imaging of the radial artery following partial sheath removal showed intimal tears in 67% and medial dissections in 36% of patients following 6F PCI.[5] Following 6F sheath insertion, this acute injury leads to chronic long-term radial narrowing (intimal hyperplasia: 15/15 patients detected by IVUS, and 11/15 patients detected histologically following radial artery harvest for CABG) and chronic loss of vasomotor function in the majority of patients.[6,7] These changes, together with radial occlusion, limit the success of repeat radial catheterization, with success rates below 50% reported following multiple previous procedures, and make a previously catheterized radial artery a poor artery graft.[8,9] Radial occlusion rates vary considerably from study to study, depending on many factors, with typical rates being 5% to 10% but with rates recently reported up to 33% following 6F sheath insertion.[10,11]

Reducing the system a single French size from 6F to 5F has been shown to significantly reduce these complications. In the former study, pain score >3 was reduced from 38% to 9%, and in two studies radial occlusion rate has been shown to be reduced by more than 50%.[11,12] Furthermore, acute and chronic radial artery injuries are limited to the distal section in contact with the radial sheath.[13,14] The reasons for the marked sensitivity to sheath size and the absence of injury proximal to the sheath can be explained by comparing sheath size to radial lumen size. In these comparisons, radial injury was significantly more frequent when the sheath outer diameter (OD) exceeded the radial lumen diameter.[4,15] This study also showed that for radial arteries larger than a 7F sheath, 7F procedures are well tolerated, with low radial occlusion rates.

Radial Artery Size

A 6F sheath is designed to accommodate guide catheters of 6F and smaller sizes and so its internal diameter is greater than the diameter of a 6F guide (2.0 mm). The OD of 6F sheaths in current use is approximately 2F larger than its inner diameter at 2.62 mm for the Terumo Glidesheath.[16] Several studies have measured the radial artery lumen size. The results using ultrasound from the first large study by Saito 1999 in 250 Japanese patients are shown in (Fig. 20-1).[15] This shows a wide variation in radial artery diameter from 1.5 mm to almost 4.5 mm, with larger sizes found in men than in women. Using current 4F, 5F, 6F, and 7F sheath diameters of 2.0, 2.29, 2.62, and 3.1 mm, it can be estimated that the radial lumen is smaller than the OD of a 7F sheath in 65% of women and 40% of men, smaller than a 6F sheath in 40% of women and 20% of men, and smaller than the ODs of 5F and 4F sheaths in 10% and 5% of patients. Subsequent studies, including our own unpublished data (Fig. 20-2), have in fact suggested that the radial artery lumen may be smaller still (Table 20-1), with lumens smaller

than 4F, 5F, 6F, and 7F sheaths in 5% to 20%, 10% to 35%, 20% to 60%, and 50% to 90% of patients, respectively, with larger arteries in men. This suggests that sheath sizes even smaller than 5F may be advantageous in terms of reducing radial injury. However, this remains to be demonstrated in practice. Correlation between radial occlusion and prior radial artery size in two studies has shown that the radial arteries that occlude are significantly smaller than the sheath size.

So, in summary, radial size is smaller than a 5F sheath in approximately one-third, smaller than a 6F sheath in one-half, and smaller than a 7F sheath in three-quarters of patients. When such oversized sheaths are used, radial injury, pain, and occlusion frequently occur. There is therefore an urgent need to find alternatives to the use of conventional sheaths.

Asahi Sheathless Eaucath

A potential solution to allow the use of 6F and larger guide catheters via transradial access while minimizing radial artery trauma is to use catheters that have been designed for insertion into the radial artery without the need for a sheath, thereby reducing catheter size within the radial artery by up to 2F sizes. The so-called sheathless guides and guiding sheaths have been available for peripheral angioplasty for many years and are inserted over a wire and central dilator directly

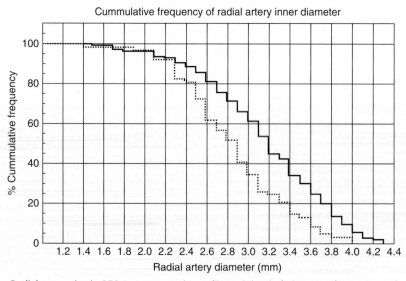

FIGURE 20-1   Radial artery size in 250 Japanese patients. (From Saito S, Ikei H, Hosokawa G, et al. Influence of the ratio between radial artery inner diameter and sheath outer diameter on radial artery flow after transradial coronary intervention. *Catheter Cardiovasc Interv.* 1999;46:173–178.)

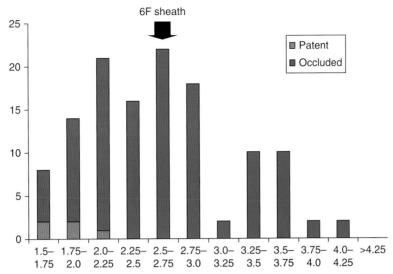

FIGURE 20-2   Radial artery size distribution and associated radial patency postprocedure in 124 Caucasian patients.

into the artery. Asahi Intecc commercialized 6.5F and 7.5F sheathless guides called Eaucath for transradial coronary intervention in Japan in 2004 and 2005, respectively. These guide catheters have ODs of 6.5F and 7.5F (2.16 and 2.49 mm), which are less than the ODs of conventional 5F and 6F sheaths (2.29 and 2.62 mm), respectively (Fig. 20-3). These catheters are thicker walled than conventional guide catheters and have the same internal diameters as conventional 6F and 7F sheaths (0.070 and 0.081 inches). These catheters can therefore be regarded as replacements for conventional 6F and 7F systems, while potentially causing less trauma than conventional 5F and 6F sheaths, respectively.

The Asahi Eaucath has a central dilator tapered onto a 0.035-inch wire that both straightens the curved catheter shape and has smooth transitions from the wire to the catheter (Fig. 20-4). The

catheter is also hydrophilically coated to allow atraumatic insertion. As the dilator is tapered onto a 0.035-inch wire, usual practice is to insert a 4F or 5F sheath, advance a 0.035-inch wire, and then remove the sheath, leaving only the wire in situ. Following advancement into the aorta, the dilator is removed, and the guide springs back into a range of popular shapes for coronary cannulation and behaves similar to a conventional guide catheter. Catheters may be exchanged over a 0.035-inch wire directly into the radial artery. The proximal end of the catheter may be fixed in position using an adhesive dressing during PCI.

The performance of these catheters has been reported in several studies. Following the European launch in 2007, we were the first to report the use of sheathless guide catheters. We described the use of the 7.5F sheathless in 17 patients undergoing complex PCI with the use

TABLE 20-1   Proportion of Patients in Whom the Radial Lumen Is Less Than the Diameter of Conventional 4F, 5F, 6F, and 7F Sheaths

| Patients (Ref.) | N | % Patients Lumen < OD Sheath | | | | | | | |
| | | <7F | | <6F | | <5F | | <4F | |
		Men	Women	Men	Women	Men	Women	Men	Women
Japanese[15]	250	50	75	20	40	8	10	5	5
Japanese[17]	135	60	90	30	50	10	30	5	20
Japanese[18]	115	86		56		35		15	
Caucasian[a]	124	79		55		35		20	

[a]Unpublished personal data.

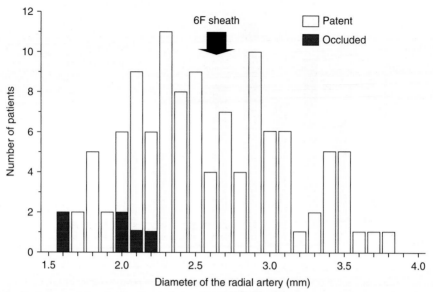

FIGURE 20-3   Radial artery size distribution and associated radial patency post procedure in 115 Japanese patients. (From Kwan TW, Cherukuri S, Huang Y, et al. Feasibility and safety of 7F sheathless guiding catheter during transradial coronary intervention. *Catheter Cardiovasc Interv.* 2012;80:274–280.)

of bifurcation techniques or adjunctive equipment requiring a larger bore size than 6F.[19] Procedural success using a sheathless guide was achieved in all cases. Several subsequent studies have similarly shown that 7.5F sheathless guides are well tolerated for complex interventional procedures requiring a large-bore guiding catheter.[20] Following this in 2010, we reported the use of the 6.5F sheathless guide in 100 patients undergoing routine PCI.[21] Procedural success was 100%, and there were no catheter-related complications reported. Casemix included 25% patients undergoing primary PCI and 50 patients undergoing urgent PCI for ACS, and procedures included a range of adjunctive equipment and techniques compatible with 6F. Radial occlusion was observed in only two patients. Our conclusion was that sheathless guides could completely replace conventional guiding catheters for both routine and complex PCI. Recently, a very large series of 7,853 procedures has confirmed the utility and safety of these devices that were used in 76% of all PCI procedures by 43 operators over an 8-year period at a single Japanese center.[22] Procedural success using sheathless guides was very high (98.9%), with a low catheter-induced coronary osteum dissection rate (0.2%).

We have subsequently compared two consecutive cohorts of patients (unpublished data). In the first sheathless cohort of 231 patients, transradial intervention (TRI) was performed using sheathless guides in 212/213 patients and crossover to conventional guide due to catheter tip dissection in one patient. In the second conventional cohort

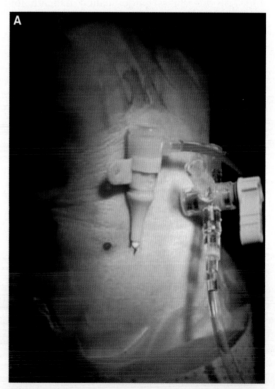

FIGURE 20-4   Method of sheathless guide insertion. **A:** Prior insertion of a 4F or 5F sheath used for prior angiography if required and for insertion of a 0.035-inch wire. **B:** Eaucath with its dilator. **C:** Dilator inserted into Eaucath. **D:** Dilator fixed at distal end of Eaucath. **E:** Eaucath advanced over a 0.035-inch wire and dilator into radial artery (after removal of sheath). **F:** Dilator removed when catheter in aorta. **G:** Proximal end connected to Y connector.

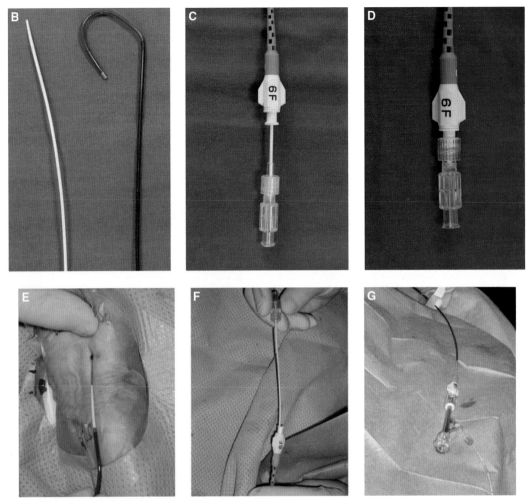

FIGURE 20-4   Continued.

of 304 patients, TRI was performed using conventional sheaths in 271/285 patients, with crossover to sheathless due to small radial artery in 14 patients. Greater pain was associated with the use of 7F conventional sheaths than with the sheathless 7.5F; however, pain scores for 6F compared to 6.5F sheathless were similar. Radial occlusion rates were also similar at 4.4% using conventional and 3.7% using sheathless guides at 2 months.

These studies, therefore, show that while Asahi sheathless guides are a very effective and safe alternative to conventional guides, the lower profile of equipment has not yet been shown to translate into reduced radial pain and injury. Further studies are needed to investigate the reasons. Furthermore, as the catheters are stiffer than conventional guides and lack the support and functionality of a sheath, they are somewhat more cumbersome to use. The need for insertion over a 0.035-inch wire as well as prior angiography in

ad hoc PCI also necessitate the prior insertion of a 4F or 5F sheath, negating some of the benefits of a sheathless system. It is difficult therefore to fully endorse the routine use of Asahi sheathless guides.

However, the selective use of sheathless guides can be fully supported. Radial artery size varies widely, and can be approximated by palpation or measured directly using ultrasound. The 6.5F sheathless guide is a good option for patients with small radial arteries, frequent in women, in whom it is likely to be much better tolerated than a 6F sheath while allowing a greater range of interventional options than 5F. Similarly, for patients with small and average-size radial arteries, 7F conventional sheaths are often poorly tolerated and 7.5F sheathless guides are a good option. Such selective use has been reported in several studies, showing very high procedural success.[16,20,23] Sciahbasi et al.[20] reported a procedural success of 100% in 79 patients with small radial arteries and 134 patients with potentially complex bifurcation transradial PCI using 6.5F and 7.5F sheathless guides, respectively. Similarly, Youn et al.[23] reported a 100% procedural success for non-CTO (chronic total occlusion) lesions in 29 patients with very small radial arteries that were all smaller than a 5F sheath (<2.3 mm) and had a mean diameter of only 1.8 mm. The 6.5F sheathless guides are particularly suited to us in small radial arteries because not only is the diameter significantly smaller than that of a 5F sheath (2.16 compared to 2.3 mm), but also the catheter is hydrophilic along its length, and the presence of the central dilator smoothes the transitions and eliminates the "razor effect" caused by the gap between the catheter and the wire.[24] An example of excellent tolerability of two separate 6.5F Eaucath guides for PCI following failure to advance a 5F catheter due to spasm is shown in (Fig. 20-5).

The commonest shapes used for left coronary interventions in our series and other series are the PB3.0 and PB3.5, which are similar to extra backup shapes of the same size. The commonest shapes for right coronary artery (RCA) interventions are JR4 and AL 0.75.[16,22] In 2008, an 8.5F sheathless guide was also commercialized in Japan and later in Europe. This has been used for CTOs and other procedures requiring an 8F guide, and has an OD smaller than that of a 7F sheath.

Medikit "Virtual" 3F Percutaneous Coronary Intervention

A second sheathless guide system by the Japanese company Medikit is available in Japan. This system has both 5F and 6.5F sheathless catheters, and the kit contains all the equipment required for use, obviating the need for an additional sheath. The catheters are thinner walled than the Asahi Eaucath, making them less stiff but with relatively larger internal lumens. The 5F version has the same internal lumen as a conventional 5F guide catheter, but the OD is equal to a 3F sheath, and so this system has been labeled as "virtual 3F PCI." The 6.5F version has a larger internal lumen than does the Asahi 6.5F Eaucath.

The radial artery is punctured with the enclosed 22G sheathed needle. A mini guidewire is then introduced through the sheathed needle

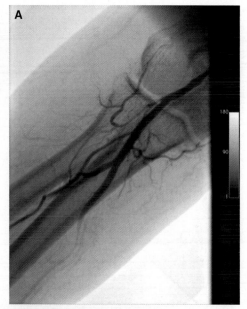
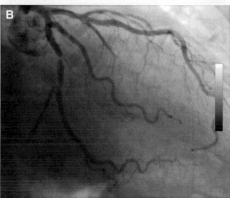
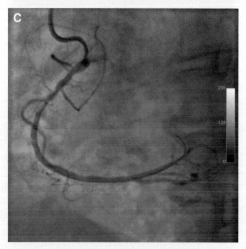

FIGURE 20-5 Small radial artery with spasm associated with introduction of 5F guide catheter. Following successful introduction of 6.5F PB3.5 Eaucath, PCI of circumflex is performed. Following exchange to a 6.5F AL 0.75 Eaucath, PCI of RCA is performed.

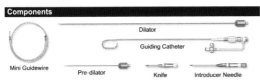

FIGURE 20-6   Medikit sheathless system "Works" includes a 22G needle, mini guidewire, minidilator, long dilator, guide catheter, and detachable valve. (From Medikit, Japan.)

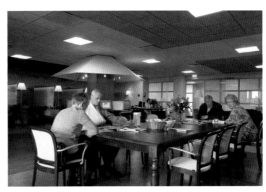

FIGURE 20-8   Same-day discharge at OLVG Amsterdam.

(via its sheath), followed by a minidilator. The short wire is then exchanged for a long wire and the minidilator removed. The guide catheter is then advanced over a full-length dilator into the radial artery over this long wire (Fig. 20-6).

There are some experiences in Japan about the feasibility and safety of "virtual" 3F PCI procedures, particularly from the cardiologists adhering to the Slender Club Japan. Mizuno et al.[25] recently reported on their experience with the "virtual" 3F PCI system. They treated 36 lesions (among which were seven CTOs) in 27 patients, with a procedural success of 92% and no access site–related complications. "Virtual" 3F procedures can be particularly advantageous in patients with small radial arteries, those who are old, those using chronic anticoagulation, or those who are planned for repeated procedures. Moreover, compression times can be reduced to 1 to 2 hours (Fig. 20-7), and patients can safely be discharged the same day (Fig. 20-8). Finally, in the case of a "virtual" 3F procedure, the chance of radial occlusion is significantly reduced, both because of the avoidance of radial/catheter mismatch and because of the very short time of hemostasis.

Procedures that are feasible with a conventional 5F guiding catheter can be accomplished with a "virtual" 3F guiding catheter, both simple interventions as direct stenting of type A lesions (Fig. 20-9A) and more complex procedures, as stenting of venous grafts (Fig. 20-9B). Indeed, the ongoing "downsizing" of stents and other devices make it possible to perform 5F PCI in the vast majority of unselected PCI populations.[26] Schobel et al.[27] performed 5F PCI procedures in 88% of a consecutive series of 1,200 all-comer patients (including bifurcations, CTOs, type C lesions, and unstable patients). In future, it is expected that the compatibility of thromboaspiration devices and bifurcation stents, which is at present set at 6F, will also extend to 5F guiding catheters. These advances will enable not only 5F conventional PCI but virtual 3F sheathless PCI to be suitable for a wide range of patients.

Alternative Systems

In many countries, including the United States, neither the Asahi nor the Medikit systems are available, leading operators to seek alternative solutions to achieve sheathless insertion of conventional guide catheters.[28,29] In place of a dedicated central dilator, an inner smaller-bore catheter, a long sheath dilator, and/or a partially inflated balloon have been used. In 116 such 7F procedures, Kwan et al.[29] described a 95% success rate and a low 2.5% 30-day radial occlusion rate. These reports show that it is possible to introduce conventional guides over unconventional inner catheter and achieve procedural success. However, it is likely that unless the transitions between wire, inner catheter, and guide catheter are smooth, procedural difficulties introducing such systems may be encountered.

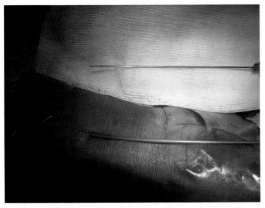

FIGURE 20-7   "Virtual" 3F PCI: details of the radial access.

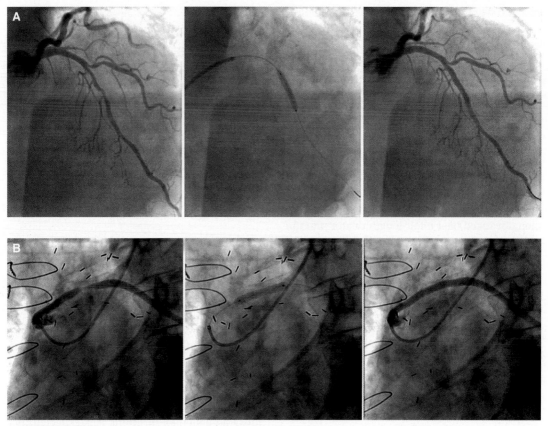

FIGURE 20-9   A: Direct stenting of mid-LAD by means of a "virtual" 3F guiding catheter. **B:** Stenting of venous graft by means of a "virtual" 3F guiding catheter.

Conclusion

Most radial PCIs are performed using 6F sheaths. While the greatest interest in sheathless systems will be to introduce 7F guides for complex PCI, there is considerable radial trauma associated with 6F conventional PCI that manifests as procedural pain and spasm at the time of the procedure and radial artery impaired endothelial function and occlusion in the long term. Sheathless solutions include the Asahi Eaucath, Medikit Works, and ad hoc techniques. These systems work well and can replace conventional catheters for PCI. The Asahi Eaucath has been the most widely evaluated, with excellent outcomes. It is likely that this will reduce radial trauma and reduce radial hemostasis times, in particular, with the use of 5F sheathless or virtual 3F PCI. However, proof of concept is awaited. Meanwhile, sheathless systems remain an excellent solution for 6F equivalent PCI in patients with small radial arteries and complex 7F PCI in remaining patients in whom conventional sheaths are poorly tolerated.

REFERENCES

1. Jolly SS, Yusuf S, Cairns J, et al. Radial versus femoral access for coronary angiography and intervention in patients with acute coronary syndromes (RIVAL): a randomised, parallel group, multicentre trial. *Lancet*. 2011;377:1409-1420.
2. Bertrand OF, Rao SV, Pancholy S, et al. Transradial approach for coronary angiography and interventions: results of the first international transradial practice survey. *JACC Cardiovasc Interv*. 2010;3:1022-1031.
3. Kiemeneij F, Vajifdar BU, Eccleshall SC, et al. Evaluation of a spasmolytic cocktail to prevent radial artery spasm during coronary procedures. *Catheter Cardiovasc Interv*. 2003;58:281-284.
4. Gwon HC, Doh JH, Choi JH, et al. A 5Fr catheter approach reduces patient discomfort during transradial coronary intervention compared with a 6Fr approach: a prospective randomized study. *J Interv Cardiol*. 2006;19:141-147.
5. Yonetsu T, Kakuta T, Lee T, et al. Assessment of acute injuries and chronic intimal thickening of the radial artery after transradial coronary intervention by optical coherence tomography. *Eur Heart J*. 2010;31:1608-1615.
6. Burstein JM, Gidrewicz D, Hutchison SJ, et al. Impact of radial artery cannulation for coronary angiography and angioplasty on radial artery function. *Am J Cardiol*. 2007;99:457-459.
7. Staniloae CS, Mody KP, Sanghvi K, et al. Histopathologic changes of the radial artery wall secondary to transradial catheterization. *Vasc Health Risk Manag*. 2009;5:527-532.

8. Kamiya H, Ushijima T, Kanamori T, et al. Use of the radial artery graft after transradial catheterization: is it suitable as a bypass conduit? *Ann Thorac Surg.* 2003;76:1505–1509.

9. Sakai H, Ikeda S, Harada T, et al. Limitations of successive transradial approach in the same arm: the Japanese experience. *Catheter Cardiovasc Interv.* 2001;54:204–208.

10. Kotowycz MA, Dzavik V. Radial artery patency after transradial catheterization. *Circ Cardiovasc Interv.* 2012;5:127–133.

11. Uhlemann M, Mobius-Winkler S, Mende M, et al. The Leipzig prospective vascular ultrasound registry in radial artery catheterization: impact of sheath size on vascular complications. *JACC Cardiovasc Interv.* 2012;5:36–43.

12. Dahm JB, Vogelgesang D, Hummel A, et al. A randomized trial of 5 vs. 6 French transradial percutaneous coronary interventions. *Catheter Cardiovasc Interv.* 2002;57:172–176.

13. Edmundson A, Mann T. Nonocclusive radial artery injury resulting from transradial coronary interventions: radial artery IVUS. *J Invasive Cardiol.* 2005;17:528–531.

14. Wakeyama T, Ogawa H, Iida H, et al. Intima-media thickening of the radial artery after transradial intervention. An intravascular ultrasound study. *J Am Coll Cardiol.* 2003;41:1109–1114.

15. Saito S, Ikei H, Hosokawa G, et al. Influence of the ratio between radial artery inner diameter and sheath outer diameter on radial artery flow after transradial coronary intervention. *Catheter Cardiovasc Interv.* 1999;46:173–178.

16. Harding SA, Shah N, Briggs N, et al. Complex transradial percutaneous coronary intervention using a sheathless guide catheter. *Heart Lung Circ.* 2013;22:188–192.

17. Fujii T, Masuda N, Toda E, et al. Analysis of right radial artery for transradial catheterization by quantitative angiography—anatomical consideration of optimal radial puncture point. *J Invasive Cardiol.* 2010;22:372–376.

18. Yokoyama N, Takeshita S, Ochiai M, et al. Anatomic variations of the radial artery in patients undergoing transradial coronary intervention. *Catheter Cardiovasc Interv.* 2000;49:357–362.

19. Mamas MA, Fath-Ordoubadi F, Fraser DG. Atraumatic complex transradial intervention using large bore sheathless guide catheter. *Catheter Cardiovasc Interv.* 2008;72:357–364.

20. Sciahbasi A, Mancone M, Cortese B, et al. Transradial percutaneous coronary interventions using sheathless guiding catheters: a multicenter registry. *J Interv Cardiol.* 2011;24:407–412.

21. Mamas M, D'Souza S, Hendry C, et al. Use of the sheathless guide catheter during routine transradial percutaneous coronary intervention: a feasibility study. *Catheter Cardiovasc Interv.* 2010;75:596–602.

22. Kahata M, Tada N, Honda T, et al. TCT-411 use of sheathless guide catheter with transradial percutaneous coronary intervention: single center experience with 7853 procedures [abstract]. *J Am Coll Cardiol.* 2012;60.

23. Youn YJ, Yoon J, Han SW, et al. Feasibility of transradial coronary intervention using a sheathless guiding catheter in patients with small radial artery. *Korean Circ J.* 2011;41:143–148.

24. Patel T, Shah S, Pancholy S. Balloon-assisted tracking of a guide catheter through difficult radial anatomy: a technical report. *Catheter Cardiovasc Interv.* 2013;81:E215–E218.

25. Mizuno S, Takeshita S, Taketani Y, et al. Percutaneous coronary intervention using a virtual 3-Fr guiding catheter. *Catheter Cardiovasc Interv.* 2010;75:983–988.

26. Masutani M, Yoschimachi F, Matsukage T, et al. Use of slender catheters for transradial angiography and interventions. *Indian Heart J.* 2008;60:A22–A26.

27. Schobel WA, Mauser M. Miniaturization of the equipment for percutaneous coronary interventions: a prospective study in 1,200 patients. *J Invasive Cardiol.* 2003;15:6–11.

28. From AM, Bell MR, Rihal CS, et al. Minimally invasive transradial intervention using sheathless standard guiding catheters. *Catheter Cardiovasc Interv.* 2011;78:866–871.

29. Kwan TW, Cherukuri S, Huang Y, et al. Feasibility and safety of 7F sheathless guiding catheter during transradial coronary intervention. *Catheter Cardiovasc Interv.* 2012;80:274–280.

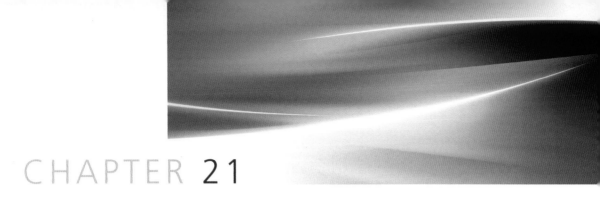

CHAPTER 21

Radial Approach in the Elderly

Eltigani Abdelaal and Warren J. Cantor

Elderly patients represent one of the most challenging subgroups of patients requiring cardiac catheterization and percutaneous coronary intervention (PCI). They are at increased risk for ischemic, hemorrhagic, and vascular complications.[1-4]

Given the proven benefit of radial access in reducing vascular access site complications,[5] it would stand to reason that elderly patients may derive the greatest benefit from radial access.

However, elderly patients have increased vascular tortuosity and calcification, which could potentially limit the success of transradial procedures[6] (Fig. 21-1). The coronary artery disease in the elderly is often more diffuse, complex, and calcified than in younger patients. The higher rates of non–access site bleeding in elderly patients[7] may obscure any benefit of radial access in reducing access site bleeding. Furthermore,

most of the studies that have documented the feasibility, safety, and efficacy of the transradial approach enrolled mainly younger patients.[5] Registries have shown selection biases in the access route chosen, with fewer elderly patients undergoing transradial procedures compared with younger patients.[8] It has therefore been questioned whether radial access is suitable for elderly patients and whether it carries the same advantages over femoral access as it does in younger patients.

Outcomes After Percutaneous Coronary Intervention for Elderly Patients versus Younger Patients

Elective Percutaneous Coronary Intervention

The decision to proceed with PCI in elderly patients is often influenced by multiple factors, including baseline functional and mental status and comorbidities. Elderly individuals presenting with coronary artery disease often have more advanced atherosclerotic vascular disease and adverse coronary morphologies, including tortuosity and calcification. Observational studies and registries of elderly patients undergoing elective PCI have shown lower rates of procedural success and higher rates of complications, including recurrent myocardial infarction (MI), stroke, vascular complications, renal failure, and in-hospital mortality[4,9,10] (Table 21-1).

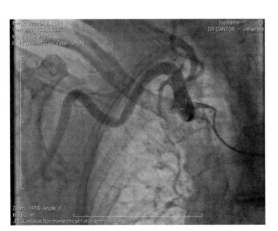

FIGURE 21-1 Tortuous brachiocephalic in a 92-year-old woman.

TABLE 21-1 Trends and Outcomes of PCI in Elderly Patients: Elective, ACS, and STEMI

Ref	Study Period and Nature	Age Cutoff	N	Radial/Femoral	Cohort	Outcome(s) Measured	Findings
Berger et al.[11]	1994–1996, CCP cohort	65	80,356	NA	Primary PTCA vs thrombolysis in elderly	30-day and 1-year survival	Primary PTCA associated with modestly lower short- and long-term mortality compared to thrombolysis
Wennberg et al.[9]	1989–1993, Single-center, registry	80	12,172	NA	PTCA in an unselected population	Impact of age on outcomes (<60, 60–69, 70–79, >80 years)	4% were octogenarians, had higher comorbidities. More often urgent PTCA in elderly. Age strongly linked to mortality and postprocedural MI
Batchelor et al.[4]	1994–1997, NCN data	80	7,472	NA	All octogenarians undergoing PCI	Risks of PCI and mortality	Octogenarians had more comorbidities and two- to fourfold increased risk of complications, including death (3.8% vs 1%), MI, stroke, and vascular complications ($P < 0.0001$). For elective PCI, mortality in octogenarians strongly influenced by comorbidities
Chauhan et al.[3]	Pooled analysis of six multicenter trials	80	6,186	NA	Mixed cohort	Procedural and clinical outcomes in elderly ≥80 (N = 301) vs young	Similar procedural success. Higher bleeding complications, in-hospital and 1-year mortality in elderly. Age-independent predictor of mortality
Klein et al.[12]	1998–2000, NCDR registry	80	8,828	NA	PCI in octogenarians	Clinical outcomes	Good success and overall mortality of 3.7%. Mortality 1.35% in absence of recent MI. PCI for STEMI or recent MI strongly predicted mortality
Kobayashi et al.[1]	Single-center, observational	80	969	NA	Multivessel stenting	In-hospital and 1-year mortality in ≥80 (N = 75) vs. <80 (N = 894)	High technical success rate in both groups. Higher in-hospital complications and 1-year mortality rate in octogenarians

Study	Year, setting	Age	N		Aim	Outcomes	Findings
Dynina et al.[10]	1998–1999, Multi-institutional PCI database	85	10,847	NA	PCI in all comers (49% were <65; 31% were 65–74; 17% were 75–84, and 3% were ≥85 years)	In-hospital outcomes by age group	The very elderly had higher post-PCI complications (stroke, renal failure) and higher mortality; Age was not an independent predictor of mortality
Mehta et al.[13]	1999–2000, GRACE study	70	2,975	NA	Effectiveness of PPCI vs thrombolysis in STEMI	In-hospital complications and clinical outcomes	Patients treated with PPCI showed lower rate of reinfarction and mortality
Halon et al.[14]	2000, Single-center, registry	70	449	NA	PCI for ACS in elderly 70–79 (group 1) and very old >80 (group 2)	Difference in presentation and outcome	Group 2 were sicker at presentation and had poorer outcomes; But a subgroup selected for angiography and PCI had a 2-year outcome similar to group 1
Zhang et al.[15]	2002–2004, Randomized	75	102	NA	Randomized PPCI for STEMI vs medical therapy	1-year MACE	Similar 30-day MACE between two groups; 1-year MACE lower in PPCI compared with conservative group (21 vs. 45%, $P = 0.029$)
Sukiennick et al.[16]	2002–2003, Single-center, retrospective	70	1,000	NA	Mixed cohort of elective, urgent, emergent PCI	In-hospital outcomes of elderly vs young	Higher comorbidities, cardiogenic shock, and MVD in elderly; High success rate in both groups; Higher mortality in elderly; Age independently predicted mortality
De Labriolle et al.[17]	1995–2005, Single-center, retrospective	75	159	NA	STEMI treated with PPCI vs thrombolysis	1-year mortality	1-year mortality higher in thrombolysis compared to primary PCI (51.4% vs 15.3%)
Merchant et al.[18]	2002–2005, Single-center, retrospective	80	179	NA	PPCI for STEMI compared to a randomly selected elective PCI in octogenarian	In-hospital outcomes	Similar procedural success in both groups; Higher bleeding, periprocedural complications, and hospital mortality in STEMI group

(continued)

TABLE 21-1 Trends and Outcomes of PCI in Elderly Patients: Elective, ACS, and STEMI (continued)

Ref	Study Period and Nature	Age Cutoff	N	Radial/ Femoral	Cohort	Outcome(s) Measured	Findings
Bagur et al.[7]	2003–2005, Randomized	70	1,348	1,348/0	Randomized SDD + GPI bolus only vs ON + GPI infusion after TR-PCI	Bleeding and MACE at 30 days; MACE 6-month, 1- and 3-year mortality	Similar bleeding and MACE at 30-days in older and younger patients Similar MACE at 6 months, 1 year, and 3 years Mortality higher in ≥70 years at 3 years Age not a predictor of bleeding or MACE
Zimmerman et al.[19]	1999–2005, Single-center, observational	75	504	218/286	STEMI	Clinical outcomes in elderly (N = 115) vs young (N = 389)	Higher comorbidities in elderly Elderly less likely to have PCI Overall higher 30-day mortality in elderly Similar mortality in those undergoing PCI Lower bleeding complications in both groups with radial
Classen et al.[20]	1997–2007, Single-center, observational	80	379	NA	Primary PCI for STEMI	30-day and 1-year mortality	Proportion of octogenarians with STEMI increased from 3.5% to 8.8% over study period Mortality in ≥80 vs in <40 years 30-day mortality = 21% vs 3.8% 1-year mortality = 28% vs 4.3%
Shelton et al.[21]	2003–2008, Two-center, retrospective	80	256	NA	Elderly patients with STEMI, treated with PPCI or lytic therapy	Short- and long-term mortality before and after inception of 24/7 PPCI	PPCI improved outcomes and significantly reduced mortality compared to lytic therapy
Liu et al.[22]	2004–2009, Single-center observational	80	16,293	All radial	In-hospital outcomes in three age groups (<65, 65–70, and ≥80)	Post-PCI clinical outcomes	Similar angiographic success Higher procedural complications in octogenarians (0.8, 1.2, 4%, $P < 0.001$) Higher MACE and in-hospital mortality in ≥80

Study	Period, Registry	Age	N	Radial/femoral	Population	Outcome	Results
Antonsen et al.[23]	2002–2008, Western Denmark PCI registry	80	3,792	NA	PCI for SA, UA, NSTEMI, and STEMI in octogenarians	30-day and 1-year mortality	Annual proportion of ≥80 years treated with PCI steadily increased. Overall mortality: 30-day 9%, 1-year 18%. Compared to SA, STEMI patients had a higher adjusted 1-year mortality
Rao et al.[24]	2004–2008, NCDR Registry	69	461,311	1.2% radial/ 97.9% femoral	Association between post-PCI bleeding, MACE and mortality in older patients	Readmission for bleeding, MACE and all-cause mortality	Overall bleeding in 3.1%. Those who bled were older, more often females, and more often comorbidities, and more often underwent PCI via femoral access. Bleeding associated with increased risk of future bleeding, MACE, and all cause mortality up to 30 months
Mandawat et al.[25]	2004–2008, Cross-sectional analysis from HCUP-NIS	90	33,644	NA	Nonagenarians admitted with STEMI	In-hospital mortality after PCI or medical therapy for >90 years	Overall PCI rate 16.9%. Rate doubled over study period. Lower mortality with PCI vs conservative therapy (15 vs 26%, P < 0.001)
Antonsen et al.[26]	2002–2009, Western Denmark PPCI registry	80	1,322	NA	PPCI for STEMI in octo- and nonagenarians	Short- and long-term outcomes	Annual proportion of octogenarians treated with PPCI doubled over study period. Acceptable 5-year survival of 40% in both octogenarians and nonagenarians
Lazzeri et al.[27]	2004–2010, Single-center, observational	75	404	NA	Elderly with STEMI, treated with PPCI	In-hospital and 1-year mortality	Proportion of elderly with STEMI increased over study period. Less bleeding. Early and late mortality unchanged

CCP, Cooperative Cardiovascular Project; GPI, glycoprotein inhibitor; GRACE, Global Registry of Acute Coronary Events; HCUP-NIS, Healthcare Cost and Utilization Project Nationwide Inpatient Sample; MACE, major adverse cardiovascular events; MVD, multivessel disease; NCDR, National Cardiovascular Database Registry; NCN, National Cardiovascular Network; ON, overnight stay; PPCI, primary PCI; SA, stable angina; SDD, same-day discharge; TR-PCI, transradial PCI; UA, unstable angina.

Batchelor et al.[4] compared in-hospital outcomes of 7,472 octogenarians (mean age, 83 years) with those of 102,236 young patients (mean age, 62 years), who underwent PCI at 22 National Cardiovascular Network database hospitals between 1994 and 1997. Octogenarians had more comorbidities, and a two- to fourfold increased risk of complications, including death (3.2% vs 1.1%), MI (1.9 vs 1.3), renal failure (3.2% vs 1%), and vascular complications ($P < 0.001$ for all comparisons). Mortality demonstrated a curvilinear relation with age, ranging from approximately 0.5% for patients <50 years old to 5% in >85 years. Age >85 years was an independent predictor of procedural mortality. For elective PCI, mortality in octogenarians was strongly influenced by the presence of comorbidities (0.79% with no risk to 7.2% with renal insufficiency and left ventricular ejection fraction < 35%). A subsequent report from the ACC-NCDR from 1998 to 2000 found that octogenarians undergoing PCI had high success rates and acceptable mortality rates,[12] with higher mortality in patients with acute or recent MI.

Percutaneous Coronary Intervention for Acute Coronary Syndromes

Elderly individuals represent the fastest growing segment of the population, are increasingly referred for PCI, and are at higher risk of both bleeding as well as thrombotic events.[28-31] Patients ≥75 years represent 10% of those who have had MI, but account for 25% of all hospital deaths.[32] Nonetheless, limited data are available on the safety of PCI in elderly patients with acute coronary syndrome (ACS) or ST-elevation MI (STEMI), as these are often underrepresented in randomized trials.[33,34] Several single-center observational and registry studies have examined the outcomes in elderly patients with ACS and STEMI treated with PCI (Table 21-1).

Percutaneous Coronary Intervention for Non-ST-Segment Elevation MI

The impact of advanced age on management, antithrombotic strategies, and clinical outcomes of ACS has been previously documented.[35,36] In an observation from the Global Registry of Acute Coronary Events (GRACE),[35] involving 24,165 patients in 102 hospitals across 14 countries stratified by age, it was found that elderly patients ≥65 years had more comorbidities, showed longer delay in seeking medical attention, and were least likely to undergo invasive treatment. Older patients were more likely to present with non-ST elevation MI (NSTEMI) than were younger patients.[35] Major bleeding rates were significantly higher with increasing age (>6% in ≥85 vs 2%-3% in <65 years; $P = <0.0001$). In-hospital mortality, adjusted for baseline characteristics, also steadily increased across age strata (odds ratio [OR]: 15.7 in patients ≥85 years, compared to <45 years).[35]

In a prespecified analysis of ACUITY trial ($N = 13,819$) of 30-day and 1-year outcomes across four age groups (<55, 55–64, 65–74, and ≥75 years), patients aged ≥75 years represented 17.7% of study population.[36] Both ischemic and bleeding complications after NSTEMI significantly increased with age. Patients who received bivalirudin alone had similar ischemic outcomes, but significantly lower bleeding complications than did those treated with heparin and glycoprotein IIb/IIIa inhibitors.[36] However, femoral access was used for the majority of these patients. The role of bivalirudin in reducing major bleeding in patients undergoing radial procedures remains uncertain.[37,38]

Few data exist on the use of radial access in PCI for ACS in the elderly. The EASY (Early Discharge After Stenting of Coronary Arteries) trial[7] compared clinical outcomes between patients ≥70 and <70 years who underwent PCI exclusively via transradial access. Patients were randomized to either same-day discharge and abciximab bolus only or overnight hospitalization and bolus, followed by 12-hour infusion of abciximab, after uncomplicated transradial stenting.[7] Among the 1,348 patients enrolled in the trial, 259 (19%) were aged ≥70 years. At 30 days, the rates of MACE (major adverse cardiovascular events) and major bleeding were similar in older and younger patients.[7] This provided a reassuring signal that the reduction in major bleeding with radial access in elderly patients is similar to that in younger patients, even when potent antithrombotic and antiplatelet agents are utilized.

Percutaneous Coronary Intervention for ST-Segment Elevation MI

Although primary PCI, combined with antithrombotic therapy, has substantially reduced morbidity and mortality associated with acute MI,[39] mortality rates in the elderly undergoing primary PCI for STEMI remain substantially higher than in younger patients.[12] Attempts to improve outcomes with more potent antithrombotic therapy are hampered by higher rates of periprocedural bleeding.[40] Furthermore, limited data are available on the safety of PCI in elderly patients with STEMI, because of underrepresentation of elderly patients in the randomized trials.[33]

Despite these shortcomings and worse outcomes, several studies have shown that elderly patients derive incrementally more benefit from primary PCI than from thrombolytic therapy.[11,41] In a recent meta-analysis of 22 randomized trials evaluating primary PCI versus thrombolytic therapy,[41] the reduction in clinical end points seen with primary PCI was not influenced by age. As such, age per se should not be an exclusion criterion for the application of primary PCI.

The use of bleeding avoidance strategies in 10,469 patients aged ≥80 years with STEMI undergoing primary PCI in an NCDR (National Cardiovascular Data Registry) study was shown to be suboptimal.[42] The use of vascular closure devices for femoral access, combined with direct thrombin inhibitors, increased over the study period (2006–2009); however, radial access was rarely used (<1%) in this age group.[42]

Radial Access in Elderly Patients versus Younger Patients

Radial Artery Size

The inner radial artery diameter, measured 1 to 2 cm proximal to the styloid process, is approximately 2.45 to 2.7 mm in the majority of individuals (2.69 in men and 2.43 in women),[43] and can therefore accommodate 6F catheters or larger. The mean radial diameter correlates significantly with body surface area.[43] In a small proportion of individuals (particularly in the elderly, females, and diabetics), it tends to be smaller in caliber. There has been no study that has specifically examined the radial diameter in the elderly population.

Tortuosity and Calcification

Elderly patients are more likely to have considerable brachiocephalic and subclavian tortuosities and advanced vascular disease. In addition, elderly subjects have a higher frequency of unfolding of the aorta and aortic root dilatation. This twists the origin of aortic arch into a posterior position, which may impede wire and catheter entry into the ascending aorta.[44] This difficulty can often be overcome with certain maneuvers such as deep inspiration to straighten the mediastinum and realign the aortic brachiocephalic trunk, allowing catheter entry and manipulation into the ascending aorta.[44] In addition to subclavian tortuosity, radial and brachial tortuosities are also more common with increasing age, as demonstrated by a two-dimensional ultrasound study of 1,191 patients undergoing transradial catheterization.[43]

The combination of diffuse atherosclerotic disease of the great vessels, tortuosity, calcification, and more complex coronary anatomy in elderly patients poses a particular challenge for transradial operators, particularly during the early phase of the learning curve. Not surprisingly, advanced age has been shown to independently predict failure of transradial approach to PCI.[45]

Right versus Left Radial Access

Despite the many advantages in favor of radial over femoral access, operators wanting to adopt the radial approach remain unclear as to which radial is better. Comparison between right and left radial accesses has, in fact, been the subject of several observational and a few randomized trials.[46-53] Such studies predominantly focused on procedural time, success rate, crossover, and radiation exposure, often with conflicting results, and as such, whether one site is superior to the other remains controversial.

A recent meta-analysis[54] pooled data from five randomized trials comparing right versus left radial access for diagnostic and interventional coronary procedures. Neither right nor left radial was significantly better than the other in terms of procedural duration, fluoroscopy time, contrast volume, or incidence of complications. However, left radial access was associated with significantly less need for crossover to the femoral approach (3.1 vs 5.2%, RR = 1.65; $P = 0.003$) compared to right radial.[54]

It is not clear whether this 2% absolute reduction in risk of access site failure with left radial is due to potential anatomical advantage with left radial, differences in operator experience, or both. It has been suggested that the left radial access provides a more natural transition into the ascending aorta, ensuring similar catheter maneuverability to that of femoral access. Some have even advocated that inexperienced operators should preferentially use left radial to minimize failure.[46] Although plausible, it remains to be proven in an adequately powered randomized trial. Until such a trial is completed, there appears to be no additional advantage to adopting the left radial access routinely, at least in the hands of an experienced operator. Indeed, in a recent international survey of transradial practice,[55] approximately 90% of operators stated that they routinely used right radial as default access.

In the only randomized trial of right versus left radial access that focused exclusively on elderly patients (octogenarians, $N = 100$),[56] both approaches were similar in procedural and fluoroscopy times. Subclavian tortuosity (as reported by the operator) was more frequent on the right than on the left side (32% vs 10%, respectively; $P = 0.002$); however, this did not translate into significantly different crossover rate.[56] In fact, there were numerically more crossovers with left (10%) than with right radial (4%), although this did not reach a statistical difference ($P = 0.24$).[56]

Radial versus Femoral Access in Elderly Patients

Observational Studies

A number of studies have compared outcomes with radial versus femoral access specifically in elderly patients (Table 21-2). Some studies included patients undergoing only coronary angiography; others included patients undergoing elective PCI, PCI for STEMI, or PCI of left

TABLE 21-2 Studies of Radial versus Femoral Access in Elderly Patients

Author Name	Age Cutoff	Population	Radial (*N*)	Femoral (*N*)	Findings
Randomized Studies					
Louvard et al.[57]	80	Angiography or PCI	192	185	Less vascular complications, slight increase in procedure duration
Achenbach et al.[58]	75	Angiography	152	155	Radial had longer total examination time, less complications
Observational Studies					
Klinke et al.[59]	80	PCI	125	128	No significant differences in MACE, trend to lower hospital stay with radial
Jaffe et al.[60]	80	Elective PCI	97	131	Radial associated with longer cannulation, more fluoro time, higher crossover, less bleeding, and access site complications
Ziakas et al.[61]	70	Primary or rescue PCI	87	68	Radial safe and effective, fewer vascular complications
Rao et al.[8]	75	PCI	7,804	585,290	Elderly have similar procedure success and trend to less bleeding with radial access
Zimmermann et al.[19]	75	STEMI	39	76	Less access site bleeding with radial
Koutouzis etal.[62]	80	Primary or rescue PCI	40	301	No difference in procedure times, clinical outcomes. Trend to less access site bleeding. Higher crossover with radial
Bertrand et al.[63]	80	PCI of left main	90	13	Feasible, same success rate
Hu et al.[64]	80	Elective PCI	112	156	Radial associated with longer cannulation, more fluoro time, higher crossover, less bleeding, and access site complications
Secco et al.[65]	75	Primary PCI for STEMI	177	106	Similar door to balloon (DTB); radial associated with significantly shorter time to arterial puncture

main. Most of these studies showed that the radial access was associated with longer procedural and fluoroscopy times, but similar success rates and lower rates of vascular and bleeding complications. The crossover rates from radial to femoral access ranged from 2% to 18%,[62,63] and were generally higher than the crossover rates from femoral to radial access. The results of these observational studies should be interpreted cautiously as there were likely many baseline differences between the radial and femoral patients. Furthermore, the relatively small number of patients in these studies limits the ability to adjust for differences between groups and the ability to generalize these results to all elderly patients.

Randomized Trials

There are two randomized trials of radial versus femoral access that focused exclusively on elderly patients.[57,58] The multicenter OCTOPLUS study[57] randomized 377 patients aged >80 years undergoing angiography or PCI to radial or femoral access. All operators were very experienced with both femoral and radial accesses. Exclusion criteria included cardiogenic shock, previous bypass surgery with bilateral internal mammary arterial grafts, and severe peripheral artery disease (PAD). The primary end point, a composite of vascular complications, transfusion, and drop in hemoglobin, was significantly lower in the radial group (1.6% vs 6.5%; $P = 0.029$). The difference in the primary end point was driven mainly by large hematomas that delayed hospital discharge, although there was also a trend to fewer drops in hemoglobin or hematocrit. The radial group had similar contrast volume but longer procedure duration and higher X-ray exposure. The access site crossover rates were similar for radial and femoral groups (8.9% and 8.1%, respectively).

Similarly, Achenbach et al.[58] randomized 307 consecutive patients aged ≥75 years undergoing coronary angiography and intervention or PCI to radial or femoral access. Exclusion criteria included cardiogenic shock, renal failure, planned right and left heart catheterization, unfavorable Allen test, and peripheral arterial disease. Primary end points were success rate and major complications. In the radial group, crossover to femoral was required in 9% of cases. Examination time was significantly longer in the radial group, but no difference was found in the fluoroscopy time. The rate of major complications (bleeding requiring surgery, transfusion, stroke) was 0% in radial versus 3.2% in femoral group ($P < 0.001$). Minor complications (defined as clinically apparent bleeding of access site, not requiring transfusion or surgical intervention) were also significantly lower with radial access (1.3 vs 5.8%, $P < 0.001$).[58]

In a meta-analysis of randomized trials comparing radial and femoral accesses,[5] the two trials (684 patients) with a mean age >70 had a similar reduction in major bleeding with radial access as the 16 trials (4,807 patients) with a mean age <70 years (OR 0.18 and 0.30, $P = 0.003$ and $P < 0.001$, respectively).[5]

The largest randomized trial comparing the radial and femoral accesses was the RIVAL trial (Fig. 21-2).[66] The primary end point of death, MI, stroke, or non-CABG major bleeding was similar in the radial and femoral groups. No significant interaction was observed in the subgroups of patients aged <75 and ≥75 years. Overall, the radial group had significantly fewer vascular complications, although the rates of this and other secondary end points have not been reported for the elderly subgroup.

Use of Radial Access for Elderly Patients in Clinical Practice

Over the past 20 years, the uptake of transradial cardiac catheterization has spread slowly across Canada, Europe, and Asia. Transradial angiography (TRA) is now used in approximately 50% of PCI procedures in Canada and 40% in Europe.[67] Although the uptake of transradial access has been slower in the United States, this is gradually changing.[68]

Recent registry data involving >590,00 procedures in the National Cardiovascular Data Registry (from 606 sites in the United States) examined the trend of radial versus femoral access for PCI between 2004 and 2007.[8] There was similar procedural success but significantly lower risk of bleeding complications with radial than with femoral access. However, in this observational data, the interaction in terms of age, gender, and indication for PCI were significant in the adjusted analysis of bleeding, such that the advantage of radial access was more pronounced among patients aged <75 years, females, and in those presenting with NSTEMI.[8] Despite potential benefits, radial access was paradoxically used less frequently in the elderly, females, and those with ACS.[8] These findings were echoed in an observational study[69] of 17,509 patients from five institutions in the United States between 2008 and 2011, in which elderly patients were less likely to be offered radial access.[69]

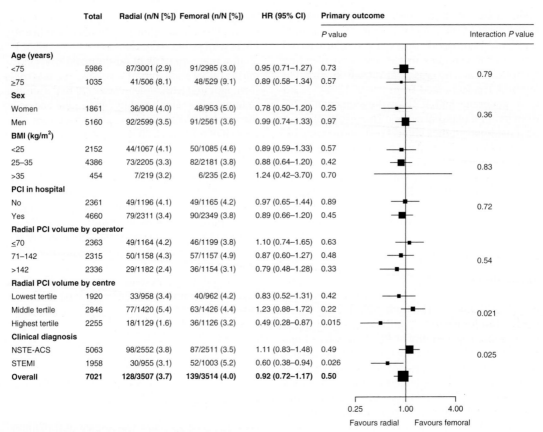

	Total	Radial (n/N [%])	Femoral (n/N [%])	HR (95% CI)	Primary outcome P value	Interaction P value
Age (years)						
<75	5986	87/3001 (2.9)	91/2985 (3.0)	0.95 (0.71–1.27)	0.73	0.79
≥75	1035	41/506 (8.1)	48/529 (9.1)	0.89 (0.58–1.34)	0.57	
Sex						
Women	1861	36/908 (4.0)	48/953 (5.0)	0.78 (0.50–1.20)	0.25	0.36
Men	5160	92/2599 (3.5)	91/2561 (3.6)	0.99 (0.74–1.33)	0.97	
BMI (kg/m²)						
<25	2152	44/1067 (4.1)	50/1085 (4.6)	0.89 (0.59–1.33)	0.57	
25–35	4386	73/2205 (3.3)	82/2181 (3.8)	0.88 (0.64–1.20)	0.42	0.83
>35	454	7/219 (3.2)	6/235 (2.6)	1.24 (0.42–3.70)	0.70	
PCI in hospital						
No	2361	49/1196 (4.1)	49/1165 (4.2)	0.97 (0.65–1.44)	0.89	0.72
Yes	4660	79/2311 (3.4)	90/2349 (3.8)	0.89 (0.66–1.20)	0.45	
Radial PCI volume by operator						
≤70	2363	49/1164 (4.2)	46/1199 (3.8)	1.10 (0.74–1.65)	0.63	
71–142	2315	50/1158 (4.3)	57/1157 (4.9)	0.87 (0.60–1.27)	0.48	0.54
>142	2336	29/1182 (2.4)	36/1154 (3.1)	0.79 (0.48–1.28)	0.33	
Radial PCI volume by centre						
Lowest tertile	1920	33/958 (3.4)	40/962 (4.2)	0.83 (0.52–1.31)	0.42	
Middle tertile	2846	77/1420 (5.4)	63/1426 (4.4)	1.23 (0.88–1.72)	0.22	0.021
Highest tertile	2255	18/1129 (1.6)	36/1126 (3.2)	0.49 (0.28–0.87)	0.015	
Clinical diagnosis						
NSTE-ACS	5063	98/2552 (3.8)	87/2511 (3.5)	1.11 (0.83–1.48)	0.49	0.025
STEMI	1958	30/955 (3.1)	52/1003 (5.2)	0.60 (0.38–0.94)	0.026	
Overall	**7021**	**128/3507 (3.7)**	**139/3514 (4.0)**	**0.92 (0.72–1.17)**	**0.50**	

0.25   1.00   4.00

Favours radial   Favours femoral

FIGURE 21-2 Subgroup analysis Forrest Plot from RIVAL.

In summary, elderly patients undergoing invasive cardiac procedures are at high risk for bleeding and ischemic complications. Although the elderly have been underrepresented in randomized trials comparing radial and femoral access, elderly patients appear to derive a benefit similar to that of younger patients in terms of reduced bleeding and access site complications with the radial approach. Anatomic considerations including smaller radial arteries, brachiocephalic and subclavian tortuosity, and unfolding of the aorta may lead to higher rates of crossover to femoral access, particularly for operators less experienced with radial access. Further research and technological advances will lead to further improvements in procedural success rates, and will help clarify the optimal antithrombotic strategy for elderly patients undergoing radial PCI. Radial access is currently very much underutilized in elderly patients, particularly in the United States. It is crucial to ensure that the benefits of radial access are extended to all patient subgroups, particularly those at higher risk of bleeding, to avoid the "risk-treatment" paradox in which interventions are used least in the patients expected to benefit the most from them.[70]

REFERENCES

1. Kobayashi Y, Mehran R, Mintz GS, et al. Comparison of in-hospital and one-year outcomes after multiple coronary arterial stenting in patients > or =80 years old versus those <80 years old. *Am J cardiol.* 2003;92(4):443–446.
2. Piper WD, Malenka DJ, Ryan TJ Jr, et al. Predicting vascular complications in percutaneous coronary interventions. *Am Heart J.* 2003;145(6):1022–1029.
3. Chauhan MS, Kuntz RE, Ho KL, et al. Coronary artery stenting in the aged. *J Am Coll Cardiol.* 2001;37(3):856–862.
4. Batchelor WB, Anstrom KJ, Muhlbaier LH, et al. Contemporary outcome trends in the elderly undergoing percutaneous coronary interventions: results in 7,472 octogenarians. National Cardiovascular Network Collaboration. *J Am Coll Cardiol.* 2000;36(3):723–730.
5. Jolly SS, Amlani S, Hamon M, et al. Radial versus femoral access for coronary angiography or intervention and the impact on major bleeding and ischemic events: a systematic review and meta-analysis of randomized trials. *Am Heart J.* 2009;157(1):132–140.
6. Cao Z, Zhou YJ, Zhao YX, et al. Transradial approach for coronary angioplasty in Chinese elderly patients. *Chin Med J (Engl).* 2008;121(12):1126–1129.
7. Bagur R, Bertrand OF, Rodes-Cabau J, et al. Comparison of outcomes in patients > or =70 years versus <70 years

after transradial coronary stenting with maximal antiplatelet therapy for acute coronary syndrome. *Am J Cardiol.* 2009;104(5):624–629.

8. Rao SV, Ou FS, Wang TY, et al. Trends in the prevalence and outcomes of radial and femoral approaches to percutaneous coronary intervention: a report from the National Cardiovascular Data Registry. *JACC Cardiovasc Interv.* 2008;1(4):379–386.

9. Wennberg DE, Makenka DJ, Sengupta A, et al.; and The Northern New England Cardiovascular Disease Study Group. Percutaneous transluminal coronary angioplasty in the elderly: epidemiology, clinical risk factors, and in-hospital outcomes. *Am Heart J.* 1999;137(4 pt 1):639–645.

10. Dynina O, Vakili BA, Slater JN, et al. In-hospital outcomes of contemporary percutaneous coronary interventions in the very elderly. *Catheter Cardiovasc Interv.* 2003;58(3): 351–357.

11. Berger AK, Schulman KA, Gersh BJ, et al. Primary coronary angioplasty vs thrombolysis for the management of acute myocardial infarction in elderly patients. *JAMA.* 1999;282(4):341–348.

12. Klein LW, Block P, Brindis RG, et al. Percutaneous coronary interventions in octogenarians in the American College of Cardiology-National Cardiovascular Data Registry: development of a nomogram predictive of in-hospital mortality. *J Am Coll Cardiol.* 2002;40(3):394–402.

13. Mehta RH, Sadiq I, Goldberg RJ, et al. Effectiveness of primary percutaneous coronary intervention compared with that of thrombolytic therapy in elderly patients with acute myocardial infarction. *Am Heart J.* 2004;147(2):253–259.

14. Halon DA, Adawi S, Dobrecky-Mery I, et al. Importance of increasing age on the presentation and outcome of acute coronary syndromes in elderly patients. *J Am Coll Cardiol.* 2004;43(3):346–352.

15. Zhang Q, Zhang RY, Zhang JS, et al. Outcomes of primary percutaneous coronary intervention for acute ST-elevation myocardial infarction in patients aged over 75 years. *Chin Med J.* 2006;119(14):1151–1156.

16. Sukiennik A, Krol A, Jachalska A, et al. Percutaneous coronary angioplasty in elderly patients: assessment of in-hospital outcomes. *Cardiol J.* 2007;14(2):143–154.

17. de Labriolle A, Giraudeau B, Pacouret G, et al. Revascularization algorithm in acute STEMI should take into account age. *Cardiovasc Revasc Med.* 2007;8(2):90–93.

18. Merchant FM, Weiner RB, Rao SR, et al. In-hospital outcomes of emergent and elective percutaneous coronary intervention in octogenarians. *Coron Artery Dis.* 2009;20(2):118–123.

19. Zimmermann S, Ruthrof S, Nowak K, et al. Outcomes of contemporary interventional therapy of ST elevation infarction in patients older than 75 years. *Clin Cardiol.* 2009;32(2):87–93.

20. Claessen BE, Kikkert WJ, Engstrom AE, et al. Primary percutaneous coronary intervention for ST elevation myocardial infarction in octogenarians: trends and outcomes. *Heart.* 2010;96(11):843–847.

21. Shelton RJ, Crean AM, Somers K, et al. Real-world outcome from ST elevation myocardial infarction in the very elderly before and after the introduction of a 24/7 primary percutaneous coronary intervention service. *Am Heart J.* 2010;159(6):956–963.

22. Liu SW, Qiao SB, Xu B, et al. Comparison of outcomes after transradial intervention in patients of different age groups. *Zhonghua Yi Xue Za Zhi.* 2010;90(40):2852–2855.

23. Antonsen L, Jensen LO, Thayssen P, et al. Comparison of outcomes of patients >/= 80 years of age having percutaneous coronary intervention according to presentation (stable vs unstable angina pectoris/

non-ST-segment elevation myocardial infarction vs ST-segment elevation myocardial infarction). *Am J Cardiol.* 2011;108(10):1395–1400.

24. Rao SV, Dai D, Subherwal S, et al. Association between periprocedural bleeding and long-term outcomes following percutaneous coronary intervention in older patients. *JACC Cardiovasc Interv.* 2012;5(9):958–965.

25. Mandawat A, Mandawat MK. Percutaneous coronary intervention after ST-segment elevation myocardial infarction in nonagenarians: use rates and in-hospital mortality. *J Am Coll Cardiol.* 2013;61(11):1207–1208.

26. Antonsen L, Jensen LO, Terkelsen CJ, et al. Outcomes after primary percutaneous coronary intervention in octogenarians and nonagenarians with ST-segment elevation myocardial infarction: from the Western Denmark heart registry. *Catheter Cardiovasc Interv.* 2013;81(6):912–919.

27. Lazzeri C, Valente S, Chiostri M, et al. Trends in mortality rates in elderly ST elevation myocardial infarction patients submitted to primary percutaneous coronary intervention: a 7-year single-center experience. *Geriatr Gerontol Int.* 2013;13(3):711–717.

28. Alexander KP, Roe MT, Chen AY, et al. Evolution in cardiovascular care for elderly patients with non-ST-segment elevation acute coronary syndromes: results from the CRUSADE National Quality Improvement Initiative. *J Am Coll Cardiol.* 2005;46(8):1479–1487.

29. Brieger D, Van de Werf F, Avezum A, et al. Interactions between heparins, glycoprotein IIb/IIIa antagonists, and coronary intervention. The Global Registry of Acute Coronary Events (GRACE). *Am Heart J.* 2007;153(6):960–969.

30. Alexander KP, Newby LK, Cannon CP, et al. Acute coronary care in the elderly, part I: non-ST-segment-elevation acute coronary syndromes: a scientific statement for healthcare professionals from the American Heart Association Council on Clinical Cardiology: in collaboration with the Society of Geriatric Cardiology. *Circulation.* 2007;115(19):2549–2569.

31. Alexander KP, Newby LK, Armstrong PW, et al. Acute coronary care in the elderly, part II: ST-segment-elevation myocardial infarction: a scientific statement for healthcare professionals from the American Heart Association Council on Clinical Cardiology: in collaboration with the Society of Geriatric Cardiology. *Circulation.* 2007;115(19):2570–2589.

32. Gilat D, Goldbourt U, Reicher-Reiss H, et al.; and SPRINT Study Group. Prognosis of acute myocardial infarction in the elderly. *Harefuah.* 1993;124(10):601–603, 668.

33. Lee PY, Alexander KP, Hammill BG, et al. Representation of elderly persons and women in published randomized trials of acute coronary syndromes. *JAMA.* 2001;286(6): 708–713.

34. Granger CB, Goldberg RJ, Dabbous O, et al. Predictors of hospital mortality in the global registry of acute coronary events. *Arch Intern Med.* 2003;163(19):2345–2353.

35. Avezum A, Makdisse M, Spencer F, et al. Impact of age on management and outcome of acute coronary syndrome: observations from the Global Registry of Acute Coronary Events (GRACE). *Am Heart J.* 2005;149(1):67–73.

36. Lopes RD, Alexander KP, Manoukian SV, et al. Advanced age, antithrombotic strategy, and bleeding in non-ST-segment elevation acute coronary syndromes: results from the ACUITY (Acute Catheterization and Urgent Intervention Triage Strategy) trial. *J Am Coll Cardiol.* 2009;53(12):1021–1030.

37. MacHaalany J, Abdelaal E, Bataille Y, et al. Benefit of bivalirudin versus heparin after transradial and transfemoral percutaneous coronary intervention. *Am J Cardiol.* 2012;110(12):1742–1748.

38. Bertrand OF, Jolly SS, Rao SV, et al. Meta-analysis comparing bivalirudin versus heparin monotherapy on ischemic and bleeding outcomes after percutaneous coronary intervention. *Am J Cardiol.* 2012;110(4):599–606.

39. Keeley EC, Boura JA, Grines CL. Primary angioplasty versus intravenous thrombolytic therapy for acute myocardial infarction: a quantitative review of 23 randomised trials. *Lancet.* 2003;361(9351):13–20.

40. Mehta RH, Granger CB, Alexander KP, et al. Reperfusion strategies for acute myocardial infarction in the elderly: benefits and risks. *J Am Coll Cardiol.* 2005;45(4): 471–478.

41. de Boer SP, Westerhout CM, Simes RJ, et al. Mortality and morbidity reduction by primary percutaneous coronary intervention is independent of the patient's age. *JACC Cardiovasc Interv.* 2010;3(3):324–331.

42. Dodson JA, Wang Y, Chaudhry SI, et al. Bleeding-avoidance strategies and outcomes in patients >/=80 years of age with ST-elevation myocardial infarction undergoing primary percutaneous coronary intervention (from the NCDR CathPCI Registry). *Am J Cardiol.* 2012;110(1):1–6.

43. Yoo BS, Yoon J, Ko JY, et al. Anatomical consideration of the radial artery for transradial coronary procedures: arterial diameter, branching anomaly and vessel tortuosity. *Int J Cardiol.* 2005;101(3):421–427.

44. Freestone B, Nolan J. Transradial cardiac procedures: the state of the art. *Heart.* 2010;96(11):883–891.

45. Dehghani P, Mohammad A, Bajaj R, et al. Mechanism and predictors of failed transradial approach for percutaneous coronary interventions. *JACC Cardiovasc Interv.* 2009;2(11):1057–1064.

46. Sciahbasi A, Romagnoli E, Burzotta F, et al. Transradial approach (left vs right) and procedural times during percutaneous coronary procedures: TALENT study. *Am Heart J.* 2011;161(1):172–179.

47. Santas E, Bodi V, Sanchis J, et al. The left radial approach in daily practice. A randomized study comparing femoral and right and left radial approaches. *Rev Esp Cardiol.* 2009;62(5):482–490.

48. Kawashima O, Endoh N, Terashima M, et al. Effectiveness of right or left radial approach for coronary angiography. *Catheter Cardiovasc Interv.* 2004;61(3):333–337.

49. Kanei Y, Nakra NC, Liou M, et al. Randomized comparison of transradial coronary angiography via right or left radial artery approaches. *Am J Cardiol.* 2011;107(2):195–197.

50. Fernandez-Portales J, Valdesuso R, Carreras R, et al. Right versus left radial artery approach for coronary angiography: Differences observed and the learning curve. *Rev Esp Cardiol.* 2006;59(10):1071–1074.

51. Norgaz T, Gorgulu S, Dagdelen S. A randomized study comparing the effectiveness of right and left radial approach for coronary angiography. *Catheter Cardiovasc Interv.* 2012;80(2):260–264.

52. Larsen P, Shah S, Waxman S, et al. Comparison of procedural times, success rates, and safety between left versus right radial arterial access in primary percutaneous coronary intervention for acute ST-segment elevation myocardial infarction. *Catheter Cardiovasc Interv.* 2011;78(1):38–44.

53. Pelliccia F, Trani C, Biondi-Zoccai GG, et al. Comparison of the feasibility and effectiveness of transradial coronary angiography via right versus left radial artery approaches (from the PREVAIL Study). *Am J Cardiol.* 2012;110(6):771–775.

54. Biondi-Zoccai G, Sciahbasi A, Bodi V, et al. Right versus left radial artery access for coronary procedures: an international collaborative systematic review and meta-analysis including 5 randomized trials and 3210 patients. *Int J Cardiol.* 2013;166(3):621–626.

55. Bertrand OF, Rao SV, Pancholy S, et al. Transradial approach for coronary angiography and interventions: results of the first international transradial practice survey. *JACC Cardiovasc Interv.* 2010;3(10):1022–1031.

56. Freixa X, Trilla M, Feldman M, et al. Right versus left transradial approach for coronary catheterization in octogenarian patients. *Catheter Cardiovasc Interv.* 2012;80(2):267–272.

57. Louvard Y, Benamer H, Garot P, et al. Comparison of transradial and transfemoral approaches for coronary angiography and angioplasty in octogenarians (the OCTOPLUS study). *Am J Cardiol.* 2004;94(9):1177–1180.

58. Achenbach S, Ropers D, Kallert L, et al. Transradial versus transfemoral approach for coronary angiography and intervention in patients above 75 years of age. *Catheter Cardiovasc Interv.* 2008;72(5):629–635.

59. Klinke WP, Hilton JD, Warburton RN, et al. Comparison of treatment outcomes in patients > or =80 years undergoing transradial versus transfemoral coronary intervention. *Am J Cardiol.* 2004;93(10):1282–1285.

60. Jaffe R, Hong T, Sharieff W, et al. Comparison of radial versus femoral approach for percutaneous coronary interventions in octogenarians. *Catheter Cardiovasc Interv.* 2007;69(6):815–820.

61. Ziakas A, Gomma A, McDonald J, et al. A comparison of the radial and the femoral approaches in primary or rescue percutaneous coronary intervention for acute myocardial infarction in the elderly. *Acute Card Care.* 2007;9(2):93–96.

62. Koutouzis M, Matejka G, Olivecrona G, et al. Radial vs. femoral approach for primary percutaneous coronary intervention in octogenarians. *Cardiovasc Revasc Med.* 2010;11(2):79–83.

63. Bertrand OF, Bagur R, Costerousse O, et al. Transradial vs femoral percutaneous coronary intervention for left main disease in octogenarians. *Indian Heart J.* 2010;62(3):234–237.

64. Hu F, Yang Y, Qiao S, et al. Comparison between radial and femoral approach for percutaneous coronary intervention in patients aged 80 years or older. *J Interv Cardiol.* 2012;25(5):513–517.

65. Secco GG, Marinucci L, Uguccioni L, et al. Transradial versus transfemoral approach for primary percutaneous coronary interventions in elderly patients. *J Invasive Cardiol.* 2013;25(5):254–256.

66. Jolly SS, Yusuf S, Cairns J, et al. Radial versus femoral access for coronary angiography and intervention in patients with acute coronary syndromes (RIVAL): a randomised, parallel group, multicentre trial. *Lancet.* 2011;377(9775):1409–1420.

67. Ratib K, Mamas MA, Routledge HC, et al. Influence of access site choice on incidence of neurologic complications after percutaneous coronary intervention. *Am Heart J.* 2013;165(3):317–324.

68. Feldman DN, Swaminathan RV, Kaltenbach L, et al. Adoption of radial access and comparison of outcomes to femoral approach in percutaneous coronary intervention: an updated report from the NCDR®. *Circulation.* 2012;126:A12423.

69. Wimmer NJ, Resnic FS, Mauri L, et al. Risk-treatment paradox in the selection of transradial access for percutaneous coronary intervention. *J Am Heart Assoc.* 2013; 2(3):e000174.

70. McAlister FA. The end of the risk-treatment paradox? A rising tide lifts all boats. *J Am Coll Cardiol.* 2011;58(17): 1766–1767.

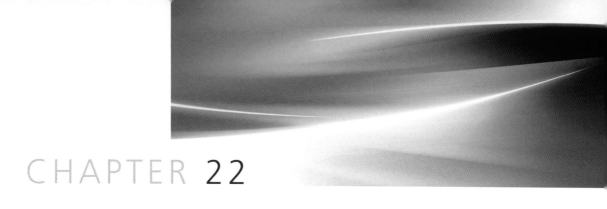

CHAPTER 22

Carotid, Femoral, Aortoiliac, and Renal Interventions

J. Tift Mann III, John T. Coppola, Ravikiran Korabathina, Tejas Patel and Rajiv Gulati

Transradial Carotid Stenting

J. Tift Mann III

Introduction

When performed by experienced operators using distal embolic protection, carotid artery stenting has been shown to be a proven alternative to carotid endarterectomy in patients with significant carotid disease.[1-6] The procedure is currently approved in the United States for patients who have an increased risk for surgery. The femoral artery is the conventional access site for carotid stent procedures, but this approach may be difficult or impossible in certain patients with anatomical variations of the aortic arch or common carotid artery. Furthermore, arteriosclerotic disease within the aortic arch may be a source of cerebral emboli liberated by transfemoral (TF) catheter manipulations.[7-10] Finally, peripheral vascular disease and the risk of femoral access-site bleeding are additional limitations to the traditional approach. Thus, an alternative access for carotid stenting is occasionally necessary.

Previous studies have demonstrated both the feasibility and safety of transradial (TR) approach for carotid artery stenting.[11-27] Indeed, Etxegoien et al.[16] have recently reported a two-center series in which TR carotid stenting was successful in 347/382 (91%) patients, with a low complication rate. Adverse events included two major strokes (0.6%), one of which lead to death, three minor strokes (1%), and no myocardial infarction at 30 days. No bleeding complications occurred.

Carotid stent procedures from both the right and left accesses have been presented in the literature. Patel et al.[23] have described a contralateral arm technique in a series of 20 patients with a success rate of 80%, and success was higher in patients presenting with right internal carotid disease. The purpose of this section is to describe the technique of carotid stenting from the right radial approach.

Transradial Carotid Angiography

From the right radial approach, initial carotid angiography is performed with 5F diagnostic catheters. It is important to initially assess the aortic arch and the configuration of the origin of the great vessels with a left anterior oblique (LAO) aortogram using a standard pigtail catheter. Subsequent catheter selection is based on the arch type as well as the appearance of the takeoff of the common carotid arteries.

For TR left carotid angiography, a wire-braided Simmons 2 diagnostic catheter is most commonly utilized. Reforming this large curve in the aorta may be problematic, and the technique described by Lee et al.[28] is recommended. The catheter is initially positioned in the transverse aorta and the guidewire withdrawn into the primary curve. Advancing the catheter into the ascending aorta with *counterclockwise* rotation creates a loop on itself that will select the origin of the left common carotid. A 0.025-inch glidewire may assist selection (Fig. 22-1). The distal limb of the catheter is positioned more deeply in the left common carotid by gently withdrawing the catheter using *clockwise* rotation (Fig. 22-2).

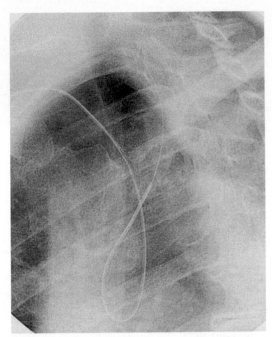

FIGURE 22-1 From the transverse aorta, the Simmons 2 catheter is prolapsed into the ascending aorta with counterclockwise rotation creating a loop on itself that will select the left common carotid artery. A 0.025-inch straight glidewire assists with selection.

Alternative catheters for left carotid angiography may also be used. A Simmons 1 diagnostic catheter works well when the distance between the innominate and the left common carotid is narrow, while a Tiger or Kimny catheter is better for wider distances. A 0.025-inch glidewire will not deform the primary curve of the diagnostic catheter and is useful in selecting the common carotid.

In the presence of bovine left carotid anatomy, the right radial approach is the preferred strategy for angiography and stenting. An Amplatz AR2 will easily select the origin of the bovine common carotid (Fig. 22-3).

For TR right carotid angiography, catheter selection is based on an initial RAO subclavian arteriogram (Fig. 22-4). The latter defines subclavian tortuosity as well as the angle of takeoff of the right common carotid artery. A Simmons 1 catheter is used in most cases (Fig. 22-5). A Tiger catheter is an alternative choice, especially when the angle of takeoff of the right common carotid is less acute.

Right Radial Access for Carotid Stenting

It is apparent from initial feasibility studies that the right TR technique for carotid stenting involves three different techniques for the three basic anatomical types of carotid disease: right internal carotid, bovine left internal carotid, and nonbovine left internal carotid. Thus, this section is subdivided to review the three basic techniques.

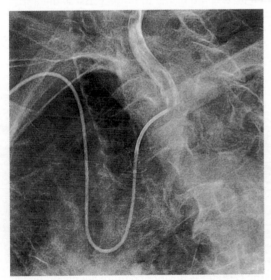

FIGURE 22-2 A Simmons 2 catheter positioned in the left common carotid artery.

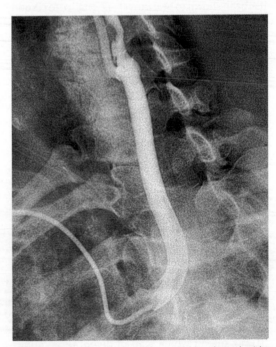

FIGURE 22-3 The bovine left carotid is selected with an Amplatz AR2 catheter.

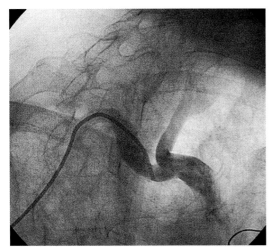

FIGURE 22-4 An RAO arteriogram of the innominate artery bifurcation.

The technique of TR insertion of a sheath for carotid stent deployment is a variation of the technique used for femoral access. Thus, a diagnostic catheter positioned in the external carotid artery is used for the insertion of an exchange-length, supportive guidewire over which the sheath is deployed. Once the sheath is in place, the technique of embolic protection device deployment and carotid stenting is precisely the same as from the femoral artery. However, deployment of the sheath from the right arm necessarily involves acute angles that must be negotiated, and different catheters are required than the ones used with the femoral approach.

Right Internal Carotid

The right carotid is selected with a 5F Simmons 1 diagnostic catheter. The original technique of right internal carotid artery stenting involves passing the Simmons 1 catheter into the external carotid artery over a glidewire or extra-support coronary guidewire (Fig. 22-6).[10] An exchange-length 0.035-inch J wire was then inserted, which serves as the platform for sheath deployment. Although an Amplatz superstiff wire is used for

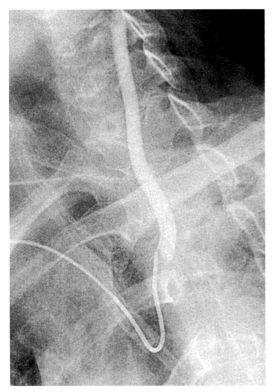

FIGURE 22-5 Simmons 1 catheter positioned in the right common carotid artery.

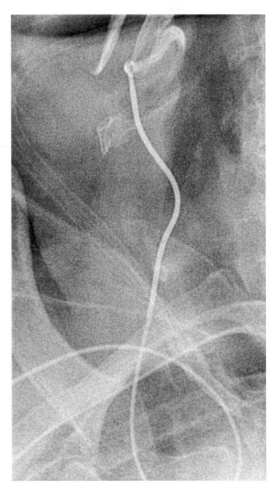

FIGURE 22-6 French Simmons 1 catheter in right external carotid artery.

this purpose from the femoral approach, excessive tension is created by the acute angles from the arm and its use should generally be avoided.

The TAD II (Covidien, Mansfield, MA) is a 0.035-inch exchange-length guidewire that tapers to a soft 0.018-inch floppy tip. The external carotid can often be directly cannulated with this guidewire, which then serves as a platform for the deployment of the shuttle sheath. Thus, the step of passing the diagnostic catheter into the external carotid artery is omitted, expediting the procedure. The Advantage (Terumo Corporation, Somerset, NJ) hybrid wire may also be used for this purpose, and the selection of the external carotid with its hydrophilic tip may be easier.

When the angle of takeoff of the right common carotid is vertical or acute (Fig. 22-7), a telescopic technique with the sheath (90 cm) over the Simmons 1 catheter (100 cm) is useful to traverse the acute angle. A 5F shuttle sheath is best used in this situation in view of its flexibility and smooth transition with no lip at the sheath/catheter junction.

An alternative strategy for right carotid acute angles involves the use of a wire-braided

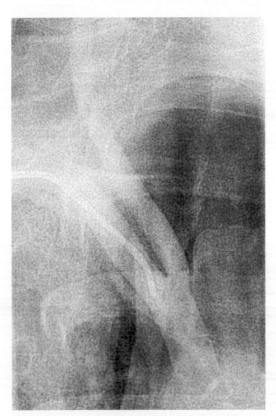

FIGURE 22-7 An RAO innominate arteriogram demonstrating a vertical takeoff of the right common carotid with no horizontal segment for support.

Simmons 2 catheter (see the previous paragraph for reforming technique). This catheter is passed into the external over a glidewire or extra-support coronary wire and then exchanged for the shuttle sheath. This catheter should not be used in women or short patients as the long distal limb may actually reach the carotid bifurcation.

When a small radial artery or acute angle necessitates the use of a 5F shuttle sheath, only lower-profile Precise stents and Wallstents are compatible. An important caveat is that suction produced by the introduction of stent can introduce air into the system. Thus, stents are positioned with roadmap fluoroscopy and/or bony landmarks. Alternatively, one can patiently wait for complete bleed-back before injecting the contrast material.

Nonbovine Left Internal Carotid

The nemesis for the development of a consistent technique for nonbovine left internal carotid stenting from the right radial artery has been the acute angle that must be traversed for the deployment of a shuttle sheath in the left common carotid. The angle results in poor inferior support for the catheter system, resulting in a tendency for catheters to prolapse into the ascending aorta. This problem is particularly ominous should prolapse occur during stent delivery.

The use of a wire-braided Simmons 2 catheter (Cook Medical, Bloomington, IN) with its relatively long distal end has been found to provide adequate support for passing a guidewire into the external carotid in the majority of cases. A Simmons 3 catheter provides even more support and is utilized in cases of type II and type III arches with particularly acute angles of takeoff of the common carotid.

The anchoring technique with a stepwise exchange of glidewire or TAD II wire and 0.035-inch J wire through the diagnostic catheter in the external is most commonly utilized. With extreme angles, a 5F or 6F multipurpose or Amplatz R2 guide catheter can be used as an intermediate transfer catheter to insert an Amplatz superstiff guidewire. In these extreme situations, kinking of the shuttle sheath may occur at the acute angle, and a heavily braided, semihydrophilic Destination sheath (Terumo Corporation, Somerset, NJ) should be substituted.

A telescopic approach with a Simmons 2 diagnostic within the sheath is preferred in most cases of nonbovine left internal carotid artery (LICA) lesions. As previously noted, a 5F shuttle sheath is more flexible without a lip at the sheath/catheter transition. If a 6F sheath is required, it should be telescoped over a 6F diagnostic Simmons 2/3 to prevent this transition lip from catching at the origin of the common carotid.

In patients with a type I arch and left internal carotid lesions, the TAD II guidewire can be passed directly into the external and usually provides sufficient support for the deployment of the shuttle sheath (Fig. 22-8). Again, a telescoped 5F shuttle sheath/Simmons 2 is better. This simple technique is successful only with less severe angles of takeoff of the left common carotid.

The catheter looping and retrograde engagement technique (CLARET) is an alternative strategy that has been described by Fang et al.[17] in a large series of patients. The unique feature of this technique is the use of the right coronary cusp to provide inferior support for the system (Fig. 22-6). The technique uses a 7F Kimny or multipurpose guide catheter placed in the carotid for the stent procedure. Because of the large external diameter of this catheter, it can be used

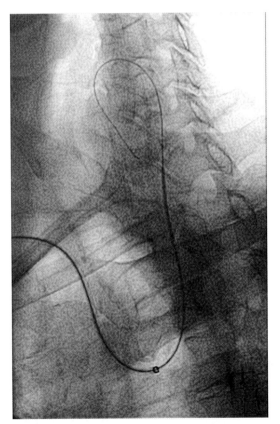

FIGURE 22-8 A shuttle sheath telescoped over a Simmons 2 diagnostic catheter introduced over a TAD II guidewire into the left internal carotid artery in a patient with a type I arch.

only in a minority of patients transradially unless inserted sheathlessly. Catheter instability also may be problematic.

Bovine Left Internal Carotid

The right TR approach may be the preferred strategy for carotid stenting of bovine left internal carotid lesions. The initial takeoff of the bovine carotid is evaluated using an LAO aortic arch arteriogram. When the initial segment of the common carotid is horizontal (Fig. 22-3), an Amplatz R2 diagnostic catheter is suitable. When the initial segment is more vertical (Fig. 22-4), a Simmons 1 or 2 is necessary to implement the exchange for the shuttle sheath. Techniques similar to the right or nonbovine left internal carotid cases for the insertion of the shuttle sheath are utilized.

Caveats

It should be emphasized that experience in the TR approach is important as these are advanced techniques. New operators are encouraged to be comfortable both with TR cerebrovascular angiography and with TF carotid stenting before undertaking these procedures.

The most important limitation of this technique is the lack of inferior support at the origin of the common carotid where sheath angulation is most extreme. This is particularly an issue with nonbovine left carotids and is the cause of most TR carotid failures. Prolapse of the shuttle sheath into the ascending aorta is most likely to occur during the initial delivery attempt, but may also occur during delivery of rigid, bulky stents. The latter situation is ominous since the embolic protection device may be pulled back across the carotid lesion while still fully deployed, increasing the risk of embolic stroke.

Finally, air introduction may occur when bulky stents are advanced through small-diameter sheaths, and stents should be positioned using roadmap fluoroscopy or bony landmarks. Contrast injections are made only after careful bleed-back.

Conclusion

The TR approach for carotid stenting is feasible and holds promise as an alternative technique to conventional femoral access. High success rates with low complications have been demonstrated with right and left carotid stenting. It is the preferred access site for bovine left carotid stenting and right carotid stenting in the presence of a "hostile" arch. However, further refinement of the technique as well as future technological improvements are necessary to simplify the procedure and optimize results.

Aorto-Iliac

John T. Coppola and Ravikiran Korabathina

Natural History

The prevalence of lower extremity peripheral artery disease (PAD) varies depending on the population studied and the criteria used to define disease. When an ankle-brachial index (ABI) measurement of <0.9 is the diagnostic standard, the overall prevalence of PAD according to the Atherosclerosis Risk in Communities study cohort for individuals between 45 and 64 years of age was 2.6%.[29,30] The Multi-Ethnic Study of Atherosclerosis study cohort showed a significant rise in prevalence with each subsequent age decade, rising to 6.44% in those between 65 and 74 years and 11.98% in those between 75 and 84 years.[29,31] Lower extremity PAD is also highly prevalent in populations with high atherosclerotic risk factor burden, as illustrated by the PAD Awareness, Risk and Treatment: New Resources for Survival (PARTNERS) study.[32] Of 6,417 patients presenting to primary care practices who were 70 years or older or aged 50 to 69 with diabetes mellitus or tobacco dependence, PAD was detected in 29%. In the population with manifest cardiovascular disease defined by a history of angina, myocardial infarction, coronary revascularization, aortic aneurysm repair, stroke, or carotid endarterectomy, the prevalence increased to over 40%. Furthermore, PAD was more common in African Americans and women without cardiovascular disease.

Aorto-iliac PAD appears to have a different epidemiology when compared to infrainguinal PAD, likely stemming from the histological differences between these arterial beds. In a retrospective analysis, atherosclerosis of the larger and more elastic aorto-iliac arteries was associated more so with smoking and to a lesser degree with diabetes.[33] When looking at patients with early-onset PAD, defined as onset before the age of 50, interestingly, 65% were shown to have aorto-iliac disease in one study, and the risk factors strongly associated with this disease location were the absence of diabetes, low HDL cholesterol, and female gender.[34] The relation of female gender to aorto-iliac disease is intriguing,

especially given that hypoplastic aortic vessels are more common in women, and an association between smaller aortic diameters and aortic atherosclerosis progression has been demonstrated.[35] Typically, PAD presents as a multilevel disease, with most surgical series reporting that up to two-thirds of individuals present with both aorto-iliac and infrainguinal disease.[36] Nevertheless, the presence of large-vessel PAD has been shown to carry greater prognostic implications, with a nearly fourfold higher risk for fatal and nonfatal cardiovascular events than is seen with small-vessel PAD.[37]

Clinical Diagnosis and Vascular Testing

Many patients with PAD have no symptoms, and a large proportion of symptomatic individuals do not present with classic intermittent claudication.[38] Typical symptoms of aorto-iliac disease include buttock, hip, and thigh pain while walking; however, patients may also present with leg fatigue, muscle weakness, erectile dysfunction, and tissue loss. As a means of uniformly describing symptoms, both the Fontaine and Rutherford classification systems have been used (Table 22-1).

Noninvasive physiologic vascular testing helps with localizing lower limb PAD. Using segmental limb pressures, a thigh-brachial index (TBI) of >1.1 is considered normal, and a value <0.9 is abnormal.[39] With the placement of a high thigh cuff, an abnormal TBI in both limbs suggests aorto-iliac disease, and an abnormal TBI in one limb may allude to ipsilateral iliac disease. Plethysmography can be used to obtain pulse volume recordings (PVR). As the normal PVR is characterized by a sharp systolic upstroke and a prominent dicrotic notch during the downslope toward the baseline, when aorto-iliac disease is present, the thigh PVR will lose the dicrotic notch and become rounded and blunted (Fig. 22-9). Furthermore, all PVRs from the bilateral limb segments would be abnormal. In unilateral iliac disease, the thigh PVR in the affected limb would be abnormal with normal-appearing waveforms in the contralateral limb.

The degree of stenosis required to exert a physiologic impact large enough to produce ischemic symptoms has been defined in older angiographic surgical series. Using an experimental iliac model, one study showed that a focal 1-cm lesion of 80% would be required in order to reduce limb flow by 20%.[40] Studies of symptomatic patients with claudication and intermediate

TABLE 22-1   Classification of Peripheral Arterial Disease: Fontaine's Stages and Rutherford's Categories

	Fontaine		Rutherford	
Stage	Clinical	Grade	Category	Clinical
I	Asymptomatic	0	0	Asymptomatic
IIa	Mild claudication	I	1	Mild
IIB	Moderate-to-severe claudication	I	2	Moderate claudication
		I	3	Severe claudication
III	Ischemic rest pain	II	4	Ischemic rest pain
IV	Ulceration or gangrene	III	5	Minor tissue loss
		III	6	Major tissue loss

lesions between 50% and 75% have shown that when an aorto-femoral peak systolic pressure gradient of 10 mmHg exists across an iliac stenosis, symptoms improve after revascularization.[41] While multiple criteria for translesional gradient assessment have been described, including the use of peak systolic gradient, mean gradient, and pulse pressure differential, the peak systolic gradient has been shown to carry the highest sensitivity.[42]

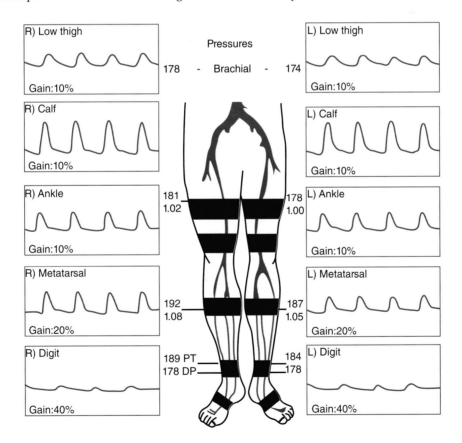

FIGURE 22-9   **A:** A normal PVR study. **B:** An abnormal PVR study in a 54-year-old female with bilateral buttock claudication with ambulation, demonstrating abnormal bilateral thigh waveforms suggesting aorto-iliac disease. (From Parks Medical Electronics, Aloha, Oregon.)

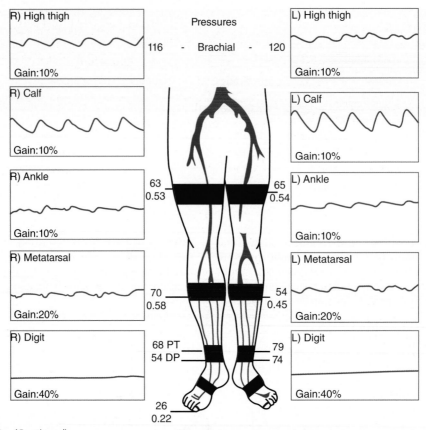

FIGURE 22-9 *(Continued)*

Treatment

Conservative

Medical Therapy. The treatment landscape of aorto-iliac PAD has changed markedly over the past two decades, especially since its recognition as a coronary heart disease risk equivalent. As such, aggressive atherosclerosis risk factor modification, including the appropriate introduction of lipid-lowering, antiplatelet, antihypertensive, and antihyperglycemic drugs has become the cornerstone of therapy. Smoking cessation therapies and following the dietary prescription as outlined in the National Cholesterol Education Program Adult Treatment Panel III guidelines are particularly important.[43] Pharmacologic drugs directed at claudication treatment have also proven useful, and in the United States, a trial with cilostazol has been given a class I indication and pentoxifylline a class IIb indication for symptom relief and functional improvement.[44]

Supervised Exercise Rehabilitation. Adjunctive to medical therapy, rehabilitation therapy for intermittent claudication is fully supported by the literature. Gardner and Poehlman[45] performed a meta-analysis of 21 studies, showing a marked 179% increase in distance to claudication onset and 122% increase in distance to maximal claudication pain, following a program of exercise rehabilitation. This meta-analysis also detailed the parameters that confer the most benefit being an exercise program that lasts 6 months and includes 30-minute exercise sessions occurring three times weekly. Moving a step further, Spronk et al.[46] recently compared supervised exercise training to angioplasty in 151 patients with mostly aorto-iliac disease. They demonstrated equal efficacy between these two treatment strategies in terms of functional capacity and quality-of-life scores 12 months following either therapy.

The effectiveness of an initial strategy of conservative therapy for aorto-iliac PAD versus immediate revascularization is supported by randomized controlled trial data. In an older study, Whyman et al.[47] compared 62 patients with ilio-femoral stenoses and claudication who were randomized to treatment by balloon angioplasty or conventional medical therapy. There was no difference in treadmill onset to claudication or maximum walking distance at 2 years. Unfortunately, the limitations of this study were the inclusion of only a small number of discrete iliac stenoses, exclusion of iliac occlusions, high screening failure rate in meeting the study criteria, and unclear but likely outdated medical therapy. Frans et al.[48] conducted a meta-analysis looking only at randomized controlled trial data in the more modern era and confirmed the equivalence of supervised exercise training with percutaneous transluminal angioplasty (PTA) in terms of improved walking distances. Unfortunately, this meta-analysis also suffered limitations owing to the inclusion of both iliac and femoral lesion types and the heterogeneity of end point definitions. Most recently, short-term data from the multicenter Claudication: Exercise versus Endoluminal Revascularization (CLEVER) study have been presented.[49] This trial randomized 119 patients with aorto-iliac disease, including almost 40% with iliac occlusions, to optimal medical care, supervised exercise, or stent placement. This is the only trial to date that has focused exclusively on large, proximal-vessel PAD, with three comparative arms: medical therapy alone, exercise training, and endovascular stenting. Supervised exercise therapy conferred a significantly greater change in peak walking time over 6 months when compared to either stent placement or optimal medical therapy alone.

Revascularization

When revascularization is deemed necessary, as when there is failure of conservative therapies, the patient's comorbidity profile and lesion anatomy help in selecting the appropriate revascularization option. An anatomic classification of aorto-iliac PAD was devised by the Trans-Atlantic Inter-society Consensus Working Group (TASC II) in an attempt to balance the risk and durability of revascularization procedures and to make suggestions regarding the choice between endovascular versus surgical revascularization options (Fig. 22-10).[50] Type A lesions are short stenoses that yield excellent endovascular results. Type B, C, and D lesions are either long stenoses or occlusions of increasing severity. The most challenging type D lesions are felt to give such poor endovascular results that a surgical strategy should be considered as the first choice. Data regarding treatment preference for type B and C lesions are limited, but type B lesions often give good

results when approached using an endovascular strategy. Type C lesions provide good long-term results from an open surgical procedure, and this should be the preferred choice unless the patient has a high operative risk.

In any regard, prior to proceeding with either surgical or endovascular treatments, imaging studies are compulsory in order to provide the blueprint for the repair strategy. Duplex ultrasonography gives both anatomic and physiologic data on stenosis severity. Magnetic resonance angiography has very high specificity and sensitivity for aorto-iliac disease and has the advantage of avoiding radiation and contrast. Computed tomographic angiography has comparatively similar sensitivity and specificity but requires the use of contrast and radiation.

Surgical Approach

Surgical bypass, mostly consisting of aorto-femoral and axillo-femoral bypasses, was formerly considered the primary revascularization route for patients with severe aorto-iliac disease, especially for TASC B-D lesions. The largest meta-analysis of surgical cases by de Vries et al.[51] showed that while the 5-year long-term patency of these procedures is high at 91%, this is countered by their high operative mortality of 3.3% and aggregate morbidity of 8.3%. It is for these reasons that interest in percutaneous therapies has grown.

Endovascular Approach

Efficacy and Safety. The polyvascular nature of atherosclerosis, and its incumbent high risk for major adverse cardiac and cerebral events, that is frequently present in the individual who manifests with PAD makes surgical repair options riskier and often precludes the use of such an aggressive approach. Remarkable advancements in the endovascular armamentarium may offer the higher-risk PAD patient a better safety margin. In fact, the most recent ACC/AHA (American College of Cardiology/American Heart Association) PAD guidelines have given a class I indication for endovascular procedures if the anatomy is suitable (i.e., TASC A lesions) in a patient with lifestyle-limiting claudication that has not responded to exercise or medication.[44] This recommendation is based on multiple series in the literature demonstrating the efficacy and safety of this approach. Bosch et al.,[52] in a large meta-analysis of studies conducted in the 1990s, demonstrated a technical success rate for iliac stenting of 96% with a durable primary patency at 4 years of 74%. Furthermore, the 30-day mortality was low at 0.8%, with a major complication rate of 5.2%. More

Type A lesions

• Unilateral or bilateral stenoses of CIA
• Unilateral or bilateral single short (≤3 cm) stenosis of EIA

Type B lesions:

• Short (≤3 cm) stenosis of infrarenal aorta
• Unilateral CIA occlusion
• Single or multiple stenosis totaling 3–10 cm involving the EIA not extending into the CFA
• Unilateral EIA occlusion not involving the origins of internal iliac or CFA

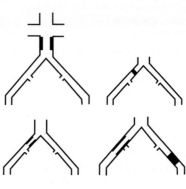

Type C lesions

• Bilateral CIA occlusions
• Bilateral EIA stenoses 3–10 cm long not extending into the CFA
• Unilateral EIA stenosis extending into the CFA
• Unilateral EIA occlusion that involves the origins of internal iliac and/or CFA
• Heavily calcified unilateral EIA occlusion with or without involvement of origins of internal iliac and/ or CFA

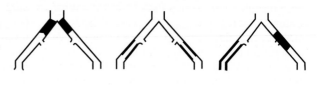

Type D lesions

• Infra-renal aortoiliac occlusion
• Diffuse disease involving the aorta and bothe iliac arteries requiring treatment
• Diffuse multiple stenoses involving the unilateral CIA, EIA, and CFA
• Unilateral occlusions of both CIA and EIA
• Bilateral occlusions of EIA
• Iliac stenoses in patients with AAA requiring treatment and not amenable to endograft placement or other lesions requiring open aortic or iliac surgery

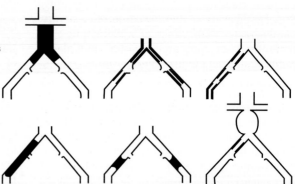

FIGURE 22-10 TASC classification of aorto-iliac lesions. (From Norgren L, Hiatt WR, Dormandy JA, et al.; TASC II Working Group. Inter-society consensus for the management of peripheral arterial disease (TASC II). *J Vasc Surg.* 2007;45 (suppl S):S5–S67.)

recently, Murphy et al.,[53] in their large single-center experience of aorto-iliac stenting, showed 8-year primary and secondary patencies of 74% and 84%, respectively, with a 30-day mortality rate of 0.5%.

The efficacy and durability of endovascular techniques when compared directly against open surgical procedures for aorto-iliac PAD have been confirmed in the literature. An earlier study by Holm et al.[54] randomized 102 patients to PTA versus surgery for short-segment iliac disease between 1983 and 1988, showing similar success rates in terms of postprocedural improvement in ABIs at discharge and at 1 year between the two strategies. More recently, a study from the Cleveland Clinic by Kashyap et al.[55] compared aorto-bifemoral bypass to endovascular therapy in patients with TASC B–D lesions, with over 75% of patients having type C or D lesions. While the primary patency rate at 3 years was higher in the surgical than in the endovascular group (93% vs 74%, respectively), the secondary patency rates were equivalent at 93%. There were no significant differences in safety when comparing the two groups, in terms of perioperative mortality or postoperative complications. Unexpectedly, female gender and smoking were not related to primary patency, whereas the presence of diabetes was related to patency loss. Interestingly, they found a high primary patency rate of 90% for type D lesions treated via an endovascular route.

More data have emerged addressing the feasibility and durability of endovascular techniques in advanced TASC groups, challenging the current AHA/ACC guideline recommendation of deferring such lesions to surgical repair only. Ichihashi et al.[56] reported their experience with 533 aorto-iliac lesions, stratified by lower versus higher TASC classification. They found no difference in technical success rates between TASC A and B lesions versus TASC C and D lesions (both were 99%). The TASC C and D lesions were characterized by significantly longer procedural times and higher complication rates (9% for TASC C and D vs 3% for TASC A and B). There were no significant differences in the 1-, 3-, 5-, and 10-year primary patency rates between the groups. Leville et al.[57] presented their experience with 92 aorto-iliac occlusions, of which three-quarters were TASC C and D lesions. The overall technical success was 91%, with successful recanalization and stenting of 86% of TASC D lesions. The primary and secondary patency rates were 76% and 90%, respectively, at 3 years, and these did not vary significantly by TASC stratification. An older series by Scheinert et al.[58] showed similar findings in 212 unilateral iliac occlusions, demonstrating a 90% technical success rate with 4-year primary and secondary patencies of 76% and 85%, respectively, and a low major complication rate of 1.4%. In summary, these retrospective studies confirm the efficacy of percutaneous strategies in effectively treating even advanced aorto-iliac lesions.

Percutaneous Transluminal Angioplasty and Stenting. The optimal technical strategy to treating aorto-iliac lesions is still being refined, especially given the availability of newer techniques and equipment. Provisional stenting, consisting of balloon angioplasty with bailout stenting only in cases of suboptimal result, or primary stenting of aorto-iliac vessels are both given class I indications by the current AHA/ACC guidelines.[44] Furthermore, it is recommended that an iliac lesion with an angiographic stenosis between 50% and 75% be further interrogated to assess for a peak systolic pressure gradient of 10 mmHg. The basis for this recommendation comes from Dutch Iliac Stent Trial Study Group that conducted a prospective, randomized, multicenter study assigning 279 patients to primary stenting of iliac lesions or provisional stenting if results were determined to be suboptimal based on a pressure gradient greater than 10 mmHg after angioplasty.[59] Fewer than half the patients in the provisional group required a stent for suboptimal outcome. There were no differences in success rates or clinical outcomes at 2 years. However, on the basis of the contemporaneous large meta-analysis by Bosch et al.[52] showing a 39% reduction in the relative risk of long-term failure with stenting versus PTA alone, many interventionalists will now perform primary stenting of aorto-iliac lesions.

Access-Site Considerations. Percutaneous peripheral interventions have historically been performed using the femoral artery as the access site. One of the major safety concerns with the use of the TF approach is the occurrence of access-site complications, including bleeding, which may be attenuated with a TR approach. Davies et al.[60] reported a 2.1% access-site complication rate in 937 patients undergoing aorto-iliac interventions using the TF route, and Johnston et al.,[61] in a review of the Toronto General Hospital experience of 984 iliac angioplasties, found a similar rate of 2.8%. Hildick-Smith et al.[62] looked at the impact of known aorto-femoral PAD on the success of diagnostic coronary angiography in 297 patients when approached from either the TF or the brachial/radial route. There was a higher failure rate when using TF access compared to arm access (79% for femoral vs 91% for brachial/radial). Significant vascular complications, including pulseless limb, false aneurysm requiring surgery, dissection, and major hematoma, occurred in 6% of the TF cases and in none of the arm cases. Given the high-risk clinical profile of the individual with PAD, the TR access option is continuously being explored as a means of improving the safety profile of endovascular procedures.

From the coronary literature, it is clear that access-site complications, especially postprocedural bleeding, are strongly associated with both higher short- and long-term mortality.[63-65] Among the many risk factors that have been shown to contribute to increased bleeding potential, only those that are procedure related, such as puncture site, are readily modifiable. While two-thirds of overall bleeding events following percutaneous coronary intervention for acute coronary syndromes are related to non–access site bleeding, in elective procedures, the majority of bleeding is from the access site. Access-site hemorrhagic complications are independently linked to an almost twofold increase in long-term mortality.[66] In this regard, data from the coronary literature have illustrated the marked reduction in bleeding and vascular complications that can be achieved with TR access than with the more traditional TF approach.[67,68]

Aorto-iliac angioplasty and stenting can be safely performed via the TR approach. de Belder et al.[69] first suggested the use of TR access in patients with PAD in 1997, and reported a 97% technical success rate, with no complications. Flachskampf et al.[70] described the first case report of TR aorto-iliac stenting, suggesting that longer catheters would be required to refine the technique. Sanghvi et al.[71] reported a series of 15 patients treated for aorto-iliac lesions via the TR approach, demonstrating successful completion in 14 patients. The one failure required additional procedures more distal in the leg, and given the limited stent shaft lengths that were available in 2006, the procedure had to be converted to a TF approach. Staniloae et al.[72] prospectively treated 27 patients with 33 iliac lesions via the TR approach and compared this to a group of 47 similar lesions treated via the TF approach. The clinical characteristics were similar, as were the preprocedure ABIs and Rutherford category; however, lesion parameters differed, as the TR group had a threefold higher presence of total occlusions and greater baseline diameter stenosis. Despite this inequality in lesion types, there was no difference in mean procedural time or contrast volume requirement. There were no major bleeding complications in either group, and the technical success rates were similar between the groups. In unsuccessful TR cases, the major barrier was either subclavian artery tortuosity or equipment shaft length limitations.

Transradial Technical Tips. The routine approach to the suprainguinal intervention starts with gaining access from the left radial artery. This has the advantage of traversing a shorter distance to the descending aorta and not crossing the aortic arch and cerebral vessels. The left subclavian artery most often directs the angiographer toward the descending aorta, so we usually begin the procedure with a 125-cm multipurpose catheter and an angle-tipped hydrophilic-coated 0.035-inch wire. Occasionally, an internal mammary shape catheter

may be required to negotiate the descending aorta due to a type III aortic arch. Regardless of the wire used, it is mandatory that its passage is carefully followed with fluoroscopy to its destination in the lower abdominal aorta. Severe complications can result from "blind" advancement of the wire into tributaries of the thoracic or abdominal aorta. We recommend that in most cases, angiography of the aorto-iliac system begins with a pigtail "power" injection of the lower abdominal aorta (typically 20 mL over 1 second in the anteroposterior projection). This initial scout film may help define any aortic aneurysms, collateral vessels, and the presence of ostial disease of the common iliac arteries. This initial view may be forgone only in the presence of renal insufficiency with the backup of excellent noninvasive imaging. Selective angiography of the entire lower extremity is then performed with the 5F 125-cm multipurpose catheter. Once the anatomy is defined, with a 0.035-inch, 260-cm guidewire positioned into the descending aorta, the entire system can be exchanged for a long 110-cm, 5F or 6F introducer sheath. The sheath can then be positioned at the ostium of the target common iliac artery (CIA) or in the distal aorta and the intervention completed in the usual manner (Fig. 22-11).

The major limitations are currently related to the severe tortuosity that can be encountered at the level of radial or subclavian arteries. Furthermore, in patients with long upper extremities or very tortuous descending aortas, introducer sheaths longer than 110 cm are required for selective cannulation of the common iliac arteries. In the authors' experience, these situations are encountered in about 5% to 10% of the cases, and the current equipment may be insufficient in terms of working shaft length, particularly when treating lesions in the distal external iliac artery.

A special consideration should be given to bilateral ostial iliac disease (Fig. 22-12). If the distal aorta is not severely diseased, both iliac lesions can be easily stented from a single TR access site in a consecutive manner. However, if protection of the contralateral iliac is desired, this will not be possible with single access. When this is deemed necessary, as in situations where the distal aorta needs to be reconstructed or the operator prefers a kissing balloon technique, a second access site is recommended. This can be achieved using a short (7–11 cm) sheath placed in the other radial artery (RA) and directing a second guidewire into the contralateral iliac using a long 4F to 5F vertebral-shape catheter. There is no need for a second long sheath since the angiography is performed via the initial long sheath.

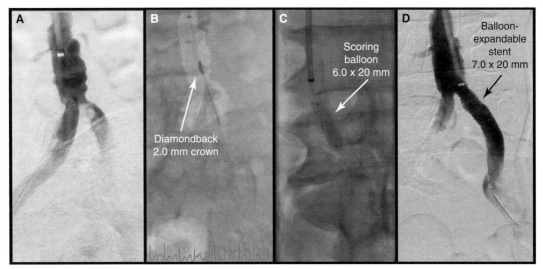

FIGURE 22-11 A: Angiography through a 6F, 110-cm Shuttle sheath from the left RA, revealing a calcified, left CIA stenosis. **B:** Orbital atherectomy of the left CIA using the Diamondback360 system. **C:** PTA of the left CIA. **D:** Final angiography of left CIA poststenting.

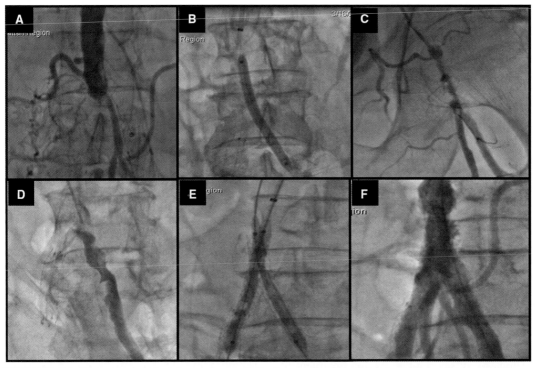

FIGURE 22-12 TR approach to Leriche syndrome. **A:** Aortogram showing distal aorta total occlusion. **B:** Balloon angioplasty of left CIA following successful wire crossing. **C:** Catheter-directed thrombolysis of left CIA. **D:** Left CIA opacification following overnight infusion of tPA. **E:** Kissing balloon inflation of bilateral CIA. **F:** Successful restoration of inflow.

Iliac angioplasty and stenting can now be performed via a 5F, 110-cm introducer sheath, because of the recent availability of a 5F stenting platform (6–10 mm diameter, 20–80 cm length, Cook Medical). However, a 6F introducer sheath should be used when facing chronic total occlusions, as the larger sheath offers better support and allows the use of eventual reentry devices. In addition, in the presence of severe calcification, a 6F sheath allows the use of an atherectomy device (Diamondback/Predator 360, Cardiovascular Systems Inc., St. Paul, MN) that facilitates good stent expansion.

Conclusion

Aorto-iliac artery angioplasty and stenting is easily and safely performed from a TR approach. There are very rare circumstances where conversion to TF access is needed. This approach allows excellent patient satisfaction as well as a rapid, same-day hospital discharge.

Transradial Femoral Intervention

Tejas Patel

With the aging of the population, the incidence of peripheral arterial disease is increasing. Diehm et al.[73] reported abnormal ABI in 19% of patients over the age of 50. Intermediate claudication was seen in 3% to 7% of patients aged between 60 and 70 years.[74] Recently conducted trials of treatment options in patients with claudication due to femoral artery lesions have compared balloon angioplasty to stenting or self-expanding to balloon-expandable stents. Wilson suggested that a control group of optimal medical therapy, including a supervised exercise program, should be included in any device trials.[75] He reviewed five studies comparing medical therapy to intervention and found that at 2 years the medical control had better functional outcomes. These studies have been criticized since the majority of patients were not treated with stents.

Dick et al.[76] randomized 73 patients to balloon angioplasty versus stenting for the treatment of superficial femoral artery (SFA) lesions from 30 to 200 mm in length with greater than a 50% stenosis. Prior studies suggested that in short lesions less than 50 mm, 1-year restenosis rates with balloon angioplasty or stenting were similar at 30%.[77] Lesions greater than 100 mm seemed to do better with stent implantation.[78] Dick et al.[79] attempted

to look at intermediate-length lesions. It appeared that long lesions when stented had better patency rates, but if restenosis occurred, treatment results were disappointing, with up to 70% recurrence rates. Their goal was to see whether stenting could be avoided in these intermediate lesions. Among patients randomized to balloon angioplasty, 26% required bailout stenting for flow-limiting dissection or significant residual stenosis. A CT angiography was performed at 6 months and an ultrasound at 1 year. The restenosis rates at 6 months were 21.9% versus 55.6%, and at 1 year the stented group was still significantly better with a 34% restenosis versus 61% for balloon angioplasty. From these studies, it appears that stenting with self-expanding stents is superior to balloon angioplasty in all but the most discrete SFA lesions. Chalmers et al.[80] randomized patients to balloon angioplasty versus stenting in complex lesions. About 93% of lesions were total occlusions with a mean lesion length close to 120 mm. The restenosis rates at 1 year were disappointingly high at 42% for stenting and 47% for balloon angioplasty. This suggested that in the subset of total occlusions, balloon angioplasty with stenting reserved for bailout is a reasonable approach.

The common femoral artery is an area that is not ideal for stenting due to flexion in the inguinal area and the desire to preserve this region for possible surgical bypass. The common femoral artery can be treated with balloon angioplasty and atherectomy if severe life-style-limiting claudication or critical limb ischemia exists. Bonvini group had a large experience with endovascular treatment of common femoral lesions.[81] The series had 360 patients, most having inflow and outflow lesions in addition to CFA disease. The series included 96 patients with isolated CFA lesions and 60 patients with total occlusion of the CFA. Almost all cases (98.6%) were treated with balloon angioplasty. The one-year target lesion revascularization rate was 20%. Dattilo et al.[82] had a retrospective review of CFA cases, some done for native disease and some for complications of femoral procedures or closure devices. The choice of devices was based on the nature of the lesions. For lesions that were heavily calcified, the Diamondback orbital atherectomy device was used. For flow-limiting dissections or complications of Angioseal device, the Silver Hawk atherectomy device was used. For lesions felt to require thrombectomy, the Pathway catheter system was used. After the use of the different atherectomy devices, balloon angioplasty was performed and stenting was avoided wherever possible. Of the various systems used, the orbital atherectomy system is the only device that can be used with a

6F introducer for burrs below 2.25 mm. They reported a success rate of 90% and a primary patency at 2 years of 83%. The greatest risk of restenosis was seen in the patients with native disease.

The major limitation in performing TR approach for femoral artery intervention is the lack of adequate length systems and small enough diameter systems to allow for the use of 5F or 6F introducers. Trani et al.[83] described their group's experience with a new over-the-wire 5 F compatible 180-cm shaft length self-expanding Nitinol stent (The Sinus SuperFlex-518 Optimed, Ettlingen, Germany). The stent system is currently not available in the United States or Canada. The current length and size limits the ability to perform many femoral procedures using radial access. The orbital atherectomy device system of Cardiovascular Systems Inc. (CSI) is the only 6F compatible atherectomy system and has a working length of 143 cm. This can allow the treatment of CFA and some very proximal SFA lesions. Several 150-cm shaft length balloon systems are available in the market. The balloon catheters allow for treatment of in-stent restenosis and de novo lesions, but if stenting is required, the current stent systems are not long enough.

The technical approach to femoral work is similar to the approach to iliac procedures.[84] The left radial artery is the preferred site to avoid passing around the aortic arch. This will give an additional 6 to 8 cm of working length. The radial artery is punctured in a standard manner and a short 5F introducer is placed, followed by the injection of a vasodilator solution. The descending aorta is entered using a diagnostic IMA or MP catheter. Using the catheter for support, the iliac artery on the ipsilateral side is entered and a 300-cm wire is passed into the CFA. The catheter is then exchanged for the long introducer sheath. A control angiogram is performed and the guidewire is advanced across the lesion to be treated. The balloon or stent can then be delivered. At the completion of the procedure, the patient is ambulatory and can be discharged safely even on outpatient basis.

Renal Artery Intervention

Rajiv Gulati

Endovascular renal artery intervention for severe renal artery stenosis may be performed as a treatment modality in patients with resistant hypertension, hypertensive urgency, renal insufficiency, and flash pulmonary edema.[85-89] Two recent randomized trials, however, have suggested that percutaneous renal artery intervention does not provide long-term clinical benefit when compared with medical therapy alone in patients with hypertension and renal artery stenosis.[90,91] Despite the findings of these studies, it remains true that carefully selected patients benefit, and benefit greatly, from renal intervention. Such patients include those with flash pulmonary edema, critically severe hypertension, and deteriorating renal function, all of whom were markedly underrepresented in randomized trials. However, it also remains true that a small number of patients experience procedure-related, clinically devastating atheroembolic complications, resulting in renal failure, limb gangrene, or death. Arguably, a significant proportion of complications reported in clinical trials may be related to the use of the femoral artery as the primary access site.

Access-Site Choice

Renal intervention has historically been performed via femoral arterial access or brachial artery access when the femoral approach is contraindicated. Femoral complications include pseudoaneurysm, hematoma, and retroperitoneal bleeding. In the ASTRAL randomized study, the femoral access complication rate was 12.8%[90] in the interventional arm, driven by large femoral bleeds. On the other hand, brachial access carries a risk of arterial occlusion, which due to the artery's status as an end-vessel can provoke limb-threatening ischemia. In addition, the proximity of the brachial artery to the median nerve confers a risk of disabling neurologic trauma, either through nerve damage or compression from hematoma.[92,93] These complications, which can occur via both percutaneous access and surgical cut-down, have dampened the enthusiasm for transbrachial approaches for endovascular intervention.[94-96]

Advantages of Radial Approach

Access-Site Complications

For coronary angiography and intervention, the TR approach is associated with marked reductions in access-site bleeding and complications and improvement in quality-of-life parameters compared with the femoral approach. Access-site comparisons have however been less well studied in peripheral angiography and intervention. TR renal angiography and intervention were first shown to be feasible in case series where a femoral approach was contraindicated.[97,98] In a retrospective study, we showed that elective TR renal artery intervention was feasible and safe. More so, in a historic comparison with matched controls undergoing transfemoral renal intervention, there were no access-site complications in the TR arm. Fluoroscopy times and contrast volumes were similar in the radial and femoral groups.[99]

Coaxial Guide Alignment

The renal artery course after arising from the aorta is typically caudal in direction, occasionally horizontal but only very rarely cranial. Thus, an approach "from above" is almost always more likely to achieve coaxial alignment of the guiding catheter compared with an approach from the femoral artery. This confers a major advantage of the radial (vs femoral approach). With coaxial alignment comes markedly more straightforward advancement of balloon and stent catheters, which is a particular advantage with the typically calcified stenoses seen in aorto-renal atherosclerotic disease.

Atheroembolic Risk

There is a marked variation in the distribution of atherosclerotic plaque between the ascending, thoracic, and abdominal aorta in humans.[100] The greatest plaque volume is located in the infrarenal abdominal aorta (Fig. 22-13). The propensity for displacement of atherosclerotic plaque would therefore appear to be much greater with

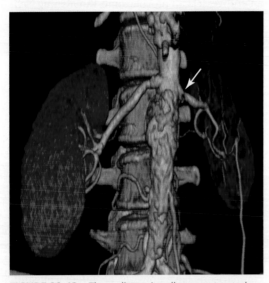

FIGURE 22-13 Three-dimensionally reconstructed CT aorto-renal angiogram. Markedly more atheroma is seen in the infrarenal aorta in comparison to the suprarenal aorta. Also noted is the horizontal takeoff of the right renal artery and caudal takeoff of the left renal artery. High-grade focal stenosis of left renal artery (arrow) supplying a shrunken left kidney.

techniques that predispose to catheter contact with the infrarenal segment of aortic wall. This is much more of concern with a femoral rather than a radial approach. While the risk of atheroembolization from a femoral approach can be mitigated by the use of "no-touch" techniques to minimize aortic wall contact, these transfemoral renal procedures can still result in limb gangrene and death, as highlighted in the ASTRAL study.

Transradial Renal Angiography and Interventional Techniques

Left versus Right Radial

We found the use of the left radial artery to be preferable to the right for three reasons. First, this avoids crossing the aortic arch and great vessel origins, theoretically reducing the risk of cerebral embolization. Second, limiting tortuosity is less frequent in the left subclavian artery compared with the innominate[101,102] Third, the distance to the renal arteries is shorter, due to not having to cross the arch. In this regard, our single failure in this series related to insufficient length of guiding catheter to reach the renal arteries from the right radial. Distance to the renal artery origins is a limitation for the length of currently available guiding catheters (100 cm) and stents (120 cm). As such, it is our current practice to avoid the radial approach for tall patients or in those with very low renal artery origins.

Catheter Selection

For individual operators performing coronary angiography and intervention, crossover to a femoral approach is more frequent in the first 100 cases.[103] However, a proportion of coronary failures from a TR approach relate to complex anatomy of the aortic root, causing difficulties with catheter engagement or support from the contralateral aortic wall, factors that are much less of a barrier from a transfemoral approach. Anatomic variation and disease of the abdominal aorta is less likely to be a limitation for a TR renal intervention. In our experience, the multipurpose or Judkins right-4 guiding catheters possess ideal curves for coaxial renal artery engagement in downwardly, horizontally, or upward angulated renal origins (Figs. 22-14 and 22-15). Catheter alignment and engagement can be more challenging when proximal aortic tortuosity is present (Fig. 22-15). In these cases, it can be difficult to predict which shaped guide may be preferable for engagement or support. In such cases, we have sometimes found that while one shape may

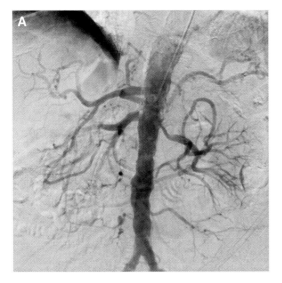

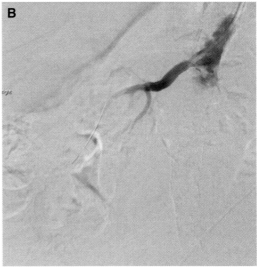

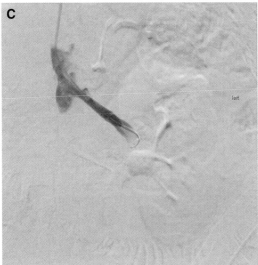

FIGURE 22-14   Nonselective left TR abdominal aortic angiogram indicating single bilateral renal arteries, both caudally directed (A). With a TR approach, a perfect coaxial alignment of 6F multipurpose guiding catheter with both left and right renal arteries was achieved. Images are following bilateral stent placement.

be ideal for one renal artery, with backup support from the tortuous contralateral wall, optimal engagement for the contralateral vessel may require a change of guiding catheter (e.g., from Judkins right to multipurpose or vice versa). Regardless, in the vast majority of cases, the use of one or both of multipurpose or Judkins right-shaped catheters almost always provide excellent fit and support.

Tips and Tricks

Despite the theoretically lower propensity for atheroembolization from a TR approach, we still advocate the use of "no-touch" techniques for catheter engagement. This entails the use of a guidewire to keep the catheter tip off the aortic wall, to direct the catheter tip toward the renal artery at the appropriate level, and then to slowly withdraw the guidewire such that the catheter tip enters the renal origin directly. In some cases, the length of commercially available guiding catheters (100 cm) is insufficient to reach the renal origins. While 125-cm guiding catheters are available, the shaft lengths of most currently available renal stents are a few centimeters too short to protrude from these guides. In these cases, the use of guide extensions such as the Guideliner (Vascular Solutions Inc., Minneapolis, MN, USA) with regular-length guiding catheters can be effective. Such devices can be used to extend the reach of a multipurpose guide by approximately 10 cm. Importantly, when this technique is to be used, a 7F guide (rather than 6F) and 6-in-7 Guideliner will be necessary for most

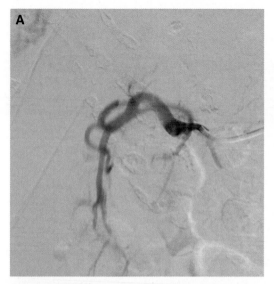

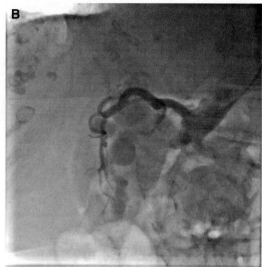

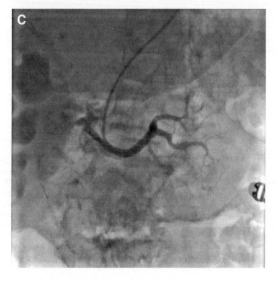

FIGURE 22-15 Selective renal artery angiography and intervention via a left TR approach. Tortuous abdominal aorta is noted with upwardly directed left renal artery but downwardly directed right renal artery. In this case, a 6F Judkins right-4–shaped guiding catheter provided excellent fit in both arteries.

cases. This is because typical renal stents are 6 or 7 mm in diameter and the lumen of the 5-in-6 Guideliner (with a 6F guide) will not accommodate such diameter stents. While the diameter of the radial artery itself will not accommodate 7F and 8F sheaths in a significant proportion of individuals, this can be mitigated by the use of sheathless techniques.[104,105]

Renal Artery Denervation

Given the broadly negative findings from the recent trials of endovascular renal angioplasty and stent placement, it seems unlikely that there will be a significant increase in volumes of renal intervention for renal artery stenosis in the near term. In stark contrast, endovascular renal artery denervation is emerging as a novel therapeutic tool for the treatment of resistant hypertension, and has the potential to hugely impact cath lab volumes in future. First-generation catheter systems are 6F to 8F sheath compatible and have mostly been designed for transfemoral access. The Symplicity catheter (Medtronic Inc.) is the most widely tested device currently available and is also the narrowest in caliber, compatible with 6F guides. Given the advantages of TR versus transfemoral access for renal interventions as already described, it makes sense that future iterations of denervation catheters will be designed for TR access. More so, it seems likely that the clinical model of renal artery denervation will rapidly evolve to high-volume, brief duration procedures performed under local anesthetic, with early (same-day) discharge. This model is markedly more compatible with a primary TR rather than a transfemoral approach. Even though most current-generation catheters are too short in length for widespread TR use and prone to kinking (e.g., at the subclavian-aortic junction), a recent case report has already demonstrated feasibility of TR renal denervation with the Symplicity device in a short patient.[106] Most recently, a dedicated TR renal denervation catheter (Iberis, Terumo Inc., Terumo, Somerset, NJ, USA) which is 4F in diameter, compatible with 6F guides and longer in length than transfemoral devices, has achieved CE mark approval. Safety and feasibility of both TR and transulnar denervation with this catheter has been reported.[107,108]

REFERENCES

1. Brott TG, et al. Stenting versus endarterectomy for treatment of carotid-artery stenosis. *N Engl J Med.* 2010;363(1): 11–23.
2. Gray WA, et al. The CAPTURE registry: predictors of outcomes in carotid artery stenting with embolic protection for high surgical risk patients in the early post-approval setting. *Catheter Cardiovasc Interv.* 2007;70(7):1025–1033.
3. Gurm HS, et al. Long-term results of carotid stenting versus endarterectomy in high-risk patients. *N Engl J Med.* 2008;358(15):1572–1579.
4. Silver FL, et al. Safety of stenting and endarterectomy by symptomatic status in the Carotid Revascularization Endarterectomy versus Stenting Trial (CREST). *Stroke.* 2011;42(3):675–680.
5. Stabile E, et al. European Registry of Carotid Artery Stenting: results from a prospective registry of eight high volume EUROPEAN institutions. *Catheter Cardiovasc Interv.* 2012;80(2):329–334.
6. White CJ, et al. Carotid stenting with distal protection in high surgical risk patients: the BEACH trial 30 day results. *Catheter Cardiovasc Interv.* 2006;67(4):503–512.
7. Barbato JE, et al. A randomized trial of carotid artery stenting with and without cerebral protection. *J Vasc Surg.* 2008;47(4):760–765.
8. Bendszus M, et al. Silent embolism in diagnostic cerebral angiography and neurointerventional procedures: a prospective study. *Lancet.* 1999;354(9190):1594–1597.
9. El-Koussy M, et al. Periprocedural embolic events related to carotid artery stenting detected by diffusion-weighted MRI: comparison between proximal and distal embolus protection devices. *J Endovasc Ther.* 2007;14(3):293–303.
10. Faggioli G, et al. Atherosclerotic aortic lesions increase the risk of cerebral embolism during carotid stenting in patients with complex aortic arch anatomy. *J Vasc Surg.* 2009;49(1):80–85.
11. Bakoyiannis C, et al. Transradial access for carotid artery stenting: a single-center experience. *Int Angiol.* 2010;29(1):41–46.
12. Bendok BR, et al. Neuroendovascular interventions for intracranial posterior circulation disease via the transradial approach: technical case report. *Neurosurgery.* 2005;56(3):E626; discussion E626.
13. Castriota F, et al. Carotid stenting using radial artery access. *J Endovasc Surg.* 1999;6(4):385–386.
14. Coroleu SF, et al. Feasibility of complex coronary and peripheral interventions by trans-radial approach using large sheaths. *Catheter Cardiovasc Interv.* 2012;79(4): 597–600.
15. Eskioglu E, Burry MV, Mericle RA. Transradial approach for neuroendovascular surgery of intracranial vascular lesions. *J Neurosurg.* 2004;101(5):767–769.
16. Etxegoien N, et al. The transradial approach for carotid artery stenting. *Catheter Cardiovasc Interv.* 2012;80(7): 1081–1087.
17. Fang HY, et al. Transradial and transbrachial arterial approach for simultaneous carotid angiographic examination and stenting using catheter looping and retrograde engagement technique. *Ann Vasc Surg.* 2010;24(5): 670–679.
18. Folmar J, Sachar R, Mann T. Transradial approach for carotid artery stenting: a feasibility study. *Catheter Cardiovasc Interv.* 2007;69(3):355–361.
19. Gan HW, Bhasin A, Wu CJ. Transradial carotid stenting in a patient with bovine arch anatomy. *Catheter Cardiovasc Interv.* 2010;75(4):540–543.
20. Layton KF, Kallmes DF, Cloft HJ. The radial artery access site for interventional neuroradiology procedures. *AJNR Am J Neuroradiol.* 2006;27(5):1151–1154.
21. Levy EI, et al. Transradial stenting of the cervical internal carotid artery: technical case report. *Neurosurgery.* 2003;53(2):448–451; discussion 451–452.
22. Mendiz OA, et al. Initial experience with transradial access for carotid artery stenting. *Vasc Endovasc Surg.* 2011;45(6):499–503.
23. Patel T, et al. Contralateral transradial approach for carotid artery stenting: a feasibility study. *Catheter Cardiovasc Interv.* 2010;75(2):268–275.
24. Pinter L, et al. Report on initial experience with transradial access for carotid artery stenting. *J Vasc Surg.* 2007;45(6): 1136–1141.
25. Shaw JA, Gravereaux EC, Eisenhauer AC. Carotid stenting in the bovine arch. *Catheter Cardiovasc Interv.* 2003;60(4): 566–569.
26. Trani C, Burzotta F, Coroleu SF. Transradial carotid artery stenting with proximal embolic protection. *Catheter Cardiovasc Interv.* 2009;74(2):267–272.
27. Yoo BS, et al. A case of transradial carotid stenting in a patient with total occlusion of distal abdominal aorta. *Catheter Cardiovasc Interv.* 2002;56(2):243–245.
28. Lee DH, et al. Routine transradial access for conventional cerebral angiography: a single operator's experience of its feasibility and safety. *Br J Radiol.* 2004;77(922):831–838.
29. Iadecola C, et al. Recommendations of the National Heart, Lung, and Blood Institute working group on cerebrovascular biology and disease. *Stroke.* 2006;37(6):1578–1581.
30. White AD, et al. Community surveillance of coronary heart disease in the Atherosclerosis Risk in Communities (ARIC) Study: methods and initial two years' experience. *J Clin Epidemiol.* 1996;49(2):223–233.
31. Bild DE, et al. Multi-ethnic study of atherosclerosis: objectives and design. *Am J Epidemiol.* 2002;156(9):871–881.
32. Hirsch AT, et al. Peripheral arterial disease detection, awareness, and treatment in primary care. *JAMA.* 2001;286(11):1317–1324.
33. Aboyans V, et al. Risk factors for progression of peripheral arterial disease in large and small vessels. *Circulation.* 2006;113(22):2623–2629.
34. Barretto S, et al. Early-onset peripheral arterial occlusive disease: clinical features and determinants of disease severity and location. *Vasc Med.* 2003;8(2):95–100.
35. Valentine RJ, et al. The influence of sex and aortic size on late patency after aortofemoral revascularization in

young adults. *J Vasc Surg.* 1995;21(2):296–305; discussion 305–306.

36. Brewster DC. Clinical and anatomical considerations for surgery in aortoiliac disease and results of surgical treatment. *Circulation.* 1991;83(2 suppl):I42–I52.

37. Aboyans V, et al., The general prognosis of patients with peripheral arterial disease differs according to the disease localization. *J Am Coll Cardiol.* 2010;55(9):898–903.

38. McDermott MM, et al. Leg symptoms in peripheral arterial disease: associated clinical characteristics and functional impairment. *JAMA.* 2001;286(13):1599–1606.

39. Gerhard-Herman M, et al. Guidelines for noninvasive vascular laboratory testing: a report from the American Society of Echocardiography and the Society of Vascular Medicine and Biology. *J Am Soc Echocardiogr.* 2006;19(8): 955–972.

40. Wesolowski SA, et al. Indications for aortofemoral arterial reconstruction: a study of borderline risk patients. *Surgery.* 1966;60(2):288–298.

41. Kinney TB, Rose SC. Intraarterial pressure measurements during angiographic evaluation of peripheral vascular disease: techniques, interpretation, applications, and limitations. *AJR Am J Roentgenol.* 1996;166(2):277–284.

42. Weismann RE, Upson JF. Intra-arterial pressure studies in patients with arterial insufficiency of lower extremities. *Ann Surg.* 1963;157:501–506.

43. Executive Summary of the Third Report of the National Cholesterol Education Program (NCEP) Expert Panel on Detection, Evaluation, and Treatment of High Blood Cholesterol in Adults (Adult Treatment Panel III). *JAMA.* 2001;285(19):2486–2497.

44. Hirsch AT, et al. ACC/AHA 2005 guidelines for the management of patients with peripheral arterial disease (lower extremity, renal, mesenteric, and abdominal aortic): executive summary a collaborative report from the American Association for Vascular Surgery/Society for Vascular Surgery, Society for Cardiovascular Angiography and Interventions, Society for Vascular Medicine and Biology, Society of Interventional Radiology, and the ACC/AHA Task Force on Practice Guidelines (Writing Committee to Develop Guidelines for the Management of Patients with Peripheral Arterial Disease) endorsed by the American Association of Cardiovascular and Pulmonary Rehabilitation; National Heart, Lung, and Blood Institute; Society for Vascular Nursing; Trans-Atlantic Inter-Society Consensus; and Vascular Disease Foundation. *J Am Coll Cardiol.* 2006;47(6):1239–1312.

45. Gardner AW, Poehlman ET. Exercise rehabilitation programs for the treatment of claudication pain: a meta-analysis. *JAMA.* 1995;274(12):975–980.

46. Spronk S, et al. Intermittent claudication: clinical effectiveness of endovascular revascularization versus supervised hospital-based exercise training—randomized controlled trial. *Radiology.* 2009;250(2):586–595.

47. Whyman MR, et al. Is intermittent claudication improved by percutaneous transluminal angioplasty? A randomized controlled trial. *J Vasc Surg.* 1997;26(4):551–557.

48. Frans FA, et al. Systematic review of exercise training or percutaneous transluminal angioplasty for intermittent claudication. *Br J Surg.* 2012;99(1):16–28.

49. Murphy TP, et al. Supervised exercise versus primary stenting for claudication resulting from aortoiliac peripheral artery disease: six-month outcomes from the claudication: exercise versus endoluminal revascularization (CLEVER) study. *Circulation.* 2012;125(1):130–139.

50. Norgren L, et al. Inter-society consensus for the management of peripheral arterial disease (TASC II). *J Vasc Surg.* 2007;45(suppl S):S5–S67.

51. de Vries SO, Hunink MG. Results of aortic bifurcation grafts for aortoiliac occlusive disease: a meta-analysis. *J Vasc Surg.* 1997;26(4):558–569.

52. Bosch JL, Hunink MG. Meta-analysis of the results of percutaneous transluminal angioplasty and stent placement for aortoiliac occlusive disease. *Radiology.* 1997;204(1): 87–96.

53. Murphy TP, et al. Aortoiliac insufficiency: long-term experience with stent placement for treatment. *Radiology.* 2004;231(1):243–249.

54. Holm J, et al. Chronic lower limb ischaemia: a prospective randomised controlled study comparing the 1-year results of vascular surgery and percutaneous transluminal angioplasty (PTA). *Eur J Vasc Surg.* 1991;5(5):517–522.

55. Kashyap VS, et al. The management of severe aortoiliac occlusive disease: endovascular therapy rivals open reconstruction. *J Vasc Surg.* 2008;48(6):1451–1457, 1457, e1-3.

56. Ichihashi S, et al. Long-term outcomes for systematic primary stent placement in complex iliac artery occlusive disease classified according to Trans-Atlantic Inter-Society Consensus (TASC)-II. *J Vasc Surg.* 2011;53(4):992–999.

57. Leville CD, et al. Endovascular management of iliac artery occlusions: extending treatment to TransAtlantic Inter-Society Consensus class C and D patients. *J Vasc Surg.* 2006;43(1):32–39.

58. Scheinert D, et al. Stent-supported recanalization of chronic iliac artery occlusions. *Am J Med.* 2001;110(9):708–715.

59. Tetteroo E, et al. Randomised comparison of primary stent placement versus primary angioplasty followed by selective stent placement in patients with iliac-artery occlusive disease. Dutch Iliac Stent Trial Study Group. *Lancet.* 1998;351(9110):1153–1159.

60. Davies MG, et al. Outcomes of reintervention for recurrent disease after percutaneous iliac angioplasty and stenting. *J Endovasc Ther.* 2011;18(2):169–180.

61. Johnston KW, et al. 5-year results of a prospective study of percutaneous transluminal angioplasty. *Ann Surg.* 1987;206(4):403–413.

62. Hildick-Smith DJ, et al. Coronary angiography in the presence of peripheral vascular disease: femoral or brachial/radial approach? *Catheter Cardiovasc Interv.* 2000;49(1):32–37.

63. Rao SV, et al. Impact of bleeding severity on clinical outcomes among patients with acute coronary syndromes. *Am J Cardiol.* 2005;96(9):1200–1206.

64. Feit F, et al. Predictors and impact of major hemorrhage on mortality following percutaneous coronary intervention from the REPLACE-2 Trial. *Am J Cardiol.* 2007;100(9):1364–1369.

65. Ndrepepa G, et al. Periprocedural bleeding and 1-year outcome after percutaneous coronary interventions: appropriateness of including bleeding as a component of a quadruple end point. *J Am Coll Cardiol.* 2008;51(7): 690–697.

66. Verheugt FW, et al. Incidence, prognostic impact, and influence of antithrombotic therapy on access and nonaccess site bleeding in percutaneous coronary intervention. *JACC Cardiovasc Interv.* 2011;4(2):191–197.

67. Agostoni P, et al. Radial versus femoral approach for percutaneous coronary diagnostic and interventional procedures: systematic overview and meta-analysis of randomized trials. *J Am Coll Cardiol.* 2004;44(2): 349–356.

68. Jolly SS, et al. Radial versus femoral access for coronary angiography or intervention and the impact on major bleeding and ischemic events: a systematic review and meta-analysis of randomized trials. *Am Heart J.* 2009;157(1):132–140.

69. de Belder AJ, et al. Transradial artery coronary angiography and intervention in patients with severe peripheral vascular disease. *Clin Radiol.* 1997;52(2):115–118.

70. Flachskampf FA, et al. Transradial stenting of the iliac artery: a case report. *Catheter Cardiovasc Interv.* 2005;65(2):193–195.

71. Sanghvi K, Kurian D, Coppola J. Transradial intervention of iliac and superficial femoral artery disease is feasible. *J Interv Cardiol.* 2008;21(5):385–387.

72. Staniloae CS, et al. Safety and efficacy of transradial aortoiliac interventions. *Catheter Cardiovasc Interv.* 2010;75(5):659–662.

73. Diehm C, et al. High prevalence of peripheral arterial disease and co-morbidity in 6880 primary care patients: cross-sectional study. *Atherosclerosis.* 2004;172(1):95–105.

74. Norgren L, et al. Inter-society consensus for the management of peripheral arterial disease (TASC II). *J Vasc Surg.* 2007;45 (suppl S):S5–S67.

75. Wilson SE. Trials of endovascular treatment for superficial femoral artery occlusive lesions: a call for medically managed control patients. *Ann Vasc Surg.* 2010;24(4):498–502.

76. Dick P, et al. Balloon angioplasty versus stenting with nitinol stents in intermediate length superficial femoral artery lesions. *Catheter Cardiovasc Interv.* 2009;74(7):1090–1095.

77. Krankenberg H, et al. Nitinol stent implantation versus percutaneous transluminal angioplasty in superficial femoral artery lesions up to 10 cm in length: the femoral artery stenting trial (FAST). *Circulation.* 2007;116(3):285–292.

78. Schillinger M, et al. Balloon angioplasty versus implantation of nitinol stents in the superficial femoral artery. *N Engl J Med.* 2006;354(18):1879–1888.

79. Dick P, et al. Conventional balloon angioplasty versus peripheral cutting balloon angioplasty for treatment of femoropopliteal artery in-stent restenosis: initial experience. *Radiology.* 2008;248(1):297–302.

80. Chalmers N, et al. Randomized trial of the SMART stent versus balloon angioplasty in long superficial femoral artery lesions: the SUPER study. *Cardiovasc Intervent Radiol.* 2013;36(2):353–361.

81. Bonvini RF, et al. Endovascular treatment of common femoral artery disease: medium-term outcomes of 360 consecutive procedures. *J Am Coll Cardiol.* 2011;58(8):792–798.

82. Dattilo PB, et al. Acute and medium-term outcomes of endovascular therapy of obstructive disease of diverse etiology of the common femoral artery. *Catheter Cardiovasc Interv.* 2013;81(6):1013–1022.

83. Trani C, Tommasino A, Burzotta F. Pushing the limits forward: transradial superficial femoral artery stenting. *Catheter Cardiovasc Interv.* 2010;76(7):1065–1071.

84. Patel T, Shah S, Pancholy SB. *Patel's Atlas of Transradial Intervention: The Basics and Beyond.* Malvern, PA: HMP Communications, 2012.

85. Gruntzig A, et al. Treatment of renovascular hypertension with percutaneous transluminal dilatation of a renal-artery stenosis. *Lancet.* 1978;1(8068):801–802.

86. Dorros G, Prince C, Mathiak L. Stenting of a renal artery stenosis achieves better relief of the obstructive lesion than balloon angioplasty. *Cathet Cardiovasc Diagn.* 1993;29(3):191–198.

87. Sapoval M, et al. Low-profile stent system for treatment of atherosclerotic renal artery stenosis: the GREAT trial. *J Vasc Interv Radiol.* 2005;16(9):1195–1202.

88. Watson PS, et al. Effect of renal artery stenting on renal function and size in patients with atherosclerotic renovascular disease. *Circulation.* 2000;102(14):1671–1677.

89. Textor SC. Revascularization in atherosclerotic renal artery disease. *Kidney Int.* 1998;53(3):799–811.

90. Wheatley K, et al. Revascularization versus medical therapy for renal-artery stenosis. *N Engl J Med.* 2009;361(20):1953–1962.

91. Cooper CJ, et al. Stenting and medical therapy for atherosclerotic renal-artery stenosis. *N Engl J Med.* 2014;370:13–22.

92. Kennedy AM, et al. Median nerve injury: an underrecognised complication of brachial artery cardiac catheterisation? *J Neurol Neurosurg Psychiatry.* 1997;63(4):542–546.

93. Otaki M. Percutaneous transradial approach for coronary angiography. *Cardiology.* 1992;81(6):330–333.

94. Wu CJ, et al. Transradial coronary angiography and angioplasty in Chinese patients. *Cathet Cardiovasc Diagn.* 1997;40(2):159–163.

95. Rao SV, et al. Trends in the prevalence and outcomes of radial and femoral approaches to percutaneous coronary intervention: a report from the national cardiovascular data registry. *JACC Cardiovasc Interv.* 2008;1(4):379–386.

96. Singh M, et al. Twenty-five-year trends in in-hospital and long-term outcome after percutaneous coronary intervention: a single-institution experience. *Circulation.* 2007;115(22):2835–2841.

97. Scheinert D, et al. Transradial approach for renal artery stenting. *Catheter Cardiovasc Interv.* 2001;54(4):442–447.

98. Kessel DO, et al. Renal stenting from the radial artery: a novel approach. *Cardiovasc Intervent Radiol.* 2003;26(2):146–149.

99. Alli O, et al. Transradial access for renal artery intervention is feasible and safe. *Vasc Endovascular Surg.* 2011;45(8):738–742.

100. McGill HC Jr, et al. Effects of coronary heart disease risk factors on atherosclerosis of selected regions of the aorta and right coronary artery. PDAY Research Group. Pathobiological determinants of atherosclerosis in youth. *Arterioscler Thromb Vasc Biol.* 2000;20(3):836–845.

101. Sciahbasi A, Romagnoli E, Burzotta F, et al. Transradial approach (left versus right) and procedural times during percutaneous coronary procedures: TALENT study. *Am Heart J.* 2011;161(1):172–179.

102. Guedes A, et al. Low rate of conversion to transfemoral approach when attempting both radial arteries for coronary angiography and percutaneous coronary intervention: a study of 1,826 consecutive procedures. *J Invasive Cardiol.* 2010;22(9):391–397.

103. Rao SV, et al. The transradial approach to percutaneous coronary intervention: historical perspective, current concepts, and future directions. *J Am Coll Cardiol.* 2010;55(20):2187–2195.

104. Mamas M, et al. Use of the sheathless guide catheter during routine transradial percutaneous coronary intervention: a feasibility study. *Catheter Cardiovasc Interv.* 2010;75(4):596–602.

105. From AM, et al. Sheathless transradial intervention using standard guide catheters. *Catheter Cardiovasc Interv.* 2010;76(7):911–96.

106. de Araujo Goncalves P, Teles RC, Raposo L. Catheter-based renal denervation for resistant hypertension performed by radial access. *J Invasive Cardiol.* 2013;25(3):147–149.

107. Jiang XJ, et al. First-in-man report of a novel dedicated radiofrequency catheter for renal denervation via the transulnar approach. *EuroIntervention.* 2013;9(6):684–686.

108. Honton B, et al. First report of transradial renal denervation with the dedicated radiofrequency Iberis catheter. *EuroIntervention.* 2014;9(12):1385–1388.

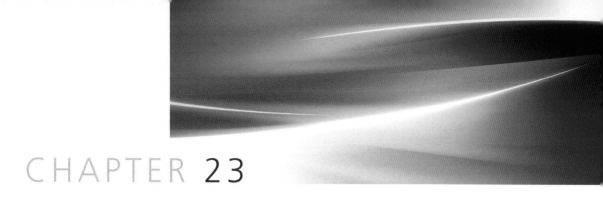

CHAPTER 23

Radiation in Transradial Access

Gurbir Bhatia, Karim Ratib, Johannes B. Dahm, and James Nolan

Introduction

Transradial diagnostic and interventional coronary procedures have been increasingly performed in the last two decades. The benefits of transradial practice in reducing vascular complications, improving clinical outcomes, and reducing economic costs[1-3] are well covered in other chapters. Yet, despite numerous advantages having been identified, transradial uptake around the cardiac world is variable: although contemporary data show increasing uptake led by committed clinicians and subgroups, transradial usage remains confined to minority clusters of enthusiasts in certain nations.[4,5]

There may be a number of reasons to account for this disparity, including training issues, reimbursement schemes, or, more simply, resistance to change long-standing practices. However, an oft-quoted disadvantage of transradial procedures is an increase in measures of X-ray exposure to patients and operators. This impression has even found its way into training curricula in emerging transradial regions.[6]

Any potential excess in radiation delivery from radial procedures would represent an important issue: if such a radiation burden were truly to exist, then it would negate the documented advantages of transradial procedures. However, this is a contentious subject, as this perceived burden stems from studies that we believe have flawed methodologies.

The aims of this chapter include revisiting basic concepts of radiation awareness, including the adverse effects of X-rays, terms used in dose measurements, and key determinants of measured doses for patients and operators. Armed with this information, we assess the available data, comparing radiation exposure between transradial and transfemoral approaches.

Adverse Effects of Radiation

Since Roentgen's discovery in the late 19th century, X-ray radiation has undoubtedly provided indisputable medical benefits. However, cardiologists must recognize that injudicious usage carries the potential for serious harm to their patients, their coworkers, and themselves.

The absolute number of recognized X-ray-induced injuries to patients is most likely underestimated: in part, this may be a function of a lack of knowledge regarding such injuries on the part of both patient and clinician. However, it should also be appreciated that there is often a latent period (which may be decades in some cases) between radiation exposure and symptoms and signs, which may prevent physicians or patients from assigning appropriate culpability.

It is vital that operators remain mindful that the X-ray procedures that they are controlling also expose them and their laboratory staff to radiation. Much of this exposure is down to scattered radiation reflected from the patient and the surroundings. Generally speaking, doses received by operators are proportional to those received by patients.[7]

Harmful effects of radiation are typically classified as being *deterministic (nonstochastic)* or *stochastic*. This classification is related to the presence or absence of a dose threshold underlying any injury.

Deterministic Effects

These are *predictable* and *dose-dependent* reactions to X-ray radiation. They have a critical threshold of exposure, below which injuries do not occur. As doses increase, so does the severity of a particular injury.

Skin injuries induced by X-ray exposure were first reported soon after the discovery of X-rays, and comprise the most frequently reported deterministic injury resulting from fluoroscopic procedures. While there is a relationship to X-ray doses, individual responses are variable, and may be influenced by inherent tissue characteristics, fractionation of doses by performing staged procedures, and even the area of skin exposed.

Skin erythema is a very early reaction to radiation exposure, typically peaking at 24 hours, and is believed to result from increased capillary permeability. Larger doses may damage the epidermal basal cell layer, resulting in an angrier inflammatory erythema (main erythema), often associated with symptoms such as discomfort and itch. More drastic injuries include ischemic dermal necrosis and frank skin ulceration, which may require skin grafting. Radiation may deplete germinal layers of hair follicles, resulting in epilation within a month of exposure. Damage to melanocytes is also recognized, and may result in skin discoloration.

There have been several reports of skin injuries after diagnostic and therapeutic coronary procedures. While such injuries are not especially frequent in relation to the number of procedures performed, severe consequences can result for all concerned parties. Painful and unsightly skin lesions and their treatment may effect a loss of patient confidence in health-care providers. For the cardiologist and health-care institution, legal consequences may be damaging.[8]

Koenig et al.[9,10] reported over 70 cases of radiation-induced skin injury from fluoroscopic (mainly coronary) procedures. Most cases developed chronic ulceration, with one quarter requiring skin grafting. A common thread among these cases appeared to be a prolonged screening time because of either procedural complications or complex anatomy.

Stochastic Effects

Stochastic effects differ from deterministic effects by not having a clear dose threshold or any relationship between severity and dose. Instead, these adverse effects are *probabilistic*; the likelihood of stimulation is proportional to the dose received.

Stochastic effects include the induction of cancer. The ionizing effect of X-ray radiation initiates free radical formation, which, in turn, can damage DNA molecules. Such effects are exemplified in the increased risk of cancer seen among survivors of atom bomb explosions and, indeed, among workers in the radiation industry.[11,12] Similarly, studies of medical X-ray workers have previously indicated increased mortality due to hematological malignancies.[13] There are more recent pointers toward an increased risk of solid tumors: for example, one study reported an increased risk of breast cancer among female technicians.[14]

Radiation Doses

As discussed above, the radiation dose delivered by a procedure has an important impact on the risks of adverse effects. Accordingly, it is vitally important that operators recognize and understand the various terms used in dose quantification. Furthermore, operators should be aware of any local regulatory requirements relating to X-ray doses, which will likely utilize such terms.

Definitions of measurements employed are provided in Table 23-1. Conceptually, for X-ray doses delivered to living tissue, quantification relates better to delivery of *energy* rather than radiation per se. Thus, *kerma* (kinetic energy released in matter) represents the energy conveyed from the X-ray beam to charged particles per unit mass in a given medium. The SI units for absorbed dose and effective dose (ED), gray (Gy) and sievert (Sv), respectively, have replaced older units.

Among these parameters, the most commonly used terms are the dose–area product (DAP), the ED, and fluoroscopy time (FT). The DAP is a function of air kerma and field size, and is measured by an ionization chamber integrated within the tube unit of most modern systems. Thus, it can be affected by the field size (i.e., the variable use of coning) used during fluoroscopic studies. It represents a useful estimate of the energy delivered to patients. The ED is the summation of equivalent doses to organs multiplied by specific tissue-weighting factors, which are influenced by the inherent sensitivity of respective tissues. This measurement provides an estimate of stochastic risk to the patient or laboratory staff. The frequently quoted FT is the total time that fluoroscopy is employed during a study. It is a simple, yet imperfect measurement of X-ray doses in coronary procedures, however, as the bulk of

TABLE 23-1	**Quantification of Radiation Delivery**	
Measurement	**Unit**	**Definition**
Absorbed dose	Gray (Gy)	The energy imparted by ionizing radiation deposited per unit mass.
Air kerma	Gray (Gy)	The unscattered dose delivered per unit volume of air.
Dose–area product (DAP)	Gy·cm^2	The air kerma integrated across the X-ray beam from the tube—a surrogate for the entire energy delivered to the patient.
Effective dose	Sievert (Sv)	The summated whole-body dose equivalent to the risk of an absorbed dose to particular body part.
Entrance skin dose	Gray (Gy)	The absorbed dose on the skin at a given location on the patient, including back-scattered radiation.
Equivalent dose	Sievert (Sv)	The radiation dose applied to a tissue allowing for the effect of that radiation on that tissue.
Fluoroscopy time	Minutes	The total time fluoroscopy is used during a procedure.

the dose is delivered during image acquisition; fluoroscopy provides only 30% to 40% of the X-ray dose of an equivalent duration of acquisition.

An alternative way of appreciating procedural doses is to consider the radiation delivered in reference to other, more basic, procedures, such as a standard chest X-ray (Table 23-2). These doses represent estimates, and it must be acknowledged that there is a good deal of variation for a given study between different institutions. Furthermore, doses can be compared to the background radiation that subjects are exposed to (e.g., by radon gas or cosmic rays): depending on geographical location, background radiation may impart a dose of 3 mSv/year.

Thus, a diagnostic coronary angiography may impart a dose equivalent to 70 chest X-rays, or just over 2 years of background radiation exposure. Moreover, when considering a frequently chartered patient journey comprising a stress-rest nuclear perfusion study, a diagnostic coronary angiography with a subsequent percutaneous coronary intervention (PCI), the cumulative radiation dose can equate to 11 years of background radiation delivered over a short period of time!

Such a journey may well predispose our patient to an increased risk of future cancer. A recent study[15] has provided some food for thought regarding cancer risk from cardiac imaging. This retrospective cohort study constructed discharge summary data looking at the incidence of cancers among a large group of Canadian patients who had undergone imaging procedures involving ionizing radiation in the context of a recent acute myocardial infarction. Radiation burden was quantified for each patient from *estimated* doses of cardiac imaging procedures. Cumulative estimated dose of radiation from cardiac procedures was an independent risk factor for cancer induction over a mean follow-up period of

TABLE 23-2	**Typical ED Estimates for Various X-ray Procedures**
Study	**Typical ED Estimate (mSv)**
Chest X-ray	0.1
Standard CT chest	7.0
Cardiac CT chest	16
Coronary angiography	7.0
Percutaneous coronary intervention	15.0
Radiofrequency arrhythmia ablation	15.0
Technetium Tc 99m heart (stress-rest)	11.4
Thallium heart (stress-rest)	16.9

Data from Cambers CE, Fetterly KA, Holzer R, et al. Radiation safety program for the cardiac catheterization laboratory. *Catheter Cardiovasc Interv.* 2011;77(4):546–556.

TABLE 23-3 **Proposed Dose Reference Levels for Diagnostic Coronary Angiography (CA) and Percutaneous Coronary Intervention (PCI)**		
Study	**CA**	**PCI**
Europe 2008[19]	FT 6.5	FT 15.5
	DAP 45	DAP 85
UK 2009[20]	FT 4.5	FT 13
	DAP 29	DAP 50
Ireland 2009[21]	FT 5	FT 18
	DAP 42	DAP 84
USA 2012[18]	FT 5.4	FT 18.5
	DAP 83	DAP 193

DAP, dose–area product in Gy·cm^2; FT, fluoroscopy time in minutes.

5 years: the authors estimated a 3% risk of cancer for every 10 mSv of radiation. However, the design of the study, coupled with the use of estimated doses without allowing for confounding factors, makes it difficult to draw firm conclusions from this study.

So, how do the doses from coronary procedures translate into a risk of cancer that we can use to counsel our patients? Unfortunately, there is a dearth of quality data to answer this question.[16] Simplistically, it can be taken that any dose of ionizing radiation has the capacity to be harmful and that the probability of cancer induction is related to total dosage, albeit without a threshold. Operators should endeavor to keep doses "as low as reasonably achievable/practicable" (ALARA/ALARP principle) while ensuring that imaging remains of a clinically acceptable standard. On top of this important ideal, a number of audits of X-ray doses during coronary procedures have been compiled with a view to providing some guidance by proposing dose reference limits (DRLs).

For example, audit data from the United Kingdom were collected in 2005 and reported in 2007.[17] For diagnostic coronary angiography, a median FT of 3.9 minutes (interquartile range [IQR], 3.3–4.5) was recorded, and median DAP was 23.5 Gy·cm^2 (IQR, 18.9–29.0); for single-stent PCI, median FT was 11.8 minutes (IQR, 10.1–13.3), and median DAP was 36 Gy·cm^2 (IQR, 29.0–50.3). Similarly, in the United States, radiographic data from the Nationwide Evaluation of X-ray Trends (NEXT) survey in 2008 to 2009 were evaluated by the Conference of Radiation Control Program Directors and the Food and Drug Administration.[18] Diagnostic angiography had a median FT of 2.9 minutes (IQR, 1.8–5.4) and a median DAP of 49 Gy·cm^2 (IQR, 27–83). Median FT for PCI was 11.0 minutes (IQR, 6.8–18.5), and median DAP was 117 Gy·cm^2 (IQR, 60.0–193).

Corresponding median DAP measurements were notably higher in this audit compared with the UK data above. It must be appreciated that the exact measurements that have been collated in a number of audits vary from study to study, and national data are not necessarily generalizable throughout a country; it is even more difficult to compare radiographic data across countries, as the data are affected by many uncontrolled variables, which are summarized in the next section. Nevertheless, the differences in the DAP measurements allows one to hypothesize that radiation protection measures in the United States may be suboptimal.

Authors of the various audits have used their data to put forward DRLs to be used as guidance for operators. Generally, the 75th percentiles have been taken as the reference levels. Table 23-3 lists DRLs for FT and DAP for diagnostic and interventional procedures, and it is apparent that there is a good deal of variation in recommended limits, indicating likely differing practices. While these figures should be regarded as guidance only, it does provide operators with a yardstick to work with when auditing their own work.

Factors Affecting Patient and Operator Doses

Patient Factors

Lesion Complexity

It should come as no surprise that the more complex coronary interventional procedures are associated with higher radiation doses. For example, attempts to recanalize chronic occlusions require more screening and acquisitions to achieve the desired goal. Dose metrics are seen to increase with the number of vessels treated as well as the total number of stents deployed. Intervention in more tortuous vessels also resulted in higher doses.[22,23]

The degree of urgency with which an intervention is performed is a further factor. Emergency PCI in the context of acute myocardial infarction was associated with significantly higher dose parameters compared to elective cases in one observational study.[22]

Patient Size

Modern fluoroscopic equipment is able to accommodate for larger patients by increasing the voltage across the cathode–anode gap in the X-ray generator: this yields higher energy photons with a better image quality, but with a resulting increased overall dose.

Measured DAP has been observed to correlate reasonably well with body mass index (BMI) and body surface area.[22] This should be considered when counseling the larger patient of potential risks prior to performing intervention, particularly when the case is likely to be complex or when the patient has already undergone recent intervention.

Operational Factors

Distances

The inverse square law dictates that increasing the distance from an X-ray source by factor x will reduce the radiation dose by factor $1/x^2$. Accordingly, if the distance from the source is doubled, the radiation dose received will drop to one quarter of the original dose. This is important when positioning the X-ray tube and the image intensifier: placing the X-ray source near to the patient will lead to higher skin doses. Operators should also minimize the source-to-image distance (SID) by ensuring that the image intensifier is as near to the patient as possible. Increasing the SID results in higher patient doses and greater scattered doses to the attending staff.

Similarly, operators and assistants should strive to position themselves as far from the X-ray tube as is possible. This will significantly reduce the scattered dose received. This can be achieved by using longer extension tubing (Fig. 23-1) to connect the manifold and the catheter.

Fluoroscopy and Acquisition

As mentioned earlier, fluoroscopy has a smaller impact on total doses imparted for a given procedure. It follows that one should focus on reducing

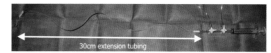

FIGURE 23-1 Extension tubing connecting the manifold and catheter reduces radiation exposure to operators.

acquisition-related doses by cutting down the number of acquisition runs, as well as their duration (frames). It should also be noted that most modern fluoroscopic units are able to alter the intensity of dose according to, for example, patient body habitus. In general, fluoroscopic intensity should be set at the lowest possible levels, with the use of the lowest frame rate that provides adequate imaging. Similarly, current models deliver fluoroscopic X-rays in quick, successive pulses, reducing the time during which radiation is released. Operators should make use of further contemporary enhancements of X-ray machines that allow for storage of the last fluoroscopic images. When image quality is not of paramount importance, fluoroscopic runs documenting, for example, balloon inflation or stent deployment can be employed in lieu of acquisition, sparing doses further.

Filtration and Collimation

X-ray tubes produce photons with a spectrum of energy levels. Lower energy photons, which would not penetrate through the patient's skin to contribute to image formation, are filtered out of the beam by aluminium and copper filters that are usually fitted as standard. Operators who are in tune with their machines can make further use of additional wedge filters, which can be employed when bordering lung tissue is exposed to the beam, resulting in lower doses and improved image quality.

Collimation, via either multiple blades or an iris diaphragm, can greatly reduce the image field of view to the region of interest. This will result in a reduced DAP as well as the dose scattered to around the laboratory.

Shielding

Most readers will be familiar with the need to religiously wear lead aprons when in the catheter laboratory. The operator's exposed areas receive about 0.05% of the patient dose; doses received beneath lead aprons are reduced to about 10% of exposed areas. Wearing leaded thyroid shields and shin guards confers further reduction in doses received by scatter. Cataract formation is another example of a deterministic injury, and this may be commoner among catheter laboratory workers.[24] The wearing of leaded glasses has been promoted to reduce ocular doses. Interventional cardiologists may be further concerned by case reports of left-sided cerebral tumors.[25] One operator had previously advocated the use of a 0.5-mm lead cap in order to reduce the doses scattered to the head.[26]

Mobile lead shielding fitted to the couch and suspended from the laboratory ceiling is commonplace, and successfully employed to reduce scattered radiation exposure to operators and staff. Additional lead flaps have been shown to augment the reduction in operator exposure,[27] principally by protecting against radiation that is scattered to the operators' midriff between the shields. The authors frequently note that the usage of these shields, particularly among trainees, can be inconsistent; the benefits of shielding should be emphasized to trainees at induction, and reiterated regularly.

Angulations

The ideal angulations are those that provide sufficient diagnostic data, but reduce doses delivered to the patient and scattered to the operator and laboratory staff.

Studies subjecting phantom patients[28] to fluoroscopic doses have reported steeper left or right anterior oblique projections ($\geq 60°$) to be particularly dose intensive (Fig. 23-2). There are likely to be benefits in changing habitual use of steep left anterior oblique (LAO) caudal views to posteroanterior (PA) caudal angulations when studying the distal left main stem. Likewise, dose reductions may be achieved by switching from the LAO cranial to a PA cranial view to study left anterior descending (LAD)/diagonal artery bifurcations. Of course, individual anatomy will dictate whether these advocated views provide complete information, but over the course of an interventional career, such altered practice may prove valuable in reducing exposure to patients and staff alike.

Operator Experience and the Transradial Learning Curve

The preceding paragraphs summarized factors that influence radiation dose delivery to patients and catheter laboratory staff. These factors, and some protective measures such as using shielding and avoiding certain angiographic projections, are applicable to all coronary procedures, and irrespective of the access site chosen. Furthermore, providing short tutorials promoting measures designed to reduce doses may well achieve these goals for operators with a wide range of experience.[29] For this subsection, we focus on

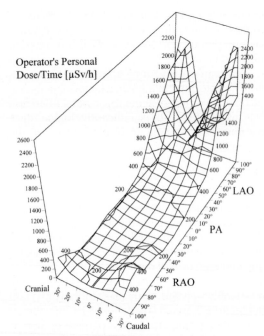

FIGURE 23-2 Calculated isodose lines in a three-dimensional graph of the operator's mean personal dose per time (μSv/h), as a function of tube angulation. LAO, left anterior oblique; PA, posteroanterior; RAO, right anterior oblique. (From Kuon E, et al. Identification of less-irradiating tube angulations in invasive cardiology. *J Am Coll Cardiol.* 2004;44(7):1420–1428.)

operator experience in transradial access procedures, highlighting the concept of a specific learning curve.

Early insights into the transradial learning curve came from operators assessing success rates for diagnostic angiography in the 1990s. For example, Spaulding et al.[30] described a learning curve for a single operator performing coronary angiography via (left) radial artery access in over 400 patients. Procedure failure occurred in 14% of the first 80 cases, but the failure rate diminished with experience, and was as low as 2% for the last 100 cases performed. Another French group[31] reported on the experiences of a single operator who performed angiography in 800 subjects. Among the first 50 cases, the failure rate was 10%, but thereafter dropped to 4% for the cohort volume between 50 and 500. After 500 cases had been performed, the failure rate settled at 1%.

For transradial PCI, a recent study has attempted to illustrate the corresponding curve for interventional rather than diagnostic procedures.[32] All nonurgent, single-vessel interventions performed with transradial access in a single Canadian institution between 1999 and 2008 ($n = 1,672$) were analyzed according to operator experience. Cohorts were stratified according to operator experience by volume: the control group was made up of operators who had performed more than 300 transradial interventions. The study groups were divided into four categories according to volumes: 1 to 50 cases, 51 to 100 cases, 101 to 150 cases, and 151 to 300 cases. Failure rates were significantly higher in the least experienced operators cohort compared to the cohort with 50 to 100 cases under their belts (7% vs 3%, $P = 0.007$). The failure rate for the experienced control group was 2%. The reasons for failure were the usual banes of the transradial operator: radial artery spasm, subclavian artery tortuosity, unsupportive guide catheters, inability to gain radial access, and radial artery loops. Nevertheless, the authors noted the positive effects of experience, recording a reduction in odds of failure of 32% for each 50 increments in procedure volume.

These studies have indicated that transradial learning curves for diagnostic and simple interventional procedures are steep, with aptitude increasing quickly with case volumes, that need to be augmented by regular practice—of course, this is also the case for transfemoral access. Traditionally, getting to grips with transradial access has been felt to be more difficult than that for the transfemoral route; many of the inherent hurdles led to procedural failures in the study described above.[32] Typically, expertise develops after a case volume of over 200 has been recorded. However, it should be noted that the case series reported by Spaulding et al.[30] and Louvard et al.[31] commenced their studies almost two decades ago, since when the transradial community has benefitted from numerous advantages in equipment and knowledge facilitating performance. When taken together with the fact that trainees are now being taught by experienced radial operators, it could be argued that the learning curve for future trainees should be a good deal smoother. Nonetheless, it is important to recognize that transradial access has its own vagaries that require experience to deal with. An appreciation of this fact is useful when evaluating studies comparing radiation doses delivered by transradial and transfemoral procedures.

Radiation in Transradial versus Transfemoral Studies

Over the last decade or so, a number of studies have evaluated compared radiation doses for transradial and transfemoral procedures. The majority of such studies have been observational in design, although there is now a sprinkling of data derived from some randomized studies.

Most observational studies that have set out to compare radiation exposure for the two access sites have been modest in size, and while many have pointed out an excess in X-ray doses to both patients and operators with transradial access, others have not. However, we believe that there are inherent methodological flaws in these studies that detract from their findings.

Observational Studies

As transradial practice was developing, early studies looking into this area were typically conducted in a single center, with varying experience between operators. It should not be forgotten that these investigators were ploughing a lone furrow in an area without the specific radial tools that have been developed to aid contemporary radial practitioners. Most studies were poorly controlled for the variables that were discussed in the previous section.

Brasselet et al.[33] conducted their prospective study of over 400 subjects in a single center over a 6-month period in 2005 to 2006. Technicians compiled dose data for transradial and transfemoral procedures for four operators blinded to these data. Radiation exposure was reported to be higher for transradial procedures for both patients and operators; these findings were consistent for diagnostic angiography alone, as well as for ad hoc PCI after angiography. The authors advised that indications for using transradial access ought to be reconsidered. These results have been frequently cited in the long debate that has ensued. On closer inspection, however, there are a number of issues with this study. First, a number of relevant factors were uncontrolled. For example, while the four operators were well versed in radiation protection, and adhered to use of lead shielding, there was no standardization for radiographic angulations. In addition, there were important differences between the subjects in the transradial and transfemoral patient groups. First, the transradial group had a significantly higher mean mass than their counterparts, and it is likely that this would be reflected in higher doses. Second, complex coronary lesions occurred more frequently in the transradial group, and could have potentially accounted for more radiation. Of course, it is difficult to control for all factors in what may have been a "real-world" study, but the results were not adjusted for these potential confounders. Another key issue was that of operator experience. The transradial procedures comprised <60% of the overall cases for all four operators during the study period, and this fact was highlighted as a marker of a relative inexperience by observers[34]; it was posited that the operators may have participated in the study in the middle of their radial learning curve, whereas they were very experienced in transfemoral work. The authors had acknowledged not only that their transradial volumes were in the "mild-moderate" category, but also that this was representative for many European centers at that time.

Our center[35] recently performed a prospective observational study with dual hypotheses to further characterize the effects of uncontrolled variables and operator experience: first, there would not be a disparity in dose measures between access sites when important variables were controlled for; second, operator experience would influence radiation exposure regardless of access site. One hundred consecutive patients undergoing their first diagnostic angiography were recruited. An experienced operator who used femoral access as his default route performed 25 cases, with a further 25 cases performed by a similarly experienced transradial counterpart. A trainee operator of intermediate experience with both modes of access performed the remaining cases, with 25 procedures by each route. Of note, imaging projections were standardized— the same views/angles were used to acquire five acquisition runs for the left coronary artery and three runs for the right coronary artery (left ventricular angiography was performed for all cases with the same projection). Furthermore, operators made similar use of available lead shielding in all cases. Among the patients, there were no differences in anthropometric measurements or comorbid conditions.

For the expert operators, there were no differences in ED, DAP, or FT. However, the operator (by 25%–30%) and patient (by 10%–15%) exposures were significantly higher for the intermediate operators than for the experts, for both the access routes. Interestingly, there were no significant differences for the trainees' dose parameters when analyzed by access route. Thus, it is likely that inadequate controlling of pertinent factors and disparities in operator experience have contributed to observational data in the past.

A Dutch group[36] has since further emphasized the need to take confounding factors into account. This team analyzed the procedural database at their high-volume unit: patient doses (as DAP) were recorded among 4,000 patients undergoing diagnostic and interventional procedures over the period 2004 to 2008. The authors constructed a predictive model in order to compare observed transradial doses with expected transfemoral doses once differences in, for example, lesion complexity were considered. From this model, diagnostic and therapeutic procedures performed transradially did not carry an increased radiation burden. In addition, when radial observed doses were stratified according to when the cases were performed, it was evident that there was a progressive fall in exposure with increasing experience. Of note, operator doses were not reported in this study.

A further single-center, retrospective study reported exposure between the two access sites for diagnostic and interventional procedures among experienced operators.[37] While FTs and DAP were increased with transradial access in both types of procedure, it is noteworthy that the differences in radiation doses delivered did not reach significances once procedures involving either trainee fellows or surgically grafted patients were excluded.

Similarly, but on a larger scale, investigators for the Swedish Coronary Angiography and Angioplasty Registry (SCAAR) conducted a study between 2008 and 2012.[38] Here, over 20,000 invasive procedures (52% diagnostic angiography and 48% coronary intervention of varying complexity) were analyzed to look at radiation exposure (also as DAP). Multivariate analysis identified patient BMI, prior history of coronary bypass graft surgery, and increased procedural complexity (e.g., >1 lesion treated, chronic total occlusions) as factors associated with higher radiation dose. After adjustment for these factors, transradial access was not associated with a higher radiation burden than was the transfemoral approach.

Randomized Studies

Clearly, randomized studies that control for the numerous variables represent the ideal way of resolving this controversy. Conducting such studies is not without difficulties. It would be desirable that individual operators should be equally adept performing procedures via either route: in reality, most operators have a default access site in daily practice, and reserve the alternative route for when difficulties arise. In addition, in the current era, given the well-documented benefits of transradial access for bleeding outcomes, patient comfort, and healthcare costs, it can be foreseen that some operators may be reluctant to enroll their patients into a study that may subject them to a femoral puncture!

The first data from any randomized study looking at the effect of access site on X-ray doses came from a single German center (and from a single, albeit, experienced operator) evaluation of almost 300 subjects.[39] Patient doses (as DAP) were significantly increased by 15% in the radial group, but, interestingly, did not differ from femoral doses for interventional procedures. Furthermore, transradial operator doses were doubled for diagnostic procedures, and were increased by 50% for in the intervention group. Underlying these findings were the facts that the operator was slightly closer during radial procedures and that the shielding used for radiation protection had not been standardized, as during the transradial cases, a side shield had not been employed as it had been for femoral cases.

A further randomized study from another experienced radial unit in Germany[40] focused its attention upon 307 elderly patients (aged >75 years), acknowledging that distorted vessel anatomy (e.g., at the proximal subclavian artery) can occur with age, and has detrimental effects for radial operators. Despite this, patient doses (DAP) and FTs were not significantly different by access site.

Another study (also German, also single-center) randomized 1,024 patients into undergoing radial or femoral coronary procedures over 18 months.[41] The aim of the study was to ascertain transradial procedure feasibility and safety in a (self-proclaimed) moderate-volume community hospital. The radial and femoral groups were well matched for baseline characteristics, and coronary disease severity was similar. In each group, around a third of patients underwent PCI. The measured patient dose metrics included FT and DAP; both were significantly higher among transradial procedures. Operator doses were not measured. One may postulate that similar issues with regard to experience may be causing this discrepancy: the four participating operators were required to have *extensive* experience in femoral procedures, with completion of at least 50 transradial catheterizations.

Finally, we come to a large, multicenter, randomized study designed to clarify the extent of any excess radiation in transradial cases. The RIVAL study[2] has been discussed in detail in other chapters. Briefly, this international, multicenter trial randomized over 7,000 subjects with acute coronary syndromes to diagnostic and/or interventional procedures performed either with radial or femoral access. Access site did not affect the composite primary outcome of death, myocardial infarction, stroke,

or non-bypass graft surgery related bleeding (although outcomes were better in the most experienced transradial centers). However, radial artery access was associated with a large reduction in vascular site complications.

A substudy comprising over 2,500 patients in whom air kerma and DAP measurements were possible (likely in units with relatively more modern equipment) was subsequently conducted and reported.[42] Operator dose measurements were not recorded. Radiation dose parameters were assessed for transradial and transfemoral procedures, and data were further analyzed according to prespecified subgroups. There was a modest, but significant, increase in FT in the radial cases (9.3 vs 8.0 minutes, $P < 0.001$). However, when stratified according to radial center volume, significant differences were only apparent in the low- and middle-volume tertiles. For air kerma measurements, there was a strong trend ($P = 0.051$) toward higher doses in all transradial cases, but again, this appeared to be driven by larger differences in the low-volume center tertile. Interestingly, there were no differences for DAP between the access sites both for the whole cohort, and also when broken down by radial center volume. The authors suggested that this might have been related to differential use of collimation to alter field size. Multivariate analysis indicated that the highest volume centers and operators were associated with lower DAP readings. The reported findings that high-volume centers are associated with lower radiation doses irrespective of access site serve to underline aforementioned thoughts regarding the importance of experience in reducing radiation exposure.

The study by Shah et al.[37] alluded to an excess risk of radiation delivery when examining coronary artery bypass graft patency among patients undergoing transradial angiography. A small study randomized previously grafted patients referred for angiography to (left) transradial or (right or left) transfemoral procedures.[43] The primary end point looked at contrast volume, with patient and operator radiation exposure among the secondary outcomes assessed. Laudably, the vast majority (80%–91%) of patients underwent their procedures with the operators aware of the graft anatomy; there was no significant difference for this between either approach. Patient and operator radiation exposure was higher (as was the primary outcome) with transradial procedures. It should be appreciated that there was a high radial-to-femoral crossover rate in this study, and that the first operator was usually a fellow in training. While the "fellow-first" approach applied to both access routes, it is possible that the fellow's aptitude favored femoral procedures.

Emerging Concepts

Which Wrist?

Experienced radial operators have been confronted by obstacles to successful procedure completion in the form of radial anomalies and subclavian/aortic tortuosity. Unfortunately, these are not rare,[44,45] and are associated with an increased risk of procedure failure. Tortuosity at the subclavian–innominate–aortic interface is commoner on the right side, perhaps more so in shorter females, and its hindrance to right radial operators has led some investigators to question whether using left radial access may be more profitable.

Data from randomized studies have recently become available. One study in a single center showed no difference in FTs among 193 patients randomized to left or right radial access.[46] Subsequently, a larger study enrolled 1,540 patients from two centers.[47] Subjects who were allocated to undergo left radial diagnostic angiography received significantly less radiation (as FT and DAP) than those randomized to right-sided access. A substudy later showed that right-sided access was associated with higher operator doses as evidenced by the dosimeters worn at the operators' left wrists.[48] Norgaz et al.[49] reported on 1,000 patients, and noted that left-sided access was associated with significant reductions in FT; this may have been related to a threefold increase in subclavian artery tortuosity reported on the right side. Lastly, a randomized study[50] was performed to assess the effect of access site on operator dose burden. The authors ensured that angiographic projections were standardized throughout. Interestingly, although there were no significant differences for fluoroscopic time or doses, operator doses were significantly reduced by 25% with left radial access. This may appear counterintuitive when procedures are performed at the patient's right side, as operators may have to stand closer to the X-ray source, and may have to occasionally move away from the protective lead shields. Nevertheless, these data appear to be reasonably consistent so far, and it will be interesting to see if future studies replicate these findings. Potential limitations to widespread use of left access include discomfort on the part of both patient and operator.

More Shields?

As discussed earlier, standard lead shielding should be in widespread use in most modern catheter laboratories. There may well be potential in using additional shielding in order to reduce X-ray scatter directed toward operators and other staff.

A randomized study[51] assessed the use of commercially available lead shielding placed over the patient's pelvis and thighs in reducing operator exposure. Over 200 patients were randomized to radial or femoral access with or without the adjunctive shielding (Fig. 23-3). The extra shielding was associated with similar, significant reductions in operator dose for radial and femoral procedures.

Operators in the United Kingdom[52] have adapted a radial arm board to accommodate a detachable 0.5-mm lead-equivalent rubber shield (Fig. 23-4). This vertical shield is designed to sit between the patient's arm and body, and serves to absorb scattered doses to reduce operator exposure from radial procedures. The designers' team performed a randomized study assessing the effects of this kit in addition to conventional lead shielding among 106 patients who underwent radial procedures. The use of this transradial radiation protection board was associated with a 30% reduction in operator doses.

Another group[53] has assessed the usefulness of a commercially available, sterile drape composed of bismuth and barium (Radpad®, Worldwide Innovations and Technologies, Overland Park, KS), which is also designed to reduce scattered X-rays.

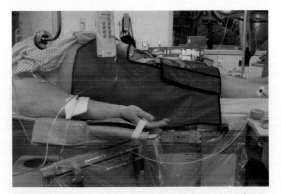

FIGURE 23-3 Patient pelvic lead shielding to reduce scatter to operators. (From Lange HW, von Boetticher H. Reduction of operator radiation dose by a pelvic lead shield during cardiac catheterization by radial access: comparison with femoral access. *JACC Cardiovasc Interv.* 2012;5(4):445–449.)

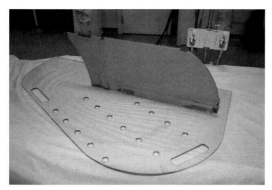

FIGURE 23-4 The transradial radiation protection board. (From Behan M, et al. Decreasing operators' radiation exposure during coronary procedures: the Transradial Radiation Protection Board. *Catheter Cardiovasc Interv.* 2010;76(1):79–84.)

The authors randomized 60 patients undergoing transradial coronary angiography by a single operator to Radpad use or not, in addition to standard shielding. Radpad use conferred extra radiation protection to the operator, significantly reducing the operator dose by almost 25%.

Fluoroscopic Frame Rate

It was noted above that the modification of the fluoroscopic frame rate affects radiation dosage: lower frame rates impart a lower dose. This will be particularly apparent in reducing cumulative doses to operators and laboratory staff over a long period of angiographic practice. A high-volume radial center in Canada has recently conducted a moderate-sized study assessing the effects of lower frame rates on operator doses.[54] The study reported sizeable and significant differences in operator doses, with rates of 7.5 frames/second compared to the standard 15 frames/second. This drop in frame rate represents a simple way to reduce one's overall exposure. It may not be possible to reduce rates to this level in every catheter laboratory, but operators should acquaint themselves with their equipment in order to potentially take advantage of this approach to radiation dose reduction. Of course, this can also be applied to transfemoral work!

Conclusion

Radiation exposure in cardiac practice is associated with important risks to patients, operators, and coworkers. While studies have highlighted possible increased radiation doses associated with radial procedures,

methodological deficiencies mean that many authors' findings need to be interpreted with caution. Taken together, the available study data are not compelling enough for transradial procedures to be denounced on the basis of excessive radiation doses. Nevertheless, the controversy that has been unfolding over the few years has served to focus attention on our need to handle radiation responsibly, irrespective of our preferred mode of access. An operator using the radial approach may encounter anatomical loops and radio-ulnar or brachio-cephalic tortuosities, which may require fluoroscopic guidance for the safe advancement of wires and catheters. For an experienced operator, once the coronary ostia are cannulated, there is no reason why operator and patient radiation exposure would differ between radial and femoral access.

Acknowledgment

The authors are grateful to Mr. Mark Wilson, Superintendent Radiographer at Birmingham Heartlands Hospital, for his assistance and review of the chapter.

REFERENCES

1. Jolly SS, Amlani S, Hamon M, et al. Radial versus femoral access for coronary angiography or intervention and the impact on major bleeding and ischemic events: a systematic review and meta-analysis of randomized trials. *Am Heart J.* 2009;157(1):132–140.
2. Jolly SS, Yusuf S, Cairns J, et al. Radial versus femoral access for coronary angiography and intervention in patients with acute coronary syndromes (RIVAL): a randomised, parallel group, multicentre trial. *Lancet.* 2011;377(9775):1409–1420.
3. Mitchell MD, Hong JA, Lee BY, et al. Systematic review and cost-benefit analysis of radial artery access for coronary angiography and intervention. *Circ Cardiovasc Qual Outcomes.* 2012;5(4):454–462.
4. Bertrand OF, Rao SV, Pancholy S, et al. Transradial approach for coronary angiography and interventions: results of the first international transradial practice survey. *JACC Cardiovasc Interv.* 2010;3(10):1022–1031.
5. Dehmer GJ, Weaver D, Roe MT, et al. A contemporary view of diagnostic cardiac catheterization and percutaneous coronary intervention in the United States: a report from the CathPCI Registry of the National Cardiovascular Data Registry, 2010 through June 2011. *J Am Coll Cardiol.* 2012;60(20):2017–2031.
6. Best PJ, Skelding KA, Mehran R, et al. SCAI consensus document on occupational radiation exposure to the pregnant cardiologist and technical personnel. *Catheter Cardiovasc Interv.* 2011;77(2):232–241.
7. Whitby M. Radiation doses to the legs of radiologists performing interventional procedures: are they a cause for concern? *Br J Radiol.* 2003;76(905):321–327.
8. Berlin L. Radiation-induced skin injuries and fluoroscopy. *AJR Am J Roentgenol.* 2001;177(1):21–25.

9. Koenig TR, Wolff D, Mettler FA, et al. Skin injuries from fluoroscopically guided procedures: part 1, characteristics of radiation injury. *AJR Am J Roentgenol.* 2001;177(1):3–11.

10. Koenig TR, Mettler FA, Wagner LK. Skin injuries from fluoroscopically guided procedures: part 2, review of 73 cases and recommendations for minimizing dose delivered to patient. *AJR Am J Roentgenol.* 2001;177(1):13–20.

11. Muirhead CR, O'Hagan JA, Haylock RG, et al. Mortality and cancer incidence following occupational radiation exposure: third analysis of the National Registry for Radiation Workers. *Br J Cancer.* 2009;100(1):206–212.

12. Nakashima M, Kondo H, Miura S, et al. Incidence of multiple primary cancers in Nagasaki atomic bomb survivors: association with radiation exposure. *Cancer Sci.* 2008;99(1):87–92.

13. Yoshinaga S, Mabuchi K, Sigurdson AJ, et al. Cancer risks among radiologists and radiologic technologists: review of epidemiologic studies. *Radiology.* 2004;233(2):313–321.

14. Doody MM, Freedman DM, Alexander BH, et al. Breast cancer incidence in U.S. radiologic technologists. *Cancer.* 2006;106(12):2707–2715.

15. Eisenberg MJ, Afilalo J, Lawler PR, et al. Cancer risk related to low-dose ionizing radiation from cardiac imaging in patients after acute myocardial infarction. *CMAJ.* 2011;183(4):430–436.

16. Einstein AJ. Effects of radiation exposure from cardiac imaging: how good are the data? *J Am Coll Cardiol.* 2012;59(6):553–565.

17. Hart D, Hillier MC, Wall BF. Doses to patients from radiographic and fluoroscopic X-ray imaging procedures in the UK-2005 review. Health Protection Agency, Radiation Protection Division, *2007.*

18. Miller DL, Hilohi CM, Spelic DC. Patient radiation doses in interventional cardiology in the U.S.: advisory data sets and possible initial values for U.S. reference levels. *Med Phys.* 2012;39(10):6276–6286.

19. Padovani R, Vano E, Trianni A, et al. Reference levels at European level for cardiac interventional procedures. *Radiat Prot Dosimetry.* 2008;129(1–3):104–107.

20. Hart D, Hillier MC, Wall BF. National reference doses for common radiographic, fluoroscopic and dental X-ray examinations in the UK. *Br J Radiol.* 2009;82(973):1–12.

21. D'Helft CJ, Brennan PC, McGee AM, et al. Potential Irish dose reference levels for cardiac interventional examinations. *Br J Radiol.* 2009;82(976):296–302.

22. Kuon E. Effective techniques for reduction of radiation dosage to patients undergoing invasive cardiac procedures. *Br J Radiol.* 2003;76(906):406–413.

23. Tsapaki V, Maniatis PN, Magginas A, et al. What are the clinical and technical factors that influence the kerma-area product in percutaneous coronary intervention? *Br J Radiol.* 2008;81(972):940–945.

24. Ciraj-Bjelac O, Rehani MM, Sim KH, et al. Risk for radiation-induced cataract for staff in interventional cardiology: is there reason for concern? *Catheter Cardiovasc Interv.* 2010;76(6):826–834.

25. Roguin A, Goldstein J, Bar O, et al. Brain and neck tumors among physicians performing interventional procedures. *Am J Cardiol.* 2013;111(9):1368–1372.

26. Kuon E. Radiation exposure benefit of a lead cap in invasive cardiology. *Heart.* 2003;89(10):1205–1210.

27. Kuon E, Schmitt M, Dahm JB. Significant reduction of radiation exposure to operator and staff during cardiac interventions by analysis of radiation leakage and improved lead shielding. *Am J Cardiol.* 2002;89(1): 44–49.

28. Kuon E, Dahm JB, Empen K, et al. Identification of less-irradiating tube angulations in invasive cardiology. *J Am Coll Cardiol.* 2004;44(7):1420–1428.

29. Kuon E, Empen K, Robinson DM, et al. Efficiency of a mini-course in radiation reducing techniques: a pilot initiative to encourage less irradiating cardiological interventional techniques (ELICIT). *Heart.* 2005;91(9):1221–1222.

30. Spaulding C, Lefèvre T, Funck F, et al. Left radial approach for coronary angiography: results of a prospective study. *Catheter Cardiovasc Interv.* 1996;39(4):365–370.

31. Louvard Y, Pezzano M, Scheers L, et al. Coronary angiography by a radial artery approach: feasibility, learning curve. One operator's experience. *Arch Mal Coeur Vaiss.* 1998;91(2):209–215.

32. Ball WT, Sharieff W, Jolly SS, et al. Characterization of operator learning curve for transradial coronary interventions. *Circ Cardiovasc Interv.* 2011;4(4):336–341.

33. Brasselet C, Blanpain T, Tassan-Mangina S, et al. Comparison of operator radiation exposure with optimized radiation protection devices during coronary angiograms and ad hoc percutaneous coronary interventions by radial and femoral routes. *Eur Heart J.* 2008;29(1):63–70.

34. Hamon M, Sourgounis A. Radiation exposure and vascular access site. *Eur Heart J.* 2008;29(7):954; author reply 954–955.

35. Lo TS, Ratib K, Chong AY, et al. Impact of access site selection and operator expertise on radiation exposure; a controlled prospective study. *Am Heart J.* 2012;164(4):455–461.

36. Kuipers G, Delewi R, Velders XL, et al. Radiation exposure during percutaneous coronary interventions and coronary angiograms performed by the radial compared with the femoral route. *JACC Cardiovasc Interv.* 2012;5(7):752–757.

37. Shah B, Bangalore S, Feit F, et al. Radiation exposure during coronary angiography via transradial or transfemoral approaches when performed by experienced operators. *Am Heart J.* 2013;165(3):286–292.

38. Delewi R, Hoebers LP, Råmunddal T, et al. Clinical and procedural characteristics associated with higher radiation exposure during percutaneous coronary interventions and coronary angiography. *Circ Cardiovasc Interv.* 2013;6(5):501–506.

39. Lange HW, von Boetticher H. Randomized comparison of operator radiation exposure during coronary angiography and intervention by radial or femoral approach. *Catheter Cardiovasc Interv.* 2006;67(1):12–16.

40. Achenbach S, Ropers D, Kallert L, et al. Transradial versus transfemoral approach for coronary angiography and intervention in patients above 75 years of age. *Catheter Cardiovasc Interv.* 2008;72(5):629–635.

41. Brueck M, Bandorski D, Kramer W, et al. A randomized comparison of transradial versus transfemoral approach for coronary angiography and angioplasty. *JACC Cardiovasc Interv.* 2009;2(11):1047–1054.

42. Jolly SS, Cairns J, Niemela K, et al. Effect of radial versus femoral access on radiation dose and the importance of procedural volume: a substudy of the multicenter randomized RIVAL trial. *JACC Cardiovasc Interv.* 2013;6(3):258–266.

43. Michael TT, Alomar M, Papayannis A, et al. A randomized comparison of the transradial and transfemoral approaches for coronary artery bypass graft angiography and intervention: the RADIAL-CABG Trial (RADIAL Versus Femoral Access for Coronary Artery Bypass Graft Angiography and Intervention). *JACC Cardiovasc Interv.* 2013;6(11):1138–1144.

44. Lo TS, Nolan J, Fountzopoulos E, et al. Radial artery anomaly and its influence on transradial coronary procedural outcome. *Heart.* 2009;95(5):410–415.

45. Burzotta F, Brancati MF, Trani C, et al. Impact of radial-to-aorta vascular anatomical variants on risk of failure in trans-radial coronary procedures. *Catheter Cardiovasc Interv.* 2012;80(2):298–303.

46. Kanei Y, Nakra NC, Liou M, et al. Randomized comparison of transradial coronary angiography via right or left radial artery approaches. *Am J Cardiol.* 2011;107(2):195–197.

47. Sciahbasi A, Romagnoli E, Burzotta F, et al. Transradial approach (left vs right) and procedural times during percutaneous coronary procedures: TALENT study. *Am Heart J.* 2011;161(1):172–179.

48. Sciahbasi A, Romagnoli E, Trani C, et al. Operator radiation exposure during percutaneous coronary procedures through the left or right radial approach: the TALENT dosimetric substudy. *Circ Cardiovasc Interv.* 2011;4(3):226–231.

49. Norgaz T, Gorgulu S, Dagdelen S. A randomized study comparing the effectiveness of right and left radial approach for coronary angiography. *Catheter Cardiovasc Interv.* 2012;80(2):260–264.

50. Dominici M, Diletti R, Milici C, et al. Operator exposure to x-ray in left and right radial access during percutaneous coronary procedures: OPERA randomised study. *Heart.* 2013;99(7):480–484.

51. Lange HW, von Boetticher H. Reduction of operator radiation dose by a pelvic lead shield during cardiac catheterization by radial access: comparison with femoral access. *JACC Cardiovasc Interv.* 2012;5(4):445–449.

52. Behan M, Haworth P, Colley P, et al. Decreasing operators' radiation exposure during coronary procedures: the Transradial Radiation Protection Board. *Catheter Cardiovasc Interv.* 2010;76(1):79–84.

53. Politi L, Biondi-Zoccai G, Nocetti L, et al. Reduction of scatter radiation during transradial percutaneous coronary angiography: a randomized trial using a lead-free radiation shield. *Catheter Cardiovasc Interv.* 2012;79(1):97–102.

54. Abdelaal E, Plourde G, MacHaalany J, et al. Effectiveness of low rate fluoroscopy at reducing operator and patient radiation dose during transradial coronary angiography and interventions. *JACC Cardiovasc Interv.* 2014;7(5):567–574.

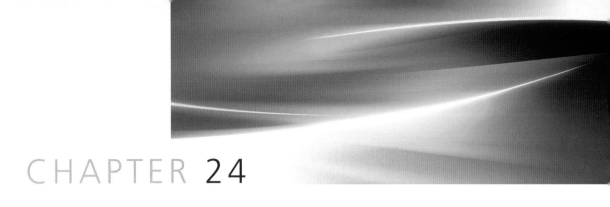

CHAPTER 24

The Radial Approach and the Risk of Periprocedural Stroke

Helen C. Routledge, Karim Ratib, and James Nolan

Why Are We Talking About It?

Neurological events are a rare but well-recognized complication of invasive coronary angiography and percutaneous coronary intervention (PCI). Clinical manifestations range from transient nonspecific symptoms to full-blown stroke with residual disability. Such events are indisputably associated with postprocedural mortality. The long-term morbidity, the implications for carers and families, and the socioeconomic costs are less well documented but make this the most devastating of all procedural complications. Although neurological events may only make up a very small proportion of our reported adverse outcomes (major adverse cardiovascular and cerebrovascular events [MACCE]) or may even escape publication altogether (major adverse cardiac events [MACE]), patients themselves rate the possibility of major stroke as an outcome worse than death.[1]

Transradial access is associated with improved patient comfort, fewer access site complications, and, in some settings, a reduced risk of mortality. Fears have been raised, however, that this choice of access site is associated with a higher risk of neurological events.

From Where Do These Fears Originate?

There are two reasons why the fear of a greater neurological risk with the transradial approach has arisen and why this possibility now requires further

discussion. The initial concerns originated following the presentation of registry data at a European meeting in 2004.[2] The Swedish Coronary Angiography and Angioplasty Registry (SCAAR) documents all percutaneous coronary procedures undertaken in 30 Swedish centers. Between 2000 and 2004, the risk of stroke following a radial procedure was observed to be double that following the femoral approach: 0.4% versus 0.2% (Table 24.1).

Aside from these data, but later used as a possible explanation for the registry findings, a hypothesis was developed concerning a number of procedural factors which might make the possibility of a stroke greater when trying to access the coronary arteries from the upper limb. The fact that transradial procedures involve the passage of catheters in proximity to the origin of the ipsilateral vertebral and carotid artery was proposed as a risk. The significance of this, as compared to that of traversing the aortic arch and origins of both carotid arteries in the transfemoral approach, however, is poorly understood. More obviously associated with the risk of neurological events are the more frequent catheter exchanges and the use of larger volumes of contrast media, which are both observed early on in the transradial learning curve for coronary procedures. These mechanistic considerations are discussed further below.

How Should We Investigate This Further?

At first thought, further investigation of this issue appears straightforward. On the basis of the hypothesis that there is a greater risk of neurological

TABLE 24-1 Results of All 30 Swedish Centers Performing Angiography and PCI, 2000 to 2004, from the SCAAR

	Radial	Femoral	*P*
N	7,962	48,682	
% PCI	44	41	
% Complications overall	5.7	4.6	<0.001
Neurological complications	0.4	0.2	0.007
Myocardial infarction	1	0.5	<0.001
Access site bleeding	1.1	1.5	

TABLE 24-2 Incidence of Stroke in Major PCI Registries

PCI Registries	*N*	Ischemic	Hemorrhagic	Total
Akkerhuis (2001)	8,555	0.22	0.14	0.37
Fuchs (2002)	9,662	0.22	0.21	0.44
Dukkipati (2004)	20,679	0.21	0.06	0.44
Wong (2005)	76,903			0.18
Sarno (2012)	339,965			0.2
Ratib (2013)	370,238			0.11

events following coronary angiography or PCI from the radial approach, a randomized controlled trial, albeit not a blinded one, could surely be undertaken. Unfortunately (or rather fortunately!), the rate of clinically detectable periprocedural neurological complications is so low as to make this virtually impossible. With an overall incidence in the order of 0.11% to 0.44% (Table 24.2), a straightforward power calculation would suggest that at least 25,000 patients would need to be randomized in order to demonstrate a difference at a significance level of 0.05. In addition, the operators would need to be those with equal experience of radial and femoral accesses and yet be willing to enter patients into the study whatever the perceived risk of access site complications.

Consequently, it is likely that our evidence base to confirm or refute this hypothesis will consist of large bodies of observational data. Further registry data are now available, and their results and limitations are discussed below. In addition, some information can be gained from the results of other randomized controlled trials, which, although not designed or powered to look at neurological end points, do at least record them.

The Mechanisms of Periprocedural Stroke

If dedicated randomized data are unavailable, perhaps we should return to basic principles and look more closely at the pathophysiological mechanisms by which adverse neurological events occur during percutaneous coronary procedures. This might improve our comprehension of the potential issue and give us important clues as to which access route is preferable. At the same time, it might be possible to determine whether there is anything that we can measure to be used as a surrogate end point in a more manageable-sized study. Small studies have indeed been undertaken, employing surrogate markers to compare the risk of neurological events from the femoral and radial approaches, and these are discussed below.

There are several mechanisms by which procedure-related neurological complications may occur: air embolus, intracerebral bleeding due to antithrombotic treatment, periprocedural hypotension leading to watershed infarcts, and contrast-induced osmolar changes affecting the blood–brain barrier. The usual presumption for those events with persistent symptoms, however, is that some embolic material has become lodged in the distal cerebral vasculature. This material is often assumed to be thrombus or thrombus containing, and in some cases responds to thrombolytic therapy. Despite flushing and intensive anticoagulation, modern imaging modalities have demonstrated that thrombus can still form inside the catheter (Fig. 24.1).

Considering all these possible mechanisms together, an increased risk of neurological sequelae

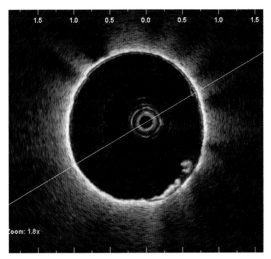

FIGURE 24-1 OCT evidence of adherent thrombus despite anticoagulation.

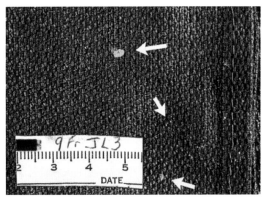

FIGURE 24-2 Debris from catheters. (From Keeley EC, Grines CL. Scraping of aortic debris by coronary guiding catheters: a prospective evaluation of 1,000 cases. *J Am Coll Cardiol.* 1998;32(7):1861–1865.)

might be assumed from those procedures undertaken transradially during the operator's learning curve. Such procedures tend to be longer and do involve more contrast injections and catheter exchanges, risking both air emboli and osmolar effects. With less experienced radial operators, catheters and wires in situ for longer periods might predispose to thrombus formation. In experienced hands or those who have been trained transradially from the outset, however, procedures are not longer than from the femoral approach and may often involve fewer catheter exchanges.

In surgical patients after cardiopulmonary bypass, cholesterol emboli with varying amounts of platelets and fibrin are found in the smaller cerebral arteries postmortem. There are no data on the composition of retrieved embolic material post-PCI, but we have long since been aware of the risk of disrupting atherosclerotic material from the aortic or femoral artery wall with guidewires and catheters. This is a frequent event and is likely to be the predominant source of periprocedural emboli and, therefore, the biggest risk for neurological events (Fig. 24.2).[3] The patient and procedural risk factors for stroke during catheterization also suggest that embolism of aortic atheroma is likely to be the predominant mechanism.[4] Outside of the catheterization laboratory and despite anticoagulation, aortic atheroma is an independent risk factor for cryptogenic stroke,[5,6] and patients known to be at highest risk of periprocedural stroke are those most likely to have aortic atheroma.[4,7,8] In a study of patients undergoing both cardiac catheterization and transesophageal echocardiographies, the vast majority (93%) of patients with coronary disease also had aortic

atheroma.[9] The distribution of aortic atheroma in this study also provides an important clue as to where the risks lie (Fig. 24.3). The fact that the majority of atheroma and the more complex "high-risk" plaques are found in the descending aorta suggests that transradial access in which the descending aorta (and in the right radial approach, much of the arch) is avoided might, in fact, be substantially safer.

Studies Using Surrogate Markers

Already employed in studies of carotid endarterectomy and cardiac surgery, transcranial Doppler measurements confirm the systematic occurrence of cerebral microemboli during cardiac catheterization (Fig. 24.4). This noninvasive measurement has been proposed as a surrogate end point with which percutaneous coronary procedures and the risk of embolic sequelae can be compared. In the first catheter study to use transcranial Doppler, emboli counts per procedure were found to be proportionate to the number of times the aortic arch was crossed with a catheter.[10] The emboli count also seemed to be related to the amount of atheroma found in the aortic arch on transesophageal echocardiography. This was a small study and certainly did not demonstrate that emboli counts were a good surrogate for clinical events, of which in fact there were none in the cohort studied.

In a subsequent study, transcranial Doppler measurements were examined alongside diffusion-weighted cerebral magnetic resonance imaging (MRI), which is currently the most sensitive tool

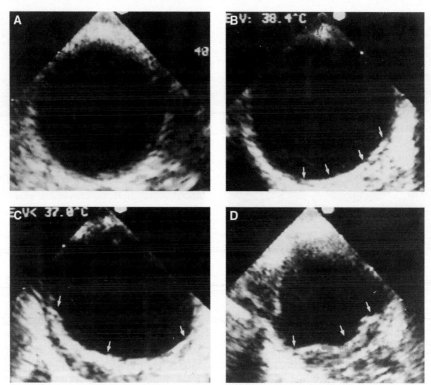

FIGURE 24-3   Location of aortic plaque at transoesophageal echocardiogram: Grade I & II (**A** & **B**): descending aorta 93%; arch 80%; ascending aorta only 37%. Complex plaque III & IV (**C** & **D**): descending aorta, 58%; arch 40%; ascending aorta, 0%. (Adapted from Khoury Z, Gottlieb S, Stern S, et al. Frequency and distribution of atherosclerotic plaques in the thoracic aorta as determined by transesophageal echocardiography in patients with coronary artery disease. *Am J Cardiol.* 1997;79(1):23–27.)

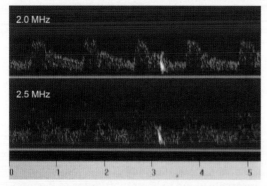

FIGURE 24-4   Solid microembolus passing through the middle cerebral artery during left heart catheterization. (From Lund C, Nes RB, Ugelstad TP, et al. Cerebral emboli during left heart catheterization may cause acute brain injury. *Eur Heart J.* 2005;26(13):1269–1275.)

available for early detection of cerebral infarction.[11] An important revelation of this study was that the majority of transcranial Doppler signals detected are caused by microbubbles and only 8% of signals recorded were actually attributable to solid microemboli. Nevertheless, there were, in a predominantly radial study, a greater number of solid emboli with radial catheterization (median number 57 vs 36, $P = 0.012$). The majority of solid microemboli occurred with the passage of a catheter from the subclavian artery into the ascending aorta. About 15% of patients undergoing transradial coronary procedures had new lesions on MRI, with no new lesions seen in the 10 femoral access patients. Whether a numerical count of the Doppler signals is a good surrogate for neurological events again remains doubtful, particularly as the three patients (or 6%) who did have transient neurological symptoms were not those with higher emboli counts, nor even those with abnormal MRI scans. In addition, some caution must be applied while interpreting a small study of patients not randomized for access site.

The SCIPION (Silent Cerebral Infarct and Percutaneous Cardiovascular Intervention EvaluatiON) trial attempted to overcome some of these limitations by randomizing patients undergoing cardiac catheterization to the radial or femoral approach. The study was powered for an end point of silent brain injury seen on diffusion-weighted

MRI. In this dedicated study, no significant difference was found in this end point or in the number of transcranial Doppler hits, when the radial and femoral approaches were compared.[12]

Overall, the data using surrogate markers to investigate access site and neurological sequelae are based on very small studies and appear inconclusive. The clinical relevance of surrogate markers for neurological complication is not clear, since microemboli are detected with transcranial Doppler during all invasive cardiac procedures. The presence of silent ischemic events demonstrated on diffusion-weighted MRI appears to be linked to more frequent catheter exchanges and prolonged procedures; however, the long-term clinical implications of these are not known.[13]

Contemporary Registry Data

Currently, PCI registries appear to be the largest source of data available, with which the incidence of neurological complications can be studied. The major limitation is that of confounding, as exemplified by the SCAAR data. Radial and femoral access groups, when examined retrospectively, are highly unlikely to be matched for the other risk factors for periprocedural stroke: age, female sex, cerebrovascular disease, intra-aortic balloon pump use, urgent PCI in acute coronary syndromes, and left ventricular and renal impairment. The original SCAAR registry data were obtained during a period when the radial approach was employed in fewer than 15% of procedures, and this approach was being chosen predominantly in higher-risk patients. Later analysis of data from subsequent years, with a significant increase in the use of radial access, has not shown this trend, and therefore, the initial differences detected are likely to represent patient selection of a higher-risk subgroup that initially underwent radial procedures (Fig. 24.5).

In a single-center 10-year retrospective study in Quebec, the notes of all patients discharged with a diagnosis of stroke or cerebrovascular accident (CVA) were reviewed. Any patient who had had a sign or symptom within 36 hours of a coronary procedure was included. Neurological complications occurred in 0.075% of 83,409 procedures collected between 1990 and 2007, and the rate was significantly lower in the transradial access group. Although baseline characteristics were similar in the radial and femoral patients, some procedural characteristics, in particular more graft cases and bigger catheters, were certainly weighted unfairly against the femoral group.[14] The PCI registry of the Euro Heart survey was recently interrogated to determine the

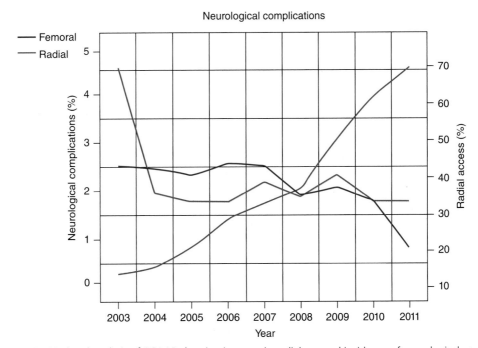

FIGURE 24-5 Updated analysis of SCAAR showing increase in radial use and incidence of neurological complications following femoral and radial access. (From Sarno G, Lagerqvist B, Frobert O, et al. Presented at EuroPCR, Paris, 2012.)

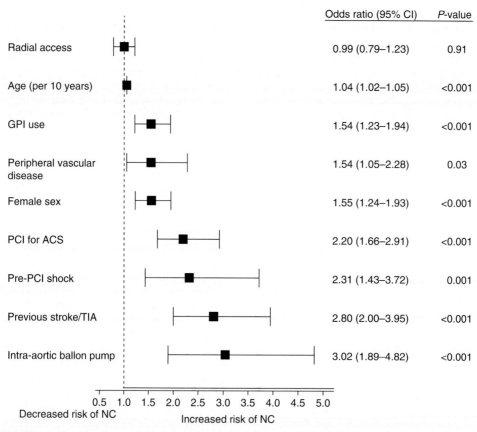

	Odds ratio (95% CI)	P-value
Radial access	0.99 (0.79–1.23)	0.91
Age (per 10 years)	1.04 (1.02–1.05)	<0.001
GPI use	1.54 (1.23–1.94)	<0.001
Peripheral vascular disease	1.54 (1.05–2.28)	0.03
Female sex	1.55 (1.24–1.93)	<0.001
PCI for ACS	2.20 (1.66–2.91)	<0.001
Pre-PCI shock	2.31 (1.43–3.72)	0.001
Previous stroke/TIA	2.80 (2.00–3.95)	<0.001
Intra-aortic ballon pump	3.02 (1.89–4.82)	<0.001

Decreased risk of NC   Increased risk of NC

FIGURE 24-6 Odds ratio of neurological complications following multivariate analysis of 370,238 procedures from the British Cardiovascular Intervention Society PCI database. (From Ratib et al. Influence of access site choice on incidence of neurologic complications after percutaneous coronary intervention. *Am Heart J.* 2013;165(3):317–324.)

incidence of PCI-related strokes in contemporary practice. Nearly 47,000 cases were included and the risk factors for stroke, which occurred in 0.4%, were determined by multivariate analysis. Patients rather than procedural factors were entered into the model, however, such that the independent influence of access site was not determined. With the same caveats as for previous registries therefore, radial access was used in just 12.3% of the patients who had neurological sequelae and 13.6% of the population overall.[15]

The most recent and largest body of data to be examined is the UK BCIS (British Cardiac Intervention Society) registry.[16] This incorporates all PCI cases over a 5-year period (370,238 cases) during which the use of radial access increased from 17% to 51%. Diagnostic catheterization is not included and neurological events are not categorized any further. The incidence of neurological complications increased over the study period, with a proportional increase in the number of higher-risk and STEMI (ST elevation myocardial infarction) patients treated. The overall incidence was in keeping with previous registry data at 0.11% but slightly lower than contemporary series with similar risk predictors.[7,17] A multivariate logistic regression analysis of the BCIS data suggests that the influence of these factors results in a similar rate of neurological complication for both access sites. This, during a phase of rapid change in access site practice when it might be expected that radial access would generate more neurological complications, is a very reassuring finding (Fig. 24.6).

Data from Randomized Controlled Trials

Large trials in which patients are randomized to the femoral or radial access site may not be powered to reveal a difference in neurological complications but are a further source that can be examined to see whether there is a signal or trend in one direction.

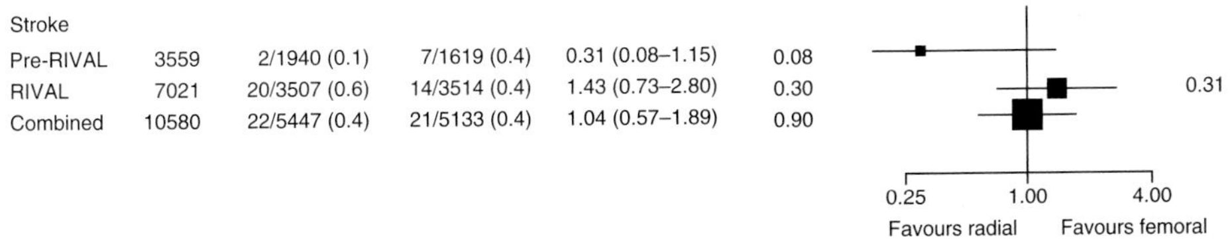

Stroke						
Pre-RIVAL	3559	2/1940 (0.1)	7/1619 (0.4)	0.31 (0.08–1.15)	0.08	
RIVAL	7021	20/3507 (0.6)	14/3514 (0.4)	1.43 (0.73–2.80)	0.30	0.31
Combined	10580	22/5447 (0.4)	21/5133 (0.4)	1.04 (0.57–1.89)	0.90	

0.25   1.00   4.00
Favours radial   Favours femoral

FIGURE 24-7   Odds ratio of stroke from the updated meta-analysis in the RIVAL publication. (From Jolly SS, Yusuf S, Cairns J, et al. Radial versus femoral access for coronary angiography in patients with acute coronary syndromes (RIVAL): a randomized, parallel group, multicenter trial. *Lancet.* 2011;377(9775):1409–1420.)

Prior to the two largest contemporary randomized controlled trials, the RIVAL (RadIal Vs femorAL access for coronary intervention trial) investigators summed up the available literature in a meta-analysis incorporating the largest body at that time of randomized radial versus femoral data.[18] No difference in the incidence of stroke was observed in the 2,535 patients where data were available (0.1% for radial access and 0.5% for femoral access, $P = 0.22$).

In the subsequent RIVAL trial,[19] all patients randomized had sustained acute coronary events and hence were already at a higher risk for neurological events than are those who undergo elective coronary intervention. The 30-day rate of stroke was included as a key secondary outcome measure. The overall rate of MACCE was 4% in the femoral arm and 3.7% in the radial arm, statistically a nonsignificant difference. Included within this was a rate of early neurological complication of 0.2%. Interestingly by 30 days, this had more than doubled (0.6% in the radial versus 0.4% in the femoral group), but this remained a statistically nonsignificant difference between the two access sites. The RIVAL publication also included an updated meta-analysis of over 10,000 patients with no difference in stroke between the radial and the femoral accesses (Fig. 24.7).

Most recently, in the RIFLE (RadIal versus FemoraL investigation in ST Elevation acute coronary syndrome) study[20] (perhaps the most convincing illustration of the benefits of radial access), although the stroke rate was somewhat higher, reflecting the higher-risk patient group with ST-elevation myocardial infarction, there was no significant difference in the rate of neurological events between the radial (0.8%) and femoral (0.6%) groups ($P = 0.725$).

Conclusion—What Is Known and Not Known

Despite early fears, the weight of observational data now suggests a slightly lower risk of adverse neurological events following transradial than transfemoral coronary procedures. Multivariate analysis suggests that the predictors of stroke are predominantly patient-associated factors. A sufficiently powered dedicated randomized trial comparing the radial and femoral approaches is unlikely ever to be undertaken, and although efforts continue to compare the two approaches using surrogate end points, these seem unlikely to truly answer the question.

There remains neither conclusive clinical data nor a convincing pathophysiological mechanism to suggest that the transradial approach to coronary angiography or intervention comes with a higher risk of stroke than that seen with the transfemoral approach.

REFERENCES

1. Solomon NA, Glick HA, Russo CJ, et al. Patient preferences for stroke outcomes. *Stroke.* 1994;25:1721–1725.
2. Sarno G, Lagerqvist B, Frobert O, et al. Outcomes of radial and femoral access for PCI over time: A report from the nationwide Swedish Coronary angiography and angioplasty registry (SCAAR). Presented at EuroPCR 2012, Paris, France, May 15, 2012.
3. Keeley EC, Grines CL. Scraping of aortic debris by coronary guiding catheters: a prospective evaluation of 1,000 cases. *J Am Coll Cardiol.* 1998;32(7):1861–1865.
4. Hoffman SJ, Routledge HC, et al. Procedural factors associated with percutaneous coronary intervention-related ischemic stroke. *JACC Cardiovasc Interv.* 2012;5:200–206.
5. Amarenco P, Cohen A, Tzourio C, et al. Atherosclerotic disease of the aortic arch and the risk of ischemic stroke. *N Engl J Med.* 1994;331(22):1474–1479.
6. Di Tullio MR, Russo C, Jin Z, et al. Aortic arch plaques and risk of recurrent stroke and death. Patent foramen ovale in cryptogenic stroke study investigators. *Circulation.* 2009;119(17):2376–2382.
7. Aggarwal A, Dai D, Rumsfeld JS, et al. American College of Cardiology National Cardiovascular Data Registry. Incidence and predictors of stroke associated with percutaneous coronary intervention. *Am J Cardiol.* 2009;104(3):349–353.
8. Fuchs S, Stabile E, Kinnaird TD, et al. Stroke complicating percutaneous coronary interventions: incidence, predictors, and prognostic implications. *Circulation.* 2002;106:86–91.
9. Khoury Z, Schwartz R, Gottlieb S, et al. Relation of coronary artery disease to atherosclerotic disease in the aorta, carotid, and femoral arteries evaluated by ultrasound. *Am J Cardiol.* 1997;80(11):1429–1433.
10. Bladin CF, Bingham L, Grigg L, et al. Transcranial Doppler detection of microemboli during percutaneous transluminal coronary angioplasty. *Stroke.* 1998;29(11):2367–2370.

11. Lund C, Nes RB, Ugelstad TP, et al. Cerebral emboli during left heart catheterization may cause acute brain injury. *Eur Heart J.* 2005;26(13):1269–1275.

12. Hamon M, Burzotta F, Oppenheim C, et al; SCIPION Investigators. Silent cerebral infarct after cardiac catheterization as detected by diffusion weighted magnetic resonance imaging: a randomized comparison of radial and femoral arterial approaches. Presented at TCT 2009, San Francisco, California.

13. Büsing KA, Schulte-Sasse C, Flüchter S, et al. Cerebral infarction: incidence and risk factors after diagnostic and interventional cardiac catheterization—prospective evaluation at diffusion-weighted MR imaging. *Radiology.* 2005;235(1):177–183.

14. Tizon-Marcus H, Barbeau GR, Dery JP, et al. Are neurological complications following percutaneous angiography or intervention more common in transfemoral versus transradial approach? Presented at ESC 2009, Barcelona, Spain.

15. Ratib K, Mamas MA, Routledge HC, et al. Influence of access site choice on incidence of neurologic complications after percutaneous coronary intervention. *Am Heart J.* 2013;165(3):317–324.

16. Werner M, Bauer T, Hochadel M, et al. Incidence and clinical impact of stroke complicating percutaneous coronary intervention: results of the Euro Heart survey PCI registry. *Circ Cardiovasc Interv.* 2013;6(4):362–369.

17. Wong SC, Minutello R, Hong MK. Neurological complications following percutaneous coronary interventions (a report from the 2000–2001 New York State Angioplasty Registry). *Am J Cardiol.* 2005;96(9):1248–1250.

18. Jolly SS, Amlani S, Hamon M, et al. Radial versus femoral access for coronary angiography or intervention and the impact on major bleeding and ischemic events: a systematic review and meta-analysis of randomized trials. *Am Heart J.* 2009;157(1):132–140.

19. Jolly SS, Yusuf S, Cairns J, et al. Radial versus femoral access for coronary angiography in patients with acute coronary syndromes (RIVAL): a randomized, parallel group, multicenter trial. *Lancet.* 2011;377:1409–1420.

20. Romagloni E, Biondi-Zoccai G, Sciahbasi A, et al. Radial versus femoral randomized investigation in ST-segment elevation acute coronary syndrome: the RIFLE-STEACS (Radial Versus Femoral Randomized Investigation in ST-Elevation Acute Coronary Syndrome) study. *J Am Coll Cardiol.* 2012;60(24):2481–2489.

CHAPTER 25

Nursing Workload

Bernadette S. Speiser and Giovanni Amoroso

Introduction

The continuing increase in the number of cardiovascular procedures (cardiac catheterizations and coronary and peripheral interventions) performed worldwide and in the United States has resulted in a shortage of adequately trained personnel (cardiology technicians, nurse specialists, and registered nurses) at interventional cardiology departments.[1]

This is compounded by the increasingly demanding escalation in the quality standards and safety components in the pre-, peri-, and postprocedural care of coronary patients.

Finally, there is intensifying pressure on health care providers to manage work within the economic constraints and increase procedural volumes. This is all couched within an expectation to maintain the standards of care, but with fewer resources (including personnel) (http://www.cardiovascularbusines.com/topics/practice-management/uncertainity-abounds-cath-lab-reimbursement).

Efficient management of the catheterization laboratory technician and nurse workload (NWL) in the catheterization laboratory areas and in the pre- and postprocedural units is a successful strategy to try and achieve these competing goals.

Transradial access (TRA) has been shown to decrease access-related complications and shorten bedrest times[2] both after diagnostic catheterizations and interventions. This approach reduces the nursing time required for postprocedural care. Moreover, the systematic adoption of TRA has facilitated the development of same-day percutaneous coronary interventions (PCI) and diagnostic catheterization discharge programs with a significant reduction in the amount of nursing workload (NML) and the quality of care provided by nursing personnel pre- and postprocedure. This chapter discusses the key aspects and the precautions related to the nursing roles and resources for TRA. This has an emphasis on optimizing efficient care delivery as well as increasing patient satisfaction.

Preprocedural Nursing

Patient Selection for TRA and Same-Day Discharge

When TRA patients are being evaluated for their procedure, there are no special needs to be addressed, compared with that required for a transfemoral procedure. It is sensible, however, to gather information about the preferred puncture site (right or left radial). This will include the evaluation of both radial and ulnar pulsations and identify special conditions (dialysis arteriovenous fistulas, previous breast surgeries with axillary lymph node removal, mammary artery grafts, etc.).

In order to facilitate same-day discharge for coronary procedures, an appropriate screening process is crucial. Patients with identified comorbidities (kidney dysfunction, heart failure, and peripheral vascular disease), the elderly, and/or those undergoing complex procedures may have a higher rate of conversion to an overnight hospital stay. These patients will require more nursing care than patients discharged the same day. Usually, the outpatient departments are neither logistically equipped nor staffed to manage the intensive and complex demand for care. Therefore, these patients should be preferably excluded from a same-day discharge program. On the other hand, if the selection criteria are too restrictive, unnecessary admission rather than same-day discharge will reduce the efficiency of care delivery. This, in turn, will overload inpatient units. Selection protocols have to be established by the facility to identify specific patient populations (age, ethnicity, and incidence of comorbidities), the specificity of the coronary procedure performed (diagnostic vs interventional, complex vs simple), and the nurse staffing full-time equivalents with training and expertise in coronary care. This protocol must take into account a process to match the best nursing care capabilities with the logistics demands. Inclusion criteria can be expanded if the nursing proficiencies and/or staffing levels of nurses can be addressed. Although the responsibility for the decision to discharge a patient home the same day will remain with the cardiologist (or a preapproved established protocol), it will be the duty of the nurses in the outpatient departments to correctly apply the selection criteria and to provide feedback on the safety and sustainability of such criteria. The level of knowledge and expertise of nursing personnel in the outpatient departments is crucially important. For this reason, nurses with certification in independent care delivery (advanced practice nurses (APNs) who can act within approved protocols are often placed in charge of these departments.

Patient Education/Preparation

As with outpatient surgeries, a team approach in the preparation of the outpatient procedures can diminish health-care expenses.[3] The patient must be fully educated and prepared for the procedure in order to decrease delays in the provision of care. Accurate patient education will allow for patient cooperation both during and after the procedure. If a patient is involved in his or her care as a partner, the patient will receive better treatment outcomes.[4] For example, appropriate patient information concerning a sterile technique and the need for patient cooperation in the maintenance of the sterile field can affect catheterization laboratory procedural time. Explaining to the patient his or her role in this endeavor will assist in avoiding the inadvertent contamination of the sterile field, thus necessitating the need for reprepping and redraping of the patient. Delays, such as this example, can increase procedural times and manpower costs.

The process of education starts before entering the outpatient or inpatient departments.

Frequently, patients have inadequate ideas or misconceptions surrounding a cardiac catheterization procedure. Many believe they are having surgery and have extreme fears because it relates to one of the most vital organs, their heart. The goal is to properly inform patients and their significant others on each step of the process, to reduce fear and anxiety. An exhaustive information process leads to greater patient satisfaction, reduces recovery time, and gives patients an overall sense of involvement.[5]

Providing handouts, booklets, videos, and webpages to visualize actual equipment such as a sheath, a coronary catheter, or a hemostatic band prior to the procedure will allow patients the time to formalize questions. It is also tremendously important to describe the transradial approach in detail (anatomy, procedure, and pros and cons). The most direct (pamphlets and newspapers) and indirect (friends and relatives) information the patients may have received may be related to the transfemoral approach. Creating written instructions that address commonly asked questions can facilitate the educational process. This approach also prevents the preprocedural staff from overlooking important teaching points. Patients can use the handouts postprocedure if questions arise. This will reduce follow-up phone calls to the institution and staffing time required to answer their questions. The materials should be short and contain pictures as reminders for the patients. However, human interactional information has been identified as the most individualized and beneficial.[6]

After patient education and information, the patient's physical preparation is the last nursing task to be performed prior to entering the procedural suite. The preparation includes reviewing the patient's chart, performing an electrocardiography (ECG or EKG), assessing pulse character and patency (radial and ulnar assessment via oximetry or Doppler) and the blood pressure, ensuring intravenous access (in the nonarterial access side), administering IV solution, obtaining blood tests (for instance, in case of anticoagulated patients), depilating the site of vascular access, and medication reconciliation. Appropriate baseline assessment of the radial/ulnar artery access can assist in detecting potential complications of radial access such as radial artery occlusion.

Patient selection, education/information, and preparation are essential tasks for optimal results of any coronary procedure, particularly when performed in a same-day setting. In this way, NML and nursing responsibilities would seem to increase rather than decrease; however, when roles are clear and protocols are standardized, there are opportunities for staff to increase professional development and autonomy. In fact, cardiologists do not need to be actively involved in these steps.

Procedural Nursing

The nursing activities and tasks during a transradial procedure do not differ significantly from those during a transfemoral procedure. Positioning the arm for puncture and preparing the sterile field could take a few more minutes, given the need for arm supports, possibly pillows or towels. The most important determinant of NWL at this time is the success of the arterial puncture procedure. A high rate of failure, and therefore crossover to another access area, may impact procedural and nursing time if the groin is not prepared in advance. Preparing the femoral access site is especially important during the laboratory's transradial learning curve. After the learning curve is completed, there are no significant differences in the NWL during a coronary procedure, except that postprocedural compression and transfer times will involve less full-time equivalent in the case of TRA.

Nursing workload and times during the peri- and procedural phases have been documented. In the Radial Access versus conventional femoral PuncTure: Outcome and Resource effectiveness in a daily routine (RAPTOR) Trial,[7] over a 1-year period, 4 patients undergoing a cardiac invasive procedure were randomized in a high-volume center to either a transfemoral access (TFA) or TRA. Approximately 75% underwent a diagnostic catheterization and 25% had coronary interventions. The variables of procedural duration, radiation times, involvement of the staff, and economic impact of the staff were

studied. Radial cannulation and diagnostic angiography required more in-laboratory time, but the overall procedural times for PCIs were similar (Table 25-1). The economic impact of nursing time by the catheterization laboratory staff was significant. For those patients who had diagnostic catheterizations, the nursing time for radial compression and immediate postcare was 31.3 minutes versus 45.2 minutes for the femoral access. For interventional procedures, the nursing time for femoral access patients was 64.4 versus 30.6 with radial access (Table 25-2). A limitation of this study was that femoral hemostasis was achieved by manual compression, which requires more time and care than the use of a femoral closure device. In this study the hospital also noted cost savings (Table 25-3).

Amoroso et al.[8] investigated the workload of nursing staff in the catheterization laboratory and the recovery area for 208 radial and 52 femoral cases. To calculate the total nursing workload for each patient, the time devoted to the different tasks and procedures was multiplied by the amount of full-time equivalents involved. It was noted that there was a significant decrease in workload in the case of radial versus femoral procedures (86 [58–126] vs 174 [134–218] minutes: $P < 0.001$) (Table 25-4 and Fig. 25-1). Multiple linear regression analysis revealed that the predictors of nursing workload included femoral access, failed radial access with crossover to femoral access, interventional procedures, and urgent versus elective procedures.[8] In addition, the radial approach was more efficient in terms of nursing workload. A study comparing the use of closure devices for femoral access versus radial access was completed by Roussanov et al.[9] The study enrolled 181 patients who underwent diagnostic cardiac catheterizations. The patients were

TABLE 25-1　Procedural Durations

N = 410	Femoral	Radial	Δ	P Value
Puncture	0.9 + 1.4	3.8 + 3	2.9 + 1.6	<0.01
Coronary angiography	8.4 + 4	10.9 + 6	1.8 + 0.3	<0.01
Coronary angiography + PCI	37.4 ± 15	33.9 ± 15	3.5	0.2
PCI with sheath exchange	23.4 ± 15	25.1 ± 15	1.7	0.5
PCI without sheath exchange	16.3 ± 13	21 ± 9	4.7 ± 4	0.3

PCI, percutaneous coronary intervention.
All values are given in minutes. P < 0.05 considered statistically significant.
Modified from Schaufele TG, Grunebaum JP, Lippe B., Breidenbach T, von Hodenbery, E. Radial access versus conventional femoral puncture: Outcome and resource effectiveness in a daily routine. The RAPTOR-Trial. Paper presented at the Scientific Sessions of the American Heart Association 2009, Orlando, FL.

TABLE 25-2 Staff Workload

	Manual Sheath Removal	Handling in Cath Lab	Time Nurse Spent with Patient
Diagnostic Cath			
Femoral	13 ± 40	14.3 ± 5	−45.2 ± 27
Radial	0.6 ± 3	17.3 ± 13	31.3 ± 18
Δ	12.4 + 37	3 + 7	13.4 + 9
P value	<0.01	0.02	0.02
Interventional Procedure			
Femoral	11.6 + 9	15.7 + 6	64.4 + 33
Radial	0 ± 0	16.6 ± 4	30.6 ± 15
Δ	11.6	0.9 ± 2	34 ± 18
P value	<0.01	0.38	<0.01

Time is given in minutes.
Modified from Schaufele TG, Grunebaum JP, Lippe B, et al. Radial access versus conventional femoral puncture: outcome and resource effectiveness in a daily routine. The RAPTOR-Trial. Paper presented at the Scientific Sessions of the American Heart Association 2009, Orlando, FL.

TABLE 25-3 Economic Impact of Staff Involvement

	Time: Diagnostic Cath + Sheath Removal	Time: Diagnostic + PCI + Sheath Removal
Femoral	72.5 + 36	91.7 + 36
Radial	54.6 ± 14	47.2 ± 12
Time saved by radial access	17.9 ± 30	47.2 ± 24
P value	<0.01	<0.01

Time is given in minutes; 3,000 procedures/yr; 1,000 PCIs change staff involvement by 1,383 hr = 36.4 wk.
Modified from Schaufele TG, Grunebaum JP, Lippe B, et al. Radial access versus conventional femoral puncture: outcome and resource effectiveness in a daily routine. The RAPTOR-Trial. Paper presented at the Scientific Sessions of the American Heart Association 2009, Orlando, FL.

divided into three groups. Seventy patients were placed in the radial group, 62 were in the femoral group without closure device utilization, and 49 were allocated to the femoral approach with closure device employment. The in-lab procedure time was nearly identical in all three groups; thus there were only minute changes in the NWL inside the procedure area. Louvard et al.[10] observed similar results on studying 210 consecutive patients who were randomized to either left or right radial approach or femoral approach. The procedure duration was longer in the left radial (14.2 ± 3.3 minutes); $P < 0.05$) access group than in with the right radial (12.4 ± 5.8 minutes) access group. The femoral group (11.2 ± 3.3 minutes) showed no significant differences when compared to the right radial access group.

Postprocedural Nursing

There are many factors that can influence the NWL after a coronary procedure:

- Care needed for compression of the arterial puncture
- Workload required for visualization and evaluation of the access site
- Supervision and management of bleeding complications
- Basic bedside needs, i.e., assistance with eating, elimination
- Baseline independence of the patient
- Type of recovery unit
- Length of stay postprocedure
- Type of coronary procedure (diagnostic vs interventional)

TABLE 25-4 Ward NWL According to Clinical, Procedural, In-hospital Variables, and Arterial Access

Variables	No (%)	Ward NWL (min)	Median	P	RC	SE	SC	P^a
All patients	174 (100)	457 [226–954]						
Sex: male vs female	130 (75)	504 [226–956]	297	0.15				
Age: >75 (vs <75)	42 (24)	394 [226–1022]	457	0.76				
BSA: >2 m² (vs <2 m²)	22 (13)	368 [226–522]	301	0.12				
Radial (vs femoral access)	118 (68)	386 [226–652]	720	0.001				
Urgent (vs elective)	78 (45)	961 [512–1255]	314	0.001				
Gp2b3a inhibitors: yes (vs no)	22 (13)	1255 [638 ± 1468]	385	0.05				
Diagnostic only (vs intervention)	46 (26)	284 [150–504]	512	0.001	0.11	0.013	0.08	<0.001
CCU (vs ward postcare)	92 (53)	891 [522–1152]	226	0.001	0.30	0.013	0.46	<0.001
Access-site complication: yes (vs no)	18 (10)	1287 [987–1647]	386	0.001	0.17	0.019	0.16	<0.001

BSA, body surface area; CCU, coronary care unit; RC, regression coefficient; SE, standard error; SC, standardized coefficient.

Modified from Amoroso G, Sarti M, Bellucci R, et al. Clinical and procedural predictors of nurse workload during and after invasive coronary procedures: the potential benefit of a systematic radial access. *Eur J Cardiovasc Nurs.* 2005;4(3):234–241.

[a]Stepwise linear regression analysis was used to define predictors of catheterization laboratory NWL ($R^2 = 0.95$ and $P = 0.001$ for model). Log transformation of data was performed before analysis. For length of hospital stay RC = 0.06, SE = 0.002, SC = 0.56, $P = 0.001$.

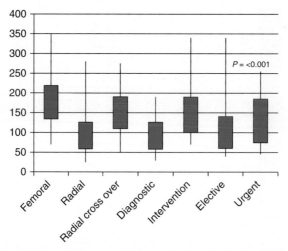

FIGURE 25-1   Differences in catheterization laboratory NWL, according to arterial access (radial vs femoral), procedure performed (diagnostic vs intervention), or procedure type (urgent vs elective). The values for nursing workload are given by the midrange (25th and 75th percentiles) by the hinges of the boxes and the 5th and 95th percentiles by the whiskers. (Modified from Amoroso G, Sarti M, Bellucci R, et al. Clinical and procedural predictors of nurse workload during and after invasive coronary procedures: the potential benefit of a systematic radial access. *Eur J Cardiovasc Nurs.* 2005;4(3):234–241.)

In the case of the transradial procedure, hemostasis is usually achieved by manual compression and maintained by means of a compression band (Fig. 25-2). In most cases a single individual can easily manage the care of one or more transradial patients. Carrington et al.[11] studied nurse engagement in the recovery area utilizing different surveillance protocols. When hemostasis was achieved utilizing the TR Band device (Terumo, Tokyo, Japan), the patients were reclassified into a lower nurse supervision level. Patients were then placed in an accelerated (1-hour) or a conventional (2-hour) weaning process. The accelerated arm showed no difference in complication rates, compared to the conventional arm. However, there was a 50% decrease in the surveillance phase because of the accelerated protocol. This decrease equates to one-quarter to one-third of the average recovery length of stay. Owing to the decreased length of stay, there is a reduction in nursing time spent in the care of the patient, thus decreasing the costs of the procedure.

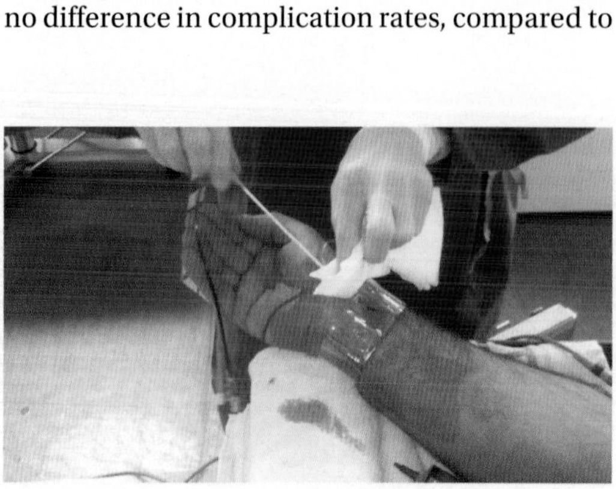

Caputo[12] supplied a cost perspective in which nurses' salaries were considered. A cardiac catheterization nurse's hourly wage was reported as $41.70 and a recovery nurse's hourly wage was reported as $36.54. The routine recovery time was 3 hours for TRA and 6 hours for TFA. For a catheterization laboratory performing 1,000 radial cases a year (versus femoral cases), this equates to a cost savings of $109,620 per year in the recovery process alone. Roussanov et al.[9] reported a similar time savings for TRA versus TFA care in the recovery period. In their study, the patients enrolled in the TRA group had a shorter recovery stay (126 ± 36 minutes) than did those in the TFA group utilizing a vascular closure device (150 ± 48 minutes: $P < 0.04$). The findings also noted that the recovery time for the TRA group was nearly half that for the TFA group in which manual pressure was utilized for hemostasis (240 ± 42 minutes: $P < 0.0001$). A cost savings of 33% was noted with TRA cases in comparison with femoral closure device cases

FIGURE 25-2   Compression of the radial artery by means of Terumo TR band.

($185 ± $52 vs $208 ± $70.4: $P < 0.001$). In cases where transradial hemostasis with a compression band is compared with transfemoral closure with a device, there is a savings of 24 minutes of nursing time. When transradial hemostasis with a compression band is compared with manual transfemoral hemostasis, a savings of 114 minutes can be gained. Nursing time represents a huge cost component of the invasive coronary procedure. Steinbrook[13] determined that a 1% to 2% change in the staffing of nurses resulted in an annual expenditure cost of $140,000 to $220,000.

Nursing workload after transfer to the ward has been quantified by Amoroso et al.[8] in a conventional overnight stay. The study identified 174 patients admitted for either a diagnostic or an interventional procedure. The nursing workload was measured in minutes and began with admission to the inpatient setting. The nursing workload with the transfemoral approach was 46% higher than that with the transradial approach. Independent predictors of NWL were identified:

- Access-site complications
- Length of in-hospital stay
- Admission to the coronary care unit
- Interventional procedures

Transfemoral access was not an independent predictor of increased NWL. However, complications such as bleeding are more frequent in transfemoral versus transradial access.[2]

Amoroso et al.[8] found that access complications required 1,287 minutes (987–1,649 minutes; $P < 0.001$) of nursing time in patients. Louvard et al.[10] found that hospital stays and bed rest periods were shorter in the radial access groups in comparison to the femoral access groups. A meta-analysis of 12 studies by Agostoni et al.[2] reviewed 3,244 patients who had either radial or femoral artery cardiac catheterizations. The radial arm of the study noted 0.3% access-site complications versus 2.8% from the femoral artery candidates ($P < 0.0001$). Vascular complications also warranted an increase in the number of treatments that require nursing time such as blood transfusions, frequent pulse assessments, ultrasound evaluation, manual compression over the access site, surgery, and postoperative recovery. A limitation of this study was that hemostasis was achieved by manual compression, and therefore, the value of transfemoral closure devices in reducing NWL could not be evaluated.

When nursing tasks were further defined and divided (by Amoroso et al.[8]) into generic and medical-care related, the generic tasks (such as feeding, toilet assistance, etc.) accounted for 138 [45–329] minutes and the medical care–related tasks for 315 [181–617] minutes. Transfemoral approach significantly increased NWL for generic tasks. This may be due in part to the limitations for patients who are constrained to bed rest and have limited ability to visualize their access site. With a transradial approach, because of the location, patients are able to watch their access site, thus providing themselves with an opportunity to participate in the care delivery. Patients may be instructed to visualize their access site and contact the nurse if they note changes. In this manner, the patient is acting as the nurse's assistant.

The physical and mental burden carried by hospital staff is difficult to quantify, but it can significantly reduce personal satisfaction. The environment of a cardiac catheterization laboratory can be stressful and demanding. The Nursing Turnover Cost Calculation Methodology ascertained a hospital pays $88,000 per nurse that leaves an institution.[14] The American Organization of Nurse Executives (AONE) has estimated that the registered nurse turnover costs hospitals in the United States 9.75 billion dollars a year.[15]

To establish projects such as Same-Day Discharge Departments or Radial Lounges, where nurses can be independently tasked per protocol, is not only a way to increase efficiency by speeding up the patients' turnover and reducing staff, but is also a way to reinforce nurse autonomy. This can assist in increasing nursing satisfaction and retain a well-trained and dedicated nursing workforce. For example, in Amsterdam, nurse specialists at the PCI lounge are responsible not only for the admission, gathering information, and preparation of the patient preprocedure, but also for the medical care and discharge after the procedure (Figs. 25-3 and 25-4). Among their tasks are checking radial compression, evaluation of radial artery patency prior to discharge, performing ECG acquisition, prescribing medications (following established protocols), consulting the procedural physicians for cases when complications develop, and providing discharge instructions and follow-up appointments. Nursing personnel are also involved in research activities and are encouraged to pursue nursing research opportunities and quality improvement activities. Appropriate triage pre-arrival to the facility and meticulous screening after the procedure are important to reduce nursing overload in the care of patients with complex care needs. At this juncture, it is important to have a

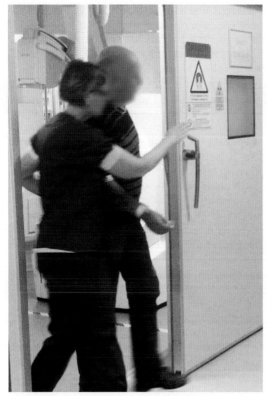

FIGURE 25-3　Patient (and nurse) walking from catheterization laboratory to PCI lounge after transradial PCI.

well-defined transfer plan to an inpatient service. This will prevent any delay in the treatment of untold events and enhance patient safety.

Follow-up Nursing

After the patient has been sent home, there is a component of nursing time spent in the follow-up process on an invasive procedure. Postprocedure phone calls are made by most institutions

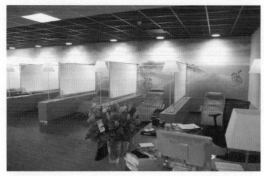

FIGURE 25-4　PCI lounge at OLVG Amsterdam.

in the United States and worldwide. Nursing staff evaluate patients for complications and answer postprocedural questions. Many of these phone assessments do provide early detection of postprocedural complications. This data must be captured and added to the NWL required for cardiac procedures. In the United States, these calls are required only for outpatient procedures, be that diagnostic or interventional cardiac catheterizations. A well-organized and thorough educational process may reduce the follow-up time by ensuring comprehensive pre- and postprocedural education. In the phone assessment, if a complication such as a pseudoaneurysm is identified, additional nursing time must be spent in arranging for further testing and care coordination. Owing to the significant reduction in complications such as major vascular hematomas in 30 days (radial = 1.2%, femoral = 3.0%; $P < 0.0001$),[16] radial access can simplify postprocedural nursing care as well.

Patient Satisfaction

There are a number of variables to be considered in determining a femoral versus a radial approach from a nursing perspective. Besides all the factors discussed, there is the component of patient satisfaction and quality of life, described by Cooper et al.[17] (Fig. 25-5). Increased patient satisfaction scores can affect hospital facility grading. Comfort measures that have identified the radial access superiority over the femoral experience[10,17-19,20,21] include the following:

- Decrease in back pain
- Early mobilization
- Ease of walking ability
- Decrease in recovery time
- Reduced need for painful femoral clamps
- Reduced sleep deprivation events
- Reduced dependency on the nursing staff for basic daily care
- Reduced frustration
- Decreased anger over unmet needs for comfort and social support
- Immediate foreign-body (sheath) removal
- Decreased hospital time and length of stay
- Reduced intrusion in physical privacy (groin exposure)
- Cost savings for families traveling with patients

Beyond that, patients are also reaping the clinical advantages of transradial approach,[2,7,8,11,13,15] in particular the following:

- Decreased mortality
- Decreased complication rates

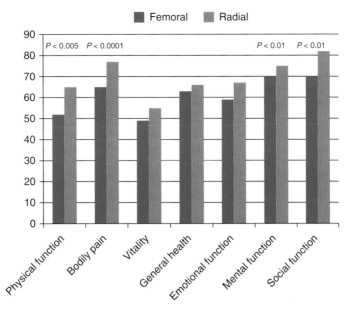

FIGURE 25-5 Quality of life measures. (Modified from Cooper CJ, El-Shiekh RA, Cohen DJ, et al. Effects of transradial access on quality of life and cost of cardiac catheterization: a randomized comparison. *Am Heart J.* 1999;138(3):430–436.)

- Simplified access for obese patients
- Simplified access for patients who cannot lie flat because of conditions such as heart failure
- Decrease in hospital-acquired infections
- Decrease in medication errors related to hospitalization
- Decreased risk of blood transfusions
- Reduced testing and procedures related to the treatment of complications
- Reduced inpatient intensive care events

Conclusion

The review of the literature provides objective evidence regarding the many facets of pre-, intra-, and postprocedural advantages of TRA. TRA supports a reduction in nursing time and workload and improves nurses' personal and professional satisfaction in the provision of care.

REFERENCES

1. Beller GA. President's page: high-quality cardiovascular care threatened by shortage of nurses and allied health professionals. *J Am Coll Cardiol.* 2000;36(5):1722–1724.
2. Agostoni P, Biondi-Zoccai GG, de Benedictis ML, et al. Radial versus femoral approach for percutaneous coronary diagnostic and interventional procedures: systematic overview and meta-analysis of randomized trials. *J Am Coll Cardiol.* 2004;44:349–356.
3. Kruzik N. Benefits of preoperative education for adult elective surgery patients. *AORN J.* 2009;90(3):381–387.
4. Roark J. When waiting-room brochures won't do: patient education requires a human touch. SURGistrategies: Solutions for Outpatient Healthcare. http://www.surgistrategies.com/articles/361feat6.html.Accessed August 7, 2012.
5. Walker, LM. Patient education: do it right and everyone wins. *Med Econ.* 1992;6(13):160–163.
6. Gilmartin J. Day surgery: patient's perceptions of a nurse-led preadmission clinic. *J Clin Nurs.* 2004;13(2):243–250.
7. Schaufele TG, Grunebaum JP, Lippe B, et al. Radial access versus conventional femoral puncture: outcome and resource effectiveness in a daily routine. The RAPTOR-Trial. Paper presented at the Scientific Sessions of the American Heart Association 2009, Orlando, FL.
8. Amoroso G, Sarti M, Bellucci R, et al. Clinical and procedural predictors of nurse workload during and after invasive coronary procedures: the potential benefit of a systematic radial access. *Eur J Cardiovasc Nurs.* 2005;4(3):234–241.
9. Roussanov O, Wilson SJ, Henley K, et al. Cost effectiveness or the radial versus femoral artery approach to diagnostic cardiac catheterization. *J Invasive Cardiol.* 2007;19(8):349–353.
10. Louvard Y, Lefevre T, Allain A, et al. Coronary angiography through the radial or the femoral approach: the CARAFE study. *Catheter Cardiovasc Interv.* 2001;52(2):181–187.
11. Carrington C, Mann R, Seif, EJ. An accelerated hemostasis protocol following transradial cardiac catheterization is safe and may shorten hospital stay: a single-center experience. *J Interv Cardiol.* 2009;22(6):571–575.
12. Caputo R. Transradial arterial access: economic considerations. *J Invasive Cardiol.* 2009;21: 18A–20A, Supplement.
13. Steinbrook R. Nursing in the crossfire. *N Engl J Med.* 2002;346:1757–1766.

14. Krsek C. Investing in nursing retention is a smart move in today's economy. Am Nurs Today. 2011;6(4). http://www.americannursetoday.com/investing-in-nursing-retention-is-a-smart-move-in-todays-economy/. Accessed October 16, 2014.

15. American Organization of Nurse Executives (AONE). RN turnover costs hospitals an estimated $9.75 billion annually. June 2010.

16. Jolly S, Yusef S, Cairns J, et al. Radial versus femoral access for coronary angiography and intervention in patients with acute coronary syndrome (RIVAL): a randomized, parallel group, multicentre trial. Lancet. 2011;337(9775):1379–1464.

17. Cooper CJ, El-Shiekh RA, Cohen DJ, et al. Effects of transradial access on quality of life and cost of cardiac catheterization: a randomized comparison. Am Heart J. 1999;138(3):430–436.

18. Amoroso G, Laarman, GJ, Kiemeneij, F. Overview of the transradial approach in percutaneous coronary intervention. J Cardiovasc Med. 2007;8(4):230–237.

19. Schussler JM. Effectiveness and safety of transradial artery access for cardiac catheterization. Bayl Univ Med Cent. 2011;24(3):205–209.

20. Tremmel JA. Launching a successful transradial program. J Invasive Cardiol. 2009;21(8) (Suppl a):5A–10A.

21. Speiser B, Bochenek-Cobb L. Abstract poster presentation. AIM Radial International Conference, Quebec City, Canada, 2012.

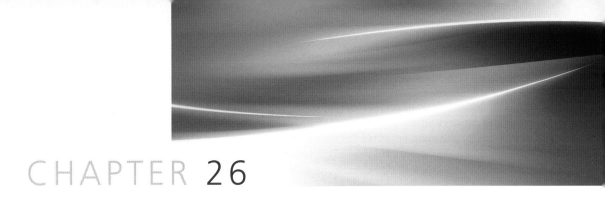

CHAPTER 26

Quality of Life and Cost-Effectiveness

Adhir Shroff and Neal Sawlani

Introduction

The clinical benefits of the transradial (TR) approach for invasive coronary procedures have been chronicled throughout this textbook. A consistent decrease in bleeding events and vascular complications are the most common themes. There may also be a mortality benefit with this approach in certain patient subsets.[1,2]

Avoiding complications will impact patient satisfaction and medical economics. However, these "soft" outcomes are not part of traditional medical literature, can be difficult to study, and are not embraced in a similar manner as traditional clinical outcomes. Nonetheless, everyday practice and the literature support a strong patient preference for the radial approach.

Similar to quality-of-life (QOL) assessments, economic analyses of health care are not as commonly reported as clinical outcomes. The current health-care environment in the United States and across the globe is creating more interest in such metrics. The primary drivers for the economic arguments in favor of the TR approach include cost savings associated with avoiding complications, decreasing staff workload, and improving efficiency by decreasing length of stay (LOS). Clearly, a community's health-care economic framework will determine its priority. In this chapter, a global focus will be the primary objective; however, many of the unique issues of the US health-care system will be discussed.

Organization of This Chapter

Initially, the chapter reviews the literature on QOL assessments with a focus on patient preference. This section also describes published clinical trials where patient preference, pain, and recovery period are mentioned. LOS is both a marker of patient preference and cost, but is covered primarily in the second part of this chapter, which will address the economics of TR access. This section is divided into two parts. The first includes a description of the main drivers of cost: complications, staff workload, and their relationship to LOS. The final section reviews the actual economic data from clinical trials.

Importance of Quality-of-Life Measures

Among the over 600,000 percutaneous coronary interventions (PCIs) performed in the United States last year,[3] the majority were performed on an elective basis. Goals of treatment in this population are primarily to improve functional status and relieve symptoms, which are known to be significant determinants of health-related QOL.[4] In recent years, health-care reform in the United States has incorporated measures of the "patient-experience" as a core quality goal. Procedure reimbursement will soon be linked to factors such as patient satisfaction. The TR approach provides a unique opportunity to combine equivalent clinical efficacy with improved comfort and patient satisfaction.

Traditionally, the impact of clinical end points such as recurrent ischemia, stroke, or repeat hospitalization has been the primary determinant of QOL in patients undergoing PCI.[5,6] A patient's subjective experience is difficult and time-consuming to measure, but is an important facet to understanding QOL. Investigators have developed several disease-specific instruments for determining QOL, including one that has been shown to have prognostic value for coronary artery disease.[7,8] The importance of patient preference and satisfaction are understudied, but are likely to impact one's perception of quality.

QOL and Cardiac Catheterization: Clinical Data

Despite the increasing prevalence of TR angiography, there has been a lack of published data with regard to its objective effects on QOL. It seems intuitive that earlier postprocedural ambulation and a reduction in access site complications would be a reliable foundation for higher patient satisfaction, but there are few studies exploring this subject. The published studies depict a clear patient preference for the TR approach over the transfemoral (TF) approach.

In one of the largest cohorts to study QOL, the investigators randomized 200 patients in a single center to TR or TF diagnostic cardiac catheterization.[9] For femoral access, 5- to 6F sheaths were used, followed by manual or mechanical compression for hemostasis, with 5 to 6 hours of bed rest. For the TR approach, 4F sheaths were utilized, followed by 1 hour of upright bed rest. QOL questionnaires and procedure-specific questions were administered to all subjects prior to the procedure, the day after the procedure, and 1 week following the procedure. Although there were no access site complications in either group, the patients expressed a preference for the TR approach as compared to the TF approach ($P < 0.0001$). Subjective assessments of bodily pain, back pain, and walking ability over the first postoperative day favored the TR group. This preference for the TR approach persisted even after 1 week and at no point did QOL favor the TF group. Among patients who had both approaches, 80% reported a preference for the TR approach.

Prolonged bed rest following PCI is a common source of dissatisfaction among patients. The growth of vascular access closure devices (VCDs) for femoral access is a testament to this fact. When compared to manual compression (MC), patients receiving a VCD report a less painful recovery.[10,11] Investigators compared patient preference between the TF approach with a VCD and the TR approach.[12] Nearly 1,500 patients underwent cardiac catheterization with one of three access strategies: TR approach, TF approach with MC, or TF approach with a VCD. QOL was assessed 1 day after the catheterization, by questionnaire.[9]

VCDs were able to reduce discomfort compared to MC, but patients found the TR approach to be significantly more comfortable (44.2% reporting no discomfort at all, $P < 0.0001$) than either of the femoral access groups. In fact, the TR approach demonstrated a significant reduction in patient discomfort for every measured indicator than did either VCDs or MC. Another group of investigators divided patients undergoing diagnostic catheterization into three groups: 6F radial access, 6F femoral access with a VCD, or 4F femoral access with MC. They noted similar postprocedure QOL but higher costs for the VCD group and lower-quality angiograms for the 4F group.[13]

A subgroup analysis of 7,021 patients randomized to either TR or TF access for acute coronary syndromes identified a large difference in patient preference between strategies.[2] In this more acute setting, 90% of patients randomized to the TR approach reported preference for the same approach if a repeat procedure was needed, compared to only 49% in the TF arm. Of those patients in the TF group, 25.6% of patients did receive a VCD.

Ambulatory Percutaneous Coronary Intervention

While there is economic and clinical data to support the feasibility of early discharge following elective PCI, ascertaining patient preference is also important. Investigators working at an ambulatory PCI unit followed 212 patients undergoing TR-PCI. These patients were asked their opinions regarding overall satisfaction, anxiety, and willingness to undergo the outpatient procedure again. Most of the patients (87%) noted being "very satisfied," with only one patient reporting "dissatisfaction." Anxiety was relatively rare: 85% reported no anxiety over the first 24 hours, and 96% would accept the ambulatory procedure again.[14] Even among selected TF patients, same-day discharge resulted in higher patient satisfaction than did an overnight stay.[15]

Although the overall number of trials is small and the end points are varied, there are a few general themes. TR access results in less pain and anxiety during the catheterization procedure. Furthermore, by decreasing time to ambulation, radial access decreases the discomfort of prolonged bed rest and allows the patient to resume normal activities sooner. QOL benefits alone are not sufficient to warrant adoption of the radial approach, but taken in combination with the clinical and economic data, radial access appears to provide benefit on multiple levels.

Cost of Complications

In the past, the quality of PCI procedures was primarily assessed by the frequency of ischemic outcomes. As technology, pharmacology, and techniques have improved, ischemic end points such as death, myocardial infarction, and urgent revascularization have seen a marked decline.[16] In the early years of PCI, bleeding and vascular complications were common.[17,18] Although these adverse events have decreased, many operators in the interventional community continue to accept such complications as an unavoidable consequence of PCI. The incremental economic burden related to adverse clinical outcomes has come to the forefront in the past 10 years and has become a focus of health-care reform in the United States.

After an analysis that suggested increased mortality among patients who experienced a bleeding event during their acute coronary syndrome,[19] the investigators assessed the economic impact of bleeding in this population.[20] Patients were divided into mild, moderate, and severe bleeding categories. The study reported that after adjusting for patient characteristics, each moderate or severe bleeding event increased costs by US$3,770 and a transfusion by US$2,080. As bleeding severity increased, the LOS and costs increased (Table 26-1).[21] The Mayo Clinic reported a significant increase in costs (US$5,883) and LOS (4.4 days) associated with PCI-related bleeding.[22]

Looking at this from another perspective, the positive economic impact of avoiding bleeding complications has been demonstrated in other areas as well. In a randomized clinical trial in patients with an acute coronary syndrome, bivalirudin monotherapy led to a net cost savings as compared to heparin and a glycoprotein inhibitor. The authors noted that despite a higher cost for antithrombotic therapy in the bivalirudin group, decreases in bleeding complications and LOS accounted for the overall cost savings with this strategy. In fact, major and minor bleedings were the most costly complications on a per-patient basis in view of their relatively common occurrence.[23]

Among Medicare beneficiaries who underwent PCI in 2002, an incremental resource utilization was reported (by Kugelmass et al.[24]) for those who experienced one or more PCI-related complications. Approximately 9.5% of patients experienced at least one complication, with vascular complications being the most common (5.47%). An uncomplicated PCI cost US$13,861 ± $9,635; however, patients who experienced any complication cost an incremental US$12,946. After multivariable adjustment, patients with a vascular complication cost an incremental US$4,830 and increased the LOS by 2.1 days.

Cost of Clinical Staff Workload

Patient preparation and recovery require nursing and technical staff. Although measurement of staff workload is not a clinical marker, it is an important process measure. By decreasing staff workload, changes to the typical workflow of patients can have a profound economic effect. Catheterization laboratory staff, holding area personnel, and recovery floor nurses will attest to the fact that TR cases require less work. Prolonged bed rest has important practical sequelae for the patient and staff, including the need for bedpans, having to feed patients, and prolonged MC. These are all time-intensive activities that occupy one or more team members. Moreover, patients are

TABLE 26-1	**Resource Use by Bleeding Severity**				
	No Bleeding (N = 780)	Mild Bleeding (N = 282)	Moderate Bleeding (N = 156)	Severe Bleeding (N = 17)	P
Total LOS (d)	5.3	6.9	15.0	16.4	<0.1
ICU LOS (d)	2.7	3.8	8.9	11.2	<0.1
Hospital costs	$11447	$17271	$36651	$56921	<0.1
Physician costs	$2835	$4403	$9147	$9643	<0.1
Total costs	$14282	$21674	$45798	$66564	<0.1

From Rao S, Kaul P, Liao L, et al. Association between bleeding, blood transfusion, and costs among patients with non–ST-segment elevation acute coronary syndromes. *Am Heart J.* 2008;155:369–374.

unable to resume caring for themselves for several hours after the procedure. In contrast, TR procedures allow patients to sit up immediately, feed themselves, ambulate, and use the bathroom once they are no longer sedated.

A German group randomly assigned patients to radial or femoral access and tracked the amount of time staff spent caring for these patients. In diagnostic cases, nursing care was needed for 13 minutes less with radial cases as compared to femoral cases ($P < 0.02$), primarily related to the time it took to perform MC of the access site. For PCI procedures, the difference was much larger, with the radial cases requiring 34 minutes less of nursing care ($P < 0.01$). They estimated that in their laboratory, where 3,000 procedures are performed annually, including 1,000 PCIs, radial cases would save them 1,383 hours of staff time.[25]

An Italian group looked at a cohort of 260 consecutive patients (52 femoral and 208 radial).[26] Catheterization laboratory nurses required less effort to care for patients who underwent TR access (86 minutes vs 174 minutes, $P < 0.001$) than for TF access patients. The ward nurses provide the bulk of postprocedure care. The investigators noted that the workload for ward nurses was 720 minutes and 386 minutes for femoral and radial procedures, respectively ($P < 0.001$). These smaller studies seem to reinforce what many radial operators, nurse managers, and hospital administrators have observed in everyday practice, namely, caring for TR patients is easier than for TF patients. In order to realize an economic benefit, the medical center or practice needs to tailor its care processes and adjust staffing ratios to account for the improved efficiency of radial access cases.

Length of Stay

In the economic substudy of GUSTO IIb, prolonged LOS was the primary driver for the increase in costs that were observed.[21] In the EASY (EArly discharge after transradial Stenting of coronarY arteries) trial (covered later in this section), the primary driver of the cost differential between the overnight observation group and the same-day discharge group was the costs related to spending the night in the hospital.[27] A group of investigators from Mexico noted that nearly 90% of the cost savings found with the radial approach were related to LOS.[28] The association between complications and LOS is complex. It stands to reason that a prolonged LOS is often a consequence of complications, but it should be clear that there are intrinsic costs to occupying a hospital bed, including the

cost of the room and staff utilization. This does not take into consideration the "opportunity cost" or the ability to use that room for another patient admission. In the United States, health-care systems are just beginning to identify hospital admissions where minimal patient care is occurring, the hospital admission is primarily for observation, or the overnight stay is based on historical standards. Government payers and private insurers are encouraging care providers to shift these admissions to same-day visits. Facilitating early discharge for low-risk, outpatient PCI patients is an opportunity to decrease LOS and costs.

TR versus TF Access: Economic Substudies of Clinical Trials

Diagnostic Catheterization

A group of French operators randomized patients to right radial, left radial, or femoral access for diagnostic angiography. Overall costs were lower for the left radial versus both the right radial and femoral access groups (French franc (FF) 4,508 $\pm$ 991, FF 4,745 $\pm$ 1,332, FF 5,213 $\pm$ 2,672, $P < 0.05$).[29] A group of US investigators conducted a retrospective analysis of patients undergoing a diagnostic catheterization procedure at a Veteran's Administration hospital. They included all equipment and procedure time that was utilized for either radial or femoral approach. Radial access cases cost less money than both femoral access with MC and femoral access when a VCD was used ($369.5 $\pm$ $74.6 vs $446.9 $\pm$ $60.2, and $553.4 $\pm$ $81.0 [both $P < 0.001$]).[30] The primary drivers of incremental cost included LOS and the cost of the VCD.

A large, single-center analysis showed that diagnostic radial procedures tended to cost about $10 more (related to costs of hemostatic bands versus MC for femoral procedures), but PCI procedures were $732 less when done from the radial route. The investigators concluded that there was $1,265 in cost savings per complication avoided in the TR group. With lower cost and less complications for the TR-PCI procedures, the radial approach was considered dominant (improved quality at a lower cost).[31]

TR-PCI

In a single-center clinical trial published in 2000, investigators collected cost data on patients undergoing PCI from both access routes. They assessed the relationship between TF-PCI with the use of a VCD and TR-PCI. In this nonrandomized study of 213 patients, they noted approximately $205 in savings favoring TR-PCI patients. Interestingly, about $122 of this difference was related to delayed discharge and complications, with the remaining $83 from differences in supply costs.[32]

In a retrospective analysis from a large database representing nearly 20% of all US hospitals, 609 TR-PCI cases were matched with over 60,000 TF cases.[33] There was a savings of $553 ($P$ = 0.033) favoring TR-PCI (total costs for TR-PCI were $11,736 ± $6,748 vs $12,288 ± $23,418 for TF-PCI). As the patient's risk of bleeding increased, there was a stronger economic argument in favor of the radial approach. Costs of care during the procedure day were similar; however, costs following the PCI until discharge were less in the radial patients, with 95% of the savings attributable to a shorter LOS (Fig. 26-1). In another study, Amin et al.[34] also compared the costs and clinical outcomes between TR-PCI and TF-PCI at five US hospitals. They found that the radial approach was associated with a cost savings exceeding $800 per patient relative to the femoral approach.

Although these studies are limited by their nonrandomized and retrospective nature, they provide a current, real-life assessment of PCI practices in the United States.

A systematic review of 14 randomized trials comparing radial and femoral accesses for diagnostic and therapeutic catheterizations employed a model to characterize the cost–benefit relationship. They included the cost of incremental procedure time and per-case costs of major complications. They noted that despite costing $1.52 more in procedure costs, radial catheterization led to an overall cost savings of $275 by decreasing the costs of complications as compared to TF procedures.[35] In their sensitivity analyses, there were no scenarios where radial cost more than femoral catheterization (Fig. 26-2). On the basis of their model, the cost advantage of radial access would disappear only if radial procedures took 20 minutes longer than femoral or if femoral complications were reduced by 60%.

Ambulatory PCI Procedures

From these earlier studies, a consistent message emerged: LOS is a major driver of cost for

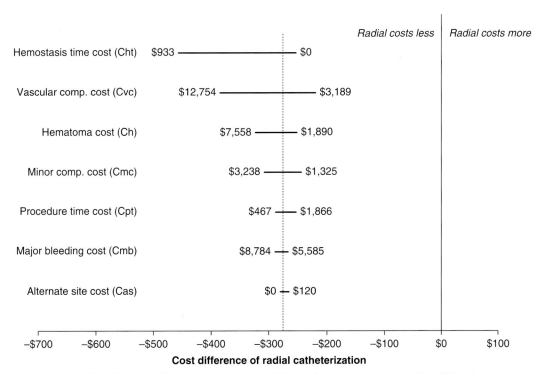

FIGURE 26-1 Effect of changes in each component variable on the net cost savings with radial catheterization as compared with femoral catheterization. (From Mitchell MD, Hong JA, Lee BY, et al. Systematic review and cost–benefit analysis of radial artery access for coronary angiography and intervention. *Circ Cardiovasc Qual Outcomes.* 2012;5:454–462.)

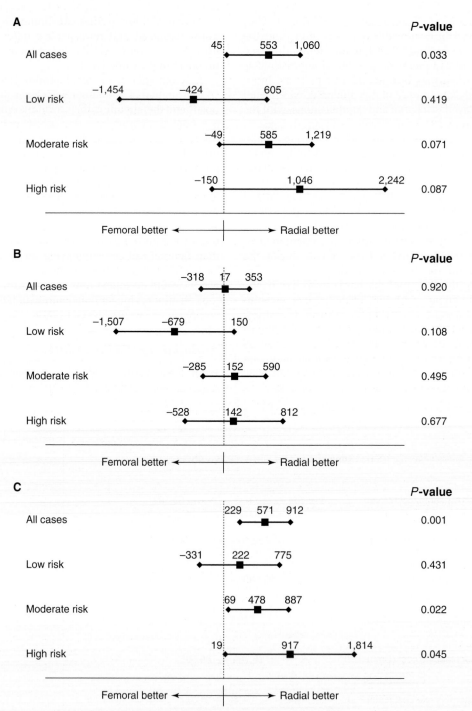

FIGURE 26-2   Costs associated with transradial and transfemoral PCIs by bleeding risk category: total direct costs of hospitalization (**A**), costs on the day of PCI (**B**), costs after PCI until discharge (**C**). (From Safley DM, Amin AP, House JA, et al. Comparison of costs between transradial and transfemoral percutaneous coronary intervention: a cohort analysis from the Premier research database. *Am Heart J.* 2013;165:303–309, e2.)

elective PCI. Strategies that can safely reduce LOS will lead to decreased costs. From a historical perspective, PCI had been considered an inpatient procedure. Owing to the technological, pharmacologic, and technical advances, PCI has become much safer. In the United States, the majority of elective PCI procedures require a 1-day LOS.[36] Several published studies have demonstrated the clinical efficacy and safety of same-day discharge in a selected group of low-risk, elective PCI patients.[16,37,38]

The clinical results of the EASY trial, published in 2006, demonstrated that complex TR-PCI in complex patients could be performed safely and that early discharge was possible.[39] In the economic analysis of this trial, the authors reported a savings of C$1,141 for the patients in the same-day-discharge cohort. The costs accumulated from the completion of the PCI (time of randomization) until discharge and then until the 30-day follow-up mark. Costs associated with the overnight stay as compared to same-day discharge accounted for nearly the entire cost differential between the groups.[27]

In a French study, among 220 patients who were eligible for discharge 4 to 6 hours after PCI for stable angina, 213 patients (96.8%) were actually discharged. After 24 hours, there were no readmissions or major adverse cardiovascular events among the patients who went home. These investigators compared the differences in costs between these patients and a group of patients undergoing PCI at other centers during this time period. The average *nonprocedural* costs of the 220 patients in this cohort was €1,230 ± €98 as compared to the control PCI patients, who cost €2,304 ± €1,814, representing a highly significant difference of €1,074 ($P < 10^{-6}$). When procedural costs were included, total costs were still lower in the ambulatory PCI patients (€3,120 ± €888 vs €4,330 ± €1,317, $P < 10^{-6}$).[15]

As was alluded to earlier in this chapter, changes in hospital processes can augment the economic advantages of using TR access. Creating an actual unit of space for ambulatory PCI is one such example. In a British hospital, Brewster et al. described the impact on bed utilization of a same-day discharge unit or "radial lounge." In one year, over 1,500 patients were managed in this unit (1,109 diagnostic and 439 PCI procedures). Nearly 85% of the PCI patients were discharged the same day and over 97% of the diagnostic procedure patients went home on the same day. The authors estimated that 595 bed days were saved.[40]

Any discussion of economics must account for reimbursement and not only cost. In the United States as of 2010, outpatient PCI procedures are reimbursed at a lower rate than inpatient procedures by about US$3,000.[36] Within the "outpatient" designation, patients can be discharged at any point within 24 hours. Therefore, discharge on the same day of the PCI as opposed to remaining in the hospital overnight will lead to a reduction in cost with no change in reimbursement. Even with lower reimbursement, some have estimated that US hospitals could save upward of US$200 million by discharging patients the same day.[41]

Conclusion

The clinical benefits of the TR approach should be the primary motivation for adopting this technique. A strong patient preference, improved satisfaction, and less pain are important secondary benefits for clinicians to consider as well. Minimizing bleeding and vascular complications, paired with a reduction in LOS, account for the majority of cost savings with the TR approach. In order for these benefits to be realized, appropriate care pathways and reimbursement need to occur.

REFERENCES

1. Romagnoli E, Biondi-Zoccai G, Sciahbasi A, et al. Radial versus femoral randomized investigation in ST-segment elevation acute coronary syndrome: The RIFLE-STEACS (Radial Versus Femoral Randomized Investigation in ST-Elevation Acute Coronary Syndrome) Study. *J Am Coll Cardiol*. 2012;60:2481–2489.
2. Jolly SS, Yusuf S, Cairns J; for the RIVAL trial group. Radial versus femoral access for coronary angiography and intervention in patients with acute coronary syndromes (RIVAL): a randomised, parallel group, multicentre trial. *Lancet*. 2011;377:1409–1420.
3. Roger VL, Go AS, Lloyd-Jones DM, et al. Heart disease and stroke statistics—2012 update: a report from the American Heart Association. *Circulation*. 2012;125:e2–e220.
4. Strauss WE, Fortin T, Hartigan P, et al. A comparison of quality of life scores in patients with angina pectoris after angioplasty compared with after medical therapy: outcomes of a randomized clinical trial. Veterans Affairs Study of Angioplasty Compared to Medical Therapy Investigators. *Circulation*. 1995;92:1710–1719.
5. Cohen DJ, Taira DA, Berezin R, et al. Cost-effectiveness of coronary stenting in acute myocardial infarction: results from the stent primary angioplasty in myocardial infarction (stent-PAMI) trial. *Circulation*. 2001;104:3039–3045.
6. Amin AP, Reynolds MR, Lei Y, et al. Cost-effectiveness of everolimus- versus paclitaxel-eluting stents for patients undergoing percutaneous coronary revascularization (from the SPIRIT-IV Trial). *Am J Cardiol*. 2012;110:765–770.
7. Spertus JA, Winder JA, Dewhurst TA, et al. Development and evaluation of the Seattle Angina Questionnaire: a new functional status measure for coronary artery disease. *J Am Coll Cardiol*. 1995;25:333–341.
8. Spertus JA, Salisbury AC, Jones PG, et al. Predictors of quality-of-life benefit after percutaneous coronary intervention. *Circulation*. 2004;110:3789–3794.
9. Cooper CJ, El-Shiekh RA, Cohen DJ, et al. Effect of transradial access on quality of life and cost of cardiac

catheterization: a randomized comparison. *Am Heart J.* 1999;138:430–436.

10. Deuling JH, Vermeulen RP, Anthonio RA, et al. Closure of the femoral artery after cardiac catheterization: a comparison of Angio-Seal, StarClose, and manual compression. *Catheter Cardiovasc Interv.* 2008;71:518–523.

11. Juergens CP, Leung DY, Crozier JA, et al. Patient tolerance and resource utilization associated with an arterial closure versus an external compression device after percutaneous coronary intervention. *Catheter Cardiovasc Interv.* 2004;63:166–170.

12. Sciahbasi A, Fischetti D, Picciolo A, et al. Transradial access compared with femoral puncture closure devices in percutaneous coronary procedures. *Int J Cardiol.* 2009;137:199–205.

13. Reddy BK, Brewster PS, Walsh T, et al. Randomized comparison of rapid ambulation using radial, 4 French femoral access, or femoral access with AngioSeal closure. *Catheter Cardiovasc Interv.* 2004;62:143–149.

14. Le Corvoisier P, Gellen B, Lesault PF, et al. Ambulatory transradial percutaneous coronary intervention: a safe, effective, and cost-saving strategy. *Catheter Cardiovasc Interv.* 2013;81:15–23.

15. Heyde GS, Koch KT, de Winter RJ, et al. Randomized trial comparing same-day discharge with overnight hospital stay after percutaneous coronary intervention: results of the elective PCI in outpatient study (EPOS). *Circulation.* 2007;115:2299–2306.

16. McGrath PD, Malenka DJ, Wennberg DE, et al. Changing outcomes in percutaneous coronary interventions: a study of 34,752 procedures in northern New England, 1990 to 1997. Northern New England Cardiovascular Disease Study Group. *J Am Coll Cardiol.* 1999;34:674–680.

17. Serruys PW, de Jaegere P, Kiemeneij F, et al. A comparison of balloon-expandable-stent implantation with balloon angioplasty in patients with coronary artery disease. Benestent Study Group. *N Engl J Med.* 1994;331:489–495.

18. Fischman DL, Leon MB, Baim DS, et al. A randomized comparison of coronary-stent placement and balloon angioplasty in the treatment of coronary artery disease. Stent Restenosis Study Investigators. *N Engl J Med.* 1994;331:496–501.

19. Rao SV, O'Grady K, Pieper KS, et al. Impact of bleeding severity on clinical outcomes among patients with acute coronary syndromes. *Am J Cardiol.* 2005;96:1200–1206.

20. A comparison of recombinant hirudin with heparin for the treatment of acute coronary syndromes. The Global Use of Strategies to Open Occluded Coronary Arteries (GUSTO) IIb investigators. *N Engl J Med.* 1996;335:775–782.

21. Rao S, Kaul P, Liao L, et al. Association between bleeding, blood transfusion, and costs among patients with non-ST-segment elevation acute coronary syndromes. *Am Heart J.* 2008;155:369–374.

22. Jacobson KM, Hall Long K, McMurtry EK, et al. The economic burden of complications during percutaneous coronary intervention. *Qual Saf Health Care.* 2007;16:154–159.

23. Pinto DS, Stone GW, Shi C, et al. Economic evaluation of bivalirudin with or without glycoprotein IIb/IIIa inhibition versus heparin with routine glycoprotein IIb/IIIa inhibition for early invasive management of acute coronary syndromes. *J Am Coll Cardiol.* 2008;52:1758–1768.

24. Kugelmass A, Cohen D, Brown P, et al. Hospital resources consumed in treating complications associated with percutaneous coronary interventions. *Am J Cardiol.* 2006;97:322–327.

25. Schäufele TG J-PG, Beate Lippe, Hodenberg TBaEv. Radial access versus conventional femoral puncture: outcome and resource effectiveness in a daily routine. The RAPTOR-Trial. American Heart Association Scientific Sessions. Orlando, FL, 2009.

26. Amoroso G, Sarti M, Bellucci R, et al. Clinical and procedural predictors of nurse workload during and after invasive coronary procedures: the potential benefit of a systematic radial access. *Eur J Cardiovasc Nurs.* 2005;4:234–241.

27. Rinfret S, Kennedy WA, Lachaine J, et al. Economic impact of same-day home discharge after uncomplicated transradial percutaneous coronary intervention and bolus-only abciximab regimen. *JACC Cardiovasc Interv.* 2010;3:1011–1019.

28. Escarcega RO, Perez-Alva JC, Jimenez-Hernandez M, et al. Transradial percutaneous coronary intervention without on-site cardiac surgery for stable coronary disease and myocardial infarction: preliminary report and initial experience in 174 patients. *Isr Med Assoc J.* 2010;12:592–597.

29. Louvard Y, Lefevre T, Allain A, et al. Coronary angiography through the radial or the femoral approach: the CARAFE study. *Catheter Cardiovasc Interv.* 2001;52:181–187.

30. Roussanov O, Wilson SJ, Henley K, et al. Cost-effectiveness of the radial versus femoral artery approach to diagnostic cardiac catheterization. *J Invasive Cardiol.* 2007;19: 349–353.

31. Applegate R, Sacrinty M, Schafer P, et al. Cost effectiveness of radial access for diagnostic cardiac catheterization and coronary intervention. *Catheter Cardiovasc Interv.* 2013;82:E375–E384.

32. Mann T, Cowper PA, Peterson ED, et al. Transradial coronary stenting: comparison with femoral access closed with an arterial suture device. *Catheter Cardiovasc Interv.* 2000;49:150–156.

33. Safley DM, Amin AP, House JA, et al. Comparison of costs between transradial and transfemoral percutaneous coronary intervention: a cohort analysis from the Premier research database. *Am Heart J.* 2013;165:303–309, e2.

34. Amin AP, House JA, Safley DM, et al. Costs of transradial percutaneous coronary intervention. *JACC Cardiovasc Interv.* 2013;6:827–834.

35. Mitchell MD, Hong JA, Lee BY, et al. Systematic review and cost-benefit analysis of radial artery access for coronary angiography and intervention. *Circ Cardiovasc Qual Outcomes.* 2012;5:454–462.

36. Cardiovascular Roundtable. The outmigration of cardiovascular services: optimizing patient selection and enhancing workflow for efficient outpatient care delivery, Washington, DC, 2010.

37. Jabara R, Gadesam R, Pendyala L, et al. Ambulatory discharge after transradial coronary intervention: preliminary US single-center experience (Same-day TransRadial Intervention and Discharge Evaluation, the STRIDE Study). *Am Heart J.* 2008;156:1141–1146.

38. Abdelaal E, Rao SV, Gilchrist IC, et al. Same-day discharge compared with overnight hospitalization after uncomplicated percutaneous coronary intervention: a systematic review and meta-analysis. *JACC Cardiovasc Interv.* 2013;6:99–112.

39. Bertrand OF, De Larochelliere R, Rodes-Cabau J, et al. A randomized study comparing same-day home discharge and abciximab bolus only to overnight hospitalization and abciximab bolus and infusion after transradial coronary stent implantation. *Circulation.* 2006;114:2636–2643.

40. Brewster S, Khimdas K, Cleary N, et al. Impact of a dedicated "radial lounge" for percutaneous coronary procedures on same-day discharge rates and bed utilization. *Am Heart J.* 2013;165:299–302.

41. Popescu AM, Weintraub WS. Outpatient percutaneous coronary interventions: hospital and health system costs saving while maintaining patient safety. *JACC Cardiovasc Interv.* 2010;3:1020–1021.

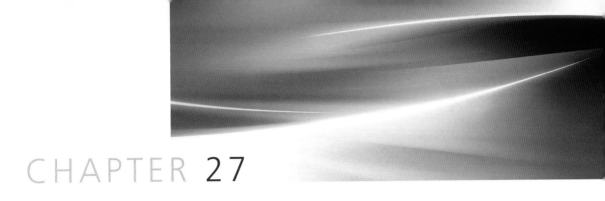

CHAPTER 27

Transradial Approach in Structural Heart Disease

Amir H. Sadrzadeh Rafie and Saibal Kar

In recent years, the volume of patients undergoing structural heart disease (SHD) interventions is rapidly increasing, and depending on the outcome of several ongoing clinical trials, this may even surpass the number of many vascular interventions performed in near future. Over the past several decades, the transradial (TR) approach has become an increasingly popular arterial access for coronary angiography and interventions. More recently, there has been a growing body of evidence suggesting that adaptation of TR approach, rather than a transfemoral one, to left heart catheterization and percutaneous coronary intervention (PCI) allows early patient mobility, significantly lowers the risk of bleeding and access site complications, and reduces hospital costs.[1-4] In this chapter, we aim to address some of the current applications of TR access as well as potential directions for future investigations of the TR realm in SHD.

Pivotal to the optimal performance of most cases of SHD interventions is precise transcatheter hemodynamic measurement and interpretation. The SHD interventions are usually long procedures and require large doses of anticoagulation, which would increase the risk of bleeding and access site complications. To this end, lack of need for large-bore vascular sheaths in the radial artery rather than transfemoral access appears to be an optimal way for left ventricular hemodynamic assessment during the procedure to minimize vascular complications. The ability to rapidly ambulate patients is a significant benefit of the TR approach, comfortable for the patient and able to lower the thromboembolic risk. Finally, in many instances, both right and left heart catheterizations are required.

Transradial Catheterization during Mitral Valve Procedures

Catheter-based hemodynamics is of critical importance during percutaneous mitral valve interventions such as transcatheter mitral valve repair for mitral regurgitation using MitraClip (Abbott Laboratories, Abbott Park, IL). The MitraClip procedure involves an echo-guided transvenous-transseptal deployment of one or more clips at the site of maximal malcoaptation of mitral leaflets. The MitraClip system is delivered to the heart through the femoral vein, and transseptal puncture of the interatrial septum is performed using a standard transseptal kit. The right internal jugular vein is cannulated for hemodynamic assessment and monitoring. A radial artery line is often obtained by the anesthesiologist for monitoring arterial pressures during these lengthy procedures under general anesthesia. The same access can be used to advance a pigtail catheter into the left ventricle and aorta for invasive hemodynamic measurements and left ventriculography. Invasive hemodynamics is complementary to echocardiographic imaging in this setting. Changes in the left atrial pressure and waveform, as well as mitral valve mean gradient and cardiac output, are important assessment parameters for both safety and efficacy.[5] As a result of this approach, only one catheter is advanced in the right femoral vein. There are no arterial access requirements in the groin. This approach minimizes the vascular complications and helps in early mobilization of the patient

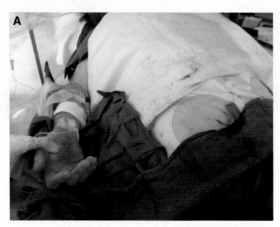
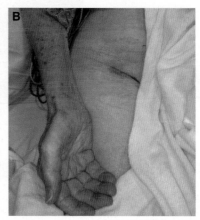

FIGURE 27-1   MitraClip procedure with a single venous access in the right groin, and right radial access for arterial pressure monitoring. **A:** Sheaths inserted just prior to procedure. **B:** Six hours postprocedure, showing no vascular issues in the groin or forearm.

after the procedure. The MitraClip procedure can often be a long procedure requiring large doses of antithrombotics. Such an approach markedly reduces the incidence of major bleeding, especially since many of these patients are high-surgical-risk patients (Fig. 27-1).

A similar approach can be used during percutaneous mitral valvuloplasty. A 4F pigtail catheter is advanced into the left ventricle via the right radial artery. The Swan Ganz catheter is advanced via the right jugular vein for measurements of right heart pressures and cardiac output assessment. Right heart catheterization can also be performed using the basilic or cephalic veins (see Chapter 13). The therapeutic valvuloplasty catheter is advanced through the right femoral vein. Such an approach allows for no catheters to be placed in the other groin and minimizes the vascular complications and allows early mobilization of the patient (Fig. 27-2).

Transradial Catheterization during Aortic Valve Procedures

Over the past decade the technique of transcatheter aortic valve implantation (TAVI) has been embraced as a novel treatment option for inoperable or high-surgical-risk patients with severe symptomatic aortic valve disease. Recent randomized studies have raised major safety concerns because of increased stroke/transient ischemic attack rates with TAVI than with medical treatment and conventional aortic valve replacement. The pathophysiology of ischemic brain

defects after TAVI is multifactorial. In addition to intrinsic patient characteristics such as age, previous stroke, atrial fibrillation, and left ventricular dysfunction, mobilization of atherosclerotic material by wire and catheter manipulations or calcified valve particles during balloon valvuloplasty or actual bioprosthesis implantation, as well as hypotension and cerebral hypoperfusion from intraprocedural tachy-pacing maneuvers during valve deployment, especially in patients with carotid disease, could also contribute toward the TAVI-associated stroke risk.[6] Embolic protection devices have been developed to reduce

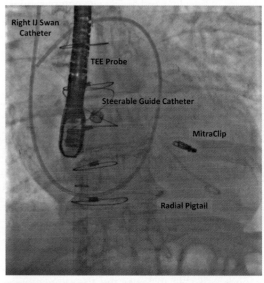

FIGURE 27-2   Fluoroscopic image of a MitraClip showing the use of pigtail catheter inserted via the right radial artery.

these events. Three different devices have been used in experimental studies to reduce the TAVI-associated stroke risk. In general, these devices use two different mechanisms of protection (capture versus deflection of the embolic material). Two of these technologies, the Claret CE Pro system (Claret Medical Inc., Santa Rosa, CA) and the Embrella (Edwards Lifesciences, Irvine, CA), are temporarily introduced via right TR or transbrachial access into the supra-aortic arteries. The SMT-Shimon Embolic protection Filter, or SHEF (SMT Medical, Herzliya Pituach, Israel), which is an embolic deflection device, requires femoral arterial access via a 9F sheath. The Claret CE ProTandem Embolic Protection Device consists of two filter baskets attached in series that capture embolic material during the procedure. This device is 6F compatible and is introduced via the right TR or transbrachial access. The proximal filter is deployed first in the truncus brachiocephalicus for the protection of the right vertebral artery as well as the right common carotid artery, followed by the distal filter in the left common carotid artery. Although there was not a systematic magnetic resonance neuroimaging at baseline and follow-up to discover new TAVI-related brain lesions, in the first-in-human experience of the Claret CE Pro system the proof of concept was at least partly illustrated by the capturing of debris in more than half of the patients, providing evidence for the potential to reduce the procedural cerebral embolic burden utilizing this dedicated filter system during TAVI.[7] The Embrella Embolic Deflector Device contains a self-expanding nitinol frame with a heparin-coated polyurethane porous membrane that does not interfere with cerebral perfusion. The system is 6F compatible and is introduced through radial or brachial access over the right side of TAVI patients. The device is designed to cover the ostia of the brachiocephalic trunk (and its right carotid branch) and the left carotid artery originating directly from the transverse aorta, thereby deflecting emboli away from the cerebral circulation. In some patients, the device might also overlie the left subclavian ostium, providing protection for the left vertebral. Because the device is not positioned within the cerebral vessels, the risk of arterial spasm, injury, thrombosis, or transiently impaired cerebral perfusion seems minimal.[8]

Post-TAVI cases of complex PCI for coronary obstructions, jailed left main or new coronary artery lesions have been described.[9] Although some cases have been performed by radial approach, the exact benefit of this access has not yet been studied in detail.[10]

Interestingly, the group of Dr. A. Colombo has also described the radial crossover techniques for secured femoral access management during TAVI procedures.[11] With this strategy, the left radial artery is cannulated at the beginning of the TAVI procedure. Using a multipurpose catheter, a 0.018-inch guidewire is positioned distal into the femoral artery, which will serve to the large introducer sheath. After valve deployment and prior to sheath removal, a 135-cm peripheral balloon is advanced over the 0.018-inch wire and is inflated prior to removal of the large sheath. This allows blood flow interruption and safe TAVI sheath removal. The same group compared their experience with the radial crossover to the previously described femoral crossover techniques. Life-threatening and major bleeding events were fewer in the radial group (9.1% vs 19.5%, $P = 0.168$, and 13.6% vs 22%, $P = 0.315$, respectively).[12]

Transradial Catheterization during Alcohol Septal Ablation

Hypertrophic cardiomyopathy (HCM) is the most frequent cause of sudden death in young adults (including trained athletes), and can lead to functional disability from heart failure and atrial fibrillation (with embolic stroke).[13] Alcohol septal ablation is a therapeutic catheter-based procedure and an alternative to surgical myectomy in the treatment of patients with HCM. On top of the bleeding hazard reduction, including groin hematoma or femoral artery injuries, the TR approach allows safe and rapid ambulation. The TRASA (Trans-Radial Alcohol Septal Ablation) trial investigators conducted a prospective study in consecutive 30 patients with symptomatic hypertrophic obstructive cardiomyopathy despite optimal medical treatment (New York Heart Association functional class III to IV).[14] All subjects demonstrated a dynamic left ventricular outflow tract gradient of at least 50 mmHg at rest or on provocation and a septal thickness >18 mm. Patients with a negative Allen test or specific contraindication for radial access were excluded. Right radial access was used in all patients, and the left main was cannulated with a 6F Judkins left 3.5 guiding catheter. After identification of the septal branches of the left anterior descending coronary artery, alcohol septal ablation was performed. A second perforator artery was cannulated and ablated if gradient reduction <50% was not achieved after the first septal ablation.

Also, to avoid transfemoral temporary pacing, a subclavian bipolar active fixation permanent pacing lead was stitched to the skin and connected to a desterilized recuperation pacemaker. Investigators showed that in this small population, procedural success was excellent (100%) and access site bleeding complications were virtually eliminated, even in the 21.4% patients with oral anticoagulation. In addition to the bleeding hazard reduction, the length of stay in the intensive care unit and the total length of hospital stay were shortened with this strategy, compared with results from other studies and registries of alcohol septal ablation in HCM.

Transradial Catheterization during Procedures for Coarctation of Aorta

Coarctation of the aorta accounts for 5% to 7% of congenital heart disease, which can be diagnosed over a wide range of ages and with varying degrees of severity. Balloon angioplasty with or without stenting has evolved as a promising treatment for coarctation, assuming appropriate anatomy and lack of other indications for cardiovascular surgery. Radial artery access is an essential component of aortic coarctation stenting in adult-sized adolescents and adults and should be employed routinely in all cases. In general, both femoral (8F) and radial artery (6F) accesses are obtained. A 6F pigtail catheter is positioned from the radial artery into the descending aorta proximal to the coarctation. The coarctation site is then crossed using a catheter from the femoral artery. Simultaneous radial artery monitoring confers several advantages. In preparing for stent delivery, it allows for accurate assessment of the gradient across the coarctation site. Performing aortography through the pigtail catheter from radial artery is useful in defining the position of the stent before deployment and clarifying the origin of the left subclavian during implantation. In addition, continuous invasive monitoring during and immediately after stent deployment permits accurate assessment of systemic blood pressure, assisting prompt recognition of hemodynamic instability because of aortic disruption. During assessment of such complications, the radial artery access obviates the need for catheter exchange of the stent balloon after deployment and nullifies the associated delay in defining the

origin of the instability. Furthermore, in cases where crossing the coarctation site is difficult, an alternative method is exchanging the pigtail catheter from the radial artery with a 4F multipurpose catheter. This in turn allows placement of a 0.035-inch extra-stiff exchange guidewire, which can be advanced across the lesion. The wire can then be snared in the descending aorta and exteriorized through the right femoral sheath. In addition, by positioning a wire from the radial approach and then exteriorizing it through the femoral access site, a "railway" is created, which allows for stent positioning and may minimize the risk of stent migration in cases with difficult anatomy.[15,16]

Although many devices for structural interventions are bulky and therefore will remain incompatible with radial artery access, radial operators performing structural-based procedures will likely continue to push the envelope. Recently, Sanghvi et al.[17] reported a perimembranous ventricular septal defect which was successfully closed using exclusively right radial artery and basilic vein access and an 8-mm Amplatzer device. Schiattarella and colleagues[18] reported the successful closure of a type I endoleak after initial successful endovascular aortic repair of an infrarenal aneurysm. The procedure was completed through right radial access with a 6F SOS omni catheter to selectively engage the aneurysmal sac. Then Onyx (Covidien, Irvine, CA) liquid embolic material formed with ethylene vinyl alcohol (EVOH) copolymer, dimethyl sulfoxide, and micronized tantalum powder was directly injected into the sac.

TR access allows for optimal hemodynamic assessment and prompt recognition of complications during or after complex structural procedures. There is a substantial economic benefit with the TR approach, which can be demonstrated with either evaluation of hospital costs or total hospital charge. Procedural morbidity is less, and patients overwhelmingly prefer the TR to the femoral approach. Radial artery access is a simple and safe technique with infrequent vascular complications that complements various diagnostic and therapeutic elements of SHD interventions.

REFERENCES

1. Agostoni P, et al. Radial versus femoral approach for percutaneous coronary diagnostic and interventional procedures; Systematic overview and meta-analysis of randomized trials. *J Am Coll Cardiol*. 2004;44(2):349–356.
2. Hildick-Smith DJ, et al. Coronary angiography from the radial artery—experience, complications and limitations. *Int J cardiol*. 1998;64(3):231–239.

3. Sciahbasi A, et al. Arterial access-site-related outcomes of patients undergoing invasive coronary procedures for acute coronary syndromes (from the ComPaRison of Early Invasive and Conservative Treatment in Patients With Non-ST-ElevatiOn Acute Coronary Syndromes [PRESTO-ACS] Vascular Substudy). *Am J Cardiol.* 2009;103(6):796–800.

4. Cooper CJ, et al. Effect of transradial access on quality of life and cost of cardiac catheterization: a randomized comparison. *Am Heart J.* 1999;138(3 pt 1):430–436.

5. Jilaihawi H, et al. Contemporary application of cardiovascular hemodynamics: transcatheter mitral valve interventions. *Cardiol Clin.* 2011;29(2):201–209.

6. Eggebrecht H, et al. Risk of stroke after transcatheter aortic valve implantation (TAVI): a meta-analysis of 10,037 published patients. *EuroIntervention.* 2012;8(1):129–138.

7. Naber CK, et al. First-in-man use of a novel embolic protection device for patients undergoing transcatheter aortic valve implantation. *EuroIntervention.* 2012;8(1):43–50.

8. Nietlispach F, et al. An embolic deflection device for aortic valve interventions. *JACC Cardiovasc Interv.* 2010;3(11): 1133–1138.

9. Ribeiro HB, et al. Coronary obstruction following transcatheter aortic valve implantation: a systematic review. *JACC Cardiovasc Interv.* 2013;6(5):452–461.

10. Greenberg G, Kornowski R. Coronary angioplasty after self-expandable transcatheter aortic valve implantation. *J Invasive Cardiol.* 2013;25(7):361–363.

11. Buchanan GL, et al. A "modified crossover technique" for vascular access management in high-risk patients undergoing transfemoral transcatheter aortic valve implantation. *Catheter Cardiovasc Interv.* 2013;81(4):579–583.

12. Curran H, et al. A comparison of the femoral and radial crossover techniques for vascular access management in transcatheter aortic valve implantation: the Milan experience. *Catheter Cardiovasc Interv.* 2014;83(1):156–161.

13. Maron BJ, Maron MS. Hypertrophic cardiomyopathy. *Lancet.* 2013;381(9862):242–255.

14. Cuisset T, et al. Transradial approach and subclavian wired temporary pacemaker to increase safety of alcohol septal ablation for treatment of obstructive hypertrophic cardiomyopathy: the TRASA trial. *Arch Cardiovasc Dis.* 2011;104(8–9):444–449.

15. Dehghani P, et al. Role of routine radial artery access during aortic coarctation interventions. *Catheter.* 2007;70(4): 622–623.

16. Gillespie MJ, Kreutzer J, Rome JJ. Novel approach to percutaneous stent implantation for coarctation of the aorta: the railway technique. *Catheter Cardiovasc Interv.* 2005;65(4):584–587.

17. Sanghvi K, Selvaraj N, Luft U. Percutaneous closure of a perimembranous ventricular septal defect through arm approach (radial artery and basilic vein). *J Interv Cardiol.* 2014;27(2):199–203.

18. Schiattarella GG, et al. Transradial approach for the endovascular treatment of type I endoleak after aortic aneurysm repair: a case report. *BMC Surg.* 2013;13(suppl 2):S47.

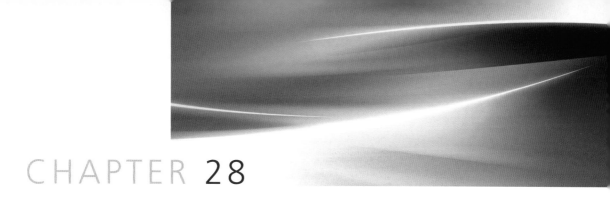

CHAPTER 28

Randomized Studies of Transradial versus Transfemoral Coronary Approach

Jimmy MacHaalany and David Meerkin

Abbreviations

- ACS: acute coronary syndrome
- AMI: acute myocardial infarction
- BMI: body mass index
- CABG: coronary artery bypass graft surgery
- CAG: coronary angiography
- DAP: dose area product
- LRA: left radial approach
- MACE: major adverse cardiovascular events
- MI: myocardial infarction
- NA: not available
- NACE: net adverse clinical events
- NS: not significant
- NSTEMI: non-ST-elevation myocardial infarction

- PCI: percutaneous coronary intervention
- PTCA: percutaneous transluminal coronary angioplasty
- QOL: quality of life
- RAO: radial artery occlusion
- RAS: radial artery spasm
- RRA: right radial approach
- SA: stable angina
- STEMI: ST-elevation myocardial infarction
- TBA: transbrachial approach
- TFA: transfemoral approach
- TLR: target lesion revascularization
- TRA: transradial approach
- TUA: transulnar approach
- TVR: target vessel revascularization
- UA: unstable angina

Right Radial Access for PTCA: A Prospective Study Demonstrates Reduced Complications and Hospital Charges

Objective	To evaluate the hypothesis that TRA angioplasty is more cost-effective than the TFA
Study Population	152 patients (76 in each group) undergoing PTCA
Follow-up	In-hospital
End Point	Procedural and cost outcomes
Procedural Success Rate/Crossover	TRA → TFA: 3; TFA → TRA: 1

(continued)

Main Results (Fig. 28-1)	• Similar primary PTCA success (TRA: 95% vs TFA: 97%), procedural and fluoroscopy times, and catheterization laboratory charge
	• TRA had fewer access site complications and lower total hospital charge (reduction of 9%; $P < 0.05$)
Conclusion	PTCA can be performed using the TRA as effectively as the TFA while avoiding clinically significant access site complications
Reference	Mann JT 3rd, Cubeddu MG, Schneider JE, et al. Right radial access for PTCA: a prospective study demonstrates reduced complications and hospital charges. *J Invasive Cardiol.* 1996;8(suppl D):40D–44D.

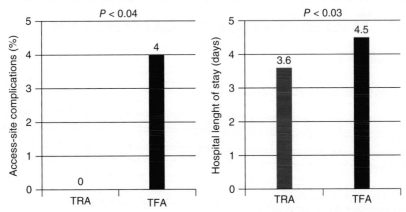

FIGURE 28-1 Access-site complications and hospital stay in transradial and transfemoral access after PTCA.

Access

Objective	To compare procedural and clinical outcomes of PTCA via the TRA, TBA, or TFA
Study Population	900 patients (300 in each group) undergoing PTCA for ACS
Follow-up	In-hospital and 1 mo
End Point	Procedural outcomes and MACE (death, MI, CABG, or repeat PTCA) at 1 mo
Procedural Success Rate/Crossover	TRA → TFA: 20; TBA → TFA: 12; TFA → TRA: 1
Main Results (Fig. 28-2)	• Successful coronary cannulation—TRA:TBA:TFA = 93.0%:95.7%:99.7% ($P < 0.001$)
	• Major entry site complications—TRA:TBA:TFA = 0%:2.3%:2.0% ($P = 0.035$)
	• Entry site complications requiring transfusion—TRA:TBA:TFA = 0%:0.7%:0.7% ($P = $ NS)
	• RAO: 9 patients (3%)
	• Similar rates of PTCA success (TRA:TBA:TFA = 88%:88%:90% [$P = $ NS]), procedural and fluoroscopy times, and MACE at 1 mo
	• No difference in length of hospital stay—TRA: 1.5 ± 2.5 d vs TBA: 1.8 ± 3.8 d vs TFA: 1.8 ± 4.2 d ($P = $ NS)
Conclusion	Procedural and clinical success of PTCA were similar for the three subgroups, with reduced entry site complications but increased access failure with transradial PTCA

Reference　Kiemeneij F, Laarman GJ, Odekerken D, et al. A randomized comparison of percutaneous transluminal coronary angioplasty by the radial, brachial and femoral approaches: the access study. *J Am Coll Cardiol.* 1997;29(6): 1269–1275.

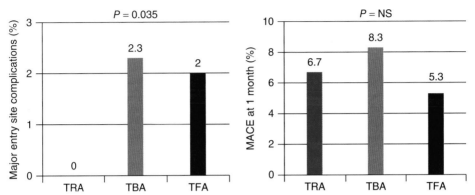

FIGURE 28-2　Major entry site complications and MACE rates in transradial, transbrachial and transfemoral access after PTCA.

Brafe Stent

Objective	To compare procedural outcomes and length of hospitalization times
Study Population	150 patients (TRA: 56; TBA: 38; TFA: 56) undergoing PTCA for ACS
Follow-up	In-hospital and 1 mo
End Point	Primary-entry site complications (bleeding, hematoma, transfusion, occlusion, surgery) and average hospitalization time post–stent implantation
Procedural Success Rate/Crossover	TRA → TFA: 1; TBA → TFA: 0; TFA → TRA: 0
Main Results (Fig. 28-3)	• Similar entry site complications • Similar in-hospital and 1 month outcomes (death, MI, revascularization, bleeding, and transfusions) • Similar hospitalization time (TBA: 77 ± 36 h vs TFA: 83 ± 33 h vs TRA: 86 ± 39 h; *P* = NS) • TRA had longer procedural times (TBA: 31.0 ± 10.0 min vs TFA: 42.2 ± 21.8 min vs TRA: 55.8 ± 31.3 min; *P* ≤ 0.001)
Conclusion	Procedural and clinical outcomes were similar for all three subgroups, with TRA having longer procedural times
Reference	Benit E, Missault L, Eeman T, et al. Brachial, radial, or femoral approach for elective Palmaz-Schatz stent implantation: a randomized comparison. *Catheter Cardiovasc Diagn.* 1997;41(2):124–130.

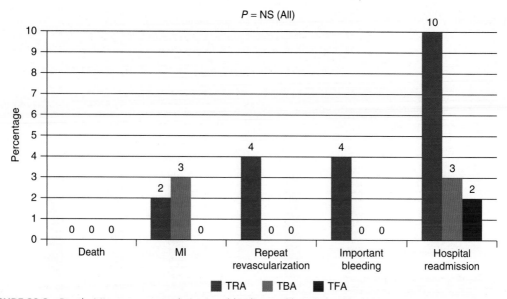

FIGURE 28-3   Death, MI, repeat revascularization, bleeding and hospital readmission rates in transradial, transbrachial and transfemoral access after PTCA.

Stenting in Acute Coronary Syndromes: A Comparison of Radial versus Femoral Access Sites

Objective	To compare TRA with TRF for coronary stenting in patients with ACS
Study Population	142 patients (TRA: 74; TRF: 68) undergoing PTCA for ACS
Follow-up	In-hospital
End Point	Hospital procedural and clinical outcomes
Procedural Success Rate/Crossover	TRA → TFA: 9; TFA → TRA: 0
Main Results (Fig. 28-4)	• Similar primary PTCA success rates (96%), death, MI, and CABG • TRA had fewer access site complications (TRA: 0% vs TRF: 4%; $P < 0.01$) • TRA had lower total hospital length of stay (TRA: 3.0 ± 0.3 d vs TRF: 4.5 ± 0.5 d; $P < 0.01$) and total hospital charge (reduction of 15%; $P < 0.01$)
Conclusion	Coronary stenting from the radial approach is efficacious in patients with ACSs. Access site bleeding complications are reduced, and early ambulation results in a shorter hospital length of stay
Reference	Mann T, Cubeddu G, Bowen J, et al. Stenting in acute coronary syndromes: a comparison of radial versus femoral access sites. *J Am Coll Cardiol*. 1998;32(3):572–576.

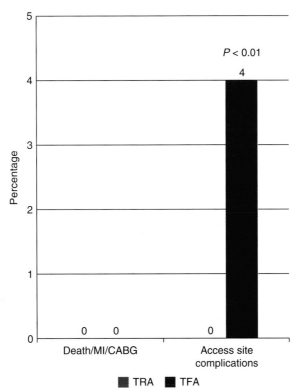

FIGURE 28-4   Death, MI, CABG and access site complications, in patients undergoing PTCA for ACS, using the transradial and transfemoral access.

Effect of Transradial Access on Quality of Life and Cost of Cardiac Catheterization: A Randomized Comparison

Objective	To assess QOL and costs of the TRA and TFA
Study Population	200 patients (TRA: 101 vs TRF: 99) undergoing catheterization
Follow-up	In-hospital and 1 wk
End Point	QOL (acute SF-36) measurements and hospitalization costs
Procedural Success Rate/Crossover	TRA → TFA: 2; TFA → TRA: 1
Main Results (Fig. 28-5)	• TFA group had longer procedural times (47 ± 2.7 min vs 31. ± 1.7 min; $P < 0.001$ • Measures of body and back pain as well as walking ability favored TRA on the first day and 1-wk follow-up ($P < 0.05$) • TRA significantly reduced duration of hospital stay (10.4 [8.3–22.7] h vs 3.6 [3.0–4.6] h; $P < 0.0001$) and total hospital costs (13%)
Conclusion	Among patients undergoing diagnostic cardiac catheterization, TRA leads to improved QOL after the procedure and reduced hospital costs
Reference	Cooper CJ, El-Shiekh RA, Cohen DJ, et al. Effect of transradial access on quality of life and cost of cardiac catheterization: a randomized comparison. *Am Heart J.* 1999;138(3 pt 1):430–436.

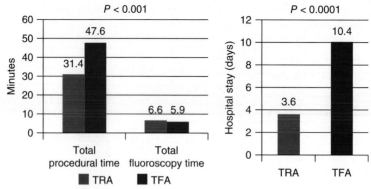

FIGURE 28-5   Total procedural and fluoroscopy time and hospital stay, in patients undergoing coronary angiogrpahy, using the transradial and transfemoral access.

CARAFE

Objective	To compare TRA and TFA with experienced radial operators
Study Population	210 (TRA: 140 vs TFA: 70) undergoing PTCA
Follow-up	In-hospital
End Point	Procedural and cost outcomes
Procedural Success Rate/Crossover	TRA → TFA: 0; TFA → TRA: 0
Main Results (Fig. 28-6)	• Procedural duration was longer with left TRA (14.2 ± 3.3 min; $P < 0.05$) than with right TRA (12.4 ± 5.8 min) and TFA (11.2 ± 3.3 min)
	• X-ray exposure was shorter in the femoral group (3.1 ± 1.7 min) than in both radial groups (right: 3.8 ± 2.2 min; left: 4.2 ± 1.7 min)
	• Higher comfort grade and preference for TRA
	• Major complications (requiring prolonged hospitalization) were more in TFA than in TRA (3% vs 0%)
	• Longer hospitalization in TFA (42.0 ± 44.8 h vs 31.4 ± 22.5 h; $P < 0.05$), causing higher hospitalization fees ($P < 0.03$)
Conclusion	After an initial learning period, TRA can be performed with a high success rate and a low complication rate. It is associated with a slight increase in procedural and fluoroscopy times, but permits earlier ambulation and discharge, improves patient comfort, and reduces costs
Reference	Louvard Y, Lefèvre T, Allain A, et al. Coronary angiography through the radial or the femoral approach: The CARAFE study. *Catheter Cardiovasc Interv.* 2001;52(2):181–187.

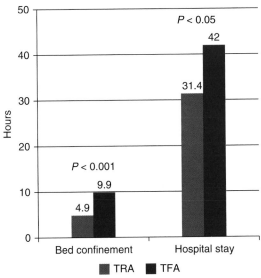

FIGURE 28-6   Bed confinement time and hospital stay, in patients undergoing PTCA, using the transradial and transfemoral access.

TEMPURA

Objective	To compare the MACE between TRA and TFA
Study Population	149 patients (TRA: 77 vs TFA: 72) with STEMI
Follow-up	In-hospital and 9 mo
End Point	In-hospital and 9 mo MACE (repeat MI, TLR, and death)
Procedural Success Rate/Crossover	TRA → TFA: 0; TFA → TRA: 1
Main Results (Fig. 28-7)	• Similar fluoroscopy times but TRA had shorter procedural times (44 ± 18 min vs 51 ± 21 min; $P = 0.033$)
	• Similar MACE, length and cost for hospital admission
Conclusion	In selected patients with AMI, PCI by TRA is feasible as compared to TFA
Reference	Saito S, Tanaka S, Hiroe Y, et al. Comparative study on transradial approach vs. transfemoral approach in primary stent implantation for patients with acute myocardial infarction: results of the TEst for Myocardial infarction by Prospective Unicenter Randomization for Access sites (TEMPURA) trial. *Catheter Cardiovasc Interv.* 2003;59(1):26–33.

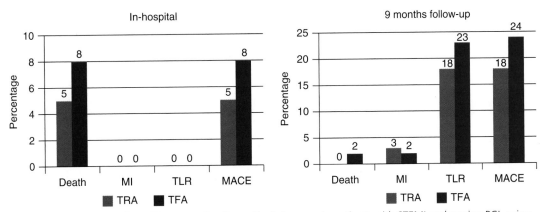

FIGURE 28-7   In-hospital MACE rates and at 9 months follow-up, in patients with STEMI undergoing PCI, using the in transradial and transfemoral access.

OCTOPLUS

Objective	To compare the incidence of significant vascular complications delaying hospital discharge in patients older than 80 yr
Study Population	377 patients (TRA: 192 vs TFA: 185) undergoing PCI for ACS or STEMI
Follow-up	In-hospital
End Point	Vascular complications
Procedural Success Rate/Crossover	TRA → TFA: 2; TFA → TRA: 0
Main Results (Fig. 28-8)	• Similar procedural success rates (96%)
	• TRA had longer fluoroscopy (4.5 ± 3.7 min vs 6.0 ± 4.4 min) and procedural times (15.9 ± 9.5 min vs radial 18.5 ± 10.5 min) during coronary angiography, with no differences observed during PCI
	• RAO: 5%
	• Vascular complications were significantly fewer in TRA (1.6% vs 6.5%; $P = 0.03$)
Conclusion	In octogenarians, the incidence of vascular complications was significantly less in the TRA group, with no reduction of efficacy
Reference	Louvard Y, Benamer H, Garot P, et al. Comparison of transradial and transfemoral approaches for coronary angiography and angioplasty in octogenarians (the OCTOPLUS study). *Am J Cardiol.* 2004;94(9):1177–1180.

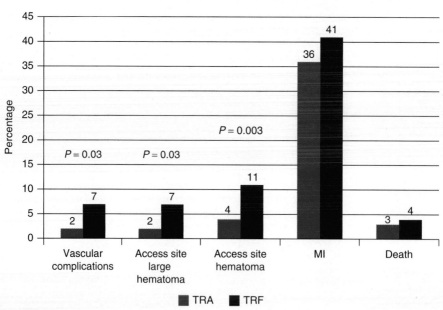

FIGURE 28-8 Vascular complications, MI and death rates, in patients >80 years old with ACS and undergoing PCI, using the transradial and transfemoral access.

OUTCLAS

Objective	To test the safety and feasibility of outpatient coronary angioplasty
Study Population	644 patients (322 in each group) undergoing PCI for SA or UA
Follow-up	In-hospital and 1 mo
End Point	MACE (cardiac death/MI/TVR), vascular complications, and major bleeding (>2 mmol/L drop)

Procedural Success Rate/Crossover	NA
Main Results (Fig. 28-9)	• Similar PCI success rates (96% vs 97%; P = NS) • Similar in-hospital and 1-mo rates of cardiac death/MI/TVR • TFA group had a higher number of patients with significant in-hospital bleeding (14.3% vs 6.3%), but no difference in transfusion rates was observed • RAO: 0.3% • A larger proportion (61% vs 55%; P = NS) of TRA patients could undergo same-day discharge (major bleeding was the sole reason for discharge delay in the TFA group)
Conclusion	PCI on an outpatient basis, performed via TRA or TFA, is safe and feasible in a considerable portion of a routine PCI population
Reference	Slagboom T, Kiemeneij F, Laarman GJ, et al. Outpatient coronary angioplasty: feasible and safe. *Catheter Cardiovasc Interv.* 2005;64(4): 421–427.

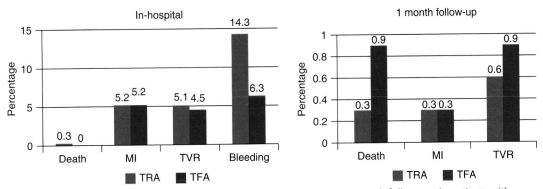

FIGURE 28-9 In-hospital MACE and bleeding rates and MACE rates at 1 month follow-up, in patients with stable or unstable angina undergoing PCI, using the transradial and transfemoral access.

RADIAL-AMI

Objective	To compare TRA with TFA for coronary stenting in patients with STEMI (primary and rescue)
Study Population	50 patients (25 in each) undergoing PCI for STEMI with the use of thrombolytics and/or glycoprotein IIb/IIIa inhibitors
Follow-up	In-hospital and 1 mo
End Point	Perfusion time, major bleeding and access site bleeding
Procedural Success Rate/Crossover	TRA → TFA: 1; TFA → TRA: 0
Main Results (Fig. 28-10)	• Similar PCI success rates (87% vs 88%) • Only difference in time intervals was greater time in TRA group from local anesthesia to first balloon inflation (32 min [26–38] vs 26 min [22–33]; P = 0.04) • No difference in fluoroscopy and procedural times • RAO: 9% • Similar death/MI/TVR at 30 d and for QOL score (walking and back pain) • No patient from either group experienced major bleeding or required blood transfusion

(continued)

Conclusion	Primary and rescue PCI can be performed, with high success rates, using either TRA or TFA. Major bleeding and vascular complications were infrequent with either access site despite the high rates of thrombolysis and glycoprotein IIb/IIIa inhibitors use
Reference	Cantor WJ, Puley G, Natarajan MK, et al. Radial versus femoral access for emergent percutaneous coronary intervention with adjunct glycoprotein IIb/IIIa inhibition in acute myocardial infarction-the RADIAL-AMI pilot randomized trial. *Am Heart J.* 2005;150(3):543–549.

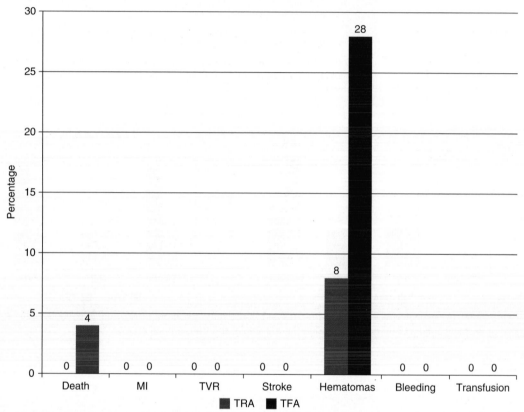

FIGURE 28-10   Thirty days clinical outcomes (MACE, procedural complications and bleeding) in STEMI patients undergoing transradial and transfemoral PCI.

Randomized Comparison of Operator Radiation Exposure during Coronary Angiography and Intervention by Radial and Femoral Approaches

Objective	To evaluate whether significant differences in operator radiation exposure can be expected in the current era during radial coronary procedures
Study Population	297 patients (TRA → 146; TFA → 151) who underwent simple coronary angiography or PCI in one noncomplicated single epicardial vessel (no left ventriculogram or aortogram and no bypass grafts)
Follow-up	In-hospital
End Point	Fluoroscopy time and radiation measurements

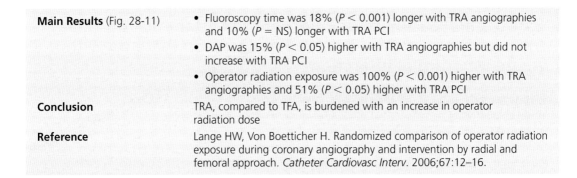

Main Results (Fig. 28-11)
- Fluoroscopy time was 18% ($P < 0.001$) longer with TRA angiographies and 10% ($P =$ NS) longer with TRA PCI
- DAP was 15% ($P < 0.05$) higher with TRA angiographies but did not increase with TRA PCI
- Operator radiation exposure was 100% ($P < 0.001$) higher with TRA angiographies and 51% ($P < 0.05$) higher with TRA PCI

Conclusion TRA, compared to TFA, is burdened with an increase in operator radiation dose

Reference Lange HW, Von Boetticher H. Randomized comparison of operator radiation exposure during coronary angiography and intervention by radial and femoral approach. *Catheter Cardiovasc Interv*. 2006;67:12–16.

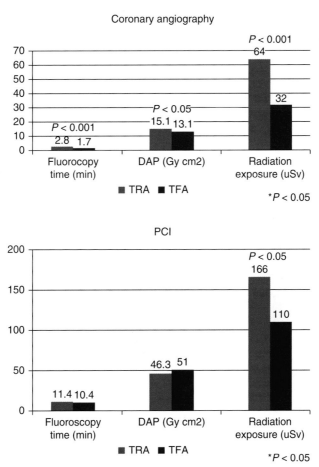

FIGURE 28-11 Fluoroscopy time, DAP and operator radiation exposure during coronary angiography and PCI in transradial and transfemoral access.

Safety and Feasibility of Emergent Percutaneous Coronary Intervention with the Transradial Access in Patients with Acute Myocardial Infarction

Objective	To study the safety and feasibility of TRA in STEMI
Study Population	370 patients (TRA: 184 vs TFA: 186) with STEMI
Follow-up	In-hospital
End Point	Procedural and hospital outcomes
Procedural Success Rate/Crossover	TRA → TFA: 3; TFA → TRA: 2
Main Results (Fig. 28-12)	• Similar PCI success rates (95% vs 94%) • Similar total procedural times (56.2 ± 12.1 min vs 54.8 ± 15.1 min; P = NS) • Vascular access site and postprocedure complications occurred less in the TRA group (local hematoma: 4% vs 1%, $P < 0.05$; vagus reflex: 8% vs 0%, $P < 0.01$; low back pain: 4% vs 0%, $P < 0.05$)
Conclusion	TRA, compared to TFA, may represent a safer technique for AMI, with similar results and a trend toward fewer local vascular complications
Reference	Li WM, Li Y, Zhao JY, et al. Safety and feasibility of emergent percutaneous coronary intervention with the transradial access in patients with acute myocardial infarction. *Chin Med J (Engl)*. 2007;120(7):598–600.

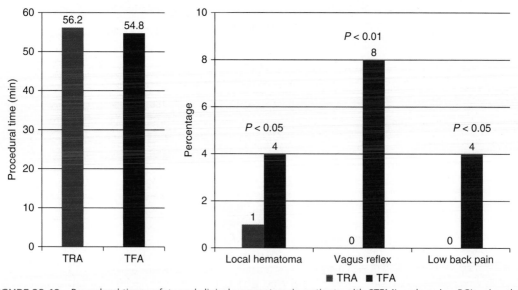

FIGURE 28-12 Procedural time, safety and clinical parameters, in patients with STEMI undergoing PCI, using the transradial and transfemoral access.

FARMI

Objective	To compare bleeding complications and PCI results in patients treated by TRA and TFA for STEMI (primary, facilitated, and rescue) using abciximab
Study Population	114 patients (57 in each) with STEMI undergoing PCI
Follow-up	In-hospital
End Point	Bleeding and PCI outcomes

Procedural Success Rate/Crossover
Main Results

TRA → TFA: 7; TFA → TRA: 1
- Similar PCI success rates (TRA: 91% vs TFA: 97%)
- TRA group had longer mean fluoroscopy times (13 ± 9 min vs 8 ± 6 min; $P < 0.01$), but no difference was seen in mean PCI times (28 ± 14 min vs 26 ± 18 min; $P = 0.72$)
- The delay between PCI and ambulation was lower in TRA group (22 ± 9 h vs 42 ± 27 h; $P < 0.001$), but this did not affect duration of hospitalization (7.2 ± 0.5 d vs 7.5 ± 0.4 d; $P = 0.59$)
- Similar in-hospital death, TIMI minor/major bleeding, and transfusion rates
- Fewer peripheral artery complications (hematoma and ecchymosis) in TRA group (14% vs 35%; $P = 0.014$)

Conclusion (Fig. 28-13)

TRA lowered peripheral arterial complication rates and allowed earlier ambulation in patients with STEMI treated with abciximab

Reference

Brasselet C, Tassan S, Nazeyrollas P, et al. Randomized comparison of femoral versus radial approach for percutaneous coronary intervention using abciximab in acute myocardial infarction: results of the FARMI trial. *Heart*. 2007;93(12): 1556–1561.

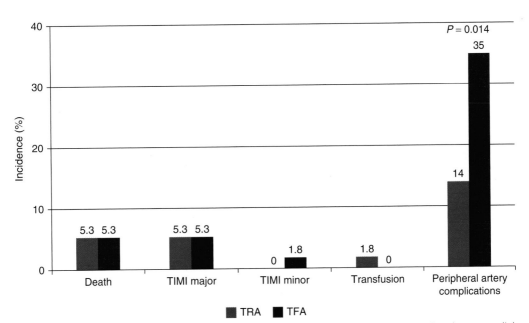

FIGURE 28-13   Death, bleeding and safety outcomes, in STEMI patients undergoing PCI, using the transradial and transfemoral access.

Transradial versus Transfemoral Approach for Coronary Angiography and Intervention in Patients Older Than 75 years

Objective	To determine success rates, procedural data, and complication rates of TRA vs TFA in patients >75 yr
Study Population	307 patients (TRA: 152 vs TFA: 155) with ACS undergoing PCI
Follow-up	In-hospital
End Point	Success rate, major adverse events (death, periprocedural MI, stroke, or vascular access complications [bleeding, aneurysms, arteriovenous fistulae] requiring intervention), and minor adverse events (symptomatic bleeding requiring no intervention)
Procedural Success Rate/ Crossover	TRA → TFA: 13; TFA → TRA: 1
Main Results (Fig. 28-14)	• Total procedural time was longer in TRA group (18.1 ± 10 min vs 15 ± 8 min; $P = 0.009$) • Similar fluoroscopy times and volumes of contrast agent used • Patients in the TFA group had higher rates of major and minor adverse events (3.2% vs 0% and 5.8% vs 1.3%, respectively; $P < 0.001$) • Patients in the TRA group had minor adverse events that resulted after crossover to femoral route due to failure to access the radial artery
Conclusion	In elderly patients, TRA has lower complication rates than does TFA
Reference	Achenbach S, Ropers D, Kallert L, et al. Transradial versus transfemoral approach for coronary angiography and intervention in patients above 75 yr of age. *Catheter Cardiovasc Interv.* 2008;72(5):629–635.

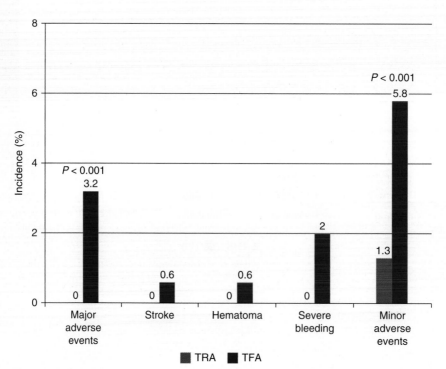

FIGURE 28-14 Major and minor adverse events rates, in patients > 75 years undergoing PCI for ACS, using the transradial and transfemoral access.

The Left Radial Approach in Daily Practice: A Randomized Study Comparing Femoral and Right and Left Radial Approaches

Objective	To compare procedural and clinical outcomes of RRA, LRA, and TFA in patients undergoing coronary angiography with/without PCI
Study Population	1,005 patients (335 in each group)
Follow-up	In-hospital
End Point	Procedures completed using the assigned approach
Procedural Success Rate	RRA: 68%; LRA: 71%; TFA: 92% ($P < 0.0001$)
Main Results (Fig. 28-15)	• Successful access site cannulation—RRA:LRA:TFA = 94.3%:87.7%:99.0% ($P < 0.001$)
	• Most common cause for crossover: RRA → anatomical difficulties at the brachiocephalic trunk; LRA → failure to canalize the radial artery; TFA → iliofemoral atherosclerosis
	• Major vascular complications—RRA:LRA:TFA = 0%:0%:1% ($P = 0.07$)
	• Minor vascular complications—RRA:LRA:TFA = 0.4%:0.8%:3.1% ($P = 0.01$)
Conclusion	The percentage of cases where LRA was successfully completed was similar to that obtained for RRA, but lower than that obtained for TFA. TRA eliminates vascular complications and enables early ambulation
Reference	Santas E, Bodi V, Sanchis J, et al. The left radial approach in daily practice: a randomized study comparing femoral and right and left radial approaches. *Rev Esp Cardiol.* 2009;62(5):482–490.

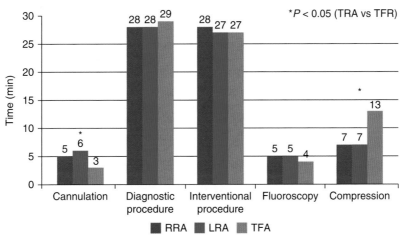

FIGURE 28-15 Procedural variables, in patients undergoing coronary angiography with/without PCI, while using the right, left transradial and transfemoral access.

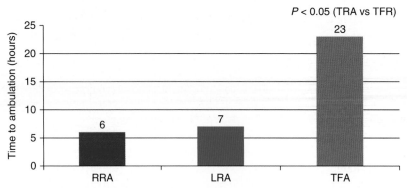

FIGURE 28-15 *(Continued)* Time to ambulation in right, left transradial and transfemoral access.

RADIAMI

Objective	To compare TRA and TFA in STEMI
Study Population	100 patients (50 in each) undergoing PCI for STEMI
Follow-up	In-hospital
End Point	Success rate and major complications
Procedural Success Rate/Crossover	TRA → TFA: 4; TFA → TRA: 1
Main Results (Fig. 28-16)	• Similar PCI success rates (88% vs 92%) • Similar total procedural time, fluoroscopy exposure. However, TRA took a longer time from arrival in the catheterization laboratory to sheath insertion (15.7 ± 7.8 min vs 11.4 ± 6.4 min; $P = 0.0028$) • No difference in death, MI, stroke, or TVR. Trend toward higher transfusion rate in TFA (6% vs 0%; $P = 0.08$) • Time to ambulation was shorter in the TRA group (22.6 ± 10.3 h vs 34.7 ± 34.6 h; $P = 0.003$) • RAO: 0.6%
Conclusion	TRA and TFA have equivalent efficacy for PCI in AMI. The use of TRA reduces the time to ambulation, with a trend toward reduction in transfusions
Reference	Chodór P, Krupa H, Kurek T, et al. RADIal versus femoral approach for percutaneous coronary interventions in patients with acute myocardial infarction (RADIAMI). *Cardiol J.* 2009;16(4):332–340.

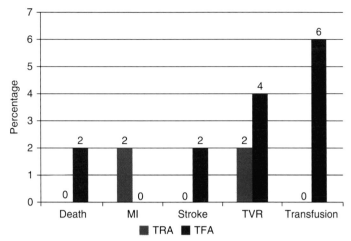

FIGURE 28-16 Death, MI, stroke, target vessel revascularization and transfusion rates in STEMI patients undergoing transradial and transfemoral access.

A Randomized Comparison of Transradial versus Transfemoral Approach for Coronary Angiography and Angioplasty

Objective	To evaluate the safety, feasibility, and procedural variables in a standard population undergoing catheterization by TRA vs TFA
Study Population	1,024 patients (512 in each) all comers undergoing catheterization
Follow-up	In-hospital
End Point	Safety, feasibility, vascular access site complications
Procedural Success Rate/ Crossover	TRA → TFA: 18; TFA → TRA: 1
Main Results (Fig. 28-17)	• Similar PCI success rates (97% vs 99%) • Higher median procedural (40.2 min [24.3–50.8] vs 37.0 min [19.6–49.1]; $P = 0.046$) and fluoroscopy times (9.0 min [3.9–10.7] vs 5.8 min [1.7–7.5]; $P = 0.001$) in the TRA group • Equivalent rates of death (0%) and reinfarction (0.6%) • More vascular access site complications in the TFA group (3.7% vs 0.6%; $P = 0.0008$) • RAO: 0.6%
Conclusion	TRA for coronary angiography and angioplasty is safe, feasible, and effective, with results similar to those obtained with the TFA. Although longer procedural time and higher radiation dose were found with TRA, it typically protects them from major vascular complications
Reference	Brueck M, Bandorski D, Kramer W, et al. A randomized comparison of transradial versus transfemoral approach for coronary angiography and angioplasty. *JACC Cardiovasc Interv.* 2009;2(11):1047–1054.

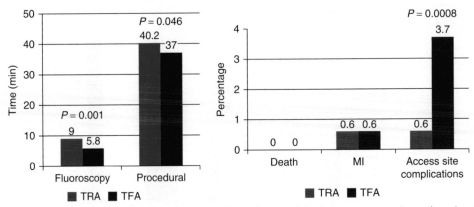

FIGURE 28-17   Procedural time and clinical outcomes in patients undergoing coronary angiography using the transradial and transfemoral access.

Comparative Study on Transradial versus Transfemoral Approach for Primary Percutaneous Coronary Intervention in Chinese Patients with Acute Myocardial Infarction

Objective	To compare TRA and TFA in Chinese STEMI patients
Study Population	200 patients (100 in each) undergoing PCI for STEMI
Follow-up	In-hospital
End Point	Safety, feasibility, complications (MACE [death/MI/TVR] and vascular complications)
Procedural Success Rate/ Crossover	TRA → TFA: 4; TFA → TRA: 0
Main Results (Fig. 28-18)	• Similar PCI success rates (96% vs 95%) • No difference in puncture, procedural and fluoroscopy times • Similar MACE rates; however, increased incidence of vascular complications in the TFA group (11% vs 3%; $P < 0.01$) • Longer hospital stay in the TFA group (12.7 ± 3.0 d vs 8.6 ± 1.8 d; $P < 0.001$) • RAO: 1%
Conclusion	TRA, compared with TFA, yields comparable procedural success, with fewer vascular access site complications in Chinese patients suffering from AMIs
Reference	Hou L, Wei YD, Li WM, et al. Comparative study on transradial versus transfemoral approach for primary percutaneous coronary intervention in Chinese patients with acute myocardial infarction. *Saudi Med J.* 2010;31(2):158–162.

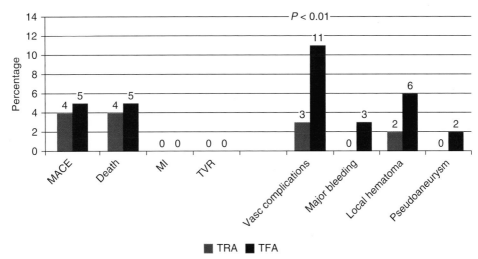

FIGURE 28-18 Clinical and vascular outcomes in Chinese patients undergoing PCI for STEMI using the transradial and transfemoral access.

TALENT

Objective	To compare the safety and efficacy of LRA with RRA for PCI
Study Population	1,540 patients (770 in each group) undergoing angiography ± PCI
Follow-up	In-hospital
End Point	Fluoroscopy time for diagnostic catheterization and PCI
Procedural Success Rate/ Crossover	RRA → TFA: 6; LRA → TFA: 9
Main Results (Fig. 28-19)	**Catheterization**

Catheterization

- LRA, compared to RRA, was associated with lower fluoroscopy time but no difference in DAP
- Similar procedural times, contrast doses, and number of catheters used

PCI

- Similar fluoroscopy times and DAP
- Similar procedural times, contrast doses, and number of catheters used
- Low rates of major vascular complications (stroke: RRA = 1 vs LRA = 0)
- No major bleeding at puncture site requiring surgical intervention or transfusion

Subgroup Analyses

- Compared with younger patients, those ≥70 yr showed longer fluoroscopy time (184 s [115–326] vs 149 s [96–232]; $P < 0.0001$), higher DAP (12.6 [7.3–25] Gy·cm^2 vs 10.5 [6.2–20.8] Gy·cm^2; $P = 0.0008$), and more contrast volume (70 ± 35 mL vs 64 ± 32 mL; $P < 0.0001$), and use of LRA was associated with lower fluoroscopy time and DAP
- Patients treated by fellows in training showed longer fluoroscopy time during diagnostic catheterization (233 s [150–366] vs 136 s [90–211]; $P < 0.0001$), higher DAP (20.1 [9.4–37.4] Gy·cm^2 vs 9.2 [6–16.6] Gy·cm^2; $P = 0.0008$), and more contrast volume (81 ± 43 mL vs 59 ± 28 mL; $P < 0.0001$)
- Use of LRA, compared to RRA, was associated with lower fluoroscopy times and DAP during diagnostic catheterization

(continued)

Conclusion	LRA for coronary diagnostic procedures, but not for PCI, is associated with lower fluoroscopy time and radiation dose, compared to RRA. This is particularly significant in older patients and for operators in training
Reference	Sciahbasi A, Romagnoli E, Burzotta F, et al. Transradial approach (left vs. right) and procedural times during percutaneous coronary procedures: TALENT study. *Am Heart J.* 2011;161(1):172–179.

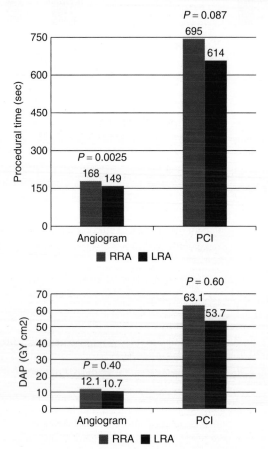

FIGURE 28-19 Procedural time and radiation exposure in patients undergoing coronary angiography with/without PCI using the left and right transradial approach.

Randomized Comparison of Transradial Coronary Angiography via Right or Left Radial Artery Approaches

Objective	To compare the procedural difficulty of the RRA and LRA in the modern era with dedicated transradial catheters
Study Population	200 patients (RRA: 101 vs LRA: 99) undergoing PCI
Follow-up	In-hospital
End Point	Procedural difficulty: (1) hydrophilic or coronary wire use for tortuosity, (2) stiff wire use for the coronary engagement, (3) multiple catheters used, or (4) nonselective injection
Procedural Success Rate/Crossover	RRA → TFA: 3; LRA → TFA: 1

Main Results (Fig. 28-20)

- Similar rates of procedural difficulty (RRA: 17% vs LRA: 20%; $P = 0.808$)
- Use of single catheter was higher in the RRA (73% vs 18%; $P < 0.001$)
- Similar fluoroscopy times and contrast volumes, but overall procedural time was longer with LRA (43.8 ± 20.6 min vs 37.7 ± 21.6 min; $P = 0.049$)
- No adverse cardiac events were seen and no major access site complications occurred

Conclusion — Procedural success and difficulty were similar in both the groups

Reference — Kanei Y, Nakra NC, Liou M, et al. Randomized comparison of transradial coronary angiography via right or left radial artery approaches. *Am J Cardiol*. 2011;107(2):195–197.

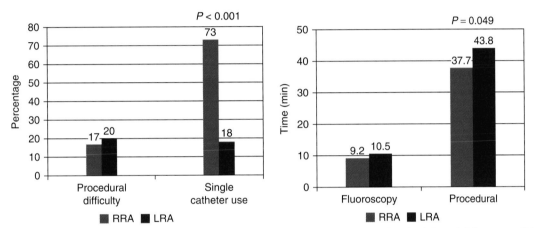

FIGURE 28-20 Comparison of procedural variables in patients undergoing PCI using the left and right transradial approach.

RADIAMI II

Objective — To compare TRA and TFA (plus STARCLOSE closure device) in STEMI patients for access site complications, patient comfort/mobilization

Study Population — 108 patients (TRA: 49 vs TFA: 59) undergoing PCI for STEMI

Follow-up — In-hospital

End Point — MACE (death/MI/stroke/TVR), access site complications, patient comfort and mobilization

Procedural Success Rate/Crossover — TRA → TFA: 2; TFA → TRA: 1

Main Results (Fig. 28-21)

- Similar PCI success rates (100% vs 98%)
- Similar total procedure and fluoroscopy times
- Similar rates of MACE (death/MI/stroke/TVR) and serious bleeding
- Similar timeline for time to upright position and time to full mobility

(continued)

Conclusion	TRA for PCI in patients with STEMI had no influence on the incidence of MACE. The duration and efficacy of PCI were comparable in both groups.
Reference	Chodór P, Kurek T, Kowalczuk A, et al. Radial vs femoral approach with StarClose clip placement for primary percutaneous coronary intervention in patients with ST-elevation. *Kardiol Pol*. 2011;69(8):763–771.

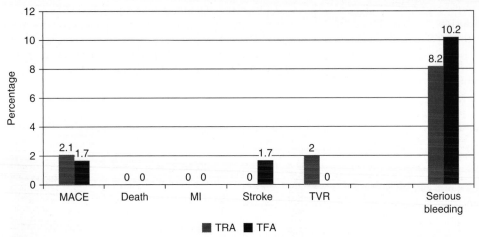

FIGURE 28-21   Clinical and safety outcomes in STEMI patients using the transradial and transfemoral access.

A Randomized Study Comparing the Effectiveness of Right and Left Radial Approaches for Coronary Angiography

Objective	To compare the effectiveness between RRA and LRA in a large unselected population undergoing diagnostic coronary angiography
Study Population	1,000 patients (RRA: 500 vs LRA: 500)
Follow-up	In-hospital
Procedural Success Rate/ Crossover	• Success—RRA: 93.8% vs LRA: 94.0%; $P = 0.96$ • Crossover—RRA → TFA: 20; LRA → TFA: 18; $P = $ NS
Main Results (Fig. 28-22)	• Similar number of catheters (2.03 ± 0.30 vs 2.06 ± 0.35; $P = $ NS) and amount of contrast (62 ± 23 mL vs 59 ± 24 mL; $P = $ NS) • Similar rates of vascular complications (hematomas and radial artery dissection or rupture) • Only fluoroscopy time was statistically different between the groups (RRA: 3.08 ± 2.62 min vs LRA: 2.76 ± 2.00 min; $P = 0.03$)
Conclusion	LRA coronary angiography is associated with similar success rate and procedural time compared to RRA. Nonetheless, fluoroscopy time is shorter in LRA
Reference	Norgaz T, Gorgulu S, Dagdelen S. A randomized study comparing the effectiveness of right and left radial approach for coronary angiography. *Catheter Cardiovasc Interv*. 2012;80:260–264.

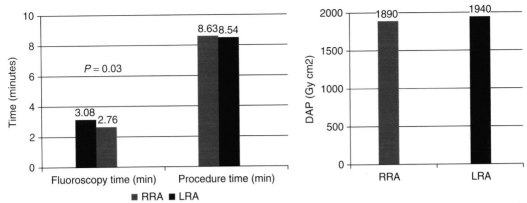

FIGURE 28-22 Comparison of procedural variables in patients undergoing coronary angiography using the left and right transradial approach.

RIVAL

Objective	To assess whether TRA was superior to TFA in patients with ACS undergoing coronary intervention
Study Population	7,021 patients (TRA: 3507 vs TFA: 3514) undergoing PCI for ACS
Follow-up	1 mo
End Point	Composite death, MI, stroke, or non-CABG-related major bleeding at 30 d
Procedural Success Rate/ Crossover	TRA → TFA: 265; TFA → TRA: 70
Main Results (Fig. 28-23)	• Similar PCI success rates (95%) • Similar total procedural times, but TRA group showed longer fluoroscopy times (9.3 min [5.8–15.0] vs 8.0 min [4.5–13.0]; $P < 0.0001$) • No difference in composite end point in the overall population • High-radial-PCI-volume (i.e., >146 radial PCI/yr/operator) centers showed a reduction in composite end point with TRA (1.6% vs 3.2%; $P = 0.015$) • Equivalent non-CABG major bleeding (TRA: 0.7% vs TFA: 0.9%; $P = 0.23$) and access site bleeding (TRA: 0.5% vs TFA: 0.6%; $P = 0.75$) • GI bleeding most common cause of non–access site bleeding • More major local vascular complications in TFA group (3.7% vs 1.4%; $P < 0.0001$) • RAO: 0.2%
Conclusion	TRA and TFA approaches are both safe and effective for PCI. However, the lower rate of local vascular complications may be a reason to use the radial approach
Reference	Jolly SS, Yusuf S, Cairns J, et al. Radial versus femoral access for coronary angiography and intervention in patients with acute coronary syndromes (RIVAL): a randomized, parallel group, multicenter trial. *Lancet.* 2011;377(9775):1409–1420.

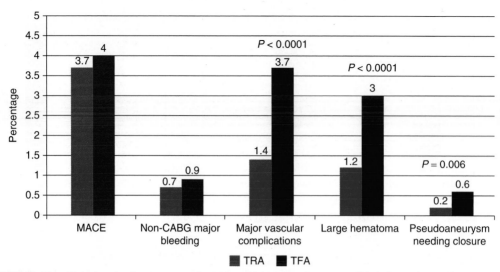

FIGURE 28-23   Clinical and safety outcomes in ACS patients using the transradial and transfemoral access.

Impact of Transradial and Transfemoral Coronary Interventions on Bleeding and Net Adverse Clinical Events in Acute Coronary Syndromes

Objective	To compare TRA and TFA on PCI-related bleeding and outcomes in ACS patients who underwent PCI in OASIS-5 trial
Study Population	7,885 patients (TRA: 872 vs TFA: 7,013) undergoing PCI for UA or NSTEMI, and using enoxaparin and fondaparinux
Follow-up	9 d, 1 and 6 mo
End Point	• MACE (composite ischemia = death/MI/refractory ischemia) • Major bleeding (according to OASIS-5 definition) • NACE (MACE + major bleeding)
Procedural Success Rate/ Crossover	NA
Main Results (Fig. 28-24)	• No difference in composite ischemic end point at 9 d, 1 and 6 mo • Lower rate of major bleeding in the TRA group at all timelines (9 d: 1.6% vs 3.5%, $P = 0.0058$; 1 mo: 2.1% vs 4.1%, $P = 0.0088$; 6 mo: 2.7% vs 5.1%, $P = 0.0086$) • A homogenous reduction in major bleeding by access site favors fondaparinux, even in patients treated with the radial approach
Conclusion	In a population of high-risk UA or NSTMEI, and using fondaparinux or enoxaparin, TRA is associated with a substantial decrease of PCI-related bleeding in comparison to TFA
Reference	Hamon M, Mehta S, Steg PG, et al. Impact of transradial and transfemoral coronary interventions on bleeding and net adverse clinical events in acute coronary syndromes. *EuroIntervention*. 2011;7(1):91–97.

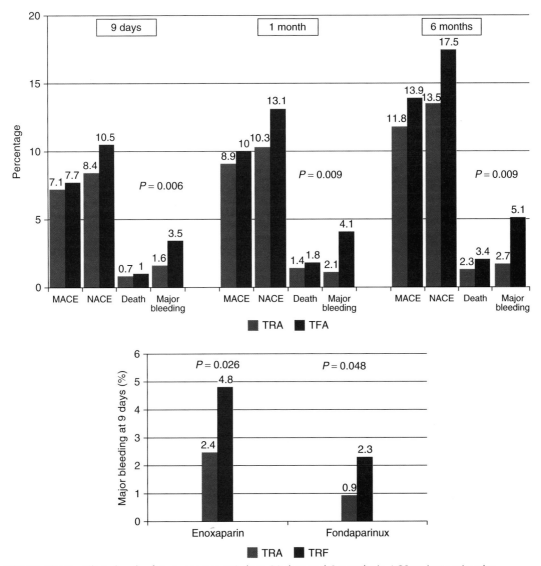

FIGURE 28-24   Clinical and safety outcomes at 9 days, 30 days and 6 months in ACS patients using the transradial and transfemoral access.

RIFLE-STEACS

Objective	To evaluate whether TRA in STEMI is associated with better outcome compared to TFA
Study Population	1,001 patients (TRA: 500 vs TFA: 501) undergoing PCI for STEMI
Follow-up	1 mo
End Point	MACE (death/MI/stroke/TLR) and NACE (MACE + non-CABG bleeding)
Procedural Success Rate/ Crossover	TRA → TFA: 47; TFA → TRA: 14

(continued)

Main Results (Fig. 28-25)
- Similar rates of PCI success (89% vs 87%)
- TRA had lower MACE (7.2% vs 11.4%; $P = 0.029$) and NACE (13.6% vs 21.0%; $P = 0.003$) and was driven by a significant reduction in mortality.
- TRA group had a shorter total hospital stay (5 [4–7] d vs 6 [5–8] d; $P = 0.008$) because of a shorter coronary care unit stay (3 [2–4] d vs 4 [3–5] d; $P < 0.001$).

Conclusion　　TRA in STEMI is associated with significant clinical benefits as it lowers both cardiac morbidity and mortality.

Reference　　Romagnoli E, Biondi-Zoccai G, Sciahbasi A, et al. Radial versus femoral randomized investigation in ST-segment elevation acute coronary syndrome: the RIFLE-STEACS (Radial versus Femoral Randomized Investigation in ST-Elevation Acute Coronary Syndrome) study. *J Am Coll Cardiol.* 2012;60(24):2481–2489.

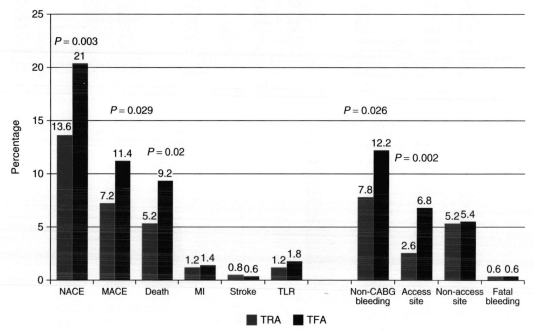

FIGURE 28-25　Clinical and safety outcomes in STEMI patients undergoing PCI and using the transradial and transfemoral access.

Randomized Comparison of Radial versus Femoral Approach in Patients with STEMI Undergoing Early PCI Following Intravenous Thrombolysis

Objective　　To evaluate the safety and efficacy of TRA for early PCI following thrombolysis in patients with STEMI

Study Population　　119 patients (TRA: 60 vs TFA: 59) undergoing PCI for STEMI

Follow-up　　In-hospital

End Point　　Vascular access site complications, bleeding, and MACE (death/MI/TVR)

Procedural Success Rate/ Crossover　　TRA → TFA: 4; TFA → TRA: 1

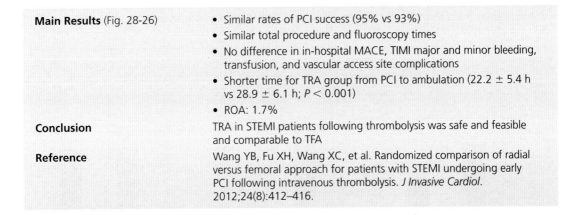

Main Results (Fig. 28-26)
- Similar rates of PCI success (95% vs 93%)
- Similar total procedure and fluoroscopy times
- No difference in in-hospital MACE, TIMI major and minor bleeding, transfusion, and vascular access site complications
- Shorter time for TRA group from PCI to ambulation (22.2 ± 5.4 h vs 28.9 ± 6.1 h; $P < 0.001$)
- ROA: 1.7%

Conclusion
TRA in STEMI patients following thrombolysis was safe and feasible and comparable to TFA

Reference
Wang YB, Fu XH, Wang XC, et al. Randomized comparison of radial versus femoral approach for patients with STEMI undergoing early PCI following intravenous thrombolysis. *J Invasive Cardiol.* 2012;24(8):412–416.

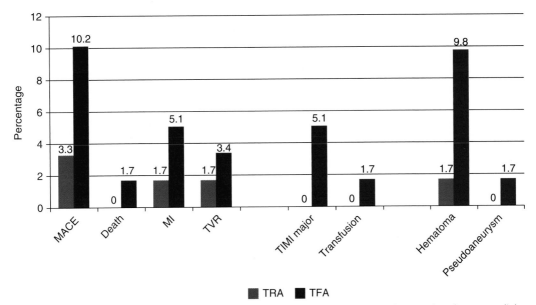

FIGURE 28-26 Clinical and safety outcomes, following facilitated PCI in STEMI patients, using the transradial and transfemoral access.

OPERA

Objective
To evaluate the dose of radiation absorbed by operators using LRA or RRA

Study Population
413 patients (RRA: 209 vs LRA: 204) undergoing diagnostic coronary angiography

Follow-up
In-hospital

End Point
Radiation dose absorbed by operators, fluoroscopy time, and DAP

Main Results (Fig. 28-27)
- Radiation dose absorbed by operators was lower in LRA (33 ± 37 μSv vs 44 ± 32 μSv; $P = 0.04$)
- No difference was observed in fluoroscopy time and DAP
- Experienced operators' radiation exposure is significantly lower than that of inexperienced operators

(continued)

| Conclusion | LRA was associated with lower radiation dose absorbed by the operator during coronary angiography |
| Reference | Dominici M, Diletti R, Milici C, et al. Operator exposure to x-ray in the left and right radial access during percutaneous coronary procedures: OPERA randomized study. *Heart*. 2013;99:480–484. |

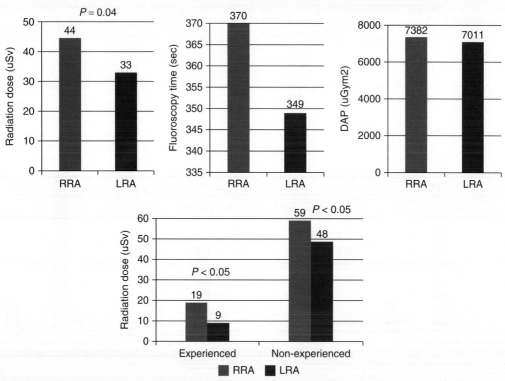

FIGURE 28-27 Comparison of procedural radiation variables in patients undergoing coronary angiography using the left and right transradial approach.

AURA

Objective	To establish noninferiority of a default TUA relative to TRA in terms of feasibility and safety
Study Population	902 patients (TRA: 440 vs TUA: 462) undergoing diagnostic coronary angiography with/without PCI
Follow-up	In-hospital and within the first 60 d
Primary End Point	Composite of crossover to another arterial access, MACE (death, MI, stroke, or urgent TVR), and major vascular events
Crossover	TRA arm: 26 (6%); TUA arm: 149 (32%)
Main Results (Fig. 28-28)	• TUA required more punctures (3 [2–6] vs 1 [1–2]; $P < 0.001$) • TUA took a longer time to obtain arterial access (6 min [3–12] vs 3 min [1–5]; $P < 0.001$), longer fluoroscopy time (4.8 min [2.5–9.3] vs 4.2 min [2.1–8.6]; $P = 0.04$), and longer total procedural time (24.5 min [15–40.3] vs 19.0 min [11.0–30.0]; $P < 0.001$)

- No difference in angiography and PCI time
- Composite end point was higher in TUA (18.0% vs 42.2%; $P < 0.001$)
- ≥3 cannulation punctures increases risk of primary end point (RR = 3.13; 95% CI [2.47–3.99]; $P < 0.001$)
- Male gender (RR = 0.68; 95% CI [0.58–0.80]; $P < 0.001$) and radial access (RR = 0.70; 95% CI [0.56–0.88]; $P = 0.002$) decrease primary outcome

Conclusion	TUA results in higher crossover rates and is inferior to TRA for the combined end point of access crossover, MACE, and major vascular events
Reference	Hahalis G, Tsigkas G, Xathopoulou I, et al. Transulnar compared with transradial artery approach as a default strategy for coronary procedures (The AURA of ARTEMIS study). *Circ Cardiovasc Interv.* 2013;6:252–261.

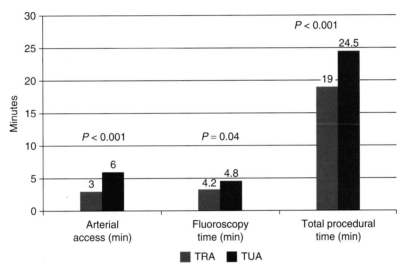

FIGURE 28-28 Comparison of procedural variables in patients undergoing coronary angiography with/without PCI using the transradial or transulnar approach.

STEMI-RADIAL

Objective	To compare radial and femoral approaches in patients presenting with STEMI and undergoing primary PCI by high-volume operators experienced in both access sites
Study Population	707 patients (TRA: 348 vs TFA: 359) undergoing primary PCI for STEMI
Follow-up	30 d and 6 mo
Primary End Point	Cumulative incidence of major bleeding (HORIZONS-AMI definition) and vascular access site complications requiring intervention at 30 d MACE: death, MI, stroke NACE: MACE + major bleeding/vascular complications
Crossover	• TRA arm: 3.7%; TFA arm: 0.6% ($P = 0.003$) • RRA → Fem: 5.0%; LRA → Fem: 1.6% ($P = 0.14$); all caused by vessel tortuosities or loops

(continued)

Main Results (Fig. 28-29)	• Primary end point was lower in TRA group (1.4% vs 7.2%; $P = 0.0001$)
	• NACE and major bleeding rates are lower in TRA group
	• ICU stay shorter in TRA group (2.5 ± 1.7 d vs 3.0 ± 2.9 d; $P = 0.004$)
	• No difference in mortality rate at 30 d (2.3% vs 3.1%; $P = 0.64$) and 6 mo (2.3% vs 3.6%; $P = 0.31$)
Conclusion	In patients undergoing primary PCI for STEMI, TRA was associated with significantly lower incidence of major bleeding, access site complications, and superior net clinical benefit
Reference	Bernat I, Horak D, Stasek J, et al. ST elevation myocardial infarction treated by radial or femoral approach in a multicenter randomized clinical trial: The STEMI-RADIAL trial. *J Am Coll Cardiol.* 2014;63(10):964–972.

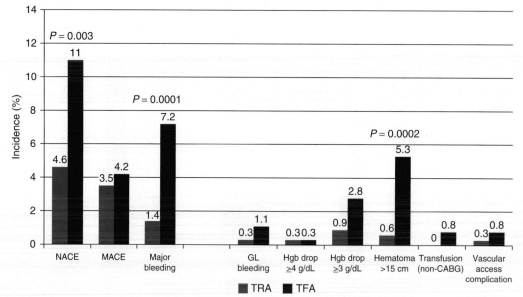

FIGURE 28-29 Clinical and safety outcomes, following primary PCI in STEMI patients, using the transradial and transfemoral access.

Comparison of Pain Levels of Transradial versus Transfemoral Coronary Catheterization: A Prospective and Randomized Study

Objective	To assess access site pain in patients undergoing coronary catheterization via the TRA compared to the TFA
Study Population	836 patients (TRA: 408 vs TFA: 428) undergoing diagnostic coronary angiography, of whom 258 (TRA: 124 vs TFA: 134) underwent PCI
Follow-up	In-hospital and at 1 mo
Main Results (Fig. 28-30)	**At end of angiography**
	• Visual analog score (VAS) was higher in the TRA after coronary angiography (3 [2–5] vs 1 [1–3]; $P < 0.0001$) or PCI (4 [2–6] vs 2 [1–3]; $P < 0.0001$)

At 30 days
- VAS was higher in the TRA after coronary angiography (1 [0–1] vs 0 [0–1]; $P < 0.0001$) or PCI (1 [0–2] vs 0 [0–1]; $P < 0.0001$)

Predictors of pain with:
- TRA: BMI < 24.3 kg/m^2 and wrist circumference < 16.7 cm
- TFA: BMI > 37 kg/m^2

Conclusion

Patients with lower BMI and small wrist circumference may experience more access site pain during TRA as compared to TFA

Reference

Akturk E, Kurtoglu E, Ermis N, et al. Comparison of pain levels of transradial versus transfemoral coronary catheterization: A prospective and randomized study. *Anadolu Kardiyol Derg.* 2014;14(2):140–146.

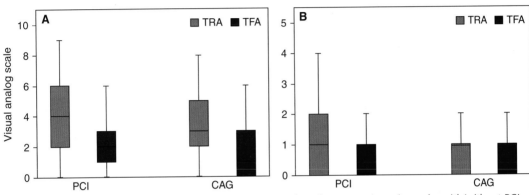

FIGURE 28-30 Comparison of access site pain in patients undergoing coronary angiography with/without PCI, using the transradial and transfemoral approach **A**- during catheterization and **B**- at 30 days.

A Randomized Trial of 5- versus 6F TRA Coronary Interventions

Objective

To investigate procedural and clinical success and vascular access complications of 5F in comparison with 6F guiding catheters

Study Population

171 patients (5F: 87 vs 6F: 84) undergoing catheterization for ACS

Follow-up

1 mo

End Point

Procedural and clinical success rate and vascular site complications

Main Results
(Fig. 28-31)

- Right radial artery was chosen in 92% of cases
- Similar procedural success rates (successful cannulation of the coronary ostia and PCI without any complications or TVR): 5F: 95.4% vs 6F: 90.5%; $P = 0.097$
- Similar clinical success rates (successful PCI without any MACE (death/MI/UA): 5F: 93.1% vs 6F: 92.9%; $P = 0.097$
- Similar vascular access site complications (loss of Hgb >2 mmol/L, need for blood transfusion or vascular repair): 0% for both
- RAS: 2.9% (5F: 1.1% vs 6F: 4.8%; $P = 0.08$)
- RAO: 3.5% (5F: 1.1% vs 6F: 5.9%; $P = 0.05$), with four patients having artery-to-catheter ratio <1

Conclusion

Selected noncomplex coronary lesions can successfully and safely be treated using a TRA strategy with either 5- or 6F guiding catheters

Reference

Dahm JB, Vogelgesang D, Hummel A, et al. A randomized trial of 5 vs. 6 French TRA coronary interventions. *Catheter Cardiovasc Interv.* 2002;57(2):172–176.

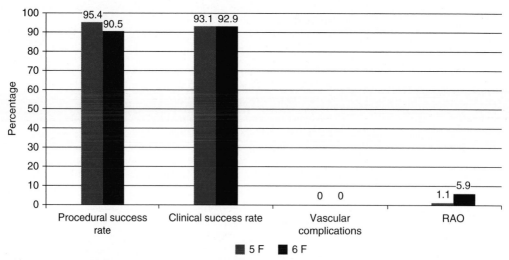

FIGURE 28-31   Procedural, clinical success rates and vascular access complications using 5F and 6F catheters during transradial catheterization for ACS.

Novel Diagnostic Catheter Specifically Designed for Both Coronary Arteries via the Right Transradial Approach: A Prospective, Randomized Trial of Tiger II versus Judkins Catheters

Objective	To assess the feasibility, safety, and performance of a novel diagnostic catheter (Tiger II vs Judkins left and right)
Study Population	160 patients (80 in each)
End Point	Time needed for procedure completion
Main Results (Fig. 28-32)	Lower total fluoroscopy time (33%; $P = 0.001$) and total procedural time (40%; $P = 0.001$) with Tiger II catheter
	Similar technical success (the randomized catheter completed the procedure without crossover to another catheter) and procedural success rates (completion of the procedure without clinical complications)
Conclusion	The Tiger II catheter, used as a multipurpose catheter during right TRA, may reduce procedural and X-ray times without affecting procedural and technical success rates
Reference	Kim SM, Kim DK, Kim DI, et al. Novel diagnostic catheter specifically designed for both coronary arteries via the right transradial approach: a prospective, randomized trial of Tiger II vs. Judkins catheters. *Int J Cardiovasc Imaging*. 2006;22(3–4): 295–303.

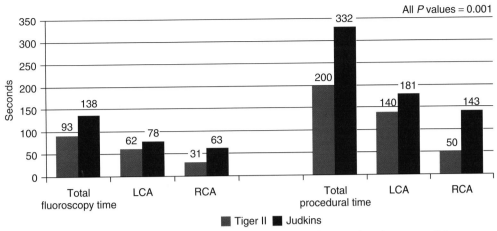

FIGURE 28-32 Comparison of procedural and fluoroscopy time in patients undergoing transradial coronary angiography using the Tiger II and the Judkins catheters.

A 5F Catheter Approach Reduces Patient Discomfort during Transradial Coronary Intervention Compared with a 6F Approach: A Prospective Randomized Study

Objective	To compare the patient's morbidity, success rate, and the operator's convenience between 5F and 6F TRA
Study Population	200 patients (100 in each group) undergoing PCI
End Point	Maximum forearm pain related to the procedure
Main Results (Fig. 28-33)	• Similar PCI success rates (5F: 99% vs 6F: 97%; $P = 0.4$), procedural time length (5F: 24.5 ± 16.4 min vs 6F: 23.2 ± 13.3 min; $P = 0.55$), and contrast volume (5F: 133 ± 60 mL vs 6F: 146 ± 60 mL; $P = 0.14$)
	• Coronary artery dissection was seen only in 1 patient (6F group)
	• Operator's convenience measurements
	• Guiding catheter support was similar
	• Vessel visualization when a balloon or stent was in the vessel was better in the 6F group ($P < 0.001$)
	• No difference in rates of local hematoma, ecchymosis, radial artery pulse loss, rebleeding or sheath pull-back difficulty
	• Overall pain scores were *lower* in the 5F group, and particularly in females and in those with low body weight and higher radial artery diameter
	• Sheath/artery ratio > 0.9 is directly correlated to pain particularly during sheath insertion, removal, and after 24 h
Conclusion	Using a 5F catheter during TRA reduces local access site pain, particularly in female patients with smaller body size, whereas the success and local complication rates were similar to those seen with a 6F approach
Reference	Gwon HC, Doh JH, Choi JH, et al. A 5Fr catheter approach reduces patient discomfort during transradial coronary intervention compared with a 6Fr approach: a prospective randomized study. *J Interv Cardiol.* 2006;19(2):141–147.

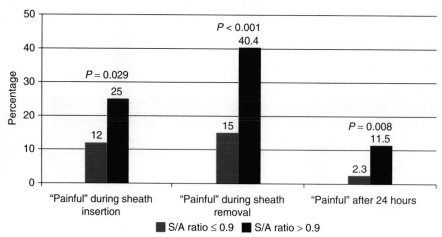

FIGURE 28-33 Comparison of access site pain during and 24 hours post transradial PCI and based on sheath/artery ratio of </= 0.9 or > 0.9.

Impact of Length and Hydrophilic Coating of the Introducer Sheath on Radial Artery Spasm during Transradial Coronary Intervention: A Randomized Study

Objective	To assess the impact of introducer length (23 vs 13 cm) and hydrophilic coating on RAS, RAO, and local vascular complications
Study Population	790 patients undergoing catheterization (long sheath: 396 vs short sheath: 394; coated: 397 vs uncoated: 393)
End Point	Incidence of operator-reported RAS and procedural success (successful completion of the intended procedure via the radial route)
Main Results (Fig. 28-34)	• Procedural success (96%), with RAS accounting for 17 of the 33 (2.2%) failed cases
	• Overall RAS was reported in 29.4% of individuals and patient discomfort due to RAS was reported in 21.8%
	At discharge
	• RAO was documented in 9.5% (73 patients) and not influenced by sheath length or coating
	At follow-up (n = 625)
	• Overall persistent RAO was documented in 6.9% (43 patients)
	• Higher incidence of local access site swelling and discomfort in patients randomized to coated sheaths (5.1% vs 0.3%; $P = 0.001$)
Conclusion	Hydrophilic sheath coating, but not sheath length, reduces the incidence of RAS during TRA procedures
Reference	Rathore S, Stables RH, Pauriah M, et al. Impact of length and hydrophilic coating of the introducer sheath on radial artery spasm during transradial coronary intervention: a randomized study. *JACC Cardiovasc Interv.* 2010;3(5):475–483.

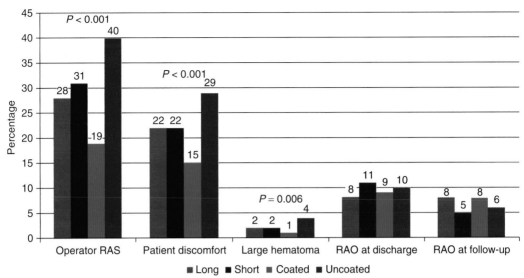

FIGURE 28-34 Comparison of radial artery spasm, patient discomfort, and radial artery clinical complications during transradial coronary catheterization using long vs. short and coated vs. uncoated sheaths.

EASY

Objective	To study whether moderate- and high-risk patients ($\pm$ abciximab infusion) can undergo same-day discharge after uncomplicated TRA
Study Population	1,005 (same-day discharge: 504 vs overnight hospitalization: 501) patients with stable ACS undergoing PCI
Follow-up	1 mo
End Point	Death/MI/urgent TVR/bleeding (REPLACE-2)/hospitalization/access site complications
Main Results (Fig. 28-35)	• Noninferiority primary end point was similar (20.4% vs 18.2% $P = 0.017$) • No death occurred at 1 mo • Very low risk of major bleeding (0.8% vs 0.2%), with transfusion given in 2 patients (0.4%) per group
Conclusion	Same-day home discharge after uncomplicated TRA PCI and bolus-only abciximab is not clinically inferior, in a wide spectrum of patients, to the standard overnight hospitalization and a bolus, followed by a 12-h infusion.
Reference	Bertrand OF, De Larochellière R, Rodés-Cabau J, et al. A randomized study comparing same-day home discharge and abciximab bolus only to overnight hospitalization and abciximab bolus and infusion after transradial coronary stent implantation. *Circulation*. 2006;114(24): 2636–2643.

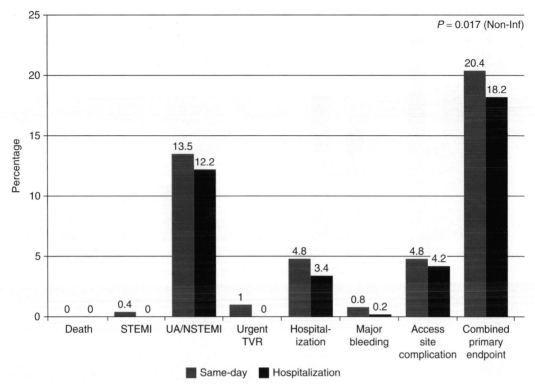

FIGURE 28-35 Clinical and safety outcomes, following transradial PCI (with/without abciximab) in stable ACS patients, using a same-day discharge vs. overnight hospitalization strategy.

PROPHET

Objective	To evaluate the efficacy of hemostasis with patency in avoiding RAO after transradial catheterization
Study Population	436 patients (conventional hemostasis: 219 vs patent hemostasis: 217) undergoing catheterization
Follow-up	24 h and 30 d
Main Results (Fig. 28-36)	• Using plethysmography, a higher rate of RAO at 24 h and 30 d was seen in the conventional hemostasis group • Higher weight and patency at the time of hemostasis were the best independent predictors for protection from RAO
Conclusion	Patent hemostasis is highly effective in reducing RAO after radial access
Reference	Pancholy S, Coppola J, Patel T, et al. Prevention of radial artery occlusion-patent hemostasis evaluation trial (PROPHET study): a randomized comparison of traditional versus patency documented hemostasis after transradial catheterization. *Catheter Cardiovasc Interv.* 2008;72(3):335–340.

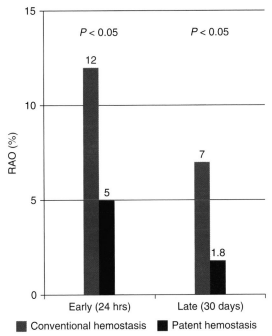

FIGURE 28-36   Radial artery occlusion rates, 24 hours and 30 days post transradial catheterization, using conventional vs. patent hemostasis strategy.

EASY—COSTS

Objective	To estimate the economic impact of same-day home discharge compared with overnight hospitalization after TRA
Study Population	1,005 (same-day discharge: 504 vs overnight hospitalization: 501) patients with stable ACS undergoing PCI
Follow-up	1 mo
Main Results (Fig. 28-37)	• Post-PCI stay was 8.9 ± 7.5 h vs 26.5 ± 14.3 h ($P < 0.001$) • At 30-day follow-up, mean difference between groups was Can $1,141, and mainly due to in-hospital stay
Conclusion	Same-day home discharge after uncomplicated TRA PCI and a bolus-only abciximab regimen resulted in a 50% relative reduction in medical costs
Reference	Rinfret S, Kennedy WA, Lachaine J, et al. Economic impact of same-day home discharge after uncomplicated transradial percutaneous coronary intervention and bolus-only abciximab regimen. *JACC Cardiovasc Interv.* 2010;3(10):1011–1019.

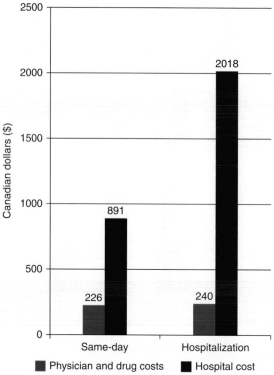

FIGURE 28-37 Medical costs comparison, following transradial PCI (with/without abciximab) in stable ACS patients, using a same-day discharge vs. overnight hospitalization strategy.

A Comparison of Two Devices for Radial Artery Hemostasis after Transradial Coronary Intervention

Objective	To evaluate the effect of two different hemostatic devices on radial artery outcomes after TRA
Study Population	600 patients (TR Band: 300 vs chitosan-based device: 300) undergoing PCI
Follow-up	In-hospital and 1 mo
End Point	Compression time, major and minor access site bleeding + complications and incidence of RAO (using 2D ultrasound)
Main Results (Fig. 28-38)	• Shorter compression time in chitosan-based pad (127.6 ± 33.0 min vs 181.6 ± 32.2 min; $P < 0.001$) • No major access site bleeding in both arms • Lower incidence of errhysis, early and late RAO in chitosan-based pad arm
Conclusion	Chitosan-based pad showed better hemostatic efficacy and a lower incidence of acute and late RAO than did the TR Band compression device
Reference	Dai N, Da-chun X, Hou L, et al. A comparison of 2 devices for radial artery hemostasis after transradial coronary intervention. *J Cardiovasc Nurs*. 2014. epub ahead of print.

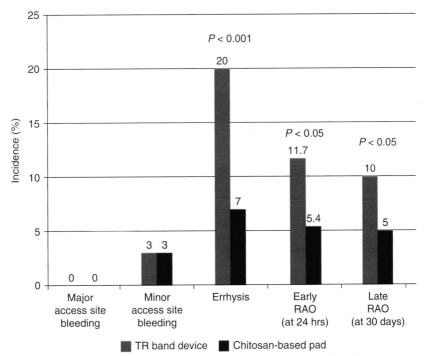

FIGURE 28-38   Radial access site outcomes, using a TR band device vs. Chitosan-based pad

CHAPTER 29

Conclusions and Future Directions

Sunil V. Rao and Olivier F. Bertrand

It should be clear from this textbook that the radial approach for cardiac and endovascular procedures is a mature field with a substantial body of evidence supporting its use over other vascular access sites. However, the transradial technique is a living science—it continues to grow and evolve, with the ultimate goal of becoming the safest, most efficient, and most cost-effective way of performing invasive percutaneous procedures. Bleeding complications remain the most common complications of any cardiac procedure, and bleeding at the vascular access site is a major source of morbidity and mortality among patients undergoing percutaneous procedures. The superficial location of the radial artery makes it ideal for reducing the risk of bleeding and vascular complications. This advantage in safety over other arterial access sites has also translated into cost savings from the societal and hospital perspectives. As outlined in this text, there are nuances to the fundamentals of transradial procedures such as arterial access, traversing the arm and chest vasculature, successfully performing a coronary, structural, or peripheral arterial procedure, and obtaining hemostasis that need to be learned and applied in order to achieve proficiency. In addition, alternative arm access such as ulnar approach and venous access for right heart procedures are feasible. The bedrock of a successful transradial program is a well-trained catheterization laboratory staff, and the information provided in this book is aimed at both physicians and nonphysician providers who are involved in transradial procedures.

As the editors of this textbook, we have recruited the world's experts in interventional cardiology and, in particular, radial access, to review the literature in its entirety. The final product is a balanced view of the role of radial approach in the armamentarium of interventional techniques. But we are not naive enough to think that the information presented here is static and will remain unchanged over time. Indeed, the adoption of radial procedures worldwide is paralleled only by the increase in the annual number of publications on this topic that support some of our firmly held beliefs and challenge others.

Although this textbook is a comprehensive and detailed overview, there are a number of areas still needing investigation. From the clinical to the technical to the political, the radial approach continues to be the topic of intense research. In the clinical realm, mechanisms involved in the association between bleeding and subsequent adverse events, including mortality, are yet to be elucidated. The inevitable decrease in the profile of interventional equipment will naturally lead to questions regarding using the veins and arteries of the arm in structural heart disease and electrophysiological procedures. The relationship between access site choice and antithrombotic therapy on ischemic and bleeding outcomes is unclear and is the subject of ongoing randomized trials. Similarly, it is not known whether the type and degree of anticoagulation affect the incidence of radial artery occlusion (RAO). Along these lines, technical aspects of transradial procedures likely have an impact on radial artery patency, and the introduction of "slender" techniques may ultimately eliminate RAO. Also from the technical perspective, iterations in equipment such as catheter shapes, sheath designs, and hemostasis devices need to be validated with respect to important radial-specific outcomes. Finally, as outlined in this textbook, the radial approach is associated with cost savings from both the societal and hospital perspectives. As reimbursement changes, the role of radial access in the economic landscape will need to be reevaluated.

The future of radial approach, like that of interventional cardiology, is bright, but tempered with the challenges of generating evidence, improving outcomes, and being economically viable. As the field continues to evolve, methods of disseminating the data and best practices will need to keep up. It is a task that we, as editors of this definitive text, welcome.

INDEX

NOTE: Page numbers followed by "*f*" and "*t*" refer to figures and tables, respectively.